Stroke in the Older Person

Stroke in the Older Person

Edited by

Sunil K. Munshi

Consultant Stroke Physician and Geriatrician, Nottingham City Hospital,
Nottingham University Hospitals NHS Trust, Nottingham, UK

Rowan H. Harwood

Professor of Palliative and End of Life Care, School of Health Sciences
University of Nottingham, Honorary Consultant Geriatrician (formerly
Consultant Stroke Physician), Nottingham University Hospitals NHS Trust,
Nottingham, UK

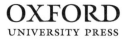

OXFORD
UNIVERSITY PRESS

OXFORD
UNIVERSITY PRESS

Great Clarendon Street, Oxford, OX2 6DP,
United Kingdom

Oxford University Press is a department of the University of Oxford.
It furthers the University's objective of excellence in research, scholarship,
and education by publishing worldwide. Oxford is a registered trade mark of
Oxford University Press in the UK and in certain other countries

© Oxford University Press 2020

The moral rights of the authors have been asserted

First Edition published in 2020

Impression: 2

Published in the United States of America by Oxford University Press
198 Madison Avenue, New York, NY 10016, United States of America

British Library Cataloguing in Publication Data

Data available

Library of Congress Control Number: 2019951492

ISBN 978-0-19-874749-9

Printed and bound by
CPI Group (UK) Ltd, Croydon, CR0 4YY

Oxford University Press makes no representation, express or implied, that the
drug dosages in this book are correct. Readers must therefore always check
the product information and clinical procedures with the most up-to-date
published product information and data sheets provided by the manufacturers
and the most recent codes of conduct and safety regulations. The authors and
the publishers do not accept responsibility or legal liability for any errors in the
text or for the misuse or misapplication of material in this work. Except where
otherwise stated, drug dosages and recommendations are for the non-pregnant
adult who is not breast-feeding

Links to third party websites are provided by Oxford in good faith and
for information only. Oxford disclaims any responsibility for the materials
contained in any third party website referenced in this work.

Dedicated to the thousands of stroke carers, the unsung heroes of stroke.........

Contents

Abbreviations

ACE	angiotensin-converting enzyme
ACEI	ACE inhibitor
ACT	acceptance and commitment therapy
ADC	apparent diffusion coefficient
ADL	activities of daily living
AF	atrial fibrillation
AHA	American Heart Association
AoS	apraxia of speech
ARB	angiotensin receptor blocker
ASA	American Stroke Association
ASPECTS	Alberta Stroke Programme Early CT Score
BP	blood pressure
BPV	blood pressure variability
CAA	cerebral amyloid angiopathy
CADASIL	cerebral autosomal dominant arteriopathy with subcortical infarcts and leukoencephalopathy
CAS	carotid angioplasty and stenting
CASES	Canadian Alteplase for Stroke Effectiveness Study
CBF	cerebral blood flow
CBT	cognitive behaviour therapy
CBV	cerebral blood volume
CCA	common carotid artery
CCB	calcium channel blocker
CDUS	carotid duplex ultrasound
CEA	carotid endarterectomy
CEMRA	contrast-enhanced MRA
CGA	comprehensive geriatric assessment
CIMT	constraint-induced movement therapy
CLAHRC	Collaborative for Leadership in Applied Health Research and Care
CNS	central nerve system
CRP	C-reactive protein
CSF	cerebrospinal fluid
CT	computed tomography
CTA	CT angiography
CVE	cerebrovascular events
CXR	chest X-ray

DAPT	dual antiplatelet therapy
DBP	diastolic blood pressure
DLB	diffuse Lewy body
DNACPR	do not attempt cardiopulmonary resuscitation
DNAR	do not attempt resuscitation
DOL	deprivation of liberty
DSA	digital subtraction angiography
DTN	dysphagia-trained nurses
DVLA	Driver and Vehicle Licensing Authority
DVT	deep venous thrombosis
DWI	diffusion-weighted imaging
ECST	European Carotid Surgery Trial
ED	emergency department
EDV	end diastolic velocity
EMST	expiratory muscle strength training
ESD	early supported discharge
ESO	European Stroke Organisation
ESR	erythrocyte sedimentation rate
FAST	face, arm, speech, time
FEES	fibreoptic endoscopic evaluation of swallowing
FI	frailty index
FOSS	Friends of Stroke Services
GCA	giant cell arteritis
GMC	General Medical Council
GRE	gradient recalled echo
GRV	gastric residual volume
HASU	hyperacute stroke unit
HDL	high-density lipoprotein
HPS	Heart Protection Study
HR	hazard ratios
HTI	haemorrhagic transformation of infarct
ICH	intracerebral haemorrhage
ICIDH	International Classification of Impairments, Disabilities, and Handicaps
ILR	implantable loop recorder
IMCA	independent mental capacity advocate
INR	international normalized ratio

IPC	intermittent pneumatic compression
IRIS	Insulin Resistance Intervention after Stroke
ISH	isolated systolic hypertension
IV	intravenous
IVC	inferior vena cava
JBDS	Joint British Diabetes Societies
LA	left atrium
LAA	left atrial appendage
LAAO	left atrial appendage occlusion
LDL	low density lipoprotein
LPA	lasting power of attorney
LPS	liberty protection safeguards
MAC	mid arm circumference
MBSR	mindfulness-based stress reduction
MCA	Mental Capacity Act
MCA	middle cerebral artery
MDT	multidisciplinary team
MI	myocardial infarction
MMI	malignant middle cerebral artery infarction
MMSE	mini-mental status examination
MNA	Mini Nutritional Assessment
MoCA	Montreal Cognitive Assessment
MR	magnetic resonance
MRA	magnetic resonance angiography
MRI	magnetic resonance imaging
MTT	mean transit time
MUST	Malnutrition Universal Screening Tool
NAA	N-acetyl-aspartate
NICE	National Institute of Clinical Excellence
NIHR	National Institute of Health Research
NIHSS	National Institutes of Health Stroke Scale
NIHSS	NIH Stroke Scale
NINDS	National Institute of Neurological Disorders and Stroke
NMDA	N-methyl-D-aspartate
NNH	number needed to harm
NNT	number needed to treat
NOMS	National Outcomes Measurement System
OCS	Oxford Cognitive Screen
OCSP	Online Certificate Status Protocol

OH	orthostatic hypotension
OHS	Oxford Handicap Score
OR	odds ratio
OT	occupational therapist
OXVASC	Oxford Vascular Study
PAS	Penetration-Aspiration Scale
PCA	posterior cerebral artery
PDS	post-traumatic diagnostic scale
PE	pulmonary embolism
PEG	percutaneous endoscopic gastrostomy
PES	peripheral electrical stimulation
PIG	per-oral image-guided
PPI	proton pump inhibitor
PRoFESS	Prevention Regimen for Effectively Avoiding Second Strokes
PRV	polycythemia rubra vera
PSCI	post-stroke cognitive impairment
PSD	post-stroke dementia
PSV	peak systolic velocity
QOL	quality of life
RCP	Royal College of Physicians
RCT	randomized controlled trial
ROM	range of motion
RR	relative risk
RUP	recurrent unexplained palpitations
SALT	speech and language therapists
SAP	stroke-associated pneumonia
SBP	systolic blood pressure
SICH	spontaneous intracerebral haemorrhage
SLT	speech and language therapist
SSRI	selective serotonin reuptake inhibitors
STEPS	Swallowing Treatment Using Pharyngeal Electrical Stimulation
STRIVE	STandards for ReportIng Vascular changes on Euroimaging
SVD	small vessel disease
SWI	susceptibility-weighted imaging
TEE	transoesophageal echocardiography
TFNE	transient focal neurological episodes
TIA	transient ischaemic attack
TICH	thrombolysis associated intracranial haemorrhage
TMS	transcranial magnetic stimulation

TOF	time of flight		VCI	vascular cognitive impairment
ToT	tip of the tongue		VEGF	vascular endothelial growth factor
TTR	time within therapeutic range		VITATOPS	VITAmins TO Prevent Stroke
TVS	transient visual symptoms		VKA	vitamin K antagonists
UL	upper limb		VNeST	verb network strengthening treatment
UTI	urinary tract infection		WMH	white matter hyperintensities
VCD	vascular cognitive disorder			

Contributors

Sandeep Ankolekar
Consultant Neurologist, King's College
Hospitals NHS Foundation Trust, London, UK

Jason P. Appleton
Clinical Research Fellow, Stroke Trials Unit,
Division of Clinical Neuroscience, University
of Nottingham, Nottingham, UK

Dorothee P. Auer
Head, Sir Peter Mansfield Imaging Centre,
School of Medicine, University of Nottingham,
Nottingham, UK

Philip M. Bath
Head of Division of Clinical Neuroscience,
Stroke Trials Unit, Division of Clinical
Neuroscience, University of Nottingham,
Nottingham, UK

Jessica Beavan
Consultant Stroke Physician, Department
of Stroke Medicine, Royal Derby Hospital,
Derby, UK

Gordon Blair
Clinical Research Fellow, Brain Research
Imaging Centre, Centre for Clinical
Brain Sciences, University of Edinburgh,
Edinburgh, UK

Adrian Blundell
Consultant Geriatrician, Nottingham
University Hospitals NHS Trust,
Nottingham, UK

Louis R. Caplan
Senior Neurologist, Department of Neurology,
Beth Israel Deaconess Medical Center, Boston,
MA, USA

Daniel Kam Yin Chan
Professor and Geriatrician, Faculty of
Medicine, University of New South Wales and
Department of Aged Care and Rehabilitation,
Bankstown Hospital, Sydney, Australia

Sushma Dhar-Munshi
Consultant Ophthalmologist, Sherwood
Forest Hospitals NHS Foundation Trust,
Sutton in Ashfield, Nottinghamshire, UK

Avril Drummond
Professor of Healthcare Research and
Occupational Therapist, University of
Nottingham, Nottingham, UK

Timothy J. England
Clinical Associate Professor of Stroke and
Honorary Consultant Physician, University
of Nottingham and Royal Derby Hospital,
Derby, UK

Amlyn L. Evans
Consultant Neuroradiologist, Nottingham
University Hospitals NHS Trust,
Nottingham, UK

Lisa Everton
Speech and Language Therapist, Speech
and Language Therapy Department,
Nottinghamshire Healthcare NHS Foundation
Trust, Nottingham, UK

Clair Finnemore
Clinical Specialist Stroke Physiotherapist,
Sandwell and West Birmingham Hospitals
NHS Trust, Birmingham, UK

Catherine Gaynor
Consultant Geriatrician, Nottingham
University Hospitals NHS Trust,
Nottingham, UK

Amy C. Gerrish
Consultant Neuroradiologist, Nottingham
University Hospitals NHS Trust,
Nottingham, UK

Adam L. Gordon
Professor of the Care of Older People,
University of Nottingham, Nottingham, UK

Paul Guyler
Lead Consultant in Stroke Medicine,
Southend University Hospital NHS
Foundation Trust, Southend-on-Sea, UK

Marissa Hagan
Senior Registrar Geriatric Medicine, Queen's
Medical Centre, Nottingham, UK

Rowan H. Harwood
Professor of Palliative and End of Life
Care, School of Health Sciences University
of Nottingham, Honorary Consultant
Geriatrician (formerly Consultant Stroke
Physician) Nottingham University Hospitals
NHS Trust, Nottingham, UK

Dawn Hicklin
Therapy Lead Stroke/Neurology
Rehabilitation: Physiotherapist, Sandwell
and West Birmingham Hospitals NHS Trust,
Birmingham, UK

Amy Hillarious
Registrar of Health Care of Older
Person, Nottingham University Hospital,
Nottingham, UK

Sally Knapp
Speech and Language Therapy Stroke Pathway
Lead, Nottinghamshire Healthcare NHS
Foundation Trust, Nottingham, UK

Ian I. Kneebone
Professor and Clinical Psychologist, Discipline
of Clinical Psychology, Graduate School of
Health, University of Technology Sydney
Sydney, Australia

Kailash Krishnan
Consultant in Stroke, School of Geriatric
Medicine, Nottingham University Hospitals
NHS Trust, Nottingham, UK

Zhe Kang Law
Clinical Research Fellow, University of
Nottingham, Nottingham, UK; Senior
Lecturer/Neurologist, National University of
Malaysia, Kuala Lumpur, Malaysia

Phillipa A. Logan
Professor of Rehabilitation Research, Faculty
of Medicine and Health Sciences, Queen's
Medical Centre, Nottingham, UK

Mohana Maddula
Consultant Stroke Physician and Geriatrician,
Tauranga Hospital, Tauranga, New Zealand

David Mangion
Consultant Stroke Medicine, Pilgrim Hospital,
United Lincolnshire Hospitals NHS Trust,
Boston, UK

Thomas McGowan
Consultant in Geriatric Medicine, King's Mill
Hospital, Sutton-in-Ashfield, UK

Jatinder S. Minhas
Postdoctoral Fellow, University of Leicester;
and Specialist Registrar in Geriatric (Stroke)
Medicine, University Hospitals of Leicester
NHS Trust, Leicester, UK

Amit K. Mistri
Consultant in Stroke Medicine, University
Hospitals of Leicester NHS Trust,
Leicester, UK

Reg C. Morris
Honorary Professor/Consultant Clinical
Psychologist, Cardiff University/Cardiff and
Vale UHB, Cardiff, UK

Sunil K. Munshi
Consultant Physician and Geriatrician,
Nottingham University Hospitals,
Nottingham, UK

Ossie Newell
Founder and Trustee of the Ossie Newell
Foundation Trust, Ambassador for Stroke
and Patient Representative, University of
Nottingham, Nottingham, UK

Declan O'Kane
Consultant Physician, Brighton and
Sussex University Hospitals,
Brighton, UK

Rowena Padamsey
School of Health Sciences, University of
Nottingham, Nottingham, UK

Deborah Plunkett
Head Orthoptist, Orthoptic Department,
King's Mill Hospital, Sutton in Ashfield,
Nottinghamshire, UK

Senthil Raghunathan
Consultant Stroke Physician, Foundation
Training Programme Director Lead, Honorary
(Consultant) Assistant Professor, University of
Nottingham, School of Medicine, Department
of Stroke Medicine, Nottingham City Hospital,
Nottingham, UK

Thompson G. Robinson
Professor of Stroke Medicine, University of
Leicester, Leicester, UK

Jagdish Sharma
Consultant Physician in Geriatric Medicine,
Stroke, and Parkinson's Disease, Lincoln
County Hospital, University of Lincoln,
Lincoln, UK

Ashit K. Shetty
Consultant Stroke Physician Honorary
(Clinical) Assistant Professor, University of
Nottingham, Nottingham University Hospital,
Nottingham, UK

Michela Simoni
Consultant Neurologist, University Hospitals
of North Midlands, Stoke on Trent, UK

Nikola Sprigg
Professor of Stroke Medicine, Stroke Trials
Unit, Division of Clinical Neuroscience,
University of Nottingham, City Hospital,
Nottingham, UK

Christopher D. Stephen
Instructor in Neurology, Massachusetts
General Hospital, Brigham and Women's
Hospital and Harvard Medical School, Boston,
MA, USA

Ganesh Subramanian
Consultant Stroke Physician, Nottingham
University Hospitals NHS Trust, Honorary
Clinical Associate Professor, University of
Nottingham, Nottingham, UK

Wayne Sunman
Consultant Stroke Physician, Nottingham
University Hospitals NHS Trust,
Nottingham, UK

Joanna M. Wardlaw
Chair of Applied Neuroimaging; Head of
Neuroimaging Sciences and Edinburgh
Imaging, Centre for Clinical Brain Sciences,
University of Edinburgh, Edinburgh, UK

Dee Webster
Highly Specialist Speech and Language
Therapist/University Teacher,
Nottinghamshire Healthcare NHS Foundation
Trust/University of Sheffield, Sheffield, UK

Chapter 1

What does it mean to have a stroke?

Ossie Newell

Introduction

I am a stroke survivor, a common term used to label those of us who have had a stroke, although I prefer the title of 'stroke conqueror'. I am 84 years old, and from my experience of life, before and after my stroke, I hope to explain what it means to have had a stroke.

Professionally I was an engineer, a Fellow of the Institutes of Mechanical Engineers and Energy, and a Fellow of the Chartered Management Institute. When I retired, I was a Director of one of the top 100 Companies quoted on the London Stock Exchange. I was responsible for 17 companies worldwide; my patch was Africa, the Middle East, Australia, New Zealand, and the West Coast of America. I was responsible for 6500 staff. In 1984, my companies generated £350 million per year, a third of the whole Group's net profit.

I retired at the age of 50, and since then did all manner of things, pursuing interests I had missed out on in my earlier life. I was in the midst of studying for an Open University degree in humanities, when, at the age of 63, I had a stroke—which changed my life forever.

My stroke

Each and every stroke is unique to the person who suffers it. Many additional factors add to the difficulties and complexities: social background, gender, and ethnicity, personal characteristics, history, relationships, and age. Growing older in years at the time of a stroke, and after it has happened, adds to the difficulties in both treatment and recovery. Generally the older a person is the greater the difficulty, related to a greater or lesser extent, to fitness or frailty. Age brings a variety of other conditions not present in younger people.

I will attempt to give a flavour of what it is like having survived a stroke, and look at the challenges faced, which in my case were 50% physical and 50% emotional and psychological. You can look at this as a journey, a unique experience, which with time becomes somewhat less daunting, and ultimately can become both acceptable and positive.

I suffered my stroke a little over 20 years ago, on Monday 9 August 1999 at 6.15pm in the evening. It is an event vividly etched into my memory. I was told that my stroke was a left-side posterior infarct. Complete paralysis to begin with, and then a severe right-sided weakness. I left hospital in a wheelchair; I could stand but could not walk. I could not dress myself properly, nor cut food or feed myself. It took a little over a year to be able walk again, albeit a short distance and very slowly, due to a complete change in the symmetry of my body, a dropped foot, and damage to muscles and tendons which affected my pelvis, leg, knee, ankle, and foot (Fig. 1.1).

It took a further year to learn to write, and 7 years to learn to draw again. I now have quite good control over my right shoulder, arm, wrist, and hand, but my ability to walk has not improved any further. I have chosen not to drive a car since my stroke; I am not safe to do so, and I use taxis to get around.

I was on a stroke ward in an acute hospital for 7 weeks. Initially the key relationship was with the nursing staff. This sets the psychological framework and motivation for absolutely everything that

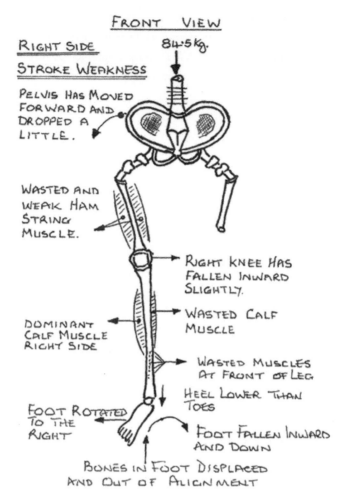

FRONT VIEW

RIGHT SIDE
STROKE WEAKNESS

84·5 Kg.

PELVIS HAS MOVED
FORWARD AND
DROPPED A
LITTLE.

WASTED AND
WEAK HAM
STRING
MUSCLE.

RIGHT KNEE HAS
FALLEN INWARD
SLIGHTLY.

WASTED CALF
MUSCLE

DOMINANT
CALF MUSCLE
RIGHT SIDE

WASTED MUSCLES
AT FRONT OF LEG

HEEL LOWER THAN
TOES

FOOT ROTATED
TO THE
RIGHT

FOOT FALLEN INWARD
AND DOWN

BONES IN FOOT DISPLACED
AND OUT OF ALIGNMENT

Fig. 1.1 'My skeletal shape as a result of my stroke.'
© O Newell.

follows in the individual's life post stroke. Then 3 months attending a day hospital, 2 days a week for half the time, then 1 day per week. Then I was discharged to my home and family. The entire process took from August 1999 until February 2000.

Once I was at home there was nothing. This was the most difficult time for me, as suddenly I was alone with my thoughts of how I had been in the past, what my capabilities had been, and with little conception of what the future might hold for me or my family. There were no rehabilitation services to help me, whatever the future would bring was entirely up to me and my family. I had been committed to the black hole of abandonment, a very, very distressing place.

Consequences and their impact

From my experience, people living after a stroke are presented with eight challenges which influence their emotional state, mental well-being, and physical recovery. This was certainly the case for me. These challenges are:

- the severity of the stroke itself and the damage it has done;
- the kind of character and personality the person had before the stroke;
- the relationships made (or not) with the doctors, nurses, and therapists who cared for them;
- the expertise delivered by the multidisciplinary therapy team;
- the environment in which this was delivered;
- the acceptance of what has happened;
- the realization that in the end it is necessary to manage your condition yourself; nobody else can do it for you;
- the hope, positivity, motivation, and painful hard work necessary to achieve recovery.

Stroke is 'nature's mugging'. My talisman is Edvard Munch's painting *The Scream*. Stroke is violent, sudden, terrifying, and devastating. Hippocrates knew this 2000 years ago. It robs you of absolutely everything. Pandora's Box is perhaps a further analogy: everything flies away except the very last thing at the bottom of the box—that was hope! (Figs. 1.2–1.4).

My journey has taken me from a wheelchair, through emotional trauma, to now, a relaxed and almost normal individual. But apart from the obvious physical difficulties, what other things have presented me with challenges to a good recovery? The most significant relate to emotions and feelings:

- In the beginning, a vivid sense of disbelief that this had happened to me, which inevitably led to panic and sheer terror in my inability to do anything.

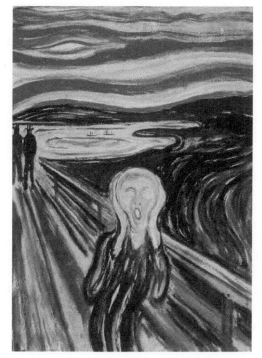

Fig. 1.2 *The Scream*, 1893.

Edvard Munch, *The Scream*, 1893. Nasjonalgalleriet, Oslo, Norway.

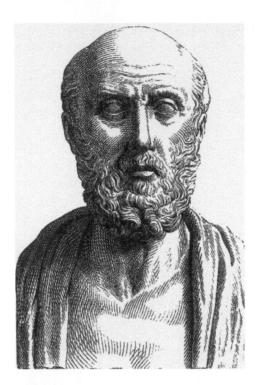

Fig. 1.3 Hippocrates.

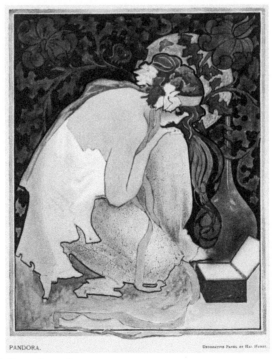

Fig. 1.4 'All that was left was hope.'

Hal Hurst, *Pandora*, 1899. Photo © Lordprice Collection/Alamy Stock Photo.

- The total devastation was all-consuming and brought an all-consuming anger.

- Communication, even though compared to many, my problems with speech and language were minor. My ability to communicate returned quickly, in a matter of weeks, but my voice remained very weak for the first year, during this period it was difficult to use a telephone.

- The worst for me by far was the loss of control and independence, common among my peers in the early days of stroke. I found the reliance on others for private and personal needs to be humiliating, and this led to sadness and depression.

- There was a strong sense of being alone, isolated, and heavy in spirit—a strange psychological state. A sense of two integrated beings; a new inferior self, who needs to be discovered and accepted, and the old self who has died, but is still there and needs to be grieved over, a real sense of bereavement and grieving.

- A distinct sense of guilt towards family and friends.

The fundamental struggle was, and remains even now, for 'normality', wanting 'to be me again'. But the simple truth is that this cannot happen, and we who have suffered a stroke are never the same again. It is extremely difficult, if not impossible to express in words the emotional pain. I know my words are inadequate, and cannot deliver the impact this has on a human being. I cannot adequately express the horrors of 'nature's mugging'; the terror of the abrupt and violent stop in a normal life, the fear of being completely broken in mind, body, and spirit, the pain, the tears, and the overwhelming emotional swings which take place, the loss of all control and dignity, self-esteem, and confidence, the loss of personal freedom, and then not knowing what the outcome might be.

The worst time for me emotionally was immediately after discharge home from hospital. I left behind what had become to me an extended family of ward staff. On return home I found myself encapsulated in desolation. On my own for long periods of time, my mind working overtime, and being unable to rationalize what had happened, and what I may have to face. I vividly recall watching *Talking Heads* on television, a series of short plays by Alan Bennett. In one particular episode, Thora Hird played a lady who had suffered a fall and was lying on the floor, alone, and unable to get up. The impact was horrendous; it reached the point where I could not bear to watch a moment longer, and I fled the room in tears, sobbing, pursued by my wife who finally caught up and held me in her arms. We both were in tears until the crisis subsided and passed.

The stress and pressure placed upon one's spouse and family is a further problem, both in the early stages in the hospital, and later when the unknown had to be faced at home. This causes feelings of guilt. The effects are never properly understood, that is, at least until someone in the family expresses their feelings and impressions at a much later date, when some insight can be gained. For me this happened through my eldest granddaughter, Sarah, who wrote an account of her feelings when she was 10 years old. The effect on me of reading it was profound and very emotional, and has stayed with me all these years. 'Woofy' is the nickname used for me by my grandchildren. In the early months after the event I sometimes felt that it would have been better for me and for my family had I not survived at all. How wrong can one be!

I remember on my birthday, as usual grandparents were coming for a party tea. Mummy and I were setting the table; as we were putting out the places we realized we had an extra plate and Mummy said 'Of course, Woofy's not here'. These few words had a big impact on me and I remember me and Mummy standing in the kitchen and crying together.

Later, we came to my birthday cake. Everyone sang 'happy birthday', and rather subdued, I blew out the candles. As I cut the cake, I decided that the first piece would be for Woofy, so

I cut it and placed it in a 'party bag' and gave it to Nan to take to him as she was going to see him later that day.

I remember clearly being given a little story book called 'Grandpa's had a stroke'. I sat and read this and afterwards I wished I hadn't because it was about a boy whose grandad used to help in the garden, as Woofy did, and now couldn't anymore. It had a picture of grandad sitting in a wheelchair using a hose to water the plants and I realized Woofy might have to do that. I knew that he would hate it and feel really frustrated because he couldn't do the things he wanted to do. That's his personality—he is very determined.

As Woofy was recovering I will always remember his determination. Now he has a good life, maybe even better than before his stroke. I think in a way, it brought our family closer and we were pretty close before. Woofy still helps with my homework and helps me to draw things, as I am not very good at art and Woofy is, even after his stroke. My cousin Connie is always asking him to draw things for her, especially dinosaur families.

Now, years later he has set up a charity, Friends of Stroke Services (FOSS). I am a member and I help as much as I can. I've helped with most of the charity events and my friends are probably fed up with hearing about FOSS. Normally grandparents are supposed to be proud of their granddaughters, but this time it's the other way round. I am really proud of Woofy for his determination, for recovering so well, and for setting up FOSS. I'm also proud of Nan for putting up with him and helping him, it must have been really hard for her. I love them both so much more than they know and hopefully as much as they deserve. They are my heroes and an inspiration to everyone.

Lessons to be learned

Sensitive issues of quality of life and the actuality, or perception of, care, dignity, and the possible end-of-life are vital to patients and their families. Excellent communication skills are needed to inform patients, families, and carers about what treatment and care is being provided and for what purpose. At the onset of stroke the patient will often literally be 'out of it' and understand nothing about what is happening around him or her, but their families will be present; distressed and needing care, guidance, and reassurance, with respect to the patient and themselves. Good communication will also address possibilities going forward, the involvement of a multidisciplinary team to provide input in goal setting, case meetings, ultimate discharge into the community and the complete pathway of care which should follow to provide good rehabilitation and recovery. A key matter for me was finding motivation and hope, leading to a positive attitude and personal responsibility for one's own condition. Lack of attention and resource in this area was disappointing; I feel the results of recovery and quality of life would be so much better if this could be improved.

I firmly believe that to be able to make these things happen it is necessary for stroke services to provide seamless, joined-up, and functional care across an entire pathway of recovery. Here in the United Kingdom, this means health and social care services acting together as one, which is not currently the case.

My motivation

My progress was made because I had excellent treatment and care in the acute hospital and day hospital rehabilitation, but nothing thereafter. This meant that I had to take personal responsibility for my recovery; in the first place this involved an acceptance of what had happened to me, and then the development of a positive attitude which led to motivation, a formidable determination, and great discipline followed by lots of hard work and pain. This has ultimately led to an unbelievable recovery and what has become an exciting and different second life and a new career working in the field of stroke.

My motivation to work for improvement was due to the fact that in the acute care setting I saw things as being inadequate in terms of environment and available resource, as far as patients were concerned. In addition, my own state and condition led to extreme frustration and to my own arrogance, and then a need to give something back for the care I had received. This allowed me to consider using the skills I had developed in my previous career. So, before I left the hospital ward I had created an organization (Friends of the Stroke Service, FOSS), with the staff, to improve conditions for the stroke wards and stroke services. Now I have a unique user knowledge and experience of healthcare and academia which has led me from the local area, to regional level and onto the national level, working to improve stroke care for the benefit of stroke survivors who will follow me.

Conclusion

The challenges faced and more or less overcome, or dealt with, following this debilitating stroke have been many and numerous, but I have made an excellent recovery. This has been partly due to good luck, partly to accessing appropriate and timely healthcare, but in large measure from sheer determination to overcome and succeed. At the same time the overall experience has been extremely positive and my post-stroke achievements have been truly amazing.

The terrible effects of my stroke related not only to my physical disability and lack of mobility, but encompassed the difficulties of safety and daily living, loss of dignity and confidence, the isolation, and the turbulent and very raw emotions and feelings which resulted from the complete experience.

When all is taken into consideration I have been extremely fortunate and very privileged to have been cared for in the good stroke facilities which were provided in my local hospital and to have been treated by professionals skilled in stroke. I was extremely lucky to be living where I was when my stroke occurred. I am acutely aware that this is not so for many people, who suffer a stroke on a global basis; much more is required to be done.

Further challenges which need serious attention on a global basis are those of age and gender. In a review of evidence relating to stroke in older people, Ruo-Li Chen et al. state:

> Stroke mostly occurs in elderly people and patient outcomes after stroke are highly influenced by age. A better understanding of the causes of stroke in the elderly might have important practical implications not only for clinical management, but also for preventive strategies and future health care policies. (*Nature Reviews Neurology* Volume 6, May 2010, pp. 256–7)

Over 80% of strokes occur in the people aged over 65 years, and patient outcomes after stroke are highly influenced by age. Improved stroke care for elderly patients is clearly an area requiring much further consideration and study.

I hope I have been able to impart a little of the drama and trauma a stroke brings, not only to the person suffering the stroke, but also to everyone in that person's family and beyond. Nothing is ever the same again; stroke is for life, but with good stroke care, determination, and good fortune, there can be a different and fulfilling life after a stroke.

The fundamental issue is, that everyone on this planet of ours should, if required, have the same opportunity and access to the best possible stroke care services should such an event ever happen to them.

Chapter 2

Epidemiology and aetiopathogenesis

Timothy J. England

Stroke: Definitions and epidemiology

The most widely accepted definition of a stroke is 'a clinical syndrome characterised by rapidly developing symptoms and/or signs of focal (and at times global) loss of cerebral function with symptoms lasting for more than 24 hours or leading to death, with no apparent cause other than that of vascular origin'.[1] This encompasses stroke secondary to its three pathological subtypes: cerebral infarction, primary intracerebral haemorrhage, and subarachnoid haemorrhage. Symptom duration of greater than 24 hours in an arbitrary cut-off point primarily developed for epidemiological purposes to distinguish a stroke from a transient ischaemic attack (TIA). While this definition is valid and useful, it is based on the assumption that TIAs are associated with complete resolution of cerebral ischaemia with no permanent brain injury. Advances in acute stroke imaging have shown this to be false and a 'tissue-based' definition is often preferred: 'a TIA is a brief episode of neurological dysfunction caused by focal brain or retinal ischaemia, with clinical symptoms typically lasting less than one hour, and without evidence of acute infarction'.[2]

Stroke is a common life-threatening condition and can be devastating to both patients and carers. Its incidence and prevalence vary according to the population studied; in the United Kingdom there are approximately 150 000 strokes each year[3] and it is the second commonest cause of death worldwide.[4] Incidence rises with age, with fewer than one-quarter of cases aged less than 65,[5,6] and, apart from the very elderly, males have a higher prevalence than females.[6] Incidence of stroke also varies according to ethnic background, for example, there is a higher incidence of stroke in black compared to white populations,[7] black people are more susceptible to stroke caused by small vessel disease[8] and far eastern countries have higher rates of spontaneous intracerebral haemorrhage.[9] Overall population prevalence of stroke is approximately 1%, which is increasing with an ageing population.[4] The risk of recurrent stroke is about 2–4% in the first month, and 9-20% within the first year, thereafter this falls to 4–5% per year, and is dependent upon stroke subtype.[10,11]

Globally, the mean age at onset of ischaemic and haemorrhagic strokes are 73 and 65, respectively;[12] in fact, age is the strongest single risk factor for developing a stroke. Despite the observed higher incidence of stroke with increasing age, datasets from the United Kingdom and elsewhere suggest that incidence is decreasing in all age groups (Table 2.1). People over 70 have seen a decrease in incidence of greater than 30% over 8 years but due to the ageing population, prevalence in this age group in the United Kingdom has increased by 6.5%. In those over 80, incidence has declined by 42% but prevalence increased by 12.5%.[13] The decline in incidence is attributed to both the use of improved preventative treatments and secular trends in risk factors.[14] This trend is not seen in lower income countries, however. In people aged ≥ 75, the incidence of ischaemic stroke increased from 23.7 per 1000 person-years in 1990 to 25.8 per 1000 person-years in 2010.[12] In the same period and age group, high-income countries observed a decrease from 28.4 to 23.4 per 1000 person-years. Similarly, haemorrhagic stroke rates in high-income countries

Table 2.1 The incidence of stroke in the United Kingdom by age group between 2000 and 2008

Age group	Approximate incidence in year (per 1000 person-years)		
	2000	**2004**	**2008**
Age 40–54	0.3	0.3	0.3
Age 55–69	1.6	1.3	1.1
Age 70+	6.4	5.8	4.4

Adapted with permission from Lee S, et al. UK stroke incidence, mortality and cardiovascular risk management 1999–2008: time-trend analysis from the General Practice Research Database. *BMJ Open*, 1, e000269. Copyright © 2011, Published by the BMJ Publishing Group Limited. doi:10.1136/bmjopen-2011-000269

have decreased (4.2 to 3.8/1000 person-years) but increased in low-income countries (7.1 to 8.6/1000 person-years).

Mortality

Stroke mortality is dependent upon aetiological subtype.[10] In the Oxford Community Stroke Project (OCSP), 675 patients were followed up for 6.5 years after their first ever stroke[15]; 19% were dead within 30 days and those who survived 30 days had an annual risk of death 2.3 times higher than the general population. After 30 days, non-stroke cardiovascular disease becomes an increasingly important cause of death. In the Oxford Vascular Study, adjusted mortality rates (survival at 1 month) due to incident stroke reduced from 0.44 to 0.28 per 1000 per year between 1981 and 2004.[16] In 2010, the worldwide average age of fatal ischaemic stroke was 79.4 and fatal haemorrhagic stroke 69.9.[12] Encouragingly, trends in mortality rates show improvements in both high and low-income countries across all age groups (Table 2.2).

The ageing brain

Physiological changes associated with ageing can alter the manner in which an elderly patient may present with a stroke. For example, increases in arterial stiffness associated with hypertension, changes in cerebral autoregulation, and the inevitable presence of multiple comorbidities, means that elderly stroke victims usually respond more adversely to minor insults, a so-called poor physiological reserve. Conversely, a cerebral infarct or haemorrhage is less likely to cause mass effect in a patient with age-related cerebral atrophy compared to a younger patient at greater risk of developing life-threatening cerebral oedema.

After the age of 60, the size and weight of the human brain decreases. Other gross changes include variable degrees of cortical atrophy, an associated increase in the volume of the ventricles and, although not an expected feature of ageing, atherosclerosis of the blood vessels. Determining whether anatomical changes in the brain are secondary to ageing or due to confounding comorbidities can be difficult. For example, in a control group of subjects without cognitive decline, cortical thickness measured at autopsy suggests only minor changes in association with age.[17] On the other hand, an 8-year longitudinal MRI based study of 66 cognitively intact individuals revealed widespread declines in cortical thickness, greater in the fronto-parietal lobes than in temporo-occipital regions.[18] These brain volume changes are not apparently associated

Table 2.2 Global stroke mortality rates (per 100 000 person-years) by age group and stroke subtype in 1990 and 2010

	High-income countries		Low-income countries	
	1990	**2010**	**1990**	**2010**
Ischaemic stroke				
Age <20	0.1	0.08	0.5	0.3
Age ≥20–64	12	9	8	7
Age 65–74	227	158	215	181
Age ≥75	1511	950	1075	950
Haemorrhagic stroke				
Age <20	0.6	0.2	2.5	1.5
Age ≥20–64	22	15	34	28
Age 65–74	163	98	435	333
Age ≥75	407	275	1073	875

Adapted with permission from Krishnamurthi RV, et al. Global and regional burden of first-ever ischaemic and haemorrhagic stroke during 1990–2010: findings from the Global Burden of Disease Study 2010. *The Lancet Global Health*, 1(5), e259–e281. Copyright © 2013, Krishnamurthi et al. Open Access article distributed under the terms of CC BY-NC-ND. Published by Elsevier Ltd. https://doi.org/10.1016/S2214-109X(13)70089-5.

with cognitive decline, but the presence of white matter hyperintensities (WMH), which do increase in an ageing brain, are associated with subsequent cognitive changes.[19] The relevance of small vessel disease and WMH is considered in further detail in a later chapter.

Pathophysiology

Stroke and TIA are merely symptoms and signs of several possible underlying disease processes. In Caucasians, 80-85% of strokes are due to cerebral infarction, 10–15% to spontaneous intracerebral haemorrhage (SICH) and 5% to subarachnoid haemorrhage (SAH).[20] Black and Southeast Asian people have a higher incidence of SICH.[21] The division in classification is important as they have implications on treatment, management, and prognosis. Ischaemic stroke and SICH are considered in turn but SAH is clinically distinct from these and will not be considered further.

Ischaemic stroke

Microscopic changes in old age and ischaemia

The human brain contains between 85 and 120 billion neurons with ten times as many glial cells. It has been estimated that there is a 10% loss of cortical neurones over a lifespan in both sexes.[22] Left untreated, a large vessel ischaemic stroke results in the loss of 1.9 million neurones and 13.8 billion synapses per minute, with 1 hour equivalent to 3.6 years of ageing.[23] The effects of only short-lived ischaemia can be devastating and the subsequent outcome of cells at risk in the ischaemic penumbra can be hampered by pre-existing age-related cellular changes. The deposition of intracellular proteins associated with ageing, such as lipofuscin, can interfere with normal cell function.[24] Lipofuscin is a granular cytoplasmic pigment, which accumulates from incompletely degraded proteins and lipids. Its role in cerebral ischaemia, however, is unclear.

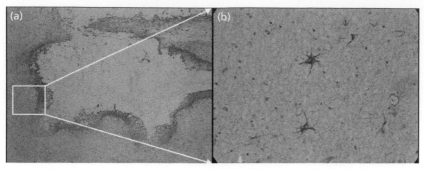

Fig. 2.1 Astrocytic gliosis surrounding a chronic cerebellar infarct. Spindle shaped astrocytes stain positively for glial fibrillary acidic protein (GFAP). Magnification (a) ×4 and (b) ×40.

Similarly, ubiquitin-positive intracellular structures are encountered in the ageing brain. Ubiquitin is a protein that normally attaches to other proteins and acts as a marker for proteasome mechanisms. Interestingly, manipulation of the ubiquitin-proteasome system with systemic proteasome inhibition has been shown to induce neuroprotection when delivered up to 9 hours post stroke, reflected by reduced infarct volume in a murine stroke model.[25] Small ubiquitin-like modifier (SUMO) peptides are also implicated in inducing ischaemic tolerance (as seen in the brains of hibernating ground squirrels).[26] Ischaemic stress increases levels of SUMO-conjugation and the presence of ubiquitin proteins in elderly brain cells may simply represent exposure to chronic hypoxia. Conversely, it may be an innate neuroprotective mechanism to ischaemia.

Ageing also causes prominent effects on glial cells, with increased deposition of glial fibrillary acidic protein (GFAP) occurring in astrocytes (Fig. 2.1); GFAP levels increase dramatically after the age of 65, especially in the hippocampus.[27] Following a stroke, astrocytes and microglia contribute to the formation of a glial scar; in preclinical stroke models of aged rats, the process of scar formation is abnormally accelerated and associated with a worse functional outcome.[28] The altered astrocytic response to ischaemia in the aged brain is considered to be one reason for worse outcomes. Other factors contributing (at the molecular level) include early upregulation of genes associated with inflammation, upregulation of proapoptotic genes, and impaired neurogenesis in both ipsilateral and contralateral hemispheres.[29] Furthermore, putative neuroprotective neurotrophic factors released by astrocytes such as insulin-like growth factor-1 (IGF-1) and vascular endothelial growth factor (VEGF) are reduced in ageing and may affect the brain's response to hypoxia and neurorecovery.

The inflammatory cascade and excitotoxic cellular damage that occurs secondary to ischaemic stroke have been well described.[30] Briefly, rapid energy and membrane failure leads to massive Na^+, Ca^{2+}, and water influx into the cell. Further toxic damage occurs secondary to mitochondrial reactive oxygen species, glutamate release, and pro-inflammatory cytokines. Neurones are more vulnerable than astrocytes to ischaemia as they have relatively little glycogen and are highly dependent on oxygen.[31] Following ischaemia, microvacuoles appear within a neuron within 1 hour. A neutrophil infiltration occurs with 24 hours, and by 2 days macrophages appear (Fig. 2.2). After around 1 week, leucocyte infiltration ceases and astrocytes accumulate around the infarct core, forming a glial scar.

Components of the inflammatory process have been targeted by multiple neuroprotective strategies[32] and yet recombinant tissue plasminogen activator (rt-PA, alteplase) is the only agent to

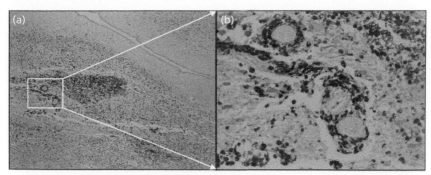

Fig. 2.2 Infiltrating CD68-positive macrophages in a chronic cortical infarct. Magnification (a) ×4 and (b) ×40.

have demonstrated clinical efficacy for treating ischaemic stroke, albeit in a narrow therapeutic time-window. Despite age-related cellular changes, clinical trials have demonstrated that older patients respond just as well to this treatment, and so age alone is not a contra-indication to alteplase administration.[33] Nonetheless, the failure to observe efficacy in clinical trials assessing neuroprotective drugs may be related to the absence of evidence in preclinical studies that mimic stroke in the older patient; i.e. most preclinical studies are conducted in healthy young rodents that yield different responses to ischaemia.

Cerebral blood flow and ischaemic thresholds

Key thresholds in cerebral blood flow (CBF) have been determined experimentally.[34,35] Normal CBF is in the region of 50 ml/100 g/min, approximately 15% of the cardiac output. This level of flow is autoregulated through mechanisms that maintain a constant CBF between mean arterial blood pressures of 50 mmHg and 150 mmHg. Following a 60–70% reduction in CBF (20 ml/100 g/min), cellular electrical failure ensues and the neurones and supporting neurovascular unit is at risk of ischaemia. Cells receiving blood flow above this threshold can compensate physiologically, and there is no clinical loss of neurological function.[36] Complete electrical failure, loss of integrity of the cellular membrane and irreversible neuronal loss occurs below a CBF of 10–12 ml/100 g/min (Fig. 2.3).

Ischaemia is not just flow dependent but also time dependent, though some neuronal regions (hippocampus, cerebellar cortex) are more vulnerable than others.[37] Ischaemic tolerance in the human brain has been observed in patients undergoing surgery for intracranial aneurysms. From a cohort of 100 patients, all of those who were subject to ischaemia for longer than 31 minutes

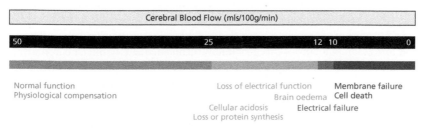

Fig. 2.3 Cerebral blood flow and its relationship with cell function.

had radiological and clinical evidence of a stroke.[38] Patients experiencing less than 14 minutes of arterial occlusion resulted in no tissue injury, and older patients (greater than 61) did not tolerate iatrogenic ischaemia as well as younger patients. This may be the consequence of cellular changes and loss of function attributable to ageing. Indeed, this abnormal tissue response to ischaemia has been observed in a number of ways. For example, spreading cortical depolarisations (recurrent deleterious electrical discharges occurring intermittently post stroke) arise less frequently in the ageing brain but with greater intensity and for more prolonged periods, potentially accelerating infarct maturation.[39] Age also has detrimental effects on other components of the neurovascular unit including degradation of the microvessels and blood brain barrier through neuroinflammation and oxidative stress.[40] Disruption of normal vasoregulatory mechanisms, coupled with an age-related reduction in the number of capillary networks and vascular density,[41] leads to a reduction in the collateral circulation which further compromises the brains response to ischaemia.

Aetiological classification

Though there are clinical indicators that might differentiate between ischaemic stroke and SICH (e.g. presence of headache and decreased conscious level in SICH), the only reliable method is with brain imaging. The aetiology of ischaemic stroke is best considered using the following subtypes,[42] which identifies the most probable pathophysiological mechanism on the basis of clinical findings and the results of investigations.

Large artery atherosclerosis

Atherosclerosis is a chronic inflammatory disorder that results in hardening and thickening of arterial walls. Though it inevitably accompanies ageing, it is not a degenerative process. A critical event in the development of atherosclerosis is the advent of endothelial dysfunction and a perpetual cycle of inflammation, usually occurring at sites of turbulent blood flow, such as the carotid bifurcation. The initial lesion, a 'fatty streak', does not cause symptoms and has been observed in the first decade of life.[43] This insult develops into an inflammatory lesion in association with increased levels of low-density lipoproteins (LDL), the lipid hypothesis. Under normal conditions, the role of LDL is to deliver cholesterol to extrahepatic cells. All cells, including those within the arterial wall, take up LDL through receptor-mediated endocytosis. En route to other extrahepatic cells, the arterial intima is exposed to excessive amounts of LDL-cholesterol secondary to slow transit through the arterial walls, the absence of lymphatic drainage in the intima and the lack of LDL receptors on intimal cells.[44] The concentration of LDL in the arterial wall is up to ten times higher compared to other interstitial fluids of the body.[45] Subsequently, injury to endothelial cells through free radicals, hypertension, toxins (smoking) and hyperglycaemia (diabetes) exacerbate further pathological accumulations of lipids. Intimal 'foam cells' are generated through the intracellular collection of cholesterol into migrating macrophages and intimal smooth muscle cells, a process of arterial plaque formation over many years.[46] Further secretion of pro-inflammatory cytokines promotes the inflammatory cascade and the production of extracellular fibrous proteins leads to the formation of a fibrous cap. Blood flow turbulence caused by the plaque itself can also contribute to progression of arterial stenosis. Over 10-20 years the arterial lumen narrows until there is a reduction in blood flow severe enough to cause neurological symptoms, or the plaque ruptures with consequential platelet activation, aggregation, and thrombus formation.[47,48]

Atherosclerosis mainly affects large and medium sized arteries at places of arterial branching (e.g. carotid bifurcation, Fig. 2.4) and it accounts for approximately 50% of ischaemic strokes in white people.[49] Many factors (such as the nature of the stroke, the presence of bruits on examination)

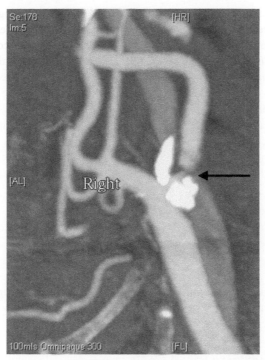

Fig. 2.4 A CT angiogram of the right internal carotid artery from an 85-year-old lady who presented with 15 minutes of left upper limb weakness. The stenosis (arrow) is heavily calcified and measures '78% narrow' by NASCET (North American Symptomatic Carotid Endarterectomy Trial) criteria. This patient also suffered with atrial fibrillation therefore making it challenging to determine whether of the primary cause of her TIA was secondary to cardioembolism or large vessel atheroma.

can implicate large artery atheroma as a cause but in reality it is often difficult to prove since there are multiple potential sites where atheroma can develop and imaging is often performed after the vessel has been given the chance to spontaneously recanalise. Nonetheless, it is known that increasing age, male sex, hypertension, lipid abnormalities, diabetes, and cigarette smoking increase the risk of atheroma formation making it reasonable to assume atherothromboembolism as a potential cause in many cases.

Cardioembolism

Embolism of cardiac origin accounts for about 20% of ischaemic strokes.[50] They are generally severe and prone to early recurrence. The most common source of embolism from the heart is from non-rheumatic atrial fibrillation (AF) with other major predisposing factors including mitral incompetence (6%), myocardial infarction within 6 weeks (5%), mitral stenosis (1%) and paradoxical embolism (1%).[51] Rarer causes include endocarditis and intracardiac tumours. In a community dwelling UK population in patients over 65, prevalence of AF was 7.2% with higher prevalence in men (7.8%) and in those over 75 (10.3%).[52] Paroxysmal AF (pAF) is challenging to diagnose but also confers significant stroke risk and is a likely cause of a proportion of cryptogenic stroke.[53] Indeed, a recent study of prolonged cardiac monitoring following acute stroke has yielded significantly higher rates of pAF; 30-day event triggered recording will detect pAF ($\geq$30 seconds) in 16% of patients compared to 3.2% in those who are investigated with a conventional

24-hour monitor.[54] The average absolute risk of ischaemic stroke in unanticoagulated non-valvular AF is 5% per annum (six times greater than those in sinus rhythm) and 12% per annum in unanticoagulated AF in patients with previous stroke or TIA.[55] Cardioembolic strokes are more prone to haemorrhagic transformation, reported in up to 71% of cases.[56] AF in older people is discussed further in Chapter 8.

Small vessel disease

Strokes caused by occlusion of the smaller arteries in the brain account for between 11% and 20% of ischaemic strokes.[49,57] These arteries arise from the leptomeningeal arteries and penetrating branches of the anterior, middle, and posterior cerebral arteries, and penetrate the parenchyma to a variable depth. They usually measure less than 900 μm in diameter. Small vessel disease (SVD) may present clinically with: lacunar strokes; diffuse white matter ischaemic change with (or without) associated cognitive decline; or with spontaneous parenchymal haemorrhage.

Lacunar infarcts are usually less than 15 mm in size and it is felt that microatheroma is the commonest underlying mechanism. The pathological basis underlying SVD was first described in 1968;[58] named 'lipohyalinosis', arteries between 40–300 μm in diameter have thickened walls and contain an eosinophilic fibrous material. Arteriosclerosis, also more prevalent with increasing age, is a term used for thickening of the arterioles (40–150 μm) prior to the later stage of fibrinoid necrosis.

Patients with a lacunar stroke have a similar risk factor profile to large vessel disease, with diabetes, hypertension, hyperlipidaemia, and current smoking most prominent.[59,60] The high risk associated with hypertension but absent risk with heart disease supports the hypothesis of a unique pathophysiologic mechanism for lacunar stroke.[60] In a recent retrospective case-control study in a Chinese population (n = 368), risk factors for lacunar stroke and non-lacunar stroke were compared[61]; lacunar stroke was more likely in those without diabetes, of female sex, and with lower fibrinogen levels. There were no differences between the groups with regards to age, blood pressure, and dyslipidaemia.

Furthermore, the initial development of SVD may be clinically silent and picked up incidentally on cerebral imaging. Silent infarcts can be found in up to 20% of healthy elderly people[62] and although, by definition, there are no overt clinical consequences, silent infarcts may be associated with more subtle changes in function or cognition that go unnoticed. This has led to more focussed research into the underlying molecular aetiological mechanisms of SVD including a search for blood-based and imaging-based biomarkers.[63]

Inflammatory arteriopathies

Inflammation of the blood vessels can be due to a primary inflammatory cause (giant cell arteritis, Takayasu's arteritis, primary angiitis), secondary to systemic inflammatory disease (such as systemic lupus erythematosus, polyarteritis nodosa, ANCA vasculitides and others) or as a consequence of infectious vasculitis. Most vasculitides occur in younger patients with the exception of giant cell arteritis (GCA) and temporal arteritis (TA) which is the commonest vasculitis in people older than 50. It is an uncommon cause of stroke, and a challenging diagnosis in the face of concomitant vascular risk factors. In a recent population-based study of 150 000 French people over a period of 11 years, biopsy-positive GCA was proven in 11 per 100 000 per year, of which only 7% (n = 4) had an associated stroke.[64] All of the cases had ≥2 vascular risk factors and all were aged ≥80. Clearly, typical symptoms associated with GCA and TA should be sought; the key symptom is headache and they are both commonly associated with polymyalgia rheumatica. While it predominantly affects the aorta and extracranial branches, several cases of GCA with intracranial involvement have been reported.[65] Unilateral blindness can occur if there is involvement of the ophthalmic arteries, or blindness can be bilateral if the vertebral arteries are affected with secondary occipital infarcts. One should be mindful that the erythrocyte sedimentation rate (ESR), which is raised in GCA, can also increase with healthy ageing: in 258 non-hospitalised patients aged 70 to 89, ESR ranged between 3 and 65 mm/hr with a mean of 13 mm/hr.[66] Further investigation including a temporal artery biopsy can be considered in an elderly stroke patient with a raised ESR and no other apparent cause. A biopsy should be at least 10 mm in length[67] (as lesions can be focal) and a negative biopsy does not rule out GCA. The characteristic histological finding is of multinucleated giant cells, an inflammatory granulomatous reaction with activated T-lymphocytes and macrophages, resulting in luminal narrowing and subsequent end-organ ischaemia.[68] Its cause remains unknown.

Haemorrhagic infarction

The presence of blood within an infarct (HTI, haemorrhagic transformation of infarct, Fig. 2.5) is common and its documented incidence depends upon the sensitivity of the modality used to detect it. Asymptomatic haemorrhage is identified in approximately 30% of computed tomography (CT) brain scans performed 10 days after the initial insult (in patients taking aspirin) and is more likely to occur in larger infarcts such as those caused by cardioembolism or large artery atheroma.[69] Autopsy studies, naturally biased towards those dying from larger strokes, also implicate that the risk of HTI is greater from cardio-embolic strokes compared to strokes secondary to other causes.[70] In serial MR imaging studies, however, haemorrhagic transformation is present in up to 85% of ischaemic stroke.[71] Intuitively, the occurrence of symptomatic HTI can adversely affect outcome; the presence of asymptomatic HTI does not.[69] The mechanisms of haemorrhagic infarct are thought to be either due to (i) reperfusion injury and blood leaking through a damaged blood vessel wall, or (ii) occlusion of venous drainage (venous infarcts are commonly haemorrhagic).

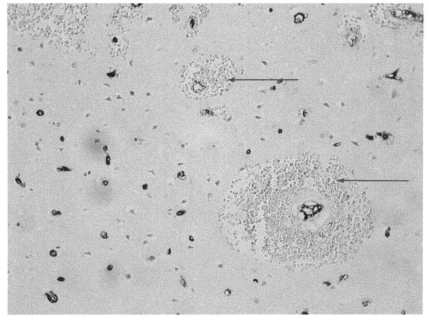

Fig. 2.5 A histological specimen from a patient with acute infarct in the hippocampus. The blood vessel walls are stained with a CD34 + antibody, and the arrows indicate extravasation of erythrocytes surrounding the endothelium signifying a haemorrhagic transformation.

Spontaneous intracerebral haemorrhage

SICH causes 10–15% of strokes in white people[72,73] and the risk of SICH appears higher in black Caribbean and black African groups compared with whites,[74] indicating a genetic causal component. Patients with SICH have a high early case fatality but survivors have a similar outcome to patients with cerebral infarction.[72] Depending on the population and duration of study, the risk of subsequent haemorrhage in patients with ICH varies between 0% and 24%.[75] Intracerebral haemorrhage may also be secondary to conditions such as intracranial tumour (primary or secondary), intracranial venous thrombosis, inherited bleeding diatheses, iatrogenic causes (e.g. thrombolysis, anticoagulation), and recreational drug use. These are not considered in further detail.

SICH can be classified into the location of the bleed, which often helps in identifying an underlying cause. Supratentorially, ICH may be lobar or deep, with most cases of deep haemorrhage relating to a history of hypertension.[76] These haemorrhages more commonly cause headache (compared to lobar bleeds), and, due to their close proximity, are more likely to extend into the ventricular system.[77] Pathophysiologically, hypertension causes early proliferation of arteriolar smooth muscle followed by smooth muscle death and collagen deposition; collagen is non-elastic and is liable to break under pressure and hence lead to haemorhage.[78] Lobar ICH suggests an alternative aetiology, and in older individuals, commonly represents amyloid angiopathy. Underlying is a progressive fibrillosis of arterioles and deposition of beta-amyloid, increasing the fragility of these vessels (described in more detail next). If the patient is younger, underlying vascular abnormalities such as an arteriovenous malformation should be suspected and investigated appropriately.

An area of increasing research and concern is the clinical impact of cerebral microbleeds (CMB). These are small foci of blood products within the cerebral tissue detected with increased sensitivity using gradient echo or susceptibility weighted MRI sequences (Fig. 2.6). They increase the risk of stroke recurrence and are frequently found in healthy elderly individuals; in a population-based longitudinal Dutch study of nearly 5000 people, the presence of CMBs increased the risk of both ischaemic and haemorrhagic stroke with a greater number of CMBs conferring a higher risk.[79] The presence of CMBs increases with age but their significance with regards to treatment with thrombolytics, anticoagulants, and antiplatelets remains controversial.[80–82]

Cerebral amyloid angiopathy

Cerebral amyloid angiopathy (CAA) occurs as a consequence of sporadic or hereditary extracellular deposition of amyloid (a fibrillary protein) and is associated with ischaemic stroke, cerebral haemorrhage, and dementia. There are over 20 forms of amyloid protein identified, several of which have been associated with CAA.[83] Amyloid Aß is seen in the walls of blood vessels in sporadic CAA independently and in association with Alzheimer's disease (AD). Sporadic CAA not associated with AD is unlikely to occur in people aged younger than 60; its prevalence in people older than 60 is more than 30% with reports indicating a degree of CAA in up to 70% of those aged greater than 85.[84] In the same population-based pathological study, which did not specifically exclude people with AD, prevalence of CAA significantly increased with age and was more severe in men. It is not known whether sporadic CAA is caused by increased cellular amyloid production, decreased amyloid clearance, or secondary to transfer of amyloid from the blood vessels.

Summary

In this chapter we have described the epidemiology, aetiological classification, and pathogenesis of stroke in the older person. We have explored the macroscopic and microscopic changes in

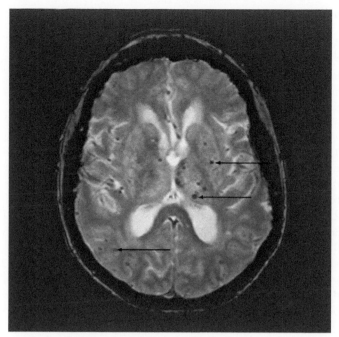

Fig. 2.6 Gradient echo MR image demonstrating multiple lobar and deep cerebral microbleeds (arrows).

the brain occurring with increasing age and their relationship with ischaemic and haemorrhagic strokes.

Acknowledgements

I would like to thank Professor James Lowe and Lucy Kerr for their help in acquiring, processing, and analysing the pathological slides used in this chapter. Consent for their use was gained when the STEMS-2 trial was performed.[85]

References

1. **Hatano S.** Experience from a multicentre stroke register: a preliminary report. *Bull World Health Organ* 1976;**54**:541–53.

2. **Albers GW, Caplan LR, Easton JD,** et al. Transient ischemic attack--proposal for a new definition. *N Engl J Med* 2002;**347**:1713–16.

3. **Bhatnagar P, Wickramasinghe K, Williams J, Rayner M, & Townsend N.** The epidemiology of cardiovascular disease in the UK 2014. *Heart* 2015;**101**:1182–9.

4. **Feigin VL, Krishnamurthi RV, Parmar P,** et al. Update on the Global Burden of Ischemic and Hemorrhagic Stroke in 1990–2013: the GBD 2013 Study. *Neuroepidemiology* 2015;**45**:161–76.

5. **Sudlow CLM, Warlow CP, & ftISIC.** Comparable studies of the incidence of stroke and its pathological types: results from an international collaboration. *Stroke* 1997;**28**:491–9.

6. **Geddes JM, Fear J, Tennant A, Pickering A, Hillman M, & Chamberlain MA.** Prevalence of self-reported stroke in a population in northern England. *J Epidemiol Community Health* 1996;**50**:140–3.

7. **Pickle LW, Mungiole M, & Gillum RF.** Geographic variation in stroke mortality in blacks and whites in the United States. *Stroke* 1997;**28**:1639–47.

8. **Markus HS, Khan U, Birns J**, et al. Differences in stroke subtypes between black and white patients with stroke: the South London Ethnicity and Stroke Study. *Circulation* 2007;**116**:2157–64.

9. **Tanaka H, Ueda Y, & Date C.** Incidence of stroke in Shibata, Japan: 1976–1978. *Stroke* 1981;**12**:460–6.

10. **Bamford J, Sandercock P, Dennis M, Burn J, & Warlow C.** Classification and natural history of clinically identifiable subtypes of cerebral infarction. *Lancet* 1991;**337**:1521–6.

11. **Hankey GJ, Jamrozik K, Broadhurst RJ**, et al. Long-term risk of first recurrent stroke in the Perth community stroke study. *Stroke* 1998;**29**:2491–500.

12. **Krishnamurthi RV, Feigin VL, Forouzanfar MH**, et al. Global and regional burden of first-ever ischaemic and haemorrhagic stroke during 1990–2010: findings from the Global Burden of Disease Study 2010. *Lancet Glob Health* 2013;**1**:e259–81.

13. **Lee S, Shafe AC, & Cowie MR.** UK stroke incidence, mortality and cardiovascular risk management 1999–2008: time-trend analysis from the General Practice Research Database. *BMJ Open* 2011;**1**:e000269.

14. **Rothwell PM, Coull AJ, Giles MF**, et al. Change in stroke incidence, mortality, case-fatality, severity, and risk factors in Oxfordshire, UK from 1981 to 2004 (Oxford Vascular Study). *Lancet* 2004;**363**:1925–33.

15. **Dennis MS, Burn JP, Sandercock PA, Bamford JM, Wade DT, & Warlow CP.** Long-term survival after first-ever stroke: the Oxfordshire Community Stroke Project. *Stroke* 1993;**24**:796–800.

16. **Rothwell PM, Coull AJ, Silver LE**, et al. Population-based study of event-rate, incidence, case fatality, and mortality for all acute vascular events in all arterial territories (Oxford Vascular Study). *Lancet* 2005;**366**:1773–83.

17. **Mouton PR, Martin LJ, Calhoun ME, Dal Forno G, & Price DL.** Cognitive decline strongly correlates with cortical atrophy in Alzheimer's dementia. *Neurobiol Aging* 1998;**19**:371–7.

18. **Thambisetty M, Wan J, Carass A, An Y, Prince JL, & Resnick SM.** Longitudinal changes in cortical thickness associated with normal aging. *Neuroimage* 2010;**52**:1215–23.

19. **Ritchie SJ, Dickie DA, Cox SR**, et al. Brain volumetric changes and cognitive ageing during the eighth decade of life. *Hum Brain Mapp* 2015;**36**:4910–25.

20. **Bamford J, Sandercock PAG, Dennis MS, & Warlow CP.** A prospective study of acute cerebrovascular disease in the community: the Oxford Community Stroke Project 1981–1986. 2. Incidence, case fatality rates and overall outcome at one year of cerebral infarction, primary intracerebral and subarachnoid haemorrhage. *J Neurol Neurosurg Psychiatry* 1990;**53**:16–22.

21. **Warlow C, Sudlow C, Dennis M, Wardlaw J, & Sandercock P.** Stroke. *Lancet* 2003;**362**:1211–24.

22. **Pakkenberg B & Gundersen HJ.** Neocortical neuron number in humans: effect of sex and age. *J Comp Neurol* 1997;**384**:312–20.

23. **Saver JL.** Time is brain—quantified. *Stroke* 2006;**37**:263–6.

24. **Sulzer D, Mosharov E, Talloczy Z, Zucca FA, Simon JD, & Zecca L.** Neuronal pigmented autophagic vacuoles: lipofuscin, neuromelanin, and ceroid as macroautophagic responses during aging and disease. *J Neurochem* 2008;**106**:24–36.

25. **Doeppner TR, Kaltwasser B, Kuckelkorn U**, et al. Systemic proteasome inhibition induces sustained post-stroke neurological recovery and neuroprotection via mechanisms involving reversal of peripheral immunosuppression and preservation of blood-brain-barrier integrity. *Mol Neurobiol* 2016;**53**(9):6332–41.

26. **Lee YJ & Hallenbeck JM.** SUMO and ischemic tolerance. *Neuromolecular Med* 2013;**15**:771–81.

27. **David JP, Ghozali F, Fallet-Bianco C**, et al. Glial reaction in the hippocampal formation is highly correlated with aging in human brain. *Neurosci Lett* 1997;**235**:53–6.

28. **Badan I, Buchhold B, Hamm A**, et al. Accelerated glial reactivity to stroke in aged rats correlates with reduced functional recovery. *J Cereb Blood Flow Metab* 2003;**23**:845–54.

29. **Buga AM, Sascau M, Pisoschi C, Herndon JG, Kessler C, & Popa-Wagner A.** The genomic response of the ipsilateral and contralateral cortex to stroke in aged rats. *J Cell Mol Med* 2008;**12**:2731–53.

30. **Dirnagl U, Iadecola C, & Moskowitz MA.** Pathobiology of ischaemic stroke: an integrated view. *Trends Neurosci* 1999;**22**:391–7.

31. **Bambrick L, Kristian T, & Fiskum G.** Astrocyte mitochondrial mechanisms of ischemic brain injury and neuroprotection. *Neurochem Res* 2004;**29**:601–8.

32. **O'Collins VE, Macleod MR, Donnan GA, Horky LL, van der Worp BH, & Howells DW.** 1,026 experimental treatments in acute stroke. *Ann Neurol* 2006;**59**:467–77.

33. **Sandercock P, Wardlaw JM, Lindley RI,** et al. The benefits and harms of intravenous thrombolysis with recombinant tissue plasminogen activator within 6 h of acute ischaemic stroke (the third international stroke trial [IST-3]): a randomised controlled trial. *Lancet* 2012;**379**:2352–63.

34. **Heiss WD.** Flow thresholds of functional and morphological damage of brain tissue. *Stroke* 1983;**14**:329–31.

35. **Heiss WD.** Experimental evidence of ischemic thresholds and functional recovery. *Stroke* 1992;**23**:1668–72.

36. **Jones TH, Morawetz RB, Crowell RM,** et al. Thresholds of focal cerebral ischemia in awake monkeys. *J Neurosurg* 1981;**54**:773–82.

37. **Garcia JH, Lassen NA, Weiller C, Sperling B, & Nakagawara J.** Ischemic stroke and incomplete infarction. *Stroke* 1996;**27**:761–5.

38. **Samson D, Batjer HH, Bowman G,** et al. A clinical study of the parameters and effects of temporary arterial occlusion in the management of intracranial aneurysms. *Neurosurgery* 1994;**34**:22–8; discussion 28–9.

39. **Farkas E & Bari F.** Spreading depolarization in the ischemic brain: does aging have an impact? *J Gerontol A Biol Sci Med Sci* 2014;**69**:1363–70.

40. **Tucsek Z, Toth P, Sosnowska D,** et al. Obesity in aging exacerbates blood-brain barrier disruption, neuroinflammation, and oxidative stress in the mouse hippocampus: effects on expression of genes involved in beta-amyloid generation and Alzheimer's disease. *J Gerontol A Biol Sci Med Sci* 2014;**69**:1212–26.

41. **Sonntag WE, Lynch CD, Cooney PT, & Hutchins PM.** Decreases in cerebral microvasculature with age are associated with the decline in growth hormone and insulin-like growth factor 1. *Endocrinology* 1997;**138**:3515–20.

42. **Adams HP, Jr., Bendixen BH, Kappelle LJ,** et al. Classification of subtype of acute ischemic stroke. Definitions for use in a multicenter clinical trial. TOAST. Trial of Org 10172 in Acute Stroke Treatment. *Stroke* 1993;**24**:35–41.

43. **Napoli C, D'Armiento FP, Mancini FP,** et al. Fatty streak formation occurs in human fetal aortas and is greatly enhanced by maternal hypercholesterolemia. Intimal accumulation of low density lipoprotein and its oxidation precede monocyte recruitment into early atherosclerotic lesions. *J Clin Invest* 1997;**100**:2680–90.

44. **Kovanen PT & Pentikainen MO.** Decorin links low-density lipoproteins (LDL) to collagen: a novel mechanism for retention of LDL in the atherosclerotic plaque. *Trends Cardiovasc Med* 1999;**9**:86–91.

45. **Smith EB.** Transport, interactions and retention of plasma proteins in the intima: the barrier function of the internal elastic lamina. *Eur Heart J* 1990;11 Suppl E:72–81.

46. **Jonasson L, Holm J, Skalli O, Bondjers G, & Hansson GK.** Regional accumulations of T cells, macrophages, and smooth muscle cells in the human atherosclerotic plaque. *Arteriosclerosis* 1986;**6**:131–8.

47. **Ross R.** Atherosclerosis--an inflammatory disease. *N Engl J Med* 1999;**340**:115–26.

48. **Kullo IJ, Edwards WD, Schwartz RS.** Vulnerable plaque: pathobiology and clinical implications. *Ann Intern Med* 1998;**129**:1050–60.

49. **Warlow CP, Dennis MS, van Gijn J,** et al. *Stroke: A Practical Guide to Management.* Oxford, UK: Blackwell Science, 1996.

50. **Palacio S & Hart RG.** Neurologic manifestations of cardiogenic embolism: an update. *Neurol Clin* 2002;**20**:179–93.

51. **Sandercock PA, Warlow CP, Jones LN, & Starkey IR.** Predisposing factors for cerebral infarction: the Oxfordshire community stroke project. *BMJ* 1989;**298**:75–80.

52. **Hobbs FD, Fitzmaurice DA, Mant J,** et al. A randomised controlled trial and cost-effectiveness study of systematic screening (targeted and total population screening) versus routine practice for the detection of atrial fibrillation in people aged 65 and over. The SAFE study. *Health Technol Assess* 2005;**9**:iii–iv, ix-x, 1–74.

53. **Weber-Kruger M, Gelbrich G, Stahrenberg R,** et al. Finding atrial fibrillation in stroke patients: randomized evaluation of enhanced and prolonged Holter monitoring--Find-AF(RANDOMISED)—rationale and design. *Am Heart J* 2014;**168**:438–45.e431.

54. **Gladstone DJ, Spring M, Dorian P,** et al. Atrial fibrillation in patients with cryptogenic stroke. *N Engl J Med* 2014;**370**:2467–77.

55. **Anonymous.** Secondary prevention in non-rheumatic atrial fibrillation after transient ischaemic attack or minor stroke. EAFT (European Atrial Fibrillation Trial) Study Group. *Lancet* 1993;**342**:1255–62.

56. **Jorgensen L & Torvik A.** Ischaemic cerebrovascular disease in an autopsy series: part prevalence, location, pathogenesis and clinical course of cerebral infarcts. *J Neurol Sci* 1969;**9**:285–320

57. **Arboix A & Marti-Vilalta JL.** New concepts in lacunar stroke etiology: the constellation of small-vessel arterial disease. *Cerebrovasc Dis* 2004;**17** Suppl 1:58–62.

58. **Fisher CM.** The arterial lesions underlying lacunes. *Acta Neuropathologica* 1968;**12**:1–15.

59. **Bogousslavsky J, Van Melle G, & Regli F.** The Lausanne Stroke Registry: analysis of 1,000 consecutive patients with first stroke. *Stroke* 1988;**19**:1083–92.

60. **You R, McNeil JJ, O'Malley HM, Davis SM, & Donnan GA.** Risk factors for lacunar infarction syndromes. *Neurology* 1995;**45**:1483–7.

61. **Chen YF, Luo CH, Liu YJ, Lu WH, & Su BR.** Distinct non-cerebrovascular risk factors for ischemic lacunar stroke and non-lacunar stroke: preliminary results. *Genet Mol Res* 2015;**14**:3170–6.

62. **Vermeer SE, Longstreth WT, Jr., & Koudstaal PJ.** Silent brain infarcts: a systematic review. *Lancet Neurol* 2007;**6**:611–19.

63. **Vilar-Bergua A, Riba-Llena I, Nafria C,** et al. Blood and CSF biomarkers in brain subcortical ischemic vascular disease: involved pathways and clinical applicability. *J Cereb Blood Flow Metab* 2015;**36**:55–71.

64. **Samson M, Jacquin A, Audia S,** et al. Stroke associated with giant cell arteritis: a population-based study. *J Neurol Neurosurg Psychiatry* 2015;**86**:216–21.

65. **Alsolaimani RS, Bhavsar SV, Khalidi NA,** et al. Severe intracranial involvement in giant cell arteritis: 5 cases and literature review. *J Rheumatol* 2016;**43**:648–56.

66. **Sharland DE.** Erythrocyte sedimentation rate: the normal range in the elderly. *J Am Geriatr Soc* 1980;**28**:346–8.

67. **Ypsilantis E, Courtney ED, Chopra N,** et al. Importance of specimen length during temporal artery biopsy. *Br J Surg* 2011;**98**:1556–60.

68. **Nordborg E & Nordborg C.** Giant cell arteritis: epidemiological clues to its pathogenesis and an update on its treatment. *Rheumatology (Oxford)* 2003;**42**:413–21.

69. **England TJ, Bath PM, Sare GM,** et al. Asymptomatic hemorrhagic transformation of infarction and its relationship with functional outcome and stroke subtype: assessment from the Tinzaparin in Acute Ischaemic Stroke Trial. *Stroke* 2010;**41**:2834–9.

70. **Lodder J, Krijne-Kubat B, & Broekman J.** Cerebral hemorrhagic infarction at autopsy: cardiac embolic cause and the relationship to the cause of death. *Stroke* 1986;**17**:626–9.

71. **Lindley RI, Joanna JM, Sandercock P,** et al. Frequency and risk factors for spontaneous hemorrhagic transformation of cerebral infarction. *J Stroke Cerebrovasc Dis* 2004;**13**:235–46.

72. **Counsell C, Boonyakarnkul S, Dennis M,** et al. Primary intracerebral haemorrhage in the Oxfordshire Community Stroke Project, 2: prognosis. *Cerebrovasc Dis* 1995;**5**:26–34.

73. **Anderson CS, Chakera TM, Stewart-Wynne EG, & Jamrozik KD.** Spectrum of primary intracerebral hemorrhage in Perth, Western Australia, 1989–90: incidence and outcome. *J Neurol Neurosurg Psychiatry* 1994;**57**:936–40.

74. **Smeeton NC, Heuschmann PU, Rudd AG, et al.** Incidence of hemorrhagic stroke in black Caribbean, black African, and white populations: the South London stroke register, 1995–2004. *Stroke* 2007;**38**:3133–8.

75. **Hanger HC, Wilkinson TJ, Fayez-Iskander N, & Sainsbury R.** The risk of recurrent stroke after intracerebral haemorrhage. *J Neurol Neurosurg Psychiatry* 2007;**78**:836–40.

76. **Thrift AG, Donnan GA, & McNeil JJ.** Epidemiology of intracerebral hemorrhage. *Epidemiol Rev* 1995;**17**:361–81.

77. **Massaro AR, Sacco RL, Mohr JP, et al.** Clinical discriminators of lobar and deep hemorrhages: the Stroke Data Bank. *Neurology* 1991;**41**:1881–5.

78. **Auer RN, Sutherland GR.** Primary intracerebral hemorrhage: pathophysiology. *Can J Neurol Sci* 2005;**32** Suppl 2:S3–12.

79. **Akoudad S, Portegies ML, Koudstaal PJ, et al.** Cerebral microbleeds are associated with an increased risk of stroke: the Rotterdam study. *Circulation* 2015;**132**:509–16.

80. **Gratz PP, El-Koussy M, Hsieh K, et al.** Preexisting cerebral microbleeds on susceptibility-weighted magnetic resonance imaging and post-thrombolysis bleeding risk in 392 patients. *Stroke* 2014;**45**:1684–8.

81. **Dannenberg S, Scheitz JF, Rozanski M, et al.** Number of cerebral microbleeds and risk of intracerebral hemorrhage after intravenous thrombolysis. *Stroke* 2014;**45**:2900–5.

82. **Gregoire SM, Jager HR, Yousry TA, Kallis C, Brown MM, & Werring DJ.** Brain microbleeds as a potential risk factor for antiplatelet-related intracerebral haemorrhage: hospital-based, case-control study. *J Neurol Neurosurg Psychiatry* 2010;**81**:679–684.

83. **Revesz T, Holton JL, Lashley T, et al.** Sporadic and familial cerebral amyloid angiopathies. *Brain Pathol* 2002;**12**:343–57.

84. **Tanskanen M, Makela M, Myllykangas L, et al.** Prevalence and severity of cerebral amyloid angiopathy: a population-based study on very elderly Finns (Vantaa 85+). *Neuropathol Appl Neurobiol* 2012;**38**:329–36.

85. **England TJ, Abaei M, Auer DP, et al.** Stem-cell trial of recovery enhancement after stroke 2 (STEMS2). Randomised placebo-controlled trial of granulocyte-colony stimulating factor in mobilising bone marrow stem cells in sub-acute stroke. *Stroke* 2012;**43**:405–11.

Chapter 3

Presentation of stroke in the older person

Jagdish Sharma

Age-related changes in central nervous system

Advancing age is associated with changes in brain parenchyma and vasculature which may have an impact on the presentation of stroke in older patients. There is a reduction in brain weight due to atrophic changes secondary to variable degree of neuronal loss in different parts of the brain. The hippocampus and cerebral cortex are most severely affected,[1] and the ventricles fill in the space released from neuronal shrinkage. The neuronal atrophy is associated with glial changes, which includes white matter degeneration and the development of periventricular leukoaraiosis.[2] While these changes may be secondary to hypoperfusion, some evidence suggests endothelial dysfunction. This can contribute to cognitive dysfunction.[3,4]

In addition there are changes to the brain microvasculature, decrease in capillary surface area but an increase in capillary diameter, volume, and total length.[5,6] These contribute to the development of leukoaraiosis.[5-7] Age-related alterations in cerebral blood vessels might reduce cerebrovascular reserve and cause disruption of focal cerebral perfusion and thus increase the susceptibility of the brain to vascular insufficiency and more severe ischaemic injury.[8-10]

Most stroke presentations in older patients are similar to those in younger patients with respect to Oxford Community Stroke Project classification. However, atypical presentations can lead to diagnostic challenges in older patients due to the interaction between age-related cerebral and circulatory changes and comorbidities.

A few studies have reported characteristics of patients presenting with stroke according to age group, describing differences in younger, older, and very old stroke patients.[11-14] These studies have investigated clinical characteristics and risk factors for stroke. The conclusion was that older stroke patients in general have similar proportions of total, or partial anterior cortical infarcts or lacunar infarcts. However, older patients had more severe neurological deficit for a given stroke syndrome, indicated by stroke severity scales or impact on activities of daily living. Older patients were also more likely to present with features of aphasia, impairment of consciousness, severity of weakness, and more frequent problems of dysarthria, dysphagia, and urinary incontinence. One study categorized patients according to computed tomography (CT) scan features in the acute phase as 'large' or 'non-large' infarcts and reported that there was no difference in mean age of the two groups of patients.[13,15]

One of the largest studies from Europe—the European BIOMED Stroke Study[11] involving 4534 consecutive patients with the first ever stroke in 12 centres in seven countries across Europe—reported that the older patients, over 80 years, were more prone to larger anterior circulation infarcts, there were fewer cerebral haemorrhages and a larger proportion of patients were in the 'unclassified' category of the 'TOAST' classification. One explanation might be the difficulty of clinical assessment of older stroke patients due to coexisting musculoskeletal pathology and cognitive impairment. The older patients were more often female, previously more dependent, and residents of care homes. The older patients presented with higher impairment of cognition and alertness, more severe paralysis, dysphasia, dysphagia, and incontinence. In addition, it is our observation that quite often the older patient presenting with a significant clinical stroke syndrome may not have any relevant findings visible on acute phase CT scan, possibly related to cerebral atrophy and chronic subcortical white matter ischaemia.

More recent data from the Dijon Stroke study further demonstrate that the rising age is associated with increasing frequency of large artery atheromatous and cardioembolic strokes and corresponding decrease in small vessel disease and undetermined causes.[16,17]

The very elderly patients

The very old patients—above the age of 85 years—are reported to be more likely to have significantly impaired level of consciousness, more severe hemiparesis, impairment of ocular movements and speech, and more likely to be confined to bed and be incontinent as compared to patients below the age of 85 years (i.e. they have more severe neurological and functional impairment).[12] These studies have reported their observations according to the neuroimaging by CT scan, and need replication using MRI. One explanation for more severe neurological and functional impairment in older patients is likely the more frequent cardioembolic strokes in the very old, reduced neuronal reserve due to cerebral atrophy and vascular changes; impaired potential for recovery related to poor adaptability in the older person would be another factor.[13]

Diagnostic difficulties

Older stroke patients often have a background of significant existing comorbidity which can affect the clinical presentation and cause difficulties in clinically examining patients. In such cases, acute phase MRI scanning may improve diagnostic accuracy.[18] There are reports of diagnostic errors in older patients for various clinical conditions including stroke.[19] A repeat examination supported by neuroimaging is frequently required to make a definitive diagnosis. For example, a paretic upper limb may be due to a fractured shoulder after a fall rather than a stroke; the presence of good hand grip in a shoulder fracture would help in differentiating the two.

There may also be gender differences in stroke presentation in older patients.[20,21] Motor and sensory deficits are similar, but elderly female patients have more impairment of speech, vision, and swallowing. It has been reported in several studies that elderly female patients have larger cortical infarcts, while men develop more lacunar infarcts.[20,21]

One complicating feature in older stroke patients is that they often have recurrent strokes on the background of previous ischaemic or haemorrhagic events. This leads to clinical uncertainties whether the patient has developed a new clinical stroke syndrome superimposed on previous stroke-related neurological deficit, which may add to the severity of total neurological deficit. The presence of periventricular and deep white matter lesions, common in older patients, increases the risk of intracerebral haemorrhage. It can be a challenge to determine what is new and what is an old stroke pathology.[22] Presence of frailty also leads to uncertainty about the diagnosis and of atypical features of stroke presentation.[23]

Stroke-related atypical presentations

One presentation of stroke patients in old age is of *seizures*, which may be a typical clinical convulsive feature but quite often has atypical presentation (i.e. the patient being found on the floor with a hemiplegic syndrome followed by recovery over the ensuing day or two, the patient often would not have any recall and neuroimaging revealing an infarct). An electroencephalogram (EEG) in such cases, performed soon after the event, is likely to support the diagnosis of a seizure recognized as *Todd's paralysis*. Non-convulsive seizure secondary to a stroke is a well-known phenomenon and should be considered in the clinical scenario of an older patient presenting with reduced Glasgow coma scale. This symptom quite often complicates vascular dementia (or rarely Alzheimer's disease),[24] but could also be caused by a tumour, mandating neuroimaging.

Headache is a common symptom at the onset of a stroke, both in ischaemic infarct and an intracerebral haemorrhage. Headache related to migraine remains a risk of stroke in older patients. Headache is also a presenting feature in cerebral infarcts particularly involving the cortical area. Although the presence of severe headache along with clinical stroke may herald other pathology such as subarachnoid haemorrhage, brain tumour, a possibility of vasculitis, and migraine-related headache should be considered as a differential diagnosis in patients presenting with stroke in older age groups[25] although new onset of migraine in the very old patient would be a rare phenomenon and should be the last on differential diagnosis.

Clinical examination of some older stroke patients may reveal bilateral brisk reflexes and extensor plantar responses in the presence of unilateral acute stroke. The explanation in some of these patients is the presence of previous *silent brain infarction* syndrome (incidental findings on neuroimaging but without known or recognized clinical stroke syndrome in the past), which is a risk factor for future strokes. Silent brain infarctions are present in 20% adults over the age of 70 years and increases the risk of stroke twofold.[26] These lesions are silent as they go undiagnosed but lead to clinical impairment of motor and cognitive function—and are thus not quite silent where functional impairment is concerned. Freezing gait syndrome is one presentation of this pathology. Previous such infarcts remain asymptomatic but may be indicated by abnormal neurological features, which may not be explained on the basis of incident stroke. These patients may also suffer from vascular dementia, which is an independent risk factor for stroke and seizures.[27]

An older patient may present with acute confusion and disorientation, and the examination may reveal only varying degree of visual impairment secondary to the usually bilateral occipital lobe infarcts without any motor neurological deficit. Hallucinations may be present. These have an impact on orientation, rehabilitation, and quality of life.[28]

One form of cerebrovascular disease encountered in older patients is of *leukoaraiosis* and cerebral white matter changes. These may present with gait impairment and examination reveals neurological abnormalities such as upper motor signs, primitive reflexes, slowing of finger tap, and extrapyramidal signs. MRI scan in such patients reveals evidence of leukoaraiosis and incident lacunar infarcts. The presence of white matter lesions is not always benign and may explain abnormal neurological clinical signs and gait and balance impairment in addition to cognitive impairment.[29] These lacunar infarcts are indicative of small vessel disease similar to leukoaraiosis.[30] In such cases investigation of the carotid artery may not be warranted.[31]

Some patients may present with features like *movement disorders* such as choreoathetosis and tremor of abrupt onset due to the lesion in extrapyramidal nigrostriatal system. Another mode of presentation is of vomiting, imbalance, and dizziness, the neuroimaging revealing the evidence of an ischaemic or a haemorrhagic lesion; lateral medullary syndrome would be one explanation.

The syndrome of *isolated vertigo and nystagmus* is now also recognized to be due to a brain stem infarct on the MRI scan rather than the non-stroke vestibular lesion. Disproportionate degree of *disorientation and personality disorder* in the presence of a hemiplegic syndrome would indicate a thalamic lesion, the hub of neurotransmission between extrapyramidal nuclei and the cortex.

Amyloid angiopathy and cortical superficial siderosis

Increasing age leads to the development of amyloid pathology of cerebral vessels. This may present as recurrent haemorrhagic strokes and the MRI scan reveals the presence of microbleeds on susceptibility weighted images.[32,33] Older patients may present with recurrent transient focal neurological symptoms such as intermittent dysphasia or limb paresis similar to the transient ischaemic attacks or minor seizures; the MRI scan may provide the explanation in the form of haemorrhagic lesions of superficial cortical siderosis. These conditions are associated with the risk of recurrent intracerebral haemorrhages and should be excluded at the time of presentation where relevant, since there is a risk of cerebral haemorrhage with thrombolysis (which otherwise is a safe and effective treatment for elderly patients presenting with ischaemic strokes).[34] Whether long-term antiplatelet therapy is safe in such patients remains a question for research.

Non-specific presentations of stroke pathology in older persons

Several clinical symptoms develop secondary to acute stroke lesions and may be the predominant presenting feature with or without the clinical evidence of a hemiplegic stroke. These may be of acute or subacute nature.

An older person with a stroke may present with a *fall* and is thus at the risk of fall-related injury and complications. A fall is more likely to be the presenting feature in a patient with non-dominant hemisphere since the patients are not quite aware of the hemiplegic limbs due to anosognosia and thus attempt to walk. The patient may present with confusion and a weak limb secondary to the hemiplegia or only the traumatic fracture without hemiplegia. Neuroimaging is essential to arrive at the diagnosis of the stroke lesion.

Older patients may accumulate a considerable number of cerebrovascular events over the years secondary to the long-term presence of risk factors. One of these is leukoaraiosis, as already mentioned; the additional presentation is with vascular *cognitive impairment* or dementia. The description by Hachinski of the stepwise deterioration in cognition and abrupt onset of dementia along with a number of parameters comprising the Hachinski ischaemic scale has been challenged but still holds true to differentiate from Alzheimer's disease.[35–39] Some of these patients may present with an insidious onset of *dysphagia* due to pseudobulbar palsy; the presence of brisk reflexes and tonic tongue movement, and the absence of diplopia and ptosis would help to differentiate from myasthenia gravis.

Older patients remain at a risk of acute confusional state in reference to any acute illness and a stroke is no exception. Delirium, an acute onset of altered level of consciousness with fluctuating course in orientation, memory, thought, or behaviour, is one mode of presentation of overt or even occult stroke, ischaemic or haemorrhagic, in older patients. Diagnosis remains a challenge since the history may not be forthcoming in the absence of a clear focal neurological deficit. Stroke patients have a higher risk of delirium than general acute medical illnesses. Presence of delirium has an unfavourable impact on recovery, mortality, and institutionalization following a stroke.[40] Patients with previous cognitive deficit, right-sided hemisphere stroke, large vessel stroke, severe stroke, and presence of cerebral atrophy are at a higher risk of developing delirium.[41] Early recognition and management may improve the outcome.

Box 3.1 Atypical and non-specific presentation of stroke pathology in older persons

Seizure

Headache

Silent infarction syndromes

Acute confusion, disorientation, delirium

Hallucinations

Syndromes of leukoaraiosis

Isolated vertigo and nystagmus

Vascular cognitive impairment

Personality disorder

Movement disorders

Fall

Freezing gait syndrome

Dysphagia—pseudobulbar palsy

Recurrent transient ischaemic attack like symptoms due to superficial cortical siderosis

Conclusion

While the majority of the older persons with stroke present with the classical stroke syndromes, some will present with atypical and non-specific presentations (Box 3.1). Stroke in the older person is not always an acute event but does present with the aftermath of long-term evolution of stroke pathology and the resultant clinical syndromes.

A detailed history and repeat examination, along with appropriate and repeat investigations of neuroimaging, general medical, and neurological nature would be required to establish the correct diagnosis and a plan of management.

References

1. **Esiri MM.** Ageing and the brain. *J Pathol* 2007;**211**:181–7.
2. **Fernando MS, Simpson JE, Matthews F, et al.** White matter lesions in an unselected cohort of elderly. Molecular pathology suggests origin from chronic hypoperfusion injury. *Stroke* 2006;**37**:1391–8.
3. **de Groot JC, de Leeuw FE, Oudkerk M, et al.** Cerebral white matter lesions and cognitive function: the Rotterdam Scan Study. *Ann Neurol* 2000;**47**:145–51.
4. **Pugh KG & Lipstiz LA.** The microvascular frontal-subcortical syndrome of ageing. *Neurobiol Aging* 2002;**23**:421–31.
5. **Farkas E, de Vos RA, Donka G, Jansen Steur EN, Mihaly A, & Luiten PGl.** Age related microvascular degeneration in the human cerebral periventricular white matter. *Acta Neuropathol* 2006;**111**:150–7.
6. **Marstrand JR, Garde E, Rostrup E, et al.** Cerebral perfusion and cerebrovascular reactivity are reduced in white matter hyperintensities. *Stroke* 2002;**33**:972–6.

7. **Bertsch K, Hagemann D, Hermes M, Walter C, Khan R, & Naumann E.** Resting cerebral blood flow, attention, and ageing. *Brain Res* 2009;**1267**:77–88.

8. **Mitchell GF.** Effects of central arterial aging on the structure and function of the peripheral vasculature: implications for end-organ damage. *J Appl Physiol* 2008;**105**:1652–60.

9. **Ueno M, Tomimoto H, Akiguchi I, Wakita H, & Sakamoto H.** Blood brain barrier disruption in white matter lesions in a rat model of chronic cerebral hypoperfusion. *J Cereb Blood Flow Metab* 2002;**22**:97–104.

10. **Qin CC, Hui RT, & Liu ZH.** Aging-related cerebral microvascular degeneration is an important cause of essential hypertension. *Med Hypotheses* 2008;**70**:643–5.

11. **Di-Carlo A, Lamassa M, Pracucci G,** et al. Stroke in the very elderly: clinical presentation and determinants of 3-month functional outcome: a European perspective. European BIOMED Study of Stroke Care Group. *Stroke* 1999;**30**:2313–19.

12. **Asplund K, Carberg B, & Sunderstrom G.** Stroke in the elderly. Observations in a population-based sample of hospitalised patients. *Cerebrovasc Dis* 1992;**2**:152–7.

13. **Sharma JC, Flecher S, & Vassallo M.** Strokes in the elderly-higher acute and 3-monthly mortality-an explanation. *Cerebrovasc Dis* 1999;**9**:2–9.

14. **Kammersgaard LP, Jorgensen HS, Nakayama H, Pedersen PM, & Oslen TS.** Short-and-long-term prognosis for very old stroke patients. The Copenhagen Stroke Study. *Age Ageing* 2004;**33**:149–54.

15. **Sharma JC, Fletcher S, Vassallo M, & Ross I.** Prognostic value of CT scan features in acute ischaemic stroke and relationship with clinical stroke syndromes. *In J Clin Practice* 2000;**54**:514–18.

16. **Bejot Y, Dauball B, Jacquin A,** et al. Trends in the ischaemic stroke in young adults between 1985 and 2011: Dijon stroke registry. *J Neurol Neurosurg Psychiatry* 2014;**85**:509–13.

17. **Ramirez L, Kim-Tenser MA, Sanossian N,** et al. Trends in acute ischaemic stroke hospitalisation in the United States. *J Am Heart Assoc* 2016;**5**(5):pii e003233.

18. **Paolini S, Burdine J, Verenes M,** et al. Rapid short MRI sequence useful in eliminating stroke mimics among acute stroke patients considered for intravenous thrombolysis. *J Neurol Disord* 2014;**1**:137.

19. **Skinner TR, Scott IA, & Martin JH.** Diagnostic errors in older patients: a systematic review of incidence and potential causes in seven prevalent diseases. *Int J Gen Med* 2016;**9**:137–46.

20. **Sharma JC, Fletcher S, & Vassallo M.** Characteristics and mortality of acute stroke patients: are there any gender differences? *J Gend Specif Med* 2002;**5**:24–7.

21. **Roquer J, Campello AR, & Gomis M.** Sex differences in first-ever acute stroke. *Stroke* 2003;**34**:1581–5.

22. **Kaffashian S, Tzourio CV, Zhu YC, Mazoyer B, & Debette S.** Differential effect of white-matter lesions and covert brain infarcts on the risk of ischemic stroke and intracerebral hemorrhage. *Stroke* 2016;**47**:1923–5.

23. **Rockwood K, Song X, Macknight C,** et al. A global clinical measure of fitness and frailty in elderly people. *CMAJ* 2005;**173**:489–95.

24. **Imfeld P, Bodmer M, Schuerch M, Jick SS, & Meier CR.** Seizures in patients with Alzheimer's disease or vascular dementia: a population-based nested case-control analysis. *Epilepsia* 2013;**54**:700–7.

25. **Monteith TS, Gardener H, Rundek T, Elkind MS, & Sacco RL.** Migraine and risk of stroke in older adults: northern Manhattan study. *Neurology* 2015;**85**:715–21.

26. **Gupta A, Giambrone AE, Gialdini G,** et al. Silent brain infarction and risk of future stroke: a systemic review and meta-analysis. *Stroke* 2016;**47**:719–25.

27. **Cook M, Baker N, Lanes S, Bullock R, Wentworth C, & Arrighi HM.** Incidence of stroke and seizure in Alzheimer's disease dementia. *Age Ageing* 2015;**44**:695–9.

28. **Sand K, Wihelmsen G, Naess H, Thomassen L, & Hoff JM.** Vision problems in ischaemic stroke patients: effects on life quality and disability. *Eur J Neurol* 2016;**23** Suppl 1:1–7.

29. **Poggesi A, Gouw A, van der Flier W,** et al. Cerebral white matter changes are associated with abnormalities on neurological examination in non-disabled elderly: the LADIS study. *J Neurol* 2013;**260**:1014–21.

30. **Ntaios G, Lip GY, Lambrou D, et al.** Leukoaraiosis and stroke recurrence risk in patients with and without atrial fibrillation. *Neurology* 2015;**84**:1213–19.

31. **Rajapakse A, Rajapakse S, & Sharma JC.** Is investigating for carotid artery disease warranted in non-cortical lacunar infarction. *Stroke* 2011;**42**:217–20.

32. **Charidimou A, Linn J, Vernooij MW, et al.** Cortical superficial siderosis: detection and clinical significance in cerebral amyloid angiopathy and related conditions. *Brain* 2015;**138**:2126–39.

33. **Zerna C, Modi J, Bilston L, Shomanesh A, Coutts B, & Smith EE.** Cerebral microbleeds and cortical superficial siderosis in patients presenting with minor cerebrovascular events. *Stroke* 2016;**47**:2236–41.

34. **Mishra NK, Ahmed N, Anderson G, et al.** Thrombolysis in very elderly people: controlled comparison of SITS International Stroke Thrombolysis Registry and Virtual International Stroke Trials Archive. *BMJ* 2010;**341**:c6046.

35. **Hachinski VC, Potter P, & Merskey H.** Leukoaraiosis. *Arch Neurol* 1987;**44**:21–8.

36. **Hachinski VC, Lassen NA, & Marshall J.** Multi-infarct dementia: a cause of mental deterioration in the elderly. *Lancet* 1974;207–10.

37. **Hachinski VC, Illiff LD, Zilkha E, et al.** Cerebral blood flow in dementia. *Arch Neurol* 1975;**32**:632–37.

38. **Denning T & Berrios GE.** The Hachinski ischaemic score: a re-evaluation. *Int J Geriatric Psychiatry* 1992;**7**:585–9.

39. **Moroney JT, Bagiella E, Desmond DW, et al.** Meta-analysis of the Hachinski score in pathologically verified dementias. *Neurology* 1997;**49**:1096–105.

40. **Shi Q, Presutti R, Selchen D, & Saponisk G.** Delirium in acute stroke. A systematic review and meta-analysis. *Stroke* 2012;**43**:645–9.

41. **Oldenbcuving AW, de Kort PLM, Jansen BPW, Algra A, Kappelle LJ, & Roks G.** Delirium in acute phase after stroke. *Neurology* 2011;**76**:993–9.

Chapter 4

Transient ischaemic attack (TIA) in the older person

Marissa Hagan and Ashit K. Shetty

Introduction

TIA has been redefined several times over the last 15 years as ongoing research helps us better understand the nature of both transient symptoms and cerebral ischaemia.

Up until 2002 the definition of TIA was 'an acute loss of focal brain or monocular function with symptoms lasting less than 24 hours and which is thought to be caused by inadequate cerebral or ocular blood supply as a result of arterial thrombosis, low flow or embolism associated with arterial, cardiac or haematological disease'.[1,2]

Advances in neuroimaging have identified that there can be brain infarction even when neurologic symptoms last less than 1 hour; thus, a proportion of patients presenting with a possible TIA may in fact have had minor strokes. Therefore, the inference that TIA is a benign event has been superseded by an understanding that even relatively brief ischaemia can cause permanent brain injury. In light of this the American Heart Association and American Stroke Association (AHA/ASA) redefined TIA as 'a transient episode of neurologic dysfunction caused by focal brain, spinal cord, or retinal ischaemia, without acute infarction'.[3] The advantages of this updated definition is that the defined end point is biologic (i.e. whether tissue infarction has or had not occurred, rather than an arbitrary 24-hour time period thus encouraging the use of neuroimaging to identify brain injury and its cause).[4]

Up to 50% of patients who meet the old criteria for TIA had evidence of acute infarction on magnetic resonance imaging (MRI) scans.[5] This may be the case for patients with the following features:

- NIHSS score <2 for hemianopia, aphasia, or limb weakness
- NIHSS score <1 for sensory inattention
- NIHSS score <5 in total[6]

Patients presenting with minor, non-disabling neurological deficits and MRI changes consistent with acute infarction should therefore receive a diagnosis of 'minor stroke'.

Incidence of TIA and implication

The age-adjusted annual incidence of TIA in the United Kingdom is about 50 cases per 100 000.[7] In the United States, the annual incidence is 200 000 to 500 000 cases depending on which clinical surveys are reviewed. However, on a worldwide basis the incidence of TIA is likely to be higher than documented due to the transient nature of symptoms and patients opting to not seek medical advice. In addition, while many people are aware of the symptoms of an acute stroke, most would not identify the symptoms or appreciate the significance of a TIA. This is significant as approximately 15% of ischaemic strokes are preceded by a confirmed TIA.[8] TIA and acute stroke lie on a spectrum of cerebrovascular ischaemia; TIA should be investigated thoroughly and preventative therapies instituted to reduce morbidity and mortality associated with stroke.

TIA pathophysiology

The pathophysiology of TIA is complex and can be split into five different groups all of which cause locally decreased blood flow to the brain.

Cardioembolic events

These account for 20–25% of TIAs. Intracardiac thrombus may form in response to stasis from impaired ejection fraction or atrial fibrillation. Occasionally, there may be a thrombogenic focus within the heart such as an artificial heart valve or infective vegetation. Infrequently, the thrombus can pass from the venous system into the arterial via a cardiac shunt causing a paradoxical embolus.

Large vessel atheroma

This accounts for 16% of TIAs. Extracranial or intracranial artery stenosis or unstable atherosclerotic plaque rupture causes *in situ* thrombosis of the vessel or artery-to-artery embolism of the thrombus.

Small vessel occlusion

This accounts for a further 16% of TIAs. Small vessel ischaemic lesions tend to be found in hypertensive patients or those with diabetes mellitus. These diseases cause microatheromas, fibrinoid necrosis, and lipohyalinosis of the small penetrating vessels.

Less common aetiologies

This affects 3% of patients with TIA. Intracranial artery or small vessel occlusion is due to hypercoagulability, dissection, vasculitis, vasospasm, or sickle cell occlusive disease.

Uncertain mechanism.

In 36% of patients the cause of TIA is never identified, despite investigation.

History, examination, and presenting symptoms

The history is key given that most patients' symptoms have resolved at the time of clinic attendance. The history should cover the following points:

- Identification of symptoms in keeping with a focal neurological deficit
- Timing of symptom onset and resolution
- Any recurrence of focal neurology and over what period. Could this be crescendo TIA?
- Presence of symptoms that may suggest a TIA mimic
- Identification of risk factors for cerebrovascular disease: diabetes mellitus, dyslipidaemia, hypertension, previous TIA, stroke, or heart disease, smoking and alcohol consumption, body weight, inactivity
- History of trauma, sudden shear stress, facial or neck pain (suggesting dissection)
- Symptoms of temporal arteritis—diplopia, visual loss, headaches, weakness, jaw pain

Key parts of the history which suggest TIA:

◆ Sudden onset—patients with gradual onset symptoms are less likely to have a TIA

◆ Intensity—maximal intensity of symptoms at onset. Gradual progression of symptoms suggests migraine

◆ Duration—most TIAs last 5–15 minutes

◆ Pattern—symptoms that correspond with a vascular territory

Cognitive impairment is a big obstacle to the correct diagnosis of TIA in the older patient. Chronology of events is sometimes vague; there may be omissions of symptoms and triggers, confabulation of events and difficulties with left–right lateralization. Time should be spent clarifying exactly what the patient meant by terms such as confusion, blurred vision, dizziness, and weakness.

Presenting symptoms of TIA vary greatly depending on the vascular territory affected and the mechanism of TIA.

The most common anterior circulation TIA symptoms are:

◆ Limb and/or facial weakness

◆ Paraesthesias or numbness

◆ Speech difficulty

◆ Headache

Posterior circulation TIAs often present with:

◆ Visual loss or double vision

◆ In-coordination

◆ Vertigo

◆ Nausea

Arterial dissections may present with:

◆ Neck or facial pain

Lacunar TIAs may present with:

◆ Limb and/or facial weakness (typically affects face, leg, and arm equally)

◆ Paraesthesias or numbness (typically affects face, leg, and arm equally)

◆ Speech difficulty

Differential diagnosis

Up to 60% of patients presenting to TIA clinic have a non-TIA diagnosis.[9,10]

Next is a list of symptoms that make the diagnosis of TIA unlikely:

◆ Gradual progression, recurrent or stereotypical symptoms

◆ Severe headache

◆ 'Confusion'

◆ Acute loss of memory

◆ Seizure

◆ Loss of consciousness

◆ Isolated dizziness, vertigo, or feeling of being lightheaded

In these cases it is important to try to identify the potential cause, as this will guide further investigation and management of the patient.

Common TIA mimics diagnosed in older patients

Migraine: migrainous aura is usually experienced as visual or speech disturbance, sensory symptoms, or motor weakness lasting from 20 to 60 minutes. Although usually followed immediately by a severe headache, there may be a delay of over an hour. Thus, patients and clinicians may not consider the aura and headache as one clinical event leading to misdiagnosis of TIA.

Seizure: Todd's paresis occurs following 1 in 10 generalized seizures and last from a few minutes to several hours. Therefore, there will be a number of patients incorrectly diagnosed with TIA due to experiencing an unwitnessed seizure, particularly in the absence of a history of epilepsy. Focal motor seizures and complex partial seizures also produce transient neurological symptoms that can be misattributed to TIA.

Vestibular disorders: peripheral vestibulopathies can cause transient dizziness. The absence of diplopia, dysarthria, cerebellar ataxia, or occipital visual field defect distinguishes simple dizziness from a posterior TIA.

Central nerve system (CNS) tumours: the first presentation of a CNS tumour may be transient neurology. Abrupt displacement of brain tissue resulting in neurological symptoms is usually caused by haemorrhage into a tumour or as a result of the tumour reaching a critical mass.

Ocular disorders: subacute angle closure glaucoma, giant cell arteritis, posterior vitreous detachment, vitreous haemorrhage, and retinal migraine can all present with transient visual symptoms (TVS), or amaurosis fugax.[11] Fundoscopy should be performed in patients presenting with monocular blindness and referred urgently to an ophthalmologist if ocular pathology is suspected (see Table 4.1 and Box 4.1).

Nerve compression: pressure or position-related peripheral nerve compression can cause transient parasthesias and numbness

Hypoglycaemia: can cause transient focal neurology that resolves with normoglycaemia.

Amyloid 'spells': Cerebral amyloid angiopathy, a cause of lobar cerebral haemorrhage in older patients, can also present with transient focal neurological episodes, or 'amyloid spells'. These are stereotyped, recurrent, transient neurological episodes of paraesthesias, numbness, or weakness of spreading onset over seconds to minutes, resolving over a similar period. Imaging with MRI is important as the risk of intracerebral bleed following an amyloid 'spell' is high.

Medications: the side effects of medications such as opiates, hypnotics, antihypertensives can simulate a myriad of neurological symptoms mimicking that of a TIA.[12]

Risk factors

Understanding the various TIA risk factors allows opportunity to develop risk reduction strategies. Risk factors can be classified into non-modifiable and modifiable:

- Non-modifiable: age, gender, race
- Modifiable: hypertension, hyperlipidaemia, current smoker, obesity, physical inactivity, atrial fibrillation, carotid stenosis, diabetes mellitus, alcohol excess

Although age is the strongest risk factor, the first five modifiable risk factors account for 82% of strokes.

Table 4.1 Summary: differential diagnosis of transient visual loss

	TIA	Seizure	Migraine	Syncope
Demography	Older patients Stroke risk factors present Men > women	Any age	Younger age Women > men	Any age, often young Women > men
CNS symptoms	Negative symptoms: numbness, visual loss, paralysis, ataxia Multiple deficits occur simultaneously	Positive symptoms: limb jerking, head turning, loss of consciousness Negative symptoms may develop post ictally	First positive symptoms then negative in the same modality: scintillating scotoma and paraesthesia most common	Light-headed, dim vision, noises distant. Transient loss of consciousness
Timing	Usually minutes, mostly <1 hour Symptoms either settle or result in completed stroke	20–120 seconds Absence, atonic seizures, and myoclonic jerks are shorter	Usually 20–30 minutes Sporadic attacks over years	Usually a few seconds Sporadic attacks over the years
Associated symptoms	Headaches may occur during the TIA event	Tongue biting, incontinence, sore muscles, headache post event	Headache after aura, nausea, vomiting, photophobia, phonophobia	Sweating, pallor, nausea

Non-modifiable

These help identify the high-risk population for TIA. If the modifiable risk factors are controlled, the overall risk of TIA can be significantly reduced.

Age

Age is a well-documented risk factor for TIA, with an incidence of 1–3 cases per 100 000 in those younger than 35 years to as many as 1500 cases per 100 000 in those older than 85 years in one study.[13]

Gender

TIA is more common in men than women. The incidence of TIAs in men (101 cases per 100 000 population) is significantly higher than that in women (70 per 100 000).[14]

Race and ethnicity

The highest incidence of TIA is seen in black men over 85 years. The incidence of TIAs in black people (98 cases per 100 000 population) is higher than that in white people (81 per 100 000 population). This is likely due to the higher prevalence of hypertension and diabetes.[15]

Modifiable

Atrial fibrillation

Atrial fibrillation causes stasis of blood in the left atrium increasing the likelihood of thrombus formation. Once the thrombus has formed in the heart it can embolize causing TIA or stroke. The

Box 4.1 A note on transient visual symptoms

TVS is a common presentation in a TIA clinic and is defined as monocular visual loss attributed to ischaemia or vascular insufficiency. Typically, the patient describes diminished or absent vision in one eye that progresses over few seconds and last for few seconds or minutes. The loss of vision usually starts in the upper field, less frequently in the periphery, and rarely in the lower field. Visual symptoms in these settings are classified as transient monocular blindness, diplopia, homonymous lateral hemianopia, bilateral positive visual phenomena, lone bilateral blindness, and others. Transient monocular blindness is the most common.[12]

Causes

Embolic	Haemodynamic
◆ Carotid bifurcation thromboembolism	◆ Extensive atheromatous occlusive disease
◆ Great vessel or distal internal carotid artery atheroembolism	◆ Inflammatory arteritis
◆ Cardiac emboli (valve, mural thrombi)	
◆ Drug abuse-related intravascular emboli	

Ocular	Neurologic
◆ Anterior ischaemic optic neuropathy	◆ Brainstem, vestibular, and oculomotor optic neuritis
◆ Central or branch retinal artery occlusion	◆ Optic nerve or chiasm compression
◆ Central or branch retinal vein occlusion	◆ Papilloedema
◆ Glaucoma	◆ Multiple sclerosis
◆ Cataracts	◆ Migraine
	◆ Psychogenic

Prognosis

In a British study, compared with cerebral TIA, patients with TVS have a similar mortality rate but a lower incidence of stroke. Patients with TVS who have an occluded or narrowed proximal internal carotid artery have a greater risk of subsequent stroke than those with a normal carotid artery (P <0.01).[11] Another study found that 20% of patients with TVS had an underlying disease associated with a high risk of stroke recurrence. This rate was lower than in patients with non-visual neurological symptoms (28.1%) but high enough to conclude that patients with TVS should undergo immediate investigation and treatment in TIA clinics.[12]

relative risk for TIA is fivefold higher in those with non-valvular atrial fibrillation compared to those in sinus rhythm. The risk significantly increases in valvular atrial fibrillation.[16,17] The 90-day risk of stroke post TIA in a patient with atrial fibrillation is approximately 11% with the risk being higher for those in persistent atrial fibrillation.

Hypertension

Hypertension is a well-known risk factor for cardiovascular and cerebrovascular disease by accelerating the atherosclerotic process. The relative risk of TIA in hypertension is two- to fivefold, with the risk increasing with higher blood pressure.[14,15] Patients diagnosed with TIA who have a blood pressure ≥140/≥90 have an increased risk of stroke with odds ratio of 2.1, 1.9, and 1.6 at 2, 7, and 90 days, respectively.[18]

Smoking history

Smoking is a risk factor for arterial disease. The effects of smoking are multiple, in raising a patient's blood pressure, increasing blood viscosity, and accelerating the rate of atherosclerosis. The risk of developing a stroke as a smoker is two- to fourfold compared to non-smokers.[19] Patients who have a high pack-year smoking history or smoke a pack of cigarettes (or more) a day are at highest risk of cerebral ischaemia.[20]

Alcohol excess

Alcohol and TIA/stroke risk has a complex relationship. There is a protective effect with moderate alcohol intake, possibly through increase of high-density lipoprotein (HDL) and decreased platelet aggregation. However, with high alcohol intake (>60 g of alcohol daily, or men consuming ≥15 drinks and women consuming ≥8 drinks per week) the risk of TIA and stroke increases by an odds ratio of 1.6.[21]

Diabetes mellitus

Diabetes is a well-known risk factor for cerebrovascular and cardiovascular disease. Hyperglycaemia in diabetes drives inflammation and slows blood flow, dramatically accelerating the development of atherosclerosis by causing abnormalities in endothelial, vascular smooth muscle cell, and platelet function. It has been suggested that up to 30% of people presenting with TIA have undiagnosed diabetes.[22] Diabetes increases the risk of TIA by an odds ratio of 1.5 to 2.[16,17] In these patients glycaemic control should achieve blood sugars of 5–15 mmol as tight control in the older patient often leads to hypoglycaemia. Given the association of diabetes with other conditions in the metabolic syndrome, diabetes, and any other identified risk factors should be aggressively managed.

Obesity

Obesity, particularly abdominal obesity, is associated with an increased risk of TIA and stroke. This is likely through a combination of poor diet and sedentary lifestyle leading to high cholesterol and diabetes.

Prognosis and risk scoring

Patients are at greatest risk of having a stroke in the hours to days post TIA. It has been documented that there is a 5% risk of stroke at 48 hours after TIA, 8% at 1 week, 12% at 1 month, and 17% at 3 months.[23,24] With appropriate intervention, approximately 10 000 recurrent strokes every year could be prevented if patients were assessed and treatment started in a timely manner.[25]

ABCD2

All patients who have had a suspected TIA (i.e. supportive history but no focal neurology at time of review) should be assessed using a validated scoring system to determine their risk of subsequent stroke. The most widely used TIA scoring system is ABCD2 (Table 4.2).[18]

The scores can then be used to determine if a patient is at low, medium, or high risk for stroke in the next 2 days:

◆ Low risk (score 0–1 0% 2-day risk, score 2–3, 1% 2-day stroke risk)

◆ Medium risk (score 4–5, 4.1% 2-day stroke risk)

◆ High risk (score 6–7, 8% 2-day score risk)[26]

Table 4.2 ABCD2 TIA risk assessment tool

Age	≥ 60 years	1 point
BP	≥ 140/90 mmHg (initial reading)	1 point
Clinical symptoms	Unilateral weakness	2 points
	Speech disturbance (no weakness)	1 point
Duration	≥ 60 minutes	2 points
	10–59 minutes	1 point
Diabetes		1 point

The use of the ABCD2 score has been incorporated into both the United Kingdom (NICE)[27] and American (AHA/ASA)[3] guidelines for the assessment of patients with TIA. Those patients with an ABCD2 score ≥4 need to be seen for specialist assessment and investigation within 24 hours and immediately commenced on high dose aspirin (e.g. 300 mg). Those with an ABCD2 score <3 should also be commenced on aspirin and reviewed by a specialist as soon as possible within 1 week of reported symptoms. Patients who report symptoms in keeping with TIA more than 1 week after symptoms occurred should be treated as low risk and managed accordingly.

ABCD3 and ABCD3-I

Patients with high ABCD2 scores are more likely to have to cerebral ischaemia on diffusion-weighted imaging. The inclusion of cerebral infarction on the ABCD2 score, scoring 3 points for ischaemia on imaging, improved the predictive power for stroke.[28] It is important to note that patients with imaging-positive transient events have a 90-day risk of stroke as high as 20%. In imaging-negative transient events the risk is 1–5%.[28,29] Colleagues from Boston have shown that risk stratification by the CIP (Clinical and Imaging Prediction) model may assist in early implementation of therapeutic measures and effective use of hospital resources (Box 4.2).

In 2010, Merwick et al.30 proposed two novel scores to predict early risk of stroke after TIA, namely, the ABCD3 and ABCD3-I scores. In the ABCD3 score, dual TIA (the presence of ≥2 TIA symptoms within 7 days) is added to the ABCD2 score. In the ABCD3-I score, the presence of abnormal findings on neuroimaging (i.e. carotid stenosis or abnormal acute diffusion-weighted image [DWI] on brain magnetic resonance imaging [MRI]) was further added to the ABCD3 score. The implication with the newer scores is that even with ABCD of 0–2, the risk of stroke may be high if DWI is positive. The ABCD2 score, or refinements

Box 4.2 Possible advantages of hospitalization

Facilitated early use of thrombolysis or thrombectomy in case patient has ischaemic stroke

Optimal medical management started

Expedited clinical evaluation and investigations

Expedited secondary prevention

Table 4.3 ABCD2 and ABCD3-I score cut off and risk stratification 90 day stroke incidence rates

Score	ABCD2 score (95% CI)	ABCD3-I (95% CI)
0–3	4.62% (1.01–8.22)	0%
4–5	20.83% (12.71–28.96)	7.53% (3.25–11.82)
6–7	23.08% (0.17–45.98)	40.91% (26.38–55.44)

Adapted with permission from Song B, et al. Validation of the ABCD3-I Score to Predict Stroke Risk After Transient Ischemic Attack. *Stroke*, 44(5), 1244–1248. Copyright © 2013, American Heart Association, Inc. https://doi.org/10.1161/STROKEAHA.113.000969.

such as the ABCD3 or ABCD3-I, is not a substitute for individualized judgement, but can aid in decision-making.

Following on from ABCD2, ABCD3, and ABCD3-I (Table 4.3), the inclusion of carotid stenosis (2 points) and ischaemia on DWI (2 points) further improved the 90-day stroke risk classification by 39%.[30] Like the ABCD2 score, the ABCD3-I score can be risk stratified into low-risk (0–3), medium-risk (4–7), and high-risk (8–13) groups.[31]

Atrial fibrillation and TIA

In addition to the various ABCD scores just mentioned, TIAs occurring in the presence of atrial fibrillation are also considered to be high risk for subsequent stroke.

Investigations

The diagnosis of TIA is largely based on the history gained from the patient and any witnesses to the event. A detailed history will help determine if the symptoms are in keeping with TIA and, if so, may help identify which vascular territory is affected and the underlying cause. While most patients who present to TIA clinic have no residual neurological features, a full clinical examination is required to rule out stroke or any TIA mimics.

Investigations are performed to identify any risk factors for TIA which can be treated.

Blood tests

The key blood tests are full blood count, coagulation profile, renal profile, lipid profile, random glucose or HbA1c, and erythrocyte sedimentation rate. These blood tests will help identify any electrolyte disturbance as a cause of transient focal neurology. A renal profile is useful when considering commencement of antihypertensive or anticoagulant medications. The HbA1c will support a diagnosis of diabetes and, in those with known diabetes, enable optimization of blood sugar control as required.

Electrocardiogram

Will identify those patients with atrial fibrillation or recent cardiac ischaemia. Left ventricular hypertrophy on voltage criteria will also support a diagnosis of hypertension. Some patients may benefit from a 24-hour electrocardiographic (ECG) recording if there is high suspicion of paroxysmal atrial fibrillation (AF). This is particularly true of older people in whom 20–25% of ischaemic strokes are due to atrial fibrillation.

Echocardiogram

If there is a history of recent myocardial ischaemia, atrial fibrillation, or heart murmur detected on auscultation, an echocardiogram may show atrial thrombus, left ventricular aneurysm with mural thrombus, atrial myxoma, or valve vegetation in cases of infective endocarditis.

Carotid duplex

Carotid doppler ultrasonography is a safe and easily accessible method of identifying internal carotid artery stenosis as an underlying cause of TIA. It should be performed on those patients presenting with carotid territory symptoms, who would be accepted for carotid endarterectomy and would consent to the surgical procedure. Patients with a carotid stenosis more than 50% may then be considered for CT angiography (CTA) or MR angiography (MRA) to further evaluate the lesion.

Unenhanced CT head

An unenhanced CT head scan should be performed in patients with suspected TIA. It is more readily accessible than MRI in most hospitals and can provide information on cerebrovascular burden, recent ischaemic events, and identify stroke mimics such as subdural haematomas or brain tumours as the cause of symptoms. A CT head is also the main form of cerebral imaging in those patients in which MRI scanning is contraindicated.

MRI

The gold-standard is diffusion-weighted MRI (DWI) as it is more sensitive than CT in identifying small areas of ischaemia in patients presenting with TIA. The use of DWI alongside the apparent diffusion coefficient (ADC) map can differentiate tissue injury very soon after the onset of symptoms. The benefit of DWI with ADC is that one can confirm early on in the presentation whether ischaemic or infarct has occurred, thus enabling diagnosis of stroke rather than TIA within a matter of hours from symptom onset.

Treatments

The treatment of TIA is aimed at preventing a further event and are the same as those given for secondary prevention following an acute stroke. Management of TIA can be split into non-pharmacological, pharmacological, and surgical treatments for immediate treatment and secondary prevention. Both the British and American stroke guidelines suggest the following treatment regime.[3,27]

Non-pharmacological

Diet

All patients should be given advice regarding a Mediterranean type diet—low saturated fat and low salt diet and high intake of fruit and vegetables. For those who drink alcohol, the safe limits of alcohol consumption (less than 21 units (1 unit = 10 g absolute alcohol) for men and less than 14 units a week for women) should be reinforced.

Exercise

All patients should be advised to increase their activity levels to at least 30 minutes of moderate intensity exercise daily.

Smoking

All patients should be advised to stop smoking. There are several over the counter and prescription treatments such as nicotine replacement therapy and bupropion to support smoking cessation.

Pharmacological treatment

Pharmacological treatment is the mainstay of stroke risk reduction following TIA. Clinicians need to be mindful that many older patients are already taking multiple prescribed medications. Side effects are more frequently reported by the older population due to drug–drug and drug–disease interactions and toxicity secondary to altered pharmacokinetics in the ageing body.

Any difficulties with taking current medications should be identified before adding 2–5 new treatments to their tablet burden. These new medications being an antiplatelet, statin, and up to three antihypertensives. One also needs to consider the patient's past medical history (e.g. cognitive impairment, peptic ulcer disease, bleeding tendency, liver or renal disease, postural hypotension, prior to prescribing secondary prevention medication). Prescribers therefore need to balance the benefit of secondary prevention against any possible side effects through slow titration of medications and close monitoring for adverse side effects.

It is reported that secondary prevention has its maximal benefit after receiving treatment for 2 or more years. Therefore, reassessment of secondary prevention treatment needs to be made to those who are in their last year of life or receiving palliative care. In these circumstances, patients may not warrant or benefit from tight blood pressure and cholesterol control and a clinician may feel it is inappropriate to prescribe such treatments. The decision not to prescribe treatment should be made on a case-by-case basis with patients and their carers involved in the decision-making process.

Antiplatelet drugs

All patients should be started on 300 mg aspirin once the diagnosis of TIA is suspected, pending clinical assessment. Three different antiplatelet regimes exist depending on patient comorbidity and drug intolerances/allergies. One can prescribe aspirin alone, aspirin plus dipyridamole or clopidogrel alone. Even though there is evidence that clopidogrel is not inferior to an aspirin-dipyridamole combination in stroke, there is no randomized controlled trial (RCT) evidence for clopidogrel in TIA. Current practice in the United Kingdom is to prescribe clopidogrel 75 mg od, based on NICE Guidelines.[32] The combination of aspirin and clopidogrel should only be used in those patients being treated for concurrent acute coronary syndrome or recent cardiac stenting. In patients with a history of gastrointestinal bleeding open discussion about the risks and benefits of antiplatelets to reduce stroke risk needs to take place and a closely monitored trial of treatment considered. Coprescribing a proton pump inhibitor (PPI) will also reduce the risk of future bleed.

Anticoagulation

Long-term anticoagulation should be prescribed to those patients with confirmed TIA who have atrial fibrillation. This should ideally be commenced once cerebral imaging has excluded intracerebral haemorrhage as a cause of the symptoms. Options include warfarin or one of the direct oral anticoagulants, also known as direct oral anticoagulant (DOACs) (e.g. rivaroxaban, apixaban, dabigatran, edoxaban). Older patients are more likely to have an underlying disease process that increases risk of bleeding or be taking medications that interact with warfarin. It should also be noted that, compared to warfarin, DOACs require significantly less monitoring which may be of benefit for those patients who find it different to attend anticoagulation clinics. Prescribers need to consider any contraindications to anticoagulants and the risk of bleeding using a tool such as HAS-BLED.[33] It is also important to consider the impact cognitive impairment may have on medication use such as multiple missed doses or accidental overdose.

Several guidelines recognize increased bleeding risk with the combination of anticoagulation and antiplatelet therapy and do not recommend this for routine use (in stable coronary artery disease with atrial fibrillation). This is particularly true for the newer DOACs. Combination therapy is recommended when a cardioembolic cerebral ischaemic event on therapeutic anticoagulation has occurred in the setting of mechanical heart valves. Routine use of combination anticoagulant and antiplatelet therapy is not recommended for cardioembolic TIAs occurring in the setting of atrial fibrillation.

Antihypertensives

In the PROGRESS trial the use of perindopril with or without indapamide in patients with confirmed TIA reduced the risk of stroke whether they were hypertensive or non-hypertensive.[34] Initiation of antihypertensive therapy is reasonable the day of, or following, the TIA as long as there are no neurological deficits. A target BP of 130/80 should be achieved in all patients as a minimum. However, in those patients with diabetes the target BP changes to 130/70. However, in extreme old age the target BP can be relaxed although there is no consensus on what this new target should be. In all patient groups the target BP should be achieved by careful titration of medications and monitoring for orthostatic hypotension and changes in renal function and cognition.

Caution should be exercised in those with postural hypotension as the inclusion of antihypertensives may significantly worsen the postural drop resulting in falls and consequent injury and lack of confidence on mobilizing. In these patients accepting a higher BP may be more appropriate as, for some, the risk of syncope and falls with harm is greater than the risk of future stroke. Caution is advised in lowering BP in patients with severe carotid stenosis prior to endarterectomy.

Statins

Following the INTERSTROKE trial all patients with confirmed TIA should be started on a statin even if their cholesterol is within target range.[35] Patients with confirmed TIA who were started on treatment with atorvastatin 80 mg daily had a reduced stroke risk of 16% compared to placebo over 4.9 years follow-up.[36] There is no documented evidence that myotoxicity and hepatotoxicity occur more frequently with increasing age. However, some advocate giving 40 mg atorvastatin to frail patients over 75 years to reduce the likelihood of myalgia and myopathy developing.[37]

Surgical

Carotid endarterectomy

Carotid endarterectomy (CEA) is beneficial in patients with an internal carotid artery stenosis of 70–99% who have had a TIA or stroke attributable to that stenosis.[38,39] There is some benefit in performing carotid endarterectomy in those with 50–69% stenosis who have had a TIA but this is very dependent on the surgical expertise at the treatment centre.[40] Suitable patients should be assessed for and undergo carotid endarterectomy as soon as possible (within 2 weeks) after TIA.

In a much-cited, influential report from the Mayo Clinic, United States, old age was listed among the poor prognostic variables.[41–46] As a result of this report, clinicians were reluctant to offer CEA to older patients with carotid stenosis. Consistent with this the North American Symptomatic Carotid Endarterectomy Trial (NASCET) excluded patients aged 80 years or above for the first 2 of its 9 years. Unfortunately this early exclusion was a mistake, as clearly shown by subsequent findings.

Studies have provided strong evidence that CEA is of benefit in older patients who tend to have a higher incidence of carotid stenosis.[41] In the prevention of ipsilateral ischaemic stroke, older patients with 50–99% symptomatic carotid stenosis benefited more from CEA than younger patients did.[44]

Among the symptomatic 2885 patients with carotid stenosis in the NASCET study, who were randomized to best medical care or best medical care and CEA, several demographic, clinical, and radiologic characteristics were identified at trial entry. Characteristics that individually altered the anticipated results included the degree of stenosis, contralateral occlusion, intracranial stenosis, gender, and widespread leukoaraiosis.[38]

In the NASCET trial a total of 2217 CEAs were carried out on 1961 patients in the registry: 334 patients aged 80 years or more underwent 360 procedures, and the remaining 1627 patients under 80 years old underwent 1857 CEAs.[38] The frequency of postoperative stroke did not differ significantly between the two age groups: 14 (0.8%) strokes occurred in patients less than 80 years vs. 4 (1.1%) in patients 80 years old or more. Operative mortality was slightly lower in the younger group, compared with the older group (0.8% vs. 1.9%, respectively, $P = 0.053$). Mortality was similar in all asymptomatic patients, but was higher in older symptomatic than older asymptomatic patients ($P = 0.007$). The combined rate of stroke, death, or both was higher in the older group than in the younger group (3.1% vs. 1.5%, respectively, $P = 0.041$), the difference arising from the significantly higher rate seen in the older symptomatic patients compared with older asymptomatic patients. The postoperative period and length of hospital stay were longer in the older group ($P = 0.001$). The groups had similar adverse event rates. Survival curve analysis demonstrated higher mortality in the older age group; however, this was similar to mortality in the normal, age-adjusted population. The number of older people needed to treat with CEA for severe stenosis in order to prevent one stroke in 2 years was reduced to three patients, compared with ten for those aged 65 years or less. Combining the NASCET study results with data from the European Carotid Surgery Trial (ECST) confirmed this special benefit of CEA for older patients.[39]

Therefore, the term 'high risk' should not be arbitrarily applied to patients reaching the 80-year threshold.[47]

However carotid endarterectomies continue to be performed less frequently in older patients. This may be due to ageism, patient frailty, comorbidity, contraindications to surgery, or patient reluctance to undergo a surgical procedure. To achieve this treatment benefit, surgeons must be skilled and patients with other life-threatening illnesses must be excluded. The general consensus is that if the survival is at least 5 years, then CEA should be undertaken. However, in high-risk symptomatic older patients this figure may be brought down to 2–3 years.

TIA in the real world

In the OXVASC (Oxford Vascular Study) and Oxfordshire Community Stroke Project (OCSP) database, about 43% of patients who suffered an ischaemic stroke retrospectively reported symptoms in keeping with TIA within 7 days before the index event.[48] Out of these, 17% had symptoms of TIA on the same day and 9% reported symptoms the day before. Therefore, TIA should be viewed as a medical emergency as it heralds high risk of ischaemic stroke just like the relationship between unstable angina and acute coronary syndrome. Thus, in order to deliver an effective stroke prevention treatment plan, the service needs to be provided quickly with expert evaluation and immediate access to investigations and treatment. There is now ample evidence that early institution of pharmacological, non-pharmacological, and surgical intervention can reduce the risk

---

Box 4.3 Indications for hospitalization

ABCD2>3

ABCD2 score 0–2 and uncertainty that diagnostic workup can be completed <2 days as outpatient ABCD2 score of 0–2 and evidence that event was caused by focal ischaemia

Crescendo TIAs—i.e. two or more attacks in 7 days

Duration of symptoms >1 hour

Symptomatic intracerebral artery (ICA) stenosis >50%

Known cardiac source of emboli such as AF

---

of stroke by 80%.[42] Most of the new clinical guidelines across the world recommend that patients with TIA should be seen within 12–24 hours of symptom onset.

In our own experience, in spite of a dedicated 7-day fast track TIA clinic, about 40% of the patients did not seek medical attention within 24 hours of symptom onset, thereby contributing to a delay in their assessment. Symptoms of TIA are frequently ignored or minimized by the patients and their carers or relatives, or underdiagnosed and not prioritized as an emergency by healthcare professionals (Box 4.3). Public education for TIA symptoms like the face, arm, speech, time (FAST) campaign in the United Kingdom can improve the public awareness. With experiences such as SOS-TIA in Paris we know that it is feasible and effective to provide urgent care, including intensive treatment, for patients with TIA, 24 hours a day with a median length of stay of 1 day and a 1.2%, 3-month stroke-event rate (although the ABCD2 score predicted it at 6%).[43]

The EXPRESS study[42] showed an 80% reduction in the 3-month stroke risk with early, intensive treatment. Health services around the world should aim at developing dedicated TIA clinics accessible 7 days a week, similar to the implementation of 'stroke units' in the past two decades. The message is that the workup of a patient with TIA should no longer be performed within days by appointment(s) to a TIA clinic or to various specialists. Evaluation and intensive treatment need to be completed within hours after symptom onset. Despite the inherent limitations of studies[40,41] related to the lack of controls, the observed stroke reduction supports the premise that TIAs should be managed as a medical emergency.

References

1. **Hatano S.** Experience from a multicentre stroke register: a preliminary report. *Bulletin of the World Health Organization* 1976;**54**:541–53.

2. **Albers GW, Caplan LR, Easton JD**, et al. Transient ischemic attack--proposal for a new definition. *N Engl J Med* 2002;**347**(21):1713–16.

3. **Easton JD, Saver JL, Albers GW**, et al. Definition and evaluation of transient ischemic attack: a scientific statement for healthcare professionals from the American Heart Association/American Stroke Association Stroke Council; Council on Cardiovascular Surgery and Anesthesia; Council on Cardiovascular Radiology and Intervention; Council on Cardiovascular Nursing; and the Interdisciplinary Council on Peripheral Vascular Disease. The American Academy of Neurology affirms the value of this statement as an educational tool for neurologists. *Stroke* 2009; **40**:2276–93.

4. **Sacco RL, Kasner SE, Broderick JP**, et al. An updated definition of stroke for the 21st century: a statement for healthcare professionals from the American Heart Association/American Stroke Association. *Stroke* 2013;**44**:2064–89.

5. **Kidwell CS, Alger JR, Di Salle F,** et al. Diffusion MRI in patients with transient ischaemic attacks. *Stroke* 1999;**30**:1174–80.

6. **Furie KL & Ay H.** Initial evaluation and management of transient ischaemic attack and minor stroke. *UpToDate* July 2016. Available from: https://www.uptodate.com/contents/initial-evaluation-and-management-of-transient-ischemic-attack-and-minor-ischemic-stroke?source=search_result&search=TIA&selectedTitle=1~150 [Accessed: 1 December 2016].

7. **Intercollegiate Stroke Working Party.** *National Clinical Guideline for Stroke*, 5th edition. London, UK: Royal College of Physicians, 2016.

8. **Hankey GJ.** Impact of treatment of people with transient ischaemic attack on stroke incidence and public health. *Cerebrovasc Dis* 1996;**6**(Suppl 1):26–33.

9. **Prabhakaran S, Silver AJ, Warrior L,** et al. Misdiagnosis of transient ischemic attacks in the emergency room. *Cerebrovasc Dis* 2008;**26**:630–5.

10. **Martin PJ, Young G, Enevoldson TP,** et al. Over diagnosis of TIA and minor stroke: experience at a regional neurovascular clinic. *QJM* 1997;**90**:759–63.

11. **Poole CJM & Ross Russell RW.** Mortality and stroke after amaurosis fugax. *Neurol Neurosurg Psychiatry* 1985;**48**:902–5.

12. **Lavallée P, Cabrejo L, Labreuche J,** et al. Spectrum of transient visual symptoms in a transient ischaemic attack cohort. *Stroke* 2013;**44**:3312–17.

13. **Kleindorfer D, Panagos P, Pancioli A,** et al. Incidence and short-term prognosis of transient ischemic attack in a population-based study. *Stroke* 2005;**36**(4):720–3.

14. **Bots ML, van der Wilk EC, Koudstaal PJ, Hofman A, & Grobbee DE.** Transient neurological attacks in the general population. Prevalence, risk factors, and clinical relevance. *Stroke* 1997;**28**(4):768–73.

15. **White H, Boden-Albala B, Wang C,** et al. Ischemic stroke subtype incidence among whites, blacks, and hispanics: the northern Manhattan study. *Circulation* 2005;**111**(10):1327–31.

16. **Sacco RL.** Risk factors for TIA and TIA as a risk factor for stroke. *Neurology* 2004;**62**(suppl 6):S7–11.

17. **Whisnant JP, Brown RD, Petty GW,** et al. Comparisons of population-based models of risk factors for TIA and ischaemic stroke. *Neurology* 1999;**53**:532–6.

18. **Johnston SC, Rothwell PM, Nguyen-Huynh MN,** et al. Validation and refinement of scores to predict very early stroke risk after transient ischaemic attack. *Lancet* 2007;**369**(9558):283–92.

19. **O'donnell MJ, Xavier D, Liu L,** et al. INTERSTROKE investigators. Risk factors for ischaemic and intracerebral haemorrhagic stroke in 22 countries (the INTERSTROKE study): a case-control study. *Lancet* 2010;**376**(9735):112–23.

20. **Furie KL, Kasner SE, Adams RJ,** et al. Guidelines for the prevention of stroke in patients with stroke or transient ischaemic attack: a guideline for healthcare professionals from the American Heart Association/American Stroke Association. *Stroke* 2011;**42**(1):227–76.

21. **Reynolds K, Lewis B, Nolen JD,** et al. Alcohol consumption and risk of stroke: a meta-analysis. *JAMA* 2003;**289**:579–88.

22. **Kernan WN, Ovbiagele B, Black HR,** et al. Guidelines for the prevention of stroke in patients with stroke and transient ischaemic attack: a guideline for healthcare professionals from the American Heart Association/American Stroke Association. *Stroke* 2014;**45**(7):2160–236.

23. **Coull AJ, Lovett JK, & Rothwell PM.** Population based study of the early risk of stroke after transient ischaemic attack or minor stroke: implications for public education and organisation of services. *BMJ* 2004;**328**(7435):326.

24. **Whisnant JP, Matsumoto N, & Elveback LR.** Transient cerebral ischemic attacks in a community. *Mayo Clin Proc* 1973;**48**:194–8.

25. **Giles MF & Rothwell PM.** Substantial underestimation of the need for outpatient services for TIA and minor stroke. *Age Ageing* 2007;**36**:676–80.

26. **Josephson SA, Sidney S, Pham TN, Bernstein AL, & Johnston SC.** Higher ABCD2 score predicts patients most likely to have true transient ischaemic attack. *Stroke* 2008;**39**(11):3096–8.

27. **National Institute for Health and Clinical Excellence (NICE).** *Stroke: The Diagnosis and Acute Management of Stroke and Transient Ischaemic Attacks.* London, UK: National Institute for Health and Clinical Excellence, 2008.

28. **Giles MF & Rothwell PM.** Systematic review and pooled analysis of published and unpublished validations of the ABCD and ABCD2 transient ischemic attack risk scores. *Stroke* 2010;**41**:667–73.

29. **Ay H, Arsava EM, Johnston SC, et al.** Clinical- and imaging-based prediction of stroke risk after transient ischaemic attack: the CIP model. *Stroke* 2009;**40**:181–6.

30. **Merwick A, Albers GW, Amarenco P, et al.** Addition of brain and carotid imaging to the ABCD^2 score to identify patients at early risk of stroke after transient ischaemic attack: a multicentre observational study. *Lancet Neurol* 2010;**9**:1060–9.

31. **Song B, Fang H, Zhao L, et al.** Validation of the ABCD^3-I score to predict stroke risk after transient ischemic attack. *Stroke* 2013;**44**(5):1244–8.

32. **National Institute for Health and Clinical Excellence (NICE).** *Transient Ischaemic Attack:* Clopidogrel, *NICE* Evidence Summary *[ESUOM23]* 2013. Available from: https://www.nice.org.uk/advice/esuom23/chapter/Key-points-from-the-evidence [Accessed: 22 July 2019].

33. **Pisters R, Lane DA, Nieuwlaat R, et al.** A novel user-friendly score (Has-Bled) to assess 1-year risk of major bleeding in patients with atrial fibrillation: the Euro Heart Survey. *Chest* 2010;**138**(5):1093–100.

34. **PROGRESS Collaborative Group.** Randomised trial of perindopril-based blood pressure lowering regimen among 6105 individuals with previous stroke or transient ischaemic attack. *Lancet* 2001;**358**:1033–41.

35. **O'Donnell MJ, Xavier D, Liu L, et al.** Risk factors for ischemic and intracerebral hemorrhagic stroke in 22 countries (the INTERSTROKE study): a case–control study. *Lancet* 2010;**376**(9735):112–23.

36. **The Stroke Prevention by Aggressive Reduction in Cholesterol Levels (SPARCL) Investigators.** High-dose atorvastatin after stroke or transient ischemic attack. *NEJM* 2006;**355**:549–59.

37. **Therapeutic Goods Administration.** Risk factors for myopathy and rhabdomyolysis with the statins. *Australian Adverse Drug Reactions Bulletin,* 2004; **23**. Available from: https://www.tga.gov.au/publication-issue/australian-adverse-drug-reactions-bulletin-vol-23-no-1 [Accessed: 22 July 2019].

38. **North American Symptomatic Carotid Endarterectomy Trial Collaborators.** Beneficial effect of carotid endarterectomy in symptomatic patients with high grade stenosis. *N Eng J Med* 1991;**325**:445–53.

39. **European Carotid Surgery Trialists' Collaborative Group.** MRC European Carotid Surgery Trial: interim results for symptomatic patients with severe (70–99%) or with mild (0–29%) carotid stenosis. *Lancet* 1991;**337**:1235–43.

40. **Sacco RL.** Extracranial carotid stenosis. *N Engl J Med* 2001;**345**:113–18.

41. **Rothwell P, Eliasziw M, Gutnikov S, Warlow C, Barnett H, for the Carotid Endarterectomy Trialists Collaboration.** Endarterectomy for symptomatic carotid stenosis in relation to clinical subgroups and timing of surgery. *Lancet* 2004;**363**:915–24.

42. **Rothwell PM, Giles MF, Chandratheva A, et al.** Effect of urgent treatment of transient ischemic attack and minor stroke on early recurrent stroke (EXPRESS study): a prospective population-based sequential comparison. *Lancet* 2007;**370**(9596):1432–42.

43. **Lavallée P, Meseguer E, Abboud H, et al.** A transient ischaemic attack clinic with round-the-clock access (SOS-TIA): feasibility and effects. *Lancet Neurol* 2007;**6**:953–6.

44. **Alamowitch S, Eliasziw M, Algra A, et al.** Risks, causes, and prevention of ischaemic stroke in elderly patients with symptomatic internal-carotid-artery stenosis. *Lancet* 2001;**357**:1154–60.

45. **Barnett HJ, Meldrum HE, Eliasziw M; North American Symptomatic Carotid Endarterectomy Trial (NASCET) Collaborators.** The appropriate use of carotid endarterectomy. *CMAJ* 2002;**166**:1169–79.

46. **Sundt TM, Sandok BA, & Whisnant JP.** Carotid endarterectomy: complications and pre-operative assessment of risk. *Mayo Clin Proc* 1975;**50**:301–6.

47. **Miller MT, Comerota AJ, Tzilinis A,** et al. Carotid endarterectomy in octogenarians: does increased age indicate 'high risk?' *J Vasc Surg* 2005;**41**(2):231–7.

48. **Rothwell PM & Warlow CP.** Timing of TIAs preceding stroke: time window for prevention is very short. *Neurology* 2005;**64**(5):817–20.

Chapter 5

Stroke mimics: Transient focal neurological events

Christopher D. Stephen and Louis R. Caplan

Introduction

An important consideration in patients who present with stroke-like symptoms is whether these symptoms are due to cerebrovascular disease or another condition, a "stroke mimic".[1-5] Stroke mimics account for up to 31% of stroke presentations,[6,7] and up to 60% of potential transient ischaemic attacks (TIAs).[8] The most common stroke mimics are seizures, migrainous auras, and functional neurological disorders.[7,9,10,11] Making an astute clinical decision based on the history and examination is particularly important, as imaging cannot definitely rule out stroke.

Seizures

An 80-year-old woman with a previous TIA presents after a motor vehicle accident hitting the left side of her car. Examination by a neurologist showed left-sided neglect and a slight left hemiparesis. MRI scan showed no acute infarct but did show significant small vessel disease. Continuous electro-encephalogram (EEG) monitoring showed marked suppression of electrical activity over the right cerebral hemisphere and occasional electrographic and clinical seizures in the right parietal region associated with rhythmic movement of the left hand.

Seizures account for up to 38% of stroke mimics.[9,10] Risk factors include prior strokes, small vessel disease, head injuries, brain tumours, subdural haematomas, vascular malformations, and space-occupying lesions. Stroke can present as, or be complicated by seizures.[1] The patient can present in any stage of the seizure or postictal period; initial ictal symptoms or signs may be unwitnessed or subtle and can go unrecognized by the patient (particularly in those who have cognitive impairment) and medical professionals. Presentation is highly variable depending on the seizure focus, both with regard to ictal and postictal semiology, as well as the duration of symptoms.

During the ictal phase, spontaneous neuronal discharge most often leads to positive phenomena including focal or generalized limb jerking or myoclonic jerks and positive sensory symptoms such as paraesthesias, or simple positive visual phenomena, such as bright colours or flashes of light. Positive phenomena are less common in cerebral ischaemia. Frequent epileptiform discharges can also interrupt speech and thought processes, resulting in brief periods of speech arrest or aphasia at times with florid paraphasic errors. Postictally, there is cortical suppression resulting in negative symptoms and signs such as weakness, numbness, or speech difficulty. The classical Todd's paresis, which often presents with hemiparesis, occurs commonly after generalized tonic-clonic or focal motor seizures.[12] Postictal dysfunction may last for days or longer. A clue to a convulsive aetiology is the tempo of onset, which evolves rapidly over several seconds with spreading focal involvement or secondary generalization. This allows differentiation from the much slower progression seen in migraine or the classically abrupt onset seen in stroke. A reduced level of consciousness is also more common in seizures than in TIAs and most territorial infarcts. Electroencephalography (EEG) can be used to identify epileptiform discharges. When attacks similar to the presenting event have occurred for years, seizures and migraine are more likely than stroke. Hyperperfusion seen in patients with seizures on computed tomography (CT) or MRI-perfusion imaging may be helpful and is different from the pattern found in stroke.[13]

Migraine

A 68-year-old woman has hypertension, hyperlipidaemia, and a long history of throbbing headaches, occasionally accompanied by right arm numbness. Today, she developed visual blurring to her right. When the blurring cleared, her right hand felt numb and weak; she then developed word-finding diffi-culties and a slight headache. A head CT and computed tomography angiography (CTA) are normal. An MRI shows no evidence of infarction. She has had several similar self-limiting episodes over the past 10 years.

Migraine is a very common stroke mimic[11] and must be differentiated from seizures and TIAs.[7] The incidence of migraine declines with age, but it is still relatively frequent in the older population.[14] A thorough history is important to detail the progression of symptoms and neurological deficits, as well as the co-occurrence of a migrainous-sounding headache.[15] In comparison to the sudden onset of symptoms in stroke, and very rapid spread in seizures, mi-graine auras have a characteristic, slow spread over several minutes, due to cortical spreading depression.[16] The sensory symptoms typically begin with positive signs that can involve dif-ferent sensory modalities. Patients may have headache before, during, or after the episode. Often, the first symptoms are a positive visual aura, a sensation of fluttering, bright flashes of light, scintillations, shimmering, or a change in perspective.[17] A migrainous visual aura is often characterized by gradual movement across the visual field, leaving behind in its trail negative phenomenon, in the form of an area of decreased vision that slowly resolves. In stroke patients, there is no clear spread, and involvement is in only one visual field, as opposed to bilaterally in migraines, and does not spread.[18] The "scintillating scotoma", a combination of both negative and positive phenomenon seen in migraine, is not seen in other conditions.[19] When the visual symptoms clear, another positive phenomenon, in the form of a tactile sensory aura, may begin. Paraesthesias most often involve the hand and face, with legs and torso much less commonly affected.[20,21] The sensation can be described as tingling, prickling, or burning sensations. The abnormal sensation starts focally, whether in a finger, leg, or on the face, and will slowly evolve and may even spread to the contralateral side. This non-anatomic distribution also provides an additional clue that the symptoms do not respect the focal anatomic confines seen in strokes. The sensory aura resolves slowly, with the first affected area clearing last and often leaves behind a feeling of decreased sensation in its wake.[20] As these positive symptoms recede, patients may then develop other 'negative' symptoms such as weakness, aphasia, or other problems. Aphasic auras generally involve paraphasic errors, in addition to word-finding difficulties.[20] Associated weakness is generally slight, in comparison to cerebrovascular causes and has a rostrocaudal typical sensory march.[22] Patients with a clear history of migraine or prior migrainous-sounding headaches with aura increase the likelihood of an atypical migrainous aura, particularly if there is a history of previous complex features.

Migrainous aura without headache, now termed acephalgic migraine, was first described in Miller Fisher's classic paper, where he detailed migraine accompaniments in individuals above age 45, most often in the absence of headache.[23] Migraine accompaniments involving sensory, motor, and aphasic symptoms almost always co-occurred with a visual aura.[23–25] Table 5.1 details features distinguishing migraine accompaniments from TIA.

Table 5.1 Features differentiating migraine accompaniments from cerebral ischaemia

Symptom type	Migraine aura	Transient ischaemic attack
Visual	Positive visual phenomena (flashes of light)	Negative symptoms (loss of vision)
	Involvement of both visual fields	Unilateral
	Slowly moving across visual field	Static
	Average duration 15–60 minutes	Average duration 3–10 minutes
		Amaurosis fugax
Sensory	Gradual build-up/evolution	Abrupt onset
	Positive phenomena (paraesthesia)	Negative symptoms (numbness)
	Cheiro-oral distribution (hand and face)	Unilateral weakness or sensory loss without slow spread
	Repetitive attacks of identical nature	Variable attacks
	Sequential progression from one modality to another (visual, sensory, speech)	Simultaneous appearance of symptom modalities (e.g. motor and sensory) and body parts (face and arm at same time)
	Sequential progression from one body part another	Symptoms appear and disappear simultaneously
	Area involved first resolves last	Flurry of stereotyped attacks uncommon
	Flurry of attacks	Average duration 5–10 minutes
	Average duration 20–30 minutes	

Adapted with permission from Vongvaivanich K, et al. Late-life migraine accompaniments: A narrative review. *Cephalalgia*, 35(10), 894–911. Copyright © 2015, © SAGE Publications. https://doi.org/10.1177/0333102414560635.

A particularly challenging mimic at any age is migraine with brainstem aura.[26] Onset is most common in youth but there are late onset cases. The onset is most often visual that may involve both positive or negative features, as well as other symptoms localizable to the brainstem including slurred speech, vertigo, tinnitus, hypacusis, diplopia, oscillopsia and gait, and appendicular ataxia. Patients may also report paraesthesias in the perioral region or in the limbs, and some may also have decreased consciousness.[27] Examination is highly variable and may reveal ophthalmoplegia, ataxia, dysarthria, or other cranial nerve abnormalities.

As a word of caution, vertebral artery dissection can also present with a similar pulsatile headache.[28,29] In addition, onset of migrainous-sounding aura late in life can be a feature of amyloid angiopathy.[30] So-called amyloid spells of transient focal neurological symptoms may be indistinguishable from an acephalgic migraine and can have both positive and negative symptoms.[31] On imaging, there is evidence of cortical superficial siderosis and cortical microbleeds.[31,32]

Transient global amnesia (TGA)

An 80-year old man has a period of acute confusion. He is perplexed and repeatedly asks questions, "Where am I? How did I get here? Who are these people with me?". On examination, he knows his identity but is disoriented to place and time. Other than amnesia for current and past events his exam is entirely normal, with normal speech and no focal neurological deficits. The memory deficit lasts for 4 hours and returns to baseline. On questioning, he had recent sexual intercourse as a treat for his 80th birthday the night before.

TGA usually occurs in older age and is characterized by the sudden onset of profound anterograde amnesia with more variable retrograde memory loss[33] followed by a gradual recovery, which may last several hours and almost always less than 24 hours.[34,35] Most cases are single events, although some patients have recurrent attacks.[36,37] Patients appear confused, and invariably ask repetitive questions about why they are here and sometimes where they are. They are unable to retain information given to them.[34,38] Patients may be anxious and can be agitated, although some become quiet and withdrawn.[34] Despite the dramatic memory loss and disorientation to place and time, patients have otherwise intact cognitive function and no other neurological symptoms. They may be able to drive safely, calculate, play a musical instrument, or even deliver a speech.[35] Following resolution of symptoms, there is permanent memory loss for the events during the attack. Caplan produced a set of criteria for TGA[39] that was later refined by Hodges and Warlow[40]:

Hodges and Warlow diagnostic criteria for TGA

1. Attacks must be witnessed and information available from a capable observer who was present for most of the attack

2. There must be a clear-cut anterograde amnesia during the attack

3. Clouding of consciousness and loss of personal identity must be absent, and the cognitive impairment limited to amnesia (i.e. no aphasia, apraxia, etc.)

4. There should be no accompanying focal neurological symptoms during the attack and no significant neurological signs afterwards

5. Epileptic features must be absent

6. Attacks must resolve within 24 hours

7. Patients with recent head injury or active epilepsy (i.e. remaining on medication or one seizure in the past 2 years) are excluded

TGA is associated with physical, sudden, or unexpected psychological stress as well as positive emotional responses; funerals as well as celebrations have been temporally related.[37] The vast majority endorse precipitating events and include: recent sexual activity,[41,42] physical exertion, swimming in cold water ('amnesia by the sea'), a hot bath, or shower.[34,35,37] These triggering events are similar to those of migraineurs and patients may have a past history of migraine.[37,43] Some attacks are related to vasoconstriction, leading to transient dysfunction of the dominant left medial temporal lobe structures.[34,35,44] TGA has been preceded in some cases by vertebral angiography.[45]

It is important to distinguish TGA from other causes of sudden onset memory loss. Strokes involving the dominant posterior cerebral artery territory may cause memory dysfunction. Compared to TGA, the deficit usually persists and there is invariably accompanying visual (hemianopia) and/or somatosensory symptoms and signs.[46,47] In transient epileptic amnesia, there are very brief, recurrent attacks of amnesia, which are starkly different from the single, long attack in TGA.[48] Psychogenic amnesia (functional global amnesia) typically affects younger people and involves profound retrograde amnesia in addition to frequent loss of personal identity but without anterograde amnesia, with preserved new learning.[49] These conditions can often be differentiated from stroke, given the lack of the characteristic repetitive questioning seen in TGA.[50-52]

Vertigo

Persistent vertigo is a common reason for presentation to emergency departments. It is often difficult to differentiate peripheral vestibulopathy from cerebrovascular lesions affecting the

Table 5.2 HINTS to INFARCT. Central patterns: (1) bilaterally normal head impulse test with spontaneous or gaze-evoked nystagmus; (2) bilateral, direction-changing, horizontal gaze-evoked nystagmus (or predominantly vertical or torsional nystagmus); (3) skew deviation

'HINTS' eye examination	Stroke findings: 'INFARCT' (any of these)
Head Impulse (right- and leftward)	Impulse Normal (bilaterally normal)
Nystagmus type (gaze testing)	Fast-phase Alternating (direction-changing nystagmus)
Test of Skew (alternate cover test)	Refixation on Cover Test (looking for skew deviation)
HINTS plus	
Presence of hearing loss. Generally on side of abnormal head impulse test (side opposite fast phase of nystagmus)	Unilateral hearing loss generally indicates an ischaemic cause (labyrinthine/lateral pontine infarction) as opposed to viral labyrinthitis

Adapted with permission from Newman-Toker DE, et al. HINTS Outperforms ABCD2 to Screen for Stroke in Acute Continuous Vertigo and Dizziness. *Academic Emergency Medicine*, 20(10), 986–996. Copyright © 2013, by the Society for Academic Emergency Medicine. https://doi.org/10.1111/acem.12223.

vestibulocerebellar pathways.[53,54] There are a variety of causes of acute dizziness including those of peripheral origin (vestibular neuritis, labyrinthitis, benign postural positional vertigo, and Meniere's disease) and central origin (mainly brain infarction and TIA and migraine with brainstem aura).[54] When vestibular disease is of cerebrovascular origin, the vast majority are due to ischaemia as opposed to haemorrhage.[55]

The acute vestibular syndrome is characterized by persistent vertigo or dizziness and can be accompanied by nausea or vomiting, worsening with head movement, as well as unsteady gait, and nystagmus.[55] Patients with posterior circulation ischaemic disease including TIA very rarely have isolated attacks of vertigo, without other accompanying symptoms attributable to brainstem or cerebellar dysfunction.[46] In peripheral causes, vertigo is often triggered by sudden movements and positional changes. Assessing features such as timing and triggers has significant clinical value.[53] CT is particularly unreliable in diagnosing acute posterior circulation infarction.[56]

Bedside examination presents an opportunity to differentiate stroke from peripheral causes of vertigo. The mnemonic HINTS (detailing the steps of eye examination) to INFARCT (the examination features favouring a stroke—Impulse Normal, Fast-phase Alternating or Refixation on Cover Test) is useful in differentiating peripheral from a central cause (see Table 5.2).[55,57] Features suggestive of a peripheral aetiology include a unilaterally abnormal head impulse test, direction-fixed, horizontal, or horizontal more than torsional nystagmus in addition to absent skew deviation by the alternate cover test. In testing nystagmus, the fast phase beats away from the abnormal side. In comparison, a central pattern may include any of the following: a normal head impulse test, bilateral direction-changing nystagmus (mainly vertical or torsional) and the presence of skew deviation. The HINTS approach was found to have a sensitivity of 96.5% and specificity 84.4% and was superior to standard risk factor analysis in differentiating a central from peripheral cause of vertigo.[57]

Metabolic disturbances

Metabolic abnormalities can result in a wide range of neurological sequelae that can be focal or global in distribution. These metabolic derangements as well as toxic consequences of drugs are increasingly prevalent in the era of significant polypharmacy in older age. *Hypoglycaemia*, in the diabetic patient taking oral hypoglycaemic medications or insulin can present in a manner similar to a stroke. Hypoglycaemia causing hemiplegia was soon recognized after the introduction of insulin.[58] Fortunately, the ubiquitous use of bedside fingerstick glucose blood testing now makes this readily detectable. There is mandatory checking of blood glucose levels prior to rTPA administration which should be routine in any potential stroke evaluation.[59] Focal deficits often resolve quickly after the administration of intravenous glucose, but in rare cases can take can take several hours.[58] *Hyperosmolar non-ketotic hyperglycaemia* can present as an abrupt onset hyperkinetic movement with hemichorea or hemiballismus and may mimic a basal ganglia stroke.[60] *Wernicke's encephalopathy*, the combination of ataxia, nystagmus, ophthalmoplegia, and confusion, often in thiamine deficient alcoholics can also be confused with other causes of an acute brainstem vascular syndrome.[61,62] The associated confusion is not present in similar cerebellar or brainstem stroke syndromes. *Hepatic encephalopathy* can also present with focal signs, although is characterized by a fluctuating picture and is associated with confusion and other signs of metabolic disturbance, such as myoclonus and asterixis.[63]

Functional neurological disorders

Although once considered rare in older age, functional neurological disorders (FND, formerly psychogenic neurological disorders or conversion disorder) are increasingly recognized in older individuals.[64,65] They are one of the most frequent stroke mimics, and account for up to 40% of non-stroke cases.[11] Most patients are younger than the usual stroke cohort (although FND can occur in old age) and patients may have repeated presentations with similar symptoms, which may result in multiple acute stroke assessments.[64,66] There is a strong female preponderance but FND can occur in both sexes[64] and risk factors include trauma (physical or psychological), psychiatric disorders, adverse life events, prior somatization, and a past history of functional neurological symptoms or other functional syndrome.[67] However, patients often may not have an identifiable trigger or psychiatric comorbidity. Due to outward clinical similarities to patients with stroke, patients with FND may be administered thrombolytics,[68] given the time constraints to adequately assess these patients, as a detailed history and clinical examination by an experienced physician (ideally a neurologist) is needed to make a diagnosis of a FND stroke mimic.[69,70] Functional weakness is characterized by inconsistent features on examination, such as variable or intermittent effort, 'give-way' or collapsing weakness, a seemingly limp arm avoiding the face when dropped from a height, or a dragging monoplegic gait. Functional weakness is more commonly hemiparetic than monoparetic[67] and a positive Hoover's sign (lack of apparent hip extension strength at baseline but found to be retained when assessed while performing concurrent contralateral hip flexion) has high diagnostic sensitivity.[71] Other features which can be more commonly seen in functional stroke mimics include midline splitting sensory loss, 'astasia abasia' uneconomical gait, or inconsistent, variable, and potentially distractible functional ataxia, although the wide spectrum of other FND symptoms may be present.[72] Treatment is multidisciplinary, involving neurology, psychiatry and the important involvement of rehabilitation specialists, physiotherapy, occupational therapy, and speech therapy as appropriate to provide FND-specific therapy based on the clinical presentation.[69,70]

Neuromuscular conditions

Myasthenia gravis

Myasthenia gravis may present with non-selective weakness of eye, face, or bulbar muscles and hence may be confused with a posterior circulation stroke.[73] A clue, is that weakness is typically generalized and fatigable. Complex ophthalmoplegia, either in isolation or in association with bulbar dysfunction and dysarthria, can also imitate a brainstem stroke; however, the variability, lack of adherence to one cranial nerve or vascular territory, as well as the diurnal variation (worse at the end of the day), and lack of generally acute onset, differentiates these conditions from an acute vascular event.

Acute compressive neuropathy

Acute focal neuropathy or plexopathy can also be confused with stroke.[74] The limitation to a single peripheral nerve territory of common compressive neuropathies is the key factor, as well as the mechanism of action of compression by prolonged abnormal posture (often postsurgery) by compression by an object or sleeping position. 'Saturday night palsy' involves compression of the radial nerve at the spiral groove, often over a bench or the armrest of a chair. This is particularly prevalent in alcohol or drug abusers, as a result of sleeping in an unusual position due to somnolence caused by the intoxicating substance.[75] Clinically, there is wrist drop with finger drop and radial distribution sensory loss. The clinical examination is complicated in this wrist dropped position. When the hand is propped up and supported, there is normal median and ulnar nerve function, pointing to a focal neuropathy as opposed to a stroke. Other compressive neuropathies include compression of the ulnar nerve at the cubital tunnel from leaning on the elbow, which can also cause an acute, generally transient ulnar neuropathy, which can be associated with ulnar hand clawing, although generally recovers rapidly after resolution of the abnormal posture. Peroneal neuropathy due to compression at the fibular head can also cause a unilateral foot drop. Although these compressive neuropathies generally resolve rapidly, they can be frightening in the older person who has not experienced similar symptoms or to family members.

Bell's palsy

Bell's palsy is another common dilemma in the emergency department, given the sudden onset of clinically obvious unilateral facial weakness.[76] The facial distortion is very distressing for patients, whose first inclination is that they have had a stroke. There may also be associated abnormal facial sensation, which may be related to the proprioceptive inputs from the facial nerve. The presence of both upper and lower facial involvement suggests a lower motor neuron (LMN) lesion, as opposed to a more central lesion, where the upper face is typically spared. Brainstem lesions may also produce an LMN-like facial palsy, so the clinician must be wary and look for the company that it keeps, namely oculomotor or other brainstem signs, or hemiparesis. Small pontine strokes can cause an isolated LMN-type facial palsy, although this is exceedingly rare.[77] The presence of eye closure weakness is rarely seen in central palsies, as seen in strokes. Other features indicative of a peripheral aetiology but not invariably present, include hyperacusis and taste disturbance. The presence of vesicles in the outer ear and tympanic membrane may indicate Ramsay Hunt syndrome.[78]

Brain tumours, subdural haematomas, and space-occupying lesions

Subdural haematomas (SDH) and brain tumours can also cause acute neurological symptoms and may be focal, depending on their location and nature.[79] In a study by Morgenstern et al., 5% of brain tumour patients at initial presentation were incorrectly diagnosed with stroke.[80] A history of recent falls or anticoagulation administration suggest SDH, which can be differentiated from stroke by CT, and symptoms may be transient.[81]

A history of current or past cancer and a progressive course suggests a brain tumour. Tumours can also be a frequent radiological differential for stroke on a CT, as hypodense cytotoxic oedema in strokes often appears similar to the vasogenic oedema seen in tumours, although the latter does not respect vascular territories. Tumours may also represent another differential for TIA. So-called transient 'tumour attacks' involve transient neurological symptoms not attributable to another cause, in the setting of brain tumours. Accounts have described such attacks in the presence of meningiomas[82] and other tumour types.[83] As part of a large multicentre TIA study, Coleman et al. identified the following features as being more consistent with a tumour than a vascular aetiology: focal jerking or shaking, pure (particularly positive) sensory symptoms, loss of consciousness, and isolated aphasia or speech arrest.[84]

Syncope and vertebrobasilar insufficiency

In a study by Kose et al., syncope accounted for 13% of stroke mimics in an old age population.[9] In patients with recurrent syncope or presyncope, there is frequent physician concern, particularly in older patients, that this may be the result of vertebrobasilar insufficiency.[85,86] However, posterior circulation TIAs only very rarely cause temporary loss of consciousness,[87] which is found only in extracranial disease of all four vessels and has been coined 'brain claudication'.[88] In practice, basilar occlusive disease invariably presents with additional motor and brainstem signs.

Primary ophthalmologic problems

Aside from the visual aura seen in migraine, transient visual loss, double vision, visual obscurations, and blurring can be caused by a number of ophthalmological conditions that are prevalent in the older person and can be confused with stroke or TIA. In light of the wide differential diagnosis, a detailed history, rapid oculomotor examination, and funduscopy conducted by a skilled practitioner is important and if possible, evaluation by ophthalmology is recommended. Diplopia is often a sudden onset phenomenon and as such, non-ischaemic causes may often be confused with stroke. Causes are best differentiated by the presence of normal eye movements or not. If eye movements are entirely normal, the most common cause is a decompensated phoria, and if abnormal include the gamut of causes of a cranial nerve palsy affecting eye movements (III, IV, and VI and internuclear ophthalmoplegia being most common), or a neuromuscular junction problem. A decompensated phoria can be elucidated by history, with a description of episodic diplopia worse in the evenings when it is dark, when the patient is tired, or after drinking alcohol. Although eye movements are normal, eye deviation can be induced on alternate cover testing.[89] Decompensated phoria is also the most common cause of post-operative diplopia, although care must be taken to differentiate it from myasthenia and other serious causes.[89]

Clues to ascertaining the causes of acute visual loss are detailed in Table 5.3 and include the tempo, duration semiology, and associated features. The characteristics of the visual loss are important, and whether they are associated with orbital pain. The presence of 'positive' symptoms, such as flashes of light, or other scintillations may be seen in migraine, retinal, or vitreous detachment. In comparison, 'negative' symptoms, including visual loss or blurred (whether in relation to a single eye or visual field distribution), central or peripheral scotoma, which include amaurosis fugax (particularly with the classic description of a curtain descending in one eyes's visual field) or a cerebral artery occlusion causing a TIA or stroke, but can also be seen in migrainous aura, optic nerve inflammation such as optic neuritis, or other primary ophthalmological causes. Retinal detachment may mimic amaurosis fugax and is more common in the older person, as well as in individuals following cataract surgery, with the severity of visual loss varies depending on the location of the detachment.[90] Of note, vitreous haemorrhage and acute cystic maculopathy are the most common causes of visual loss following cataract surgery. Glaucoma can also cause acute visual blurring, lasting minutes to hours and should be investigated in the absence of other causes. Although it is usually associated by orbital pain, glaucoma can be painless[91] and in causes of optic nerve head swelling (vascular, inflammatory, etc.), the visual loss is generally very brief but can be persistent and progressive. Cataracts can also produce visual obscurations, although this is rarely acute in nature.[92]

Table 5.3 Presentation and causes of sudden visual loss

Duration	Potential causes	Associated findings
Seconds	Dry eye or other tear film abnormalities	Foreign body sensation, lacrimation
	Papilloedema*	Headache (may be worse in morning), may have nausea/vomiting (particularly in elevated intracranial pressure [ICP]), change with Valsalva, pulsatile tinnitus, increased farsightedness; fundoscopy reveals unilateral (if compressive) or bilateral (raised ICP, etc.) disc oedema and can have haemorrhage if severe; requires head imaging
	Compressive optic neuropathy (orbit)	Vision loss in certain positions of gaze, extraocular muscle restriction, proptosis; abnormal imaging
	Orthostatic hypotension	Presyncopal symptoms (light headedness, pallor, sweating) and may have tunnel vision; orthostasis on postural vital signs measurement
1–10 minutes	Amaurosis fugax	Unilateral; cardiovascular and stroke risk factors
	Other transient ischaemic attack	Homonymous hemianopia or other visual field loss, extremity numbness or weakness, abnormality of speech, ataxia, cranial nerve abnormalities; cardiovascular and stroke risk factors
	Ocular stroke**—central retinal artery occlusion, ophthalmic artery occlusion, branch retinal artery occlusion, cilioretinal artery occlusion	Painless, variable loss of vision; cardiovascular and stroke risk factors
	Central retinal vein occlusion**	Painless vision loss; fundoscopic examination presence of retinal haemorrhages, venous engorgement, and tortuosity, cotton wool spots, optic disc oedema; risk factors for hypercoagulable state; ophthalmology review
	Giant cell arteritis (arthritic ischaemic optic neuropathy)**	Variable visual loss, headache, jaw claudication, temporal artery tenderness, myalgia, weight loss; elevated ESR/CRP may be present
10–60 minutes	Migrainous aura	Scintillating scotoma, other generally positive or later negative visual phenomena, associated headache with photophobia, phonophobia, nausea/vomiting; history of migraine and similar prior episodes
Minutes to hours	Transient angle-closure glaucoma	Halos around lights, nausea, eye pain, or headache, narrow anterior chamber angle, conjunctival injection, corneal oedema; high intraocular pressure
Days or longer	Vitreous haemorrhage	Painless vision loss, floaters, hazy vision; obscured view of the retina on fundoscopy
	Acute maculopathy	Metamorphopsia (distorted vision in which a grid of straight lines appears wavy), central scotoma; requires ophthalmology review and optical coherence tomography

(*continued*)

Table 5.3 Continued

Duration	Potential causes	Associated findings
	Retinal detachment	Unilateral, increase in floaters, photopsias (flashes of light), visual field defect
	Optic neuritis	Pain with eye movement, variable visual loss, later relative afferent pupillary defect (RAPD) and abnormal colour vision, vision starts to improve by 2–4 weeks; history of demyelination or previous optic neuritis
	Non-arteritic ischaemic optic neuropathy#	Unilateral painless visual loss and may be acute or evolve over days; fundoscopy reveals disc oedema acutely, with peripapillary retinal haemorrhages evolving over weeks to diffuse or segmental optic disc pallor; cardiovascular risk factors

* Papilloedema may have many underlying aetiologies and will need to be appropriately investigated.

** all causes of ocular stroke can initially present as transient or crescendo events.

May present acutely or evolve over several hours to days.

Any older patient with transient visual loss, particularly those with a history of polymyalgia rheumatic, should also be evaluated for giant cell arteritis, a potentially serious but treatable cause of vision loss. Evaluation should include a detailed history, assessing for symptoms including new or different headaches, scalp tenderness and jaw claudication, examination for temporal artery pulsation and tenderness, as well as laboratory evaluation with erythrocyte sedimentation rate (ESR) and C-reactive protein (CRP).[93] Further workup, including temporal artery biopsy is dependent on the degree of suspicion. If the index of suspicion is high, patients should be treated withoral steroids.[93]

Rare causes

Demyelinating disorders are less common but do occur in old age.[94] Although this usually does not have the acute onset suggestive of a stroke, they can rarely present with sudden onset deficits, as well as with brief repeated transient episodes, most often involving ataxia with dysarthria.[95,96] Autoimmune neurological disorders such as Miller Fisher syndrome can also present in older patients, and the triad of ataxia, areflexia, and complex ophthalmoplegia may be confused with a posterior circulation or brainstem stroke.[97,98] The fluctuating and complex ophthalmoplegia with decreased, as opposed to increased reflexes and in the absence of weakness or sensory abnormalities, may point towards the correct diagnosis. Fluctuations are also frequent in neurodegenerative disorders, such as dementia with Lewy bodies, but would rarely be confused with a stroke.[99] A spinal epidural haematoma can also mimic hemiparesis from stroke in older individuals, although it is almost always accompanied by neck or other pain or myelopathic symptoms.[100]

References

1. Caplan L (ed.). *Caplan's Stroke: A Clinical Approach*, 5th edition. Cambridge, UK: Cambridge University Press, 2016.

2. **Lioutas VA, Sonni S,** & **Caplan LR.** Diagnosis and misdiagnosis of cerebrovascular disease. *Curr Treat Options Cardiovasc Med* 2013;**15**(3):276–87.

3. **Libman RB, Wirkowski E, Alvir J,** et al. Conditions that mimic stroke in the emergency department. Implications for acute stroke trials. *Arch Neurol* 1995;**52**:1119–22.

4. **Kose A, Inal T, Armagan E, Kıyak R, & Demir AB.** Conditions that mimic stroke in elderly patients admitted to the emergency department. *J Stroke Cerebrovasc Dis* 2013;**22**(8):e522–7.

5. **Harbison J, Hossain O, Jenkinson D, et al.** Diagnostic accuracy of stroke referrals from primary care, emergency room physicians, and ambulance staff using the face arm speech test. *Stroke* 2003;**34**:71–6.

6. **Merino JG, Luby M, Benson RT, et al.** Predictors of acute stroke mimics in 8187 patients referred to a stroke service. *J Stroke Cerebrovasc Dis* 2013;**22**(8):e397–403.

7. **Hand PJ, Kwan J, Lindley RI, et al.** Distinguishing between stroke and mimic at the bedside: the brain attack study. *Stroke* 2006;**37**:769–75.

8. **Prabhakaran S, Silver AJ, Warrior L, McClenathan B, & Lee VH.** Misdiagnosis of transient ischemic attacks in the emergency room. *Cerebrovasc Dis* 2008;**26**(6):630–5.

9. **Kose A, Inal T, Armagan E, Kıyak R, & Demir AB.** Conditions that mimic stroke in elderly patients admitted to the emergency department. *J Stroke Cerebrovasc Dis* 2013;**22**(8):e522–7.

10. **Chernyshev OY, Martin-Schild S, Albright KC, et al.** Safety of tPA in stroke mimics and neuroimaging-negative cerebral ischemia. *Neurology* 2010;**74**:1340–5.

11. **Vroomen PC, Buddingh MK, Luijckx GJ, & De Keyser J.** The incidence of stroke mimics among stroke department admissions in relation to age group. *J Stroke Cerebrovasc Dis* 2008;**17**(6):418–22.

12. **Todd RB.** Clinical lectures on paralysis, certain diseases of the brain, and other affections of the nervous system. London, UK: John Churchill, 1854, pp. 284–307.

13. **Hedna VS, Shukla PP, Waters MF.** Seizure mimicking stroke: role of CT perfusion. *J Clin Imaging Sci* 2012;**2**:32.

14. **Prencipe M, Casini AR, Ferretti C, et al.** Prevalence of headache in an elderly population: attack frequency, disability, and use of medication. *J Neurol Neurosurg Psychiatry* 2001;**70**:377–81.

15. **Pascual J & Berciano J.** Experience in the diagnosis of headaches that start in elderly people. *J Neurol Neurosurg Psychiatry* 1994;**57**:1255–7.

16. **Pietrobon D & Moskowitz MA.** Pathophysiology of migraine. *Annu Rev Physiol* 2013;**75**:365–91.

17. **Wijman C, Wolf PA, Kase CS, et al.** Migrainous visual accompaniments are not rare in late life: the Framingham study. *Stroke* 1998;**29**:1539–43.

18. **Hansen JM, Baca SM, Vanvalkenburgh P, et al.** Distinctive anatomical and physiological features of migraine aura revealed by 18 years of recording. *Brain* 2013;**136**:3589–95.

19. **Panayiotopoulos CP, Sharoqi IA, & Agathonikou A.** Occipital seizures imitating migraine aura. *J R Soc Med* 1997;**90**:255–7.

20. **Russell MB & Olesen J.** A nosographic analysis of the migraine aura in a general population. *Brain* 1996;**119**(Pt 2):355–61.

21. **Freedom T & Jay WM.** Migraine with and without headache. *Semin Ophthalmol* 2003;**18**:210–17.

22. **Young WB, Gangal KS, Aponte RJ, et al.** Migraine with unilateral motor symptoms: a case-control study. *J Neurol Neurosurg Psychiatry* 2007;**78**:600–4.

23. **Fisher CM.** Late-life migraine accompaniments—further experience. *Stroke* 1986;**17**(5):1033–42.

24. **Vongvaivanich K, Lertakyamanee P, Silberstein SD, & Dodick DW.** Late-life migraine accompaniments: a narrative review. *Cephalalgia* 2015;**35**(10):894–911.

25. **Donnet A, Daniel C, Milandre L, et al.** Migraine with aura in patients over 50 years of age: the Marseille registry. *J Neurol* 2012;**259**:1868–73.

26. **Headache Classification Committee of the International Headache Society (IHS).** The International Classification of Headache Disorders, 3rd edition (beta version). *Cephalalgia* 2013;**33**:629–808.

27. **Kirchmann M, Thomsen LL, & Olesen J.** Basilar-type migraine: clinical, epidemiologic, and genetic features. *Neurology* 2006;**66**(6):880–6.

28. **Teodoro T, Ferreira J, Franco A, et al.** Vertebral artery dissection mimicking status migrainosus. *Am J Emerg Med* 2013;**31**(12):1721.e3–5.

29. **Metso TM, Tatlisumak T, Debette S, D et al.** Migraine in cervical artery dissection and ischemic stroke patients. *Neurology* 2012;**78**(16):1221–8.

30. **Samanci B, Coban O, & Baykan B.** Late onset aura may herald cerebral amyloid angiopathy: a case report. *Cephalalgia* 2015;**36**(10):998–1001.

31. **Charidimou A, Peeters A, Fox Z, et al.** Spectrum of transient focal neurological episodes in cerebral amyloid angiopathy: multicentre magnetic resonance imaging cohort study and meta-analysis. *Stroke* 2012;**43**:2324–30.

32. **Greenberg SM, Vonsattel JP, Stakes JW, et al.** The clinical spectrum of cerebral amyloid angiopathy: presentations without lobar hemorrhage. *Neurology* 1993; **43**:2073–9.

33. **Jager T, Bazner H, Kliegel M, Szabo K, & Hennerici MG.** The transience and nature of cognitive impairments in transient global amnesia: a meta-analysis. *J Clin Exp Neuropsychol* 2009;**31**:8–19.

34. **Caplan LR.** Transient global amnesia. In: Vinken PJ, Bruyn GW, & Klawans H (eds.) *Handbook of Clinical Neurology* (**revised series**) Vol I (45) *Clinical Neuropsychology*, Frederiks JAM (ed.), pp. 205–18. Amsterdam, the Netherlands: Elsevier Science, 1985.

35. **Caplan LR.** Transient global amnesia: characteristic features and overview. In: Markowitsch HJ (ed.) Transient Global Amnesia and Related Disorders, pp. 15–27. Toronto, Canada: Hogrgrefe & Huber, 1990.

36. **Agosti C, Akkawi NM, Borroni B, & Padovani A.** Recurrence in transient global amnesia: a retrospective study. *Eur J Neurol* 2006;**13**:986–9.

37. **Quinette P, Guillery-Girard B, Dayan J, et al.** What does transient global amnesia really mean? Review of the literature and thorough study of 142 cases. *Brain* 2006;**129**:1640–58.

38. **Fisher CM.** Transient global amnesia. Precipitating activities and other observations. *Arch Neurol* 1982;**39**:605–8.

39. **Caplan LR.** Transient global amnesia: criteria and classification. *Neurology* 1986;**36**:441.

40. **Hodges JR & Warlow CP.** The aetiology of transient global amnesia. A case-control study of 114 cases with prospective follow-up. *Brain* 1990;**113**:639–57.

41. **Dang CV & Gardner LB.** Transient global amnesia after sex. *Lancet* 1998; **352**:1557–8.

42. **Lane RJ.** Recurrent coital amnesia. *J Neurol Neurosurg Psychiatry* 1997;**63**:260.

43 **Caplan LR, Chedru F, Lhermitte F, & Mayman C.** Transient global amnesia and migraine. *Neurology* 1981;**31**:1167–70.

44. **Tong DC & Grossman M.** What causes transient global amnesia? New insights from DWI. *Neurology* 2004;**62**:2154–5.

45. **Haas DC.** Transient global amnesia after cerebral angiography. *Arch Neurol* 1983;**40**:258–9.

46. **Caplan LR.** *Posterior Circulation Disease: Clinical Findings, Diagnosis, and Management.* Boston, MA: Blackwell Science, 1996.

47. **von Cramon DY, Hebel N, & Schuri U.** Verbal memory and learning in unilateral posterior cerebral infarction. A report on 30 cases. *Brain* 1988;111:1061–77.

48. **Bartsch T, Alfke K, Stingele R, et al.** Selective affection of hippocampal CA-1 neurons in patients with transient global amnesia without long-term sequelae. *Brain* 2006;**129**:2874–84.

49. **Markowitsch HJ.** Functional retrograde amnesia—amnestic block syndrome. *Cortex* 2002;**38**:651–4.

50. **Bartsch T, Alfke K, Stingele R, et al.** Selective affection of hippocampal CA-1 neurons in patients with transient global amnesia without long-term sequelae. *Brain* 2006;**129**:2874–84.

51. **Sedlaczek O, Hirsch JG, Grips E, et al.** Detection of delayed focal MR changes in the lateral hippocampus in transient global amnesia. *Neurology* 2004;**62**:2165–70.

52. **Eustache F, Desgranges B, Petit-Taboué MC, et al.** Transient global amnesia: implicit/explicit memory dissociation and PET assessment of brain perfusion and oxygen metabolism in the acute stage. *J Neurol Neurosurg Psychiatry* 1997;**63**:357–67.

53. **Kerber KA & Newman-Toker DE.** Misdiagnosing dizzy patients—common pitfalls in clinical practice. *Neurol Clin* 2015;**33**:565–75.

54. **Kerber KA, Meurer WJ, West BT, et al.** Dizziness presentations in U.S. emergency departments, 1995–2004. *Acad Emerg Med* 2008;**15**:744–50.

55. **Tarnutzer AA, Berkowitz AL, Robinson KA, Hsieh YH, & Newman-Toker DE.** Does my dizzy patient have a stroke? A systematic review of bedside diagnosis in acute vestibular syndrome. *CMAJ* 2011;**183**:E571–92.

56. **Hwang DY, Silva GS, Furie KL, & Greer DM.** Comparative sensitivity of computed tomography vs. magnetic resonance imaging for detecting acute posterior fossa infarct. *J Emerg Med* 2012; **42**: 559–65.

57. **Newman-Toker DE, Kerber KA, Hsieh Y-H, et al.** HINTS outperforms ABCD2 to screen for stroke in acute continuous vertigo and dizziness. *Acad Emerg Med* 2013;**20**:987–96.

58. **Wallis WE, Donaldson I, Scott RS, & Wilson J.** Hypoglycemia masquerading as cerebrovascular disease (hypoglycemic hemiplegia). *Ann Neurol* 1985;**18**(4):510–12.

59. **Mehta S, Vora N, Edgell RC, et al.** Stroke mimics under the drip-and-ship paradigm. *J Stroke Cerebrovasc Dis* 2014;**23**(5):844–9.

60. **Postuma RB & Lang AE.** Hemiballism: revisiting a classic disorder. *Lancet Neurol* 2003;**2**:661–8.

61. **Bhan A, Advani R, Kurz KD, Farbu E, & Kurz MW.** Wernicke's encephalopathy mimicking acute onset stroke diagnosed by CT perfusion. *Case Rep Neurol Med* 2014;**2014**:673230.

62. **Sechi G & Serra A.** Wernicke's encephalopathy: new clinical settings and recent advances in diagnosis and management. *Lancet Neurol* 2007;**6**(5):442–55.

63. **Atchison JW, Pellegrino M, Herbers P, Tipton B, & Matkovic V.** Hepatic encephalopathy mimicking stroke. A case report. *Am J Phys Med Rehabil* 1992;**71**(2):114–18.

64. **Stone J & Aybek S.** Functional limb weakness and paralysis. *Handb Clin Neurol* 2016;**139**:213–28.

65. **Nazir FS, Lees KR, & Bone I.** Clinical features associated with medically unexplained stroke-like symptoms presenting to an acute stroke unit. *Eur J Neurol* 2005;**12**:81–5.

66. **Stone J, Warlow C, & Sharpe M.** Functional weakness: clues to mechanism from the nature of onset. *J Neurol Neurosurg Psychiatry* 2012;**83**:67–9.

67. **Stone J, Warlow C, & Sharpe M.** The symptom of functional weakness: a controlled study of 107 patients. *Brain* 2010:133;1537–51.

68. **Scott PA & Silbergleit R.** Misdiagnosis of stroke in tissue plasminogen activator-treated patients: characteristics and outcomes. *Ann Emerg Med* 2003;**42**(5):611–18.

69. **Anderson J, Nakhate V, Stephen CD, & Perez DL.** Functional (psychogenic) neurological disorders: assessment and acute management in the emergency department. *Semin Neurol* 2019;**39**(1):102–14.

70. **McKee K, Glass S, Adams C, et al.** The inpatient assessment and management of motor functional neurological disorders: an interdisciplinary perspective. *Psychosomatics* 2018;**59**(4):358–68.

71. **McWhirter L, Stone J, Sandercock P, & Whiteley W.** Hoover's sign for the diagnosis of functional weakness: a prospective unblinded cohort study in patients with suspected stroke. *J Psychosom Res* 2011;**71**:384–6.

72. **Stone J, Carson A, & Sharpe M.** Functional symptoms and signs in neurology: assessment and diagnosis. *J Neurol Neurosurg Psychiatry* 2005;**76**(Suppl I):i2–i12.

73. **Libman R, Benson R, & Einberg K.** Myasthenia mimicking vertebrobasilar stroke. *J Neurol* 2002;**249**(11):1512–14.

74. **Edlow JA & Selim MH.** Atypical presentations of acute cerebrovascular syndromes. *Lancet Neurol* 2011;**10**:550–60.

75. **Spinner RJ, Poliakoff MB, & Tiel RL.** The origin of 'Saturday night palsy'? *Neurosurgery* 2002;**51**:737–41.

76. **Fahimi J, Navi BB, & Kamel H.** Potential misdiagnoses of Bell's palsy in the emergency department. *Ann Emerg Med* 2014;**63**(4):428–34.

77. **Novy J, Michael P, Poncioni L, & Carota A.** Isolated nuclear facial palsy, a rare variant of pure motor lacunar stroke. *Clin Neurol Neurosurg* 2008;**110**:420–1.

78. **Costa A & Veiga A.** Ramsay-Hunt syndrome in the differential diagnosis of stroke. *Rev Soc Bras Med Trop* 2013;**46**(5):663.

79. **Snyder H, Robinson K, Shah D, Brennan R, & Handrigan M.** Signs and symptoms of patients with brain tumors presenting to the emergency department. *J Emerg Med* 1993;**11**(3):253–8.

80. **Morgenstern LB & Frankowski RF.** Brain tumor masquerading as stroke. *J Neurooncol* 1999;**44**:47–52.

81. **Moster ML, Johnston DE, & Reinmuth OM.** Chronic subdural hematoma with transient neurological deficits: a review of 15 cases. *Ann Neurol* 1983;**14**(5):539–42.

82. **Daly DD, Svein HJ, & Yoss RE.** Intermittent cerebral symptoms with meningiomas. *Arch Neurol* 1961;**5**:287–93.

83. **Ross RT.** Transient tumor attacks. *Arch Neurol* 1983;**40**:633–6.

84. **Coleman RJ, Bamford JM, Warlow CP, & The UK TIA Study Group.** Intracranial tumours that mimic transient cerebral ischaemia: lessons from a large multicentre trial. *J Neurol Neurosurg Psychiatr* 1993;**56**:563–6.

86. **Bassetti CL.** Transient loss of consciousness and syncope. *Handb Clin Neurol* 2014;**119**:169–91.

85. **Savitz SI & Caplan LR.** Vertebrobasilar disease. *N Engl J Med* 2005;**352**(25):2618–26.

87. **Davidson E, Rotenberg Z, Fuchs J,** et al. Transient ischemic attack-related syncope. *Clin Cardiol* 1991;**14**:141–4.

88. **Kimura K, Minematsu K, Yasaka M,** et al. The duration of symptoms in transient ischemic attacks. *Neurology* 1999;**52**:976–80.

89. **Wray SH.** *Eye Movement Disorders in Clinical Practice: Signs and Syndromes.* New York, NY: Oxford University Press, 2014, pp. 142–6.

90. **Banker AS & Freeman WR.** Retinal detachment. *Ophthalmol Clin North Am* 2001;**14**(4):695–704.

91. **Abe A, Nishiyama Y, Kitahara I,** et al. Painless transient monocular loss of vision resulting from angle-closure glaucoma. *Headache* 2007;**47**(7):1098–9.

92. **Glaser J.** *The Retina in Neuro-Ophthalmology,* 3rd edition. Baltimore, MD: Lippincott Williams & Wilkins, 1999, pp. 102–8.

93. **Dejaco C, Brouwer E, Mason JC, Buttgereit F, Matteson EL, Dasgupta B.** Giant cell arteritis and polymyalgia rheumatica: current challenges and opportunities. *Nat Rev Rheumatol* 2017 Oct;**13**(10):578–592.

94. **Martinelli V, Rodegher M, Moiola L,** et al. Late onset multiple sclerosis: clinical characteristics, prognostic factors and differential diagnosis. *Neurol Sci* 2004;**25** (Suppl 4):S350–5.

95. **Delgado MG, Santamarta E, Sáiz A, Larrosa D, García R, & Oliva P.** Fluctuating neurological symptoms in demyelinating disease mimicking an acute ischaemic stroke. *BMJ Case Rep* 2012;**2012**:pii: bcr1120115079.

96. **Cowan J, Ormerod IE, & Rudge P.** Hemiparetic multiple sclerosis. *J Neurol Neurosurg Psychiatr* 1990;**53**:675–80.

97. **Cher LM & Merory JM.** Miller Fisher syndrome mimicking stroke in immunosuppressed patient with rheumatoid arthritis responding to plasma exchange. *J Clin Neuroophthalmol* 1993;**13**(2):138–40.

98. **Hasan S, Stanslas J, Hin LP, & Basri HB.** A young lady with thalamic stroke mimicking acute Miller Fisher syndrome. *Neurosciences (Riyadh)* 2012;**17**(4):380–1.

99. **McKeith IG, Dickson DW, Lowe J,** et al. Diagnosis and management of dementia with Lewy bodies: third report of the DLB Consortium. *Neurology* 2005;**65**:1863–72.

100. **Schmidley JW, Mallenbaum S, & Broyles K.** Spinal epidural hematoma: an important stroke mimic. *Acute Med* 2013;**12**(1):36–9.

Chapter 6

Diagnostic investigations for stroke in older people: A practical approach

Senthil Raghunathan

Introduction

Diagnosis of stroke in older people may be challenging due to its varied and atypical presentations. The typical symptoms of stroke may not be apparent and stroke may present with one of the 'geriatric giants' including falls, confusion, and immobility. Hence diagnostic investigation plays an important role along with a comprehensive history and thorough clinical examination in assessing severity, prognosis, and initiating appropriate management.

Though diagnosis of stroke is primarily a clinical one, stroke mimics account for nearly 20% of suspected stroke presentations and diagnostic accuracy has been increased considerably by improvement in imaging techniques to confirm or refute diagnosis of stroke.[1]

Diagnostic investigations of acute stroke in elderly people can be categorized into the following four sections:

1. Emergency investigation of the patient—to confirm refute or categorize the diagnosis of stroke

2. Investigation of the aetiology of stroke

3. Investigation of risk factors

4. Anticipation of complication of stroke

Emergency investigation

It is impossible to distinguish between infarction and haemorrhage on clinical grounds alone. Therefore urgent brain imaging is essential.

Brain imaging

Imaging studies are used to exclude haemorrhage in the acute stroke patient, to assess the extent of brain injury, to identify the vascular lesion responsible for the ischaemic deficit, and to exclude stroke mimics. Computed tomography (CT) and Magnetic Resonace Imaging (MRI) perfusion studies can potentially distinguish irreversible brain tissue damage and salvageable 'penumbra', thereby allowing better selection of patients likely to benefit from reperfusion therapy. These imaging modalities are dependent upon their availability and its role in treatment decision-making is still under study.

Computed tomography (CT)

A non-contrast CT scan is generally all that is required to investigate acute stroke in older patients. It reliably excludes intracerebral haemorrhage, tumour, and subdural haematoma, but may not show the site of infarction.

A non-contrast CT is the recommended first line brain imaging to be done immediately after hospital admission and is usually ordered to exclude or confirm haemorrhage. The main advantages of CT are widespread access, speed of acquisition, and its high sensitivity to rule out haemorrhage.

The sensitivity of standard non-contrast CT for brain ischaemia increases after 24 hours. However only 61% had early CT signs of brain infarction where CT scans were performed within 6 hours of stroke onset (Fig. 6.1).[2]

Early signs of infarction on CT brain include the following:

♦ Cortical sulcal effacement

♦ Obscuration of lentiform nucleus

♦ Focal parenchymal hypoattenuation

♦ Loss of insular ribbon or obscuration of the Sylvian fissure

♦ Hyperattenuation of large vessels (e.g. 'hyperdense middle cerebral artery (MCA) sign')

♦ Loss of grey-white matter differentiation of basal ganglia

Presence of early CT signs of infarction is associated with a worse prognosis for survival and poor functional outcome.[3] However, it is important to be aware that patients with early CT signs of infarction have a net treatment benefit from thrombolysis.[4]

The sooner reperfusion treatment is initiated, the more likely it is to be beneficial, and benefit extends to treatment started within 4.5 hours of stroke onset.[5] In addition, the results show that alteplase is beneficial regardless of patient age, stroke severity, or the associated increased risk of symptomatic or fatal intracranial haemorrhage in the first days after alteplase treatment.

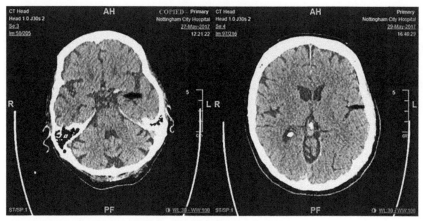

Fig. 6.1 Early radiological features of left middle cerebral artery (MCA) infarct on CT brain performed within 2 hours of symptom onset.

CT brain (left) shows hyperdensity (arrow) within left distal internal carotid artery extending to proximal left M1 segment of MCA in keeping with acute thrombus in a patient presenting with right-sided weakness and aphasia 'hyperdense MCA sign'. CT brain (right) shows hyperdensity in left sylvian fissure MCA branches suggesting a small intravascular thrombus 'Sylvian dot sign'.

Images courtesy of Department of Stroke Medicine, Nottingham City Hospital, UK.

Hence the most important factor in successful thrombolytic treatment of acute ischaemic stroke is early treatment; robust local thrombolysis policies should be in place providing for immediate CT scanning to enable rapid 'door-to-needle' times.

Non-contrast CT brain can detect acute intracerebral haemorrhage (ICH) immediately and can also define the size and location of the haematoma (although if done very early the haematoma may still be growing; see Fig. 6.2). It also provides information about extension into ventricular system, presence of surrounding oedema, and shifts in brain contents (including herniation). Acute bleeding will appear hyperdense and over weeks, the blood becomes isodense and may have a 'ring-enhancement' appearance. Chronically, the site of bleeding becomes hypodense.

No further diagnostic tests are necessary in the hypertensive patient with a well-circumscribed and homogenous haematoma that is located in a typical location for hypertensive ICH (i.e. putamen/internal capsule, caudate nucleus, thalamus, pons, or cerebellum); the clinician can be confident that the patient has a hypertensive haemorrhage. Similarly, a traumatic aetiology can usually be diagnosed with confidence, with an appropriate history and lesions in typical locations with the appearance of contusion or traumatic bleeding (e.g. anterior and/or orbital frontal lobes and temporal lobes at the surface).

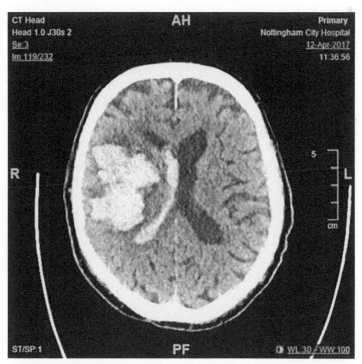

Fig. 6.2 CT brain scan showing large parenchymal haematoma in the right basal ganglia/subinsular region with extension into right lateral ventricle in a 65-year-old poorly controlled hypertensive patient.

Image courtesy of Department of Stroke Medicine, Nottingham University Hospital, UK.

An interval MRI/magnetic resonance angiography (MRA) in 4–6 weeks may be appropriate in some patients to look for other causes of ICH—amyloid angiopathy or underlying vascular malformations.

Magnetic resonance imaging

Where readily available, it makes sense to use MRI first as abnormalities on diffusion-weighted images are so apparent and make diagnosis of stroke relatively easy.

With more access to MRI than before, it is being increasing used in older stroke patients to diagnose (or rule out) strokes, exclude mimics, and has the potential for defining stroke sub-group populations that may benefit from intravenous thrombolysis or interventional vascular treatments.[5]

MRI is superior in visualizing the posterior fossa and is more sensitive to small infarcts, particularly lacunar infarcts and very small lesions in the brainstem. MRI sequences such as gradient echo (GRE) are equivalent to CT for detection of acute intracerebral haemorrhage and better than CT for detection of chronic haemorrhage.[6]

Brain MRI protocols that combine conventional T1 and T2 sequences with diffusion-weighted imaging (DWI), perfusion-weighted imaging, and GRE can reliably diagnose both acute ischaemic stroke and acute haemorrhagic stroke. These MRI techniques obviate the need for emergency CT in centres where brain MRI is readily available. New ultrafast MRI imaging protocols can reduce acquisition times from 15 to 20 minutes required by conventional MRI to 5 minutes or less, but the utility of these newer methods is not yet established.[7]

Cerebral amyloid angiopathy (CAA), although usually asymptomatic, is an important cause of primary lobar intracerebral haemorrhage in older people. While the diagnosis of CAA is made definitely by pathologic examination, a probable diagnosis of CAA can be made when MRI with GRE sequence demonstrates presence of two or more haemorrhages or microhaemorrhages restricted to regions typical for CAA (cortex or 'grey-white' junction) and entirely sparing regions typical of hypertensive haemorrhage (basal ganglia, thalamus, or pons). Haemorrhage involving cortical sulci (superficial siderosis) also suggests CAA (Fig. 6.3).

Hypertensive bleeds are typically seen in elderly patients presenting with high blood pressure and with a well-circumscribed and homogenous haematoma located at putamen/internal capsule,

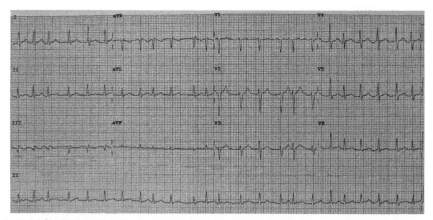

Fig. 6.3 Atrial fibrillation. Ventricular rate varies from 130 to 168 beats per minute. Rhythm is irregularly irregular. P waves are not discernible.

Image courtesy of Department of Stroke Medicine, Nottingham City Hospital, UK.

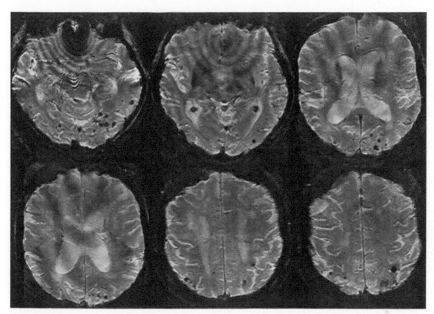

Fig. 6.4 Axial MRI GRE (gradient ECHO) shows multiple foci of signal loss in cortical–subcortical locations in an 80-year-old patient with diagnosis of probable CAA (cerebral amyloid angiopathy).

Image courtesy of Department of Stroke Medicine, Nottingham City Hospital, UK.

caudate nucleus, thalamus, pons, or cerebellum. GRE MRI may reveal evidence of micro-bleeds in deep grey and infratentorial regions such as the pons, thalamus, and basal ganglia characteristic of hypertensive bleeding prone microangiopathy.

However, there is often an overlap of radiological features of these two conditions and it is not uncommon for hypertensive bleeds to be present in typical amyloid bleed locations and vice versa.

In older patients MRI may pose a challenge if the patient is critically ill, unable to lie supine, is agitated, or has claustrophobia, an MRI-incompatible pacemaker, or ferromagnetic implants. About 10% of patients cannot tolerate MRI (Fig. 6.4).

Cardiac tests

Electrocardiography (ECG)

A baseline ECG should always be performed and may identify atrial fibrillation, myocardial infarction, or left ventricular hypertrophy.

ECG abnormalities are present in 92% of patients with acute stroke. Cardiac arrhythmias and repolarization abnormalities occur in approximately 60–70% of patients and have prognostic implications.[8]

ECG changes predominately reflect ischaemia in the subendocardium of the left ventricle, most likely the result of a centrally medicated release of catecholamines. ECG abnormalities are also common in intracerebral haemorrhage; however, most of these appear to be minor and do not require medical intervention or impact prognosis.

The most common stroke-related ECG abnormality is QT prolongation, found in 71% of patients with subarachnoid haemorrhage, 64% of patients with intraparenchymal haemorrhage, and 38% of patients with ischaemic stroke.[9] QT prolongation, a marker of abnormal cardiac repolarization, is associated with increased mortality in patients with acute intracranial haemorrhage.[10]

New T-wave abnormalities appear in approximately 15% of patients with acute stroke, even in the absence of electrolyte disturbances or primary ischaemic heart disease.[11] The characteristic large T waves, previously known as 'cerebral T waves', have been noted in 50% of patients with intracranial haemorrhage and appear particularly common following left frontal haemorrhage.[12]

Non-specific ST changes occur in 22% of patients with stroke. Stroke patients have a 7–10-fold higher incidence of ST segment depression when compared with controls, particularly if the left MCA territory has been affected.[13] In older patients with diabetes mellitus, ST segment changes are more likely to represent true myocardial ischaemia and do not necessarily present with chest pain (Table 6.1).[14]

Aberrant Q waves identical to those observed in acute myocardial infarction are well-recognized after acute stroke.[15] It is unlikely that the ischaemic changes seen on ECG in patients with acute stroke result entirely from the coincidence of acute cerebrovascular and cardiac events, as the prevalence of acute myocardial infarction among stroke patients is lower than the incidence of pathologic Q waves.

Atrial fibrillation Atrial fibrillation (AF) is an independent risk factor for ischaemic stroke, with a relative risk of about 5, and is the most prevalent chronic arrhythmia in older patients—5.9% of general population and its prevalence doubles every 10 years from age of 50 years.

Patient with AF who have a stroke are likely to have had a cardioembolic aetiology. On the other hand, AF is common in older adults, who often are at risk for other types of stroke. Thus, the presence of AF in an older stroke patient does not always mean that there is a causal relationship.[16] Therefore, even in the setting of AF, all patients with stroke need consideration of other causes of stroke, especially if they would result in different treatment.

Table 6.1 Rates of ECG abnormalities and arrhythmias following stroke (%)[1]

Type of arrhythmia	Goldstein et al.[8]	Ramani et al.[60]
Prolonged QT	37	28
U waves/Tall U waves	25	9
ST depression/changes	25	25
T-wave inversion/changes	24	34
Tachycardia/sinus tachycardia	22	15
Left ventricular hypertrophy	22	4
Q waves	22	9
Atrial fibrillation	13	0
Premature ventricular contractions	13	0
Decreased heart rate/sinus bradycardia	9	11
Right bundle branch block	7	NR
First degree heart block	6	2
Premature atrial contractures	6	NR
ST elevation	3	NR
Left bundle branch block	0	NR

Source: data from *Pract Neurol.*, 13(1), Fernandes PM, Whiteley WN, Hart SR, et al., Strokes: mimics and Chameleons, pp. 21–8, Copyright (2013), *British Medical Journal.*
[1] NR, not reported.

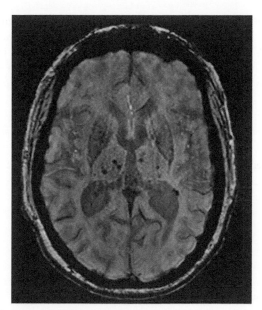

Fig. 6.5 Axial MRI GRE (gradient ECHO) sequence shows microhaemorrhages affecting the basal ganglia in a chronic hypertensive patient.

Image courtesy of Department of Stroke Medicine, Nottingham City Hospital, UK.

When AF is suspected during clinical examination, request a 12-lead ECG for confirmation (Fig. 6.5).

AF is associated with more severe ischaemic strokes and longer transient ischaemic attacks (TIAs) than emboli from carotid disease, presumably due to embolization of larger particles with AF.[17] The ratio of hemispheric events to retinal events is 25:1 with AF compared with 2:1 with carotid disease. As a result, patients with AF who suffer an ischaemic stroke appear to have a worse outcome (more disability, greater mortality) than those who have an ischaemic stroke in the absence of AF, even after adjustment for the advanced age of patients with AF-related stroke.[18]

AF is also associated with silent cerebral infarctions and TIAs.[19]

Early detection of AF is important in acute stroke and for those in sinus rhythm with a suspicion of cardio embolic stroke. Cardiac monitoring is recommended for at least the first 24 hours after the onset of ischaemic stroke to identify AF or atrial flutter.[20]

Some older patients have brain ischaemia not attributable to a definite source of cardioembolism, large artery atherosclerosis, or small artery disease despite extensive vascular and cardiac evaluation, including lack of evidence of AF on standard 12-lead ECG and 24-hour cardiac monitoring. The problem is that paroxysmal AF, if transient and asymptomatic, may be undetected on standard cardiac monitoring such as continuous telemetry and 24- or 48-hour Holter monitors.

Prolonged cardiac monitoring can increase the detection of occult AF in patients with TIA or acute ischaemic stroke who present with sinus rhythm.[21,22] Such monitoring may reduce the risk of recurrent ischaemic stroke by prompting the use of long-term anticoagulation.

Radiology tests

A chest X-ray is not routinely indicated, but is sometimes useful to diagnose associated pulmonary oedema or (aspiration) pneumonia.

Investigation into the aetiology of stroke

Around 80% of strokes are due to ischaemic pathology of which 60–80% are due to emboli. Haemorrhagic strokes constitute the remaining 20%. When investigating ischaemic strokes, it is important to look for a source of embolism or site of thrombosis.

The common sites of emboli in older people are shown in Box 6.1.

Potential embolic sources can be detected by:

- Imaging of the extracerebral vessels with carotid duplex ultrasound, transcranial ultrasound, CT angiography (CTA), or MRA
- Imaging of intracerebral vessels with CTA, MRA, digital subtraction angiography (DSA)
- Cardiac investigation
    - ECG
    - Ambulatory ECG monitoring
    - Echocardiography

These are not our normal practice to routinely carry out imaging for suspected aortic arch embolism but this may become an investigation in future, especially in patients with strong suspicion of embolic stroke with undetected source after extensive investigations.

Box 6.1 Common sources of embolism in older people

- Carotid artery bifurcation
- Vertebral artery origin
- Intracranial vessels (esp. in Chinese, South Asian population)
- Heart
    - Thrombus
    - Left ventricle
    - Prior myocardial infarction
    - Dilated cardiomyopathy with reduced cardiac output
    - Left atrium
    - Atrial fibrillation or atrial flutter
    - Valvular heart disease—mitral stenosis, prosthetic valve thrombosis
    - Non-thrombotic masses
    - Tumour—myxoma, papillary fibroelastoma
    - Vegetation—infectious endocarditis
    - Non-infectious endocarditis (malignancy, sepsis, burns, systemic inflammatory disease)
- Aortic—complex atheroma (protruding >4 mm, mobile component, and/or plaque ulceration)

Carotid duplex ultrasound

Carotid duplex ultrasound (CDUS) is a non-invasive, safe, and relatively inexpensive technique for evaluation of the carotid arteries.

CDUS is up to 98% sensitive and 89% specific in detecting a significant stenosis of the internal carotid artery.[21]

CDUS uses B-mode ultrasound imaging and Doppler ultrasound to detect focal increases in blood flow velocity indicative of high-grade carotid stenosis (Fig. 6.6). The peak systolic velocity is the most frequently used measurement to gauge the severity of the stenosis, but the end-diastolic velocity, spectral configuration, and the carotid index provide additional information.[22]

In our stroke unit at Nottingham, we screen older stroke patients for carotid stenosis with CDUS who are able to transfer from bed to chair with minimal assistance, so they may be eligible for carotid intervention if found to have significant symptomatic stenosis (>50%).

Hairline residual lumens can be missed on CDUS, but these are low risk for subsequent embolism. Several studies have found that CDUS overestimates degree of stenosis.[23] CDUS imaging can also be limited by features such as calcific carotid lesions, tortuous or kinked carotid arteries, and patient body habitus. Furthermore, CDUS must be interpreted carefully in patients with contralateral carotid occlusion to avoid overestimation of an ipsilateral carotid stenosis, since peak systolic velocity is often increased in the presence of a contralateral internal carotid occlusion.[24]

The accuracy of CDUS relies heavily upon the experience and expertise of the ultrasonographer. Measurement threshold properties vary widely between laboratories and the magnitude of the variation can be clinically important.[25] Therefore, it is suggested that high-grade stenosis should be confirmed by both anatomic (e.g. MRA, CTA, conventional angiography) and physiologic (CDUS) imaging before intervention, with CDUS performed in an accredited vascular laboratory. However, some surgeons disagree about the need for additional imaging, and carotid revascularization is performed in many centres using CDUS as sole preoperative modality for the cervical carotid artery in symptomatic patients.[26]

Relative to MRI, CDUS has limited utility in obtaining information about plaque composition and intraplaque haemorrhage, which are factors that may affect the risk of embolism.[27] However, a meta-analysis of seven studies with over 7500 subjects found that predominantly echo-lucent

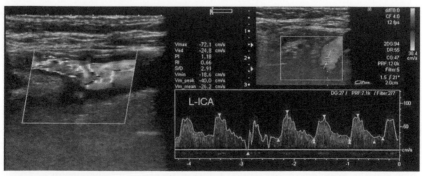

Fig. 6.6 The high peak systolic flow velocity indicates the presence of 80–90% stenosis in the left internal carotid artery proximal to the measurement.

Image courtesy of Department of Stroke Medicine, Nottingham City Hospital, UK.

plaques were associated with an increased risk of ipsilateral stroke compared with predominantly echogenic plaques across all degrees of carotid stenosis.[28]

Newer modalities such as contrast enhanced ultrasound, three-dimensional ultrasound, and compound B-mode ultrasound may offer improved carotid plaque imaging compared with CDUS. They provide a means of assaying carotid plaque features that are markers for different stages and phenotypes of atherosclerosis.

Transcranial Doppler

Transcranial Doppler (TCD) examines the major intracerebral arteries through the orbit and at base of the brain. TCD is often used in conjunction with CDUS to evaluate the haemodynamic significance of internal carotid artery stenosis and it can be used to improve the accuracy of CDUS in identifying surgical carotid disease.[29]

TCD can be used for detection of MCA microemboli that arise from the heart or carotid artery. These are visualized as high-intensity signal transients within the Doppler spectrum. There is mounting evidence from observational studies that asymptomatic cerebral embolism detected by TCD is associated with an increased risk of ischaemic stroke in patients with asymptomatic carotid atherosclerotic occlusive disease.[30]

TCD is possibly useful for the evaluation of severe extracranial internal carotid artery stenosis or occlusion, but in general CDUS and MRA are the tests of choice for older patients.[31]

CT angiography (CTA)

CTA is performed by administering a rapid bolus of standard intravenous CT contrast through a large bore intravenous cannula in the antecubital fossa. Dye can then be seen in the great vessels on the raw CT images and these can be used to reconstruct three-dimensional images of circle of Willis and extracranial cerebral arteries. Impaired renal function is a relative contraindication for its use.

CTA in elderly patients is useful to triage patients between intravenous thrombolysis, mechanical thrombectomy, and intra-arterial thrombolysis. It is also valuable in diagnosing stroke mimics; if CTA is normal, an alternative diagnosis should be sought.

CTA should be considered in older patients with acute ischaemic stroke and a proximal large artery occlusion in the anterior circulation and who present early enough for mechanical thrombectomy to be considered. Recent trials provide compelling evidence that quick, early thrombectomy with second-generation stent retriever devices is safe and effective for reducing disability when used to treat patients with stroke caused by proximal large artery anterior circulation occlusions.[32]

The finding of a 'spot sign' on CTA in intracerebral haemorrhage has been found to be associated with a high risk of haematoma expansion (Fig. 6.7).

CTA or MRA of the intracranial circulation is a useful diagnostic test for vascular malformations and aneurysms underlying intracranial bleeding in atypical locations.

CTA may also be useful when CDUS is not able to detect carotid stenosis (e.g. in cases with severe kinking, severe calcification, short neck, or high bifurcation) or when an overall view of the vascular field is required.[33] CTA is an accurate method for detection of severe carotid artery disease, particularly for detection of carotid occlusion, where CTA has sensitivity and specificity of 97% and 99%, respectively.

Magnetic resonance angiography (MRA)

MRA techniques are most often employed for evaluation the extracranial carotid arteries and utilize either two- or three-dimensional time-of-flight (TOF) MRA or gadolinium-enhanced

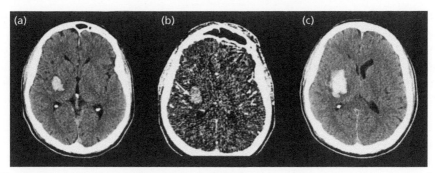

Fig. 6.7 CTA demonstrating spot sign (arrow) unifocal contrast enhancement within acute right basal ganglia haemorrhage. It corresponds to a site of active dynamic haemorrhage and is an independent predictor of ICH growth and poor outcome.

Image courtesy of Department of Stroke Medicine, Nottingham City Hospital, UK.

MRA (also known as contrast-enhanced MRA or CEMRA). Both techniques are accurate for identification of high-grade carotid artery stenosis and occlusion, but appear to be less accurate for detecting moderate stenosis.[34]

MRA is less operator-dependent than CDUS and produces a hard image of the artery. However, MRA is more expensive and time-consuming than CDUS and is less readily available.

Advanced MRA techniques are being studied to assess whether changes in carotid plaque characteristics, such as rupture of fibrous cap and intraplaque haemorrhage, are reliably associated with an increased risk of subsequent stroke in patients with asymptomatic carotid atherosclerosis.[35]

Cerebral angiography

Conventional catheter cerebral angiography is the gold standard for imaging the cerebral vasculature, however, the development of intra-arterial DSA reduces the dose of contrast, uses smaller catheters, and shortens the length of procedure. Although there is lower spatial resolution, DSA has largely replaced conventional angiography.[36]

Cerebral angiography permits an evaluation of the entire cerebral vascular anatomy including the carotid system, providing information about tandem atherosclerotic disease, plaque morphology, and collateral circulation which may affect management.[37]

In relation to older stroke patients, cerebral angiography is rarely used due to its invasive nature and risk of morbidity and mortality, and the existence of suitable alternatives.

The risk of neurologic complications is approximately 4% and risk of serious complications and death is approximately 1%. This risk increased with cerebrovascular symptoms, advanced age, diabetes, hypertension, elevated serum creatinine, and peripheral vascular disease.[38]

Cardiac studies

A cardiac evaluation is important in most patients with brain ischaemia as cardiac and aortic emboli are very common in older age groups.[39] Most older stroke patients have concurrent coronary artery disease that can lead to significant morbidity and mortality.[40]

All older patients with ischaemic stroke should have an ECG as a minimum and further cardiological investigations such as transthoracic echocardiography and 24-hour ambulatory ECG monitoring should be decided on a case to case basis if felt relevant to management of patient.

Ambulatory ECG monitoring

In contrast to the standard ECG, which provides a fixed picture of cardiac electrical activity over a brief duration, ambulatory ECG monitoring provides a view of electrocardiographic data over an extended period of time, thereby permitting evaluation of dynamic cardiac electrical phenomena that are often transient and of brief duration. Ambulatory ECG monitoring, which can be performed using a variety of techniques for as short as 24 to 48 hours and as long as months to years, offers the opportunity to review cardiac ECG data during normal routine activity.

Continuous ambulatory ECG (Holter) monitors

This continuous ambulatory ECG system is commonly performed for patients with frequent (daily) symptoms of palpitations. Continuous ambulatory ECG monitoring includes a continuous recording of all electrocardiographic data for a period of 24 or 48 hours. This technology uses a small, lightweight, battery-operated recorder that records two or three channels of electrocardiographic data from electrodes placed on the patient's chest

Once the monitoring period is over, the patient returns the device, and all of the acquired data are analysed (usually by a trained technician) and a summary report is generated for clinician review.

For those in sinus rhythm without a history of AF, prolonged cardiac monitoring is recommended for at least the first 24 hours after the onset of ischaemic stroke to identify AF or atrial flutter.[41] This approach is supported by findings of a systematic review of five prospective studies that included a total of 588 hospitalized patients with ischaemic stroke who had Holter monitoring for 21 to 72 hours.[42] Monitoring detected new AF or atrial flutter in 4.6% of these patients.

Holter monitoring is found to most useful in patients with a history of palpitations or evidence of spontaneous echo contrast on transoesophageal echocardiography (TEE), and multiple cryptogenic transient ischaemic attack.[43]

Event (loop) monitors

Event monitors, historically called loop monitors because the recording device continuously looped its recording tape, are most commonly used for patients with less frequent (i.e. weekly to monthly) symptoms. Typically utilized for 2–4 weeks, event monitors are small, lightweight devices carried by the patient with electrodes to be applied when symptoms arise. Alternatively, event monitors may be worn continuously and activated by patient trigger when symptoms arise.

Event recorders are ideal for patients who have intermittent or rare symptoms since the device may be carried for long periods of time and ECG data can be recorded during symptomatic episodes. Furthermore, they are excellent for documenting transient symptomatic or incapacitating events, and displaying the antecedent onset and subsequent offset of a paroxysmal cardiac arrhythmia.[44]

Implantable loop recorder (ILR)

An ILR is a subcutaneous monitoring device for detection of cardiac arrhythmias and are most commonly used when symptoms are infrequent (e.g. less than once per month) or other ambulatory monitoring has been unrevealing or inconclusive.[45]

Cardiac rhythm monitoring summary

So applying these principles of good screening into practice, Holter or prolonged monitoring should be considered in patients with large vessel occlusions involving anterior and posterior circulation territories and bilateral ischaemic strokes.

Table 6.2 General principles of good screening (after Wilson and Jungner)

Atrial fibrillation in acute ischaemic stroke	
1. The condition should be an important problem	✓
2. The condition should be common	+/–
3. The condition should have a readily available and acceptable treatment	✓
Holter monitoring	
4. The screening test should be accurate	✓
5. The screening procedure should have a reasonable cost	✓
6. The screening procedure should be acceptable to the patient and society	✓

Source: data from Wilson JMG, Jungner G, *Principles and practice of screening for disease*, Paper Number 34. World Health Organization, Geneva, 1968.

In summary, identifying paroxysmal atrial fibrillation/flutter is an important part of the aetiological workup of patients with ischaemic stroke.

Screening patients with ischaemic stroke with routine Holter monitoring will identity new atrial fibrillation/flutter in approximately one in 20 patients.[46] The optimal cardiac monitoring method is uncertain, though longer durations of monitoring are likely to obtain the highest diagnostic yield (Table 6.2).

Brain natriuretic peptide

Measurements of B-type (brain) natriuretic protein (BNP) and the N-terminal fragment of BNP indicate that these markers elevated in patients with AF who have cardiogenic embolism, even in those with normal ventricular function, when compared with patients who have non-cardiogenic stroke.[47] They may help identify those who have intermittent AF or are prone to develop it.

Echocardiography

Intracardiac sources of emboli account for 15–20% of strokes. Echocardiography plays an important role in the diagnosis of cardioaortic sources of embolism. All patients suspected of having an embolic stroke should have an echocardiogram to identify appropriate source.

Transthoracic echocardiography (TTE) remains the preferred non-invasive cardiac imaging especially in older stroke patients although TEE has been shown to be a superior method for identification of most cardiac sources of emboli (Table 6.3).[48]

The choice between TTE and TEE as the initial imaging test to identify a source of embolism needs to be individualized on a case-by-case basis. TTE would be initial test for the majority of older stroke patients with a suspected cardiac or aortic source of emboli, including:

◆ Patients with suspicion of left ventricular thrombus

◆ Patients in whom TEE is contraindicated (e.g. oesophageal stricture, unstable hemodynamic status) or who decline TEE

◆ Initial evaluation of suspected endocarditis, or mechanical value prostheses

TEE should be considered as the initial test to localize the source of embolism in younger patients without known cardiovascular disease, in patients with a mechanical heart valve, and in patients with suspected aortic pathology as it is the best test to examine the atria, atrial septal region, and the aorta.

Table 6.3 Non-invasive cardiac monitoring for detecting paroxysmal atrial fibrillation or flutter after acute ischaemic stroke[21]

Study, Year	N	Intervention	Duration of monitoring	Definition of atrial fibrillation	New atrial fibrillation/ flutter	Initiation of monitoring
Barthelemy et al., 2003	60	Cardiac event recorder (n* = 52)	4 days (70.1 hours)	≥30 seconds	7.7%	10 days from stroke event
		Holter monitor (n = 55)	24 hours		5.5%	Admission to neurology ward
Jabaudon et al., 2004	149	Holter monitor (n = 139)	21 hours	Not stated	5.0%	8 days after admission
		Event loop recorder (n = 88)	159 hours	AF detected by manual review	5.7%	55 days after admission
Hornig et al., 1996	261	Holter monitor (n = 261)	24 hours	Not stated; evaluated by cardiologist	3.8%	ND
Rem et al., 1985	184	Continuous cardiac monitoring (n = 159)	48 hours	Not stated; evaluated by neurology resident	2.5%	ND
		Holter monitor (n = 51)	24–48 hours		3.9%	ND
Schuchert et al., 1999	82	Holter monitor (n = 82)	72 hours	At least 1 minute	6.1%	2–3 weeks after acute stroke

Left atrial spontaneous echo contrast Spontaneous echo contrast seen during echocardiography is believed to represent erythrocyte aggregation in conditions with low shear rate or with high blood viscosity.[49] Spontaneous echo contrast or 'smoke-like' echoes seen within the left atrium (LA) during TEE is a common finding, especially in those with AF or left atrial enlargement and should raise concern about the possibility of an underlying thrombus. This finding is an independent predictor of thromboembolic risk and in patients with AF is associated with an increase in embolic rate from 3% to 12% per year.

While TTE and TEE have advantages and disadvantages, both are effective diagnostic tests with a role in the evaluation of suspected cardio aortic source of embolism. In most patients TEE yields higher quality images and has a greater sensitivity and specificity than TTE, but a few conditions (e.g. left ventricular thrombus) are better seen on TTE.

However, because it is less invasive and readily available in most institutions, TTE is often reasonable as the initial test of choice. In patients with adequate imaging windows, TTE can have a sensitivity and specificity approaching that of TEE.

Blood tests

On admission to most stroke units, it is routine practice for patients to have a routine set of blood tests as per their local departmental guidelines. However, some blood test results may be of relevance, especially to elderly people (Box 6.2).

Box 6.2 Useful blood investigations for the elderly stroke patient

Full blood count

ESR

Urea and electrolytes

Glucose

Liver function tests

Thyroid function

Lipid profile

Clotting profile

Low or high haemoglobin

A simple full blood count result showing severe anaemia or polycythemia might give a clue to underlying aetiology of stroke and help in prognosis.

Severe anaemia (Hb less than 80 g/litre) in an older patient at hospital admission for ischaemic stroke is a stronger predictor of death 1 year later than a history of heart disease, cancer, or severe stroke. Even moderate anaemia (Hb between 80 and 109 g/litre) is associated with an increased risk of death in the first year after stroke.[50] The link between anaemia and post-stroke mortality seem to be due to the fact that patients with a lower haematocrit are already getting less oxygen to the brain and an ischaemic stroke is likely to compound that effect.

Patients with polycythemia (Hb >18.5 g/dl in men and 16.5 g/dl in women) are at high risk for vaso-occlusive events including cerebral ischaemia. Although unusual, acute ischaemic stroke may be an initial presentation of polycythemia rubra vera (PRV). They may need further testing with JAK2 V617F or other functionally similar mutation and a low serum erythropoietin level. They may also need a bone marrow biopsy to confirm hypercellularity with trilineage growth with prominent erythroid, granulocytic, and megakaryocytic proliferation.

The increased haematocrit of PRV is the main determinant of blood viscosity. As the viscosity increases, cerebral blood flow decreases, platelet marginalization with increased contact to vessel walls occur, along with local effect of a high haematocrit on vessel walls.[51] This fulfils all three components of Virchow's triad and is consistent with the thought that many strokes in polycythemia patients are due to propagation of a local thrombus.

Erythrocyte sedimentation rate (ESR)

Raised ESR in patients presenting with new onset headache over 50 years of age should always raise the suspicion of giant cell arteritis (GCA), especially when associated with visual disturbances, jaw claudication, neck pain, and scalp tenderness.

Permanent visual impairment may occur in as many as 20% of patients and in some cases, GCA can cause bilateral blindness[52]. Hence newly recognized GCA should be considered a true neuro-ophthalmic emergency and need urgent treatment with high-dose steroids and referral for temporal artery biopsy, which remains the gold standard to confirm diagnosis of this granulomatous vasculitis.

Raised ESR may be associated with carotid atherosclerosis and herald increased risk of ischaemic stroke. Previous observational studies have shown significant association between ESR and degree of carotid atherosclerosis specifically carotid artery intima media thickness and carotid plaque.[53]

Glucose

Blood glucose is the single most important blood investigation post stroke as it may reveal a potentially reversible mimic.

Hypoglycaemia can cause focal neurologic deficits mimicking stroke, and severe hypoglycaemia alone can cause neuronal injury. It is important to check the blood sugar and rapidly correct low serum glucose (3.3 mmol/litre or <60 mg/dl). Normoglycemia is the desired goal while avoiding marked elevation of serum glucose.[54]

Hyperglycaemia, defined as blood glucose level more than 7.0 mmol/litre (>126 mg/dl), is common in patients with acute stroke and is associated with poor functional outcome.[55] Stress hyperglycaemia due to stroke is a common cause, although newly diagnosed diabetes is also important to be borne in mind.[56]

Hyperglycaemia may augment brain injury by several mechanisms including increased tissue acidosis from anaerobic metabolism, free radical generation, and increased blood brain barrier permeability. In light of these observations, it is reasonable to treat severe hyperglycaemia in the setting of acute stroke. The European Stroke Initiative guidelines recommend treatment for glucose more than 10 mmol/litre (>180 mg/dl).[57]

Clotting profile

Evaluation for a bleeding disorder (platelet count, prothrombin time, international normalized ratio (INR), activated partial thromboplastin time for all patients and thrombin time if patient is known or suspected to be taking a direct thrombin inhibitor or a direct factor Xa inhibitor) should be performed in every patient with an intracranial haemorrhage, especially if the cause is not immediately clear.

Anticoagulant use is the most common cause of brain haemorrhages. Compared with spontaneous intracerebral haemorrhages, anticoagulant-related haemorrhages are larger and associated with greater haematoma expansion and mortality.[58]

A patient on warfarin presenting with ischaemic stroke and subtherapeutic INR (<1.7) can be administered thrombolysis within the stipulated time-window with a slightly increased risk of symptomatic ICH but with no difference in functional outcome and death.[59]

Conclusion

The investigations listed in this chapter need to be tailored to the individual older patient with stroke. For example, when treating an older frail care home resident with severe stroke, cardiac investigations and carotid Doppler may not be appropriate and focus should be aimed at nutritional support with realistic rehabilitation goal planning with a multidisciplinary team. It is also not uncommon for a frail older patient to have a massive functional decline after stroke, both in term of physical and cognitive reserve, and may well need appropriate planning towards end-of-life care after consultation with family members and multidisciplinary team members. However, there is a considerable cohort of older stroke patients in whom thorough investigation into aetiology of stroke and instituting the right management (e.g. starting on anticoagulation after detecting paroxysmal AF on cardiac monitoring studies, carotid endarterectomy after detection of significant carotid stenosis on CDUS) would make a significant difference to their functional outcome, stroke recurrence, and quality of life.

References

1. **Fernandes PM, Whiteley WN, Hart SR, & Al-Shahi Salman R.** Strokes: mimics and Chameleons. *Pract Neurol* 2013;**13**:21–8.

2. **Wijdicks EF & Diringer MN.** Middle cerebral artery territory infarction and early brain swelling: progression and effect of age on outcome. *Mayo Clin Proc* 1998;**73**:829–36.

3. **Wardlaw JM & Mielke O.** Early signs of brain infarction at CT: observer reliability and outcome after thrombolytic treatment—systematic review. *Radiology* 2005; **235**:444–53.

4. **Patel SC, Levine SR, Tilley BC, et al.** Lack of clinical significance of early ischemic changes on computed tomography in acute stroke. *JAMA* 2001;**286**:2830–8.

5. **Köhrmann M & Schellinger PD.** Acute stroke triage to intravenous thrombolysis and other therapies with advanced CT or MR imaging: pro MR imaging. *Radiology* 2009;**251**:627–33.

6. **Fiebach JB, Schellinger PD, Gass A, et al.** Stroke magnetic resonance imaging is accurate in hyperacute intracerebral hemorrhage: a multicenter study on the validity of stroke imaging. *Stroke* 2004; **35**:502–6.

7. **U-King-Im JM, Trivedi RA, Graves MJ, et al.** Utility of an ultrafast magnetic resonance imaging protocol in recent and semi-recent strokes. *J Neurol Neurosurg Psychiatry* 2005;**76**:1002–5.

8. **Goldstein DS.** The electrocardiogram in stroke: relationship to pathophysiological type and comparison with prior tracings. *Stroke* 1979;**10**:253–9.

9. **Oppenheimer SM, Cechetto DF, & Hachinski VC.** Cerebrogenic cardiac arrhythmias. Cerebral electrocardiographic influences and their role in sudden death. *Arch Neurol* 1990;**47**:513–19.

10. **Huang CH, Chen WJ, Chang WT, et al.** QTc dispersion as a prognostic factor in intracerebral hemorrhage. *Am J Emerg Med* 2004;**22**:141–4.

11. **Lavy S, Yaar I, Melamed E, & Stern S.** The effect of acute stroke on cardiac functions as observed in an intensive stroke care unit. *Stroke* 1974;**5**:775–80.

12. **Byer E, Ashman R, & Toth LA.** Electrocardiograms with large, upright T waves and long Q-T intervals. *Am Heart J* 1947;**33**:796–806.

13. **Dimant J & Grob D.** Electrocardiographic changes and myocardial damage in patients with acute cerebrovascular accidents. *Stroke* 1977;**8**:448–55.

14. **Lavy S, Yaar I, Melamed E, & Stern S.** The effect of acute stroke on cardiac functions as observed in an intensive stroke care unit. *Stroke* 1974;**5**:775–80.

15. **Goldstein DS.** The electrocardiogram in stroke: relationship to pathophysiological type and comparison with prior tracings. *Stroke* 1979;**10**:253–9.

16. **Hart RG, Pearce LA, Miller VT, et al.** Cardioembolic vs. noncardioembolic strokes in atrial fibrillation: frequency and effect of antithrombotic agents in the stroke prevention in atrial fibrillation studies. *Cerebrovasc Dis* 2000;**10**:39–43.

17. **Anderson DC, Kappelle LJ, Eliasziw M, et al.** Occurrence of hemispheric and retinal ischemia in atrial fibrillation compared with carotid stenosis. *Stroke* 2002;**33**:1963–8.

18. **Lin HJ, Wolf PA, Kelly-Hayes M, et al.** Stroke severity in atrial fibrillation. The Framingham Study. *Stroke* 1996; **27**:1760–4.

19. **Ezekowitz MD, James KE, Nazarian SM, et al.** Silent cerebral infarction in patients with nonrheumatic atrial fibrillation. The Veterans Affairs Stroke Prevention in Nonrheumatic Atrial Fibrillation Investigators. *Circulation* 1995;**92**:2178–82.

20. **Jauch EC, Saver JL, Adams HP Jr, et al.** Guidelines for the early management of patients with acute ischemic stroke: a guideline for healthcare professionals from the American Heart Association/ American Stroke Association. *Stroke* 2013;**44**:870–947.

21. **Sabeti S, Schillinger M, Mlekusch W, et al.** Quantification of internal carotid artery stenosis with duplex US: comparative analysis of different flow velocity criteria. *Radiology* 2004; **232**:431–9.

22. **Hunink MG, Polak JF, Barlan MM, & O'Leary DH.** Detection and quantification of carotid artery stenosis: efficacy of various Doppler velocity parameters. *AJR Am J Roentgenol* 1993;**160**:619–25.

23. Sabeti S, Schillinger M, Mlekusch W, et al. Quantification of internal carotid artery stenosis with duplex US: comparative analysis of different flow velocity criteria. *Radiology* 2004; **232**:431–9.

24. Fujitani RM, Mills JL, Wang LM, & Taylor SM. The effect of unilateral internal carotid arterial occlusion upon contralateral duplex study: criteria for accurate interpretation. *J Vasc Surg* 1992;**16**:459–68.

25. Criswell BK, Langsfeld M, Tullis MJ, & Marek J. Evaluating institutional variability of duplex scanning in the detection of carotid artery stenosis. *Am J Surg* 1998;**176**:591–7.

26. Grant EG, Benson CB, Moneta GL, et al. Carotid artery stenosis: orer-scale and Doppler US diagnosis—Society of Radiologists in Ultrasound Consensus Conference. *Radiology* 2003;**229**:340–6.

27. O'Donnell TF Jr, Erdoes L, Mackey WC, et al. Correlation of B-mode ultrasound imaging and arteriography with pathologic findings at carotid endarterectomy. *Arch Surg* 1985;**120**:443–9.

28. Gupta A, Kesavabhotla K, Baradaran H, et al. Plaque echolucency and stroke risk in asymptomatic carotid stenosis: a systematic review and meta-analysis. *Stroke* 2015;**46**:91–7.

29. Wilterdink JL, Furie KL, Benavides J, et al. Combined transcranial and carotid Duplex ultrasound optimizes screening for carotid artery stenosis. *Can J Neurol Sci* 1993; **20**:S205.

30. Siebler M, Kleinschmidt A, Sitzer M, et al. Cerebral microembolism in symptomatic and asymptomatic high-grade internal carotid artery stenosis. *Neurology* 1994;**44**:615–18.

31. Sloan MA, Alexandrov AV, Tegeler CH, et al. Assessment: transcranial Doppler ultrasonography: report of the Therapeutics and Technology Assessment Subcommittee of the American Academy of Neurology. *Neurology* 2004;**62**:1468–81.

32. Goyal M, Menon BK, van Zwam WH, et al. Endovascular thrombectomy after large-vessel ischaemic stroke: a meta-analysis of individual patient data from five randomised trials. *Lancet* 2016;**387**:1723–31.

33. Corti R, Ferrari C, Roberti M, et al. Spiral computed tomography: a novel diagnostic approach for investigation of the extracranial cerebral arteries and its complementary role in duplex ultrasonography. *Circulation* 1998;**98**:984–9.

34. Debrey SM, Yu H, Lynch JK, et al. Diagnostic accuracy of magnetic resonance angiography for internal carotid artery disease: a systematic review and meta-analysis. *Stroke* 2008;**39**:2237–48.

35. Watanabe Y & Nagayama M. MR plaque imaging of the carotid artery. *Neuroradiology* 2010;**52**:253–74.

36. Hankey GJ, Warlow CP, & Sellar RJ. Cerebral angiographic risk in mild cerebrovascular disease. *Stroke* 1990;**21**:209–22.

37. Wolpert SM & Caplan LR. Current role of cerebral angiography in the diagnosis of cerebrovascular diseases. *AJR Am J Roentgenol* 1992;**159**:191–7.

38. Edwards JH, Kricheff II, Riles T, & Imparato A. Angiographically undetected ulceration of the carotid bifurcation as a cause of embolic stroke. *Radiology* 1979;**132**:369.

39. Wilterdink JL, Furie KL, & Easton JD. Cardiac evaluation of stroke patients. *Neurology* 1998;**51**:S23–6.

40. Adams RJ, Chimowitz MI, Alpert JS, et al. Coronary risk evaluation in patients with transient ischemic attack and ischemic stroke: a scientific statement for healthcare professionals from the Stroke Council and the Council on Clinical Cardiology of the American Heart Association/American Stroke Association. *Stroke* 2003;**108**:1278–90.

41. Jauch EC, Saver JL, Adams HP Jr, et al. Guidelines for the early management of patients with acute ischemic stroke: a guideline for healthcare professionals from the American Heart Association/American Stroke Association. *Stroke* 2013;**44**:870–947.

42. Liao J, Khalid Z, Scallan C, et al. Noninvasive cardiac monitoring for detecting paroxysmal atrial fibrillation or flutter after acute ischemic stroke: a systematic review. *Stroke* 2007;**38**:2935–40.

43. Flemming KD, Brown RD Jr, Petty GW, et al. Evaluation and management of transient ischemic attack and minor cerebral infarction. *Mayo Clin Proc* 2004;**79**:1071.

44. Zimetbaum PJ & Josephson ME. The evolving role of ambulatory arrhythmia monitoring in general clinical practice. *Ann Intern Med* 1999;**130**:848.

45. **Giada F, Gulizia M, Francese M**, et al. Recurrent unexplained palpitations (RUP) study comparison of implantable loop recorder versus conventional diagnostic strategy. *J Am Coll Cardiol* 2007;**49**:1951–6.

46. **Liao J, Khalid Z, Scallan C**, et al. Noninvasive cardiac monitoring for detecting paroxysmal atrial fibrillation or flutter after acute ischemic stroke. *Stroke* 2007;**38**:2935–40.

47. **de Lemos JA, McGuire DK, & Drazner MH.** B-type natriuretic peptide in cardiovascular disease. *Lancet* 2003;**362**:316–22.

48. **Pearson AC, Labovitz AJ, Tatineni S, & Gomez CR.** Superiority of transesophageal echocardiography in detecting cardiac source of embolism in patients with cerebral ischemia of uncertain etiology. *J Am Coll Cardiol* 1991;**17**:66–72.

49. **Black IW, Hopkins AP, Lee LC, & Walsh WF.** Left atrial spontaneous echo contrast: a clinical and echocardiographic analysis. *J Am Coll Cardiol* 1991;**18**:398–404.

50. **Anderson P.** Severe anemia potent predictor of death after stroke. Medscape 2 Feb 2012. Available from: https://www.medscape.com/viewarticle/757987 [Accessed: 23 July 2019].

51. **Spivak JL.** The optimal management of polycythemia vera. *Br J Haematol* 2002;**116**(2):243–54.

52. **Liozon E, Ly KH, & Robert PY.** [Ocular complications of giant cell arteritis]. *Rev Med Interne* 2013;**34**(7):421–30.

53. **Singh AS, Atam V, Yathish BE, Das L, & Koonwar S.** Role of erythrocyte sedimentation rate in ischemic stroke as an inflammatory marker of carotid atherosclerosis. *J Neurosci Rural Pract* 2014;**5**(1):40–5.

54. **Jauch EC, Saver JL, Adams HP Jr**, et al. Guidelines for the early management of patients with acute ischemic stroke: a guideline for healthcare professionals from the American Heart Association/ American Stroke Association. *Stroke* 2013;**44**:870–947.

55. **Weir CJ, Murray GD, Dyker AG, & Lees KR.** Is hyperglycaemia an independent predictor of poor outcome after acute stroke? Results of a long-term follow up study. *BMJ* 1997;**314**:1303–6.

56. **Dave JA, Engel ME, Freercks R**, et al. Abnormal glucose metabolism in non-diabetic patients presenting with an acute stroke: prospective study and systematic review. *QJM* 2010;**103**:495–503.

57. **European Stroke Initiative Executive Committee, EUSI Writing Committee, Olsen TS**, et al. European Stroke Initiative Recommendations for Stroke Management update 2003. *Cerebrovasc Dis* 2003;**16**:311–37.

58. **Flaherty ML, Tao H, Haverbusch M**, et al. Warfarin use leads to larger intracerebral hematomas. *Neurology* 2008;**71**:1084–9.

59. **Miedema L, Luijcks GJ, De Keyser J, Koch M, & Uyttenboogaart M.** Thrombolytic therapy for ischemic stroke in patients using warfarin: a systematic review and meta-analysis. *J Neurol Neurosurg Psychiatry* 2012;**83**(5);537–40.

60. **Ramani A, Shetty U, & Kundaje GN.** Electrocardiographic abnormalities in cerebrovascular accidents. *Angiology* 1990;**41**:681–6.

Chapter 7

A practical approach to neuroimaging in stroke

Amy C. Gerrish, Dorothee P. Auer, and Amlyn L. Evans

Imaging of acute infarction

Imaging is undoubtedly the most important investigation in patients with acute stroke, primarily to differentiate haemorrhagic from ischaemic tissue damage, which will define management. Any patient with suspected acute stroke should have urgent imaging, at most within 1 hour of arrival at hospital.[1]

Computed tomography (CT)

CT is usually the investigation of choice in acute stroke, due to its ready availability and rapid scan acquisition time. Its main purpose is to differentiate haemorrhagic from ischaemic stroke. Haemorrhage is easily visualized on CT, especially when acute. In contrast, the early signs of acute infarction on CT can be very subtle, and when CT is performed very soon after symptom onset, the infarct itself may not be visualized. In these cases, CT is more useful for excluding haemorrhage or an intracranial mass lesion, which may provide an alternative explanation for the patient's symptoms, and which would contraindicate thrombolysis.[2,3] It is important to bear in mind that CT involves the use of ionizing radiation; however, this is not as great a concern in the older population as it is in younger patients.

Before discussing the imaging features of acute infarction, it is useful to recap the pathophysiology. In regions of ischaemia, energy-dependent sodium-potassium cell membrane pumps fail. This causes accumulation of sodium within cells, which draws in water and chloride along an osmotic gradient. Intracellular swelling occurs, and the extracellular space becomes depleted. This is known as cytotoxic oedema. Once this has occurred, a sodium concentration gradient between the capillaries and the extracellular space develops. Sodium moves from the capillaries into the extracellular space, again drawing water and chloride with it. This second process is known as ionic oedema, although in practice the term cytotoxic oedema is used to describe the combination of the two processes. It is the movement of water from the capillaries into the extracellular space which is responsible for the volume increase and low attenuation changes seen on CT imaging. Cytotoxic oedema involves both grey and white matter, but due to the lower ischaemic tolerance of grey matter it results in the loss of their normal density contrast, thereby reducing their visual differentiation. This is in contrast to vasogenic oedema, which is a purely extracellular oedema resulting from disruption of the blood–brain barrier (i.e. leaky vessels), usually associated with tumour or infection (Fig. 7.1). This preferentially involves the white matter, and therefore accentuates, rather than obscures, the grey–white matter interface.

Thromboembolism is the most common cause of infarction, and most often affects the middle cerebral artery (MCA) territory, due to the direct route for thromboembolism from the internal carotid artery, and the size of the territory. Within the MCA territory, the insular

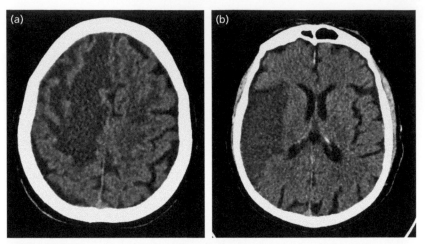

Fig. 7.1 Differentiating vasogenic from cytotoxic oedema.

Image (a) demonstrates vasogenic oedema within the right frontal lobe, which spares the grey matter and accentuates the grey–white matter boundary. Postcontrast imaging revealed a metastatic lesion within the right superior frontal gyrus. Image (b) demonstrates cytotoxic oedema within the right insular region and temporal operculum, secondary to right MCA territory infarction. This is sharply demarcated, and involves both grey and white matter, with loss of their differentiation. Note the associated mass effect and sulcal effacement present in both images.

cortex and the basal ganglia are particularly vulnerable to ischaemia due to their underlying arterial architecture. In contrast with the abundant collaterals seen over the cerebral convexities, there is a relative lack of collateral circulation of the insular cortex, and the lenticulostriate arteries supplying the basal ganglia are end arteries, which explains why the anterior insula and basal ganglia are often the first areas to show radiological abnormalities in MCA territory infarcts. This has led to the description of two radiological signs: the 'insular ribbon sign', also called 'loss of the insular ribbon', refers to loss of differentiation of the insular cortex from the adjacent white matter, with cortical swelling (Fig. 7.2(b)). 'Obscuration' or 'disappearance' of the basal ganglia refers to the loss of differentiation of the caudate and lentiform nuclei from the surrounding white matter on CT due to a relative reduction in density of the infarcted grey matter (Fig. 7.2(a)). These so-called early CT signs may be seen as early as 1 hour after symptom onset.

Another early sign of MCA territory infarction is the hyperdense MCA, which is visualization of the thrombus itself as focally increased attenuation within the MCA (Fig. 7.3). This is best demonstrated in the horizontal M1 segment, but can also be seen more distally within the M2 or M3 segments. When the hyperdense artery is seen 'end-on' in the Sylvian fissure, it may be referred to as the 'hyperdense dot sign'. The 'hyperdense MCA' is a useful positive sign; however, its absence does not exclude the possibility of vessel thrombus. In terms of vessel occlusion, it has insufficient predictive value and cannot replace CT angiography. It is also important to be aware of potential pitfalls, such as vascular calcification and the generalized hyperdensity of the vessels seen in patients with a raised haematocrit, which may lead to a false positive diagnosis.

The superficial MCA territories have the benefit of collateral networks which delay the onset of infarction. The CT features of hypoattenuation and swelling take longer to develop, and are not usually seen before 3 hours after symptom onset. When the entire MCA territory is infarcted, there can be significant mass effect, which in its most extreme form is termed 'malignant MCA territory infarction'. This can cause midline shift, transtentorial herniation, and brainstem compression.

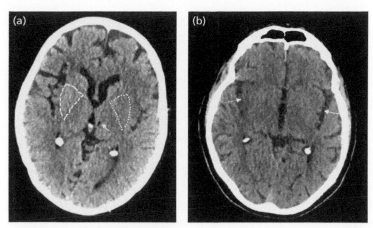

Fig. 7.2 Early signs of MCA territory infarction.

Image (a) demonstrates obscuration of the left lentiform nucleus in a patient with early left MCA territory infarction. The dashed line on the right outlines the normal lentiform nucleus, which is the same density as the brain cortex. The dotted line on the left outlines the infarcted left lentiform nucleus, which has become hypodense and now blends in with the surrounding white matter. Note also the old lacunar infarct within the left thalamus (arrow). Image (b) demonstrates the insular ribbon sign (dashed arrow) in a patient with early right MCA territory infarction. Compare the hypodense, swollen insular cortex with the normal insular cortex on the left side (solid arrow).

Infarcts within other arterial territories are less common, but demonstrate the same imaging features of hypoattenuation and swelling. Equivalent to the hyperdense MCA, a hyperdense posterior cerebral artery (PCA) or basilar artery may be identified in posterior circulation stroke. An infarct involving more than one arterial territory may be due to an incomplete circle of Willis, with absence of communicating arteries. Small cortical infarcts within multiple arterial territories are more likely due to emboli from a proximal source. 'Watershed' infarcts involve the border zone between arterial territories, which are most susceptible to episodes of hypoperfusion, for example

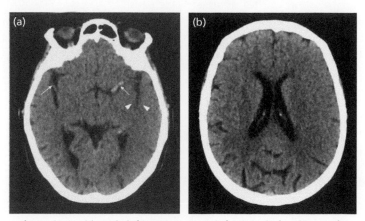

Fig. 7.3 Images of a patient with early left MCA territory infarction (a few hours after symptom onset).

Image (a) demonstrates a hyperdense left MCA (dashed arrow). Compare this with the density of the right MCA within the Sylvian fissure (solid arrow). There are features of early infarction within the insular cortex and temporal operculum (arrowheads). Image (b) demonstrates subtle generalized sulcal effacement within the left cerebral hemisphere, due to early parenchymal swelling.

during cardiac surgery. An understanding of the different patterns of infarction may therefore support the identification of different stroke aetiologies and hence aid decisions regarding further investigation and management.

Alberta Stroke Programme Early CT Score (ASPECTS)

ASPECTS was developed in the early 2000s as a reproducible, quantitative tool for the grading of acute MCA territory infarction on pretreatment CT.[4] The MCA territory is divided into ten topographic areas (Fig. 7.4), and 1 point is deducted from a total of 10 for each region which displays early ischaemic change (parenchymal swelling or hypoattenuation). A normal CT would therefore receive an ASPECT score of 10, and complete MCA territory infarction a score of 0. ASPECTS is widely used in research setting as a useful tool for standardizing the assessment of the extent of infarct, obviating the need for volumetry. It is also used in patient selection for mechanical thrombectomy, with a score of 6 as the lower threshold for inclusion.[1] Outside of these scenarios, ASPECTS is not generally used in clinical management decisions, and hence is not widely employed in current routine CT reporting.

CT perfusion

The role of CT perfusion in acute stroke is to differentiate the infarct core (irreversibly infarcted tissue) from the surrounding so-called penumbra (ischaemic but potentially salvageable tissue). The relative sizes of the infarct core and the penumbra determine the potential benefit of reperfusion therapy. A patient with a relatively large infarct core is unlikely to gain significant benefit from reperfusion therapy, and will be at higher risk of haemorrhagic reperfusion injury, in contrast with a patient who has a large, potentially salvageable penumbra.[2,3]

CT perfusion is performed by continually imaging the first pass of an iodinated contrast bolus through the brain tissue, which causes transient hyperattenuation of the tissue. Time-attenuation

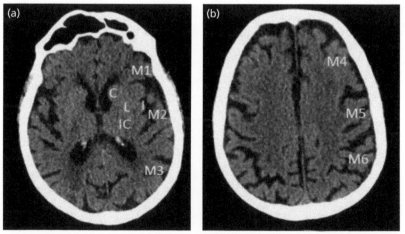

Fig. 7.4 Illustration of the ten MCA territory regions defined by ASPECTS. C (caudate nucleus), L (lentiform nucleus), IC (internal capsule), I (insular cortex), and M1–M3 are evaluated at the level of the basal ganglia. M4–M6 are evaluated at supraganglionic level.

Source: Warwick Pexman JH, Barber PA, Hill MD, et al. Use of the Alberta Stroke Program Early CT Score (ASPECTS) for assessing CT scans in patients with acute stroke. *AJNR Am J Neuroradiol* 2001;22:1534–42.

curves are produced on a voxel-by-voxel basis and kinetic modelling algorithms employed to produce perfusion maps. Three perfusion parameters are typically derived: mean transit time (MTT), cerebral blood flow (CBF), and cerebral blood volume (CBV). The infarct core will demonstrate prolonged MTT, with markedly reduced CBF and CBV. The surrounding ischaemic penumbra will also demonstrate prolonged MTT and a reduction in CBF, but will maintain normal or even elevated CBV (due to autoregulation). While CT perfusion provides an accurate haemodynamic assessment at the point of CT scanning, clinical utility is limited by the fact that tissue fate depends on both the length and the extent of hypoperfusion over the entire duration of the ischaemic period.

In practice, CT perfusion is not widely used in routine stroke imaging, and is not part of the standard selection criteria for reperfusion therapy. There may be a role for its use in patients who present outside of the time window for thrombolysis, or who present with 'wake up stroke' and therefore unknown time of symptom onset, when reperfusion treatment is being considered.

Magnetic resonance imaging (MRI)

MRI, in particular diffusion-weighted imaging (DWI), is more sensitive than CT for the detection of acute infarction.[5] In comparison with CT, which is based on a single radiodensity contrast, MRI offers multiple sequences with different imaging contrasts; however, it does have the disadvantages of restricted availability and longer scan times. MRI may also be contraindicated in some patients due to pacemakers and other metal implants, although this is becoming less of a problem as more modern devices are becoming MRI compatible. Use of MRI in acute stroke is varied across centres and countries depending on the local set-up, but is widely used in diagnostically challenging situations that cannot be addressed by CT (e.g. identification of acute or chronic infarction, detection, and age estimation of small lacunar and cortical infarcts, as well as highly sensitive diagnosis of microhaemorrhages). Moreover, MRI affords detailed tissue characterization, including metabolic and functional assessment with potential to predict patients' functional outcome, which is not currently part of routine investigation.

MRI may be used in patients with transient ischaemic attack (TIA) to confirm the presence or location of an ischaemic lesion; however, it has a high false negative rate, and there are many TIA mimics. It is not cost-effective to image all patients that present to a TIA clinic, and MRI should only be performed after assessment by a specialist physician, if the results are likely to influence management.[1,6] A basic TIA protocol should include at least T2-, T2*-, and diffusion-weighted sequences. The T2-weighted sequence provides detailed structural information, and will demonstrate areas of oedema and mass effect. T2*-weighted sequences and particularly susceptibility-weighted imaging (SWI) sequences are sensitive to paramagnetic blood products, which cause magnetic field inhomogeneity, and appear as areas of signal dropout, or 'black holes'. T2*-weighted sequences will detect both acute haemorrhage and old blood products, and SWI sequences have become the method of choice to demonstrate microhaemorrhages that show increasing prevalence in old age and index small vessel disease (Fig. 7.5). In TIA patients presenting over 7 days after symptom onset, blood-sensitive MR sequences are the preferred method for excluding haemorrhage.[1,5]

DWI is the most sensitive and specific MRI sequence for detecting acute infarction.[5] Cytotoxic oedema induced by acute tissue infarction results in cell swelling and a reduction in extracellular space. This restricts the random Brownian motion of water molecules that normally occurs within the extracellular space, and which can be detected by standard diffusion-sensitive MRI sequences. On diffusion-weighted sequences, signal is attenuated commensurate to the extent of random molecular motion of water protons. The darkest parts of the brain therefore represent

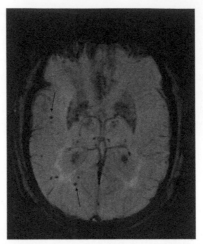

Fig. 7.5 Maximum intensity projection susceptibility-weighted imaging (SWI) at 1.5 T. The small foci of signal dropout (see arrows) represent microhaemorrhages, which cannot be seen on other imaging sequences.

areas with greatest diffusion, namely unrestricted free diffusion in the ventricular cerebrospinal fluid (CSF) (black on Fig. 7.6(b)). Normal brain parenchyma displays less signal attenuation than CSF due to barriers from cell walls, myelin sheaths, and size of the extracellular space (grey on Fig. 7.6(b)). However, acute infarcted tissue shows further restricted diffusion of water molecules due to additional diffusion barriers and lengthened diffusion paths (increased tortuosity of extracellular space) resulting from cytotoxic oedema. This reduces signal attenuation compared to the healthy brain, resulting in higher DWI signal, therefore the infarcted areas appear 'bright' (Fig. 7.6(b)).

It is important to be aware of the phenomenon of 'T2 shine through' when interpreting DWI. The diffusion-weighted sequence is inherently T2 weighted, therefore any region of T2 hyperintensity (e.g. vasogenic oedema), may appear bright on the DWI, even if it is not truly diffusion restricting.

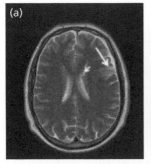 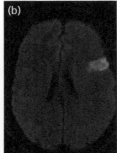 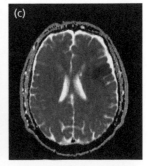

Fig. 7.6 a) T2 weighted b) DWI and c) ADC map demonstrating an area of diffusion restriction within the left frontal lobe, in keeping with acute infarction (dashed arrow). Note the old lacunar infarct within the left caudate nucleus (arrowhead), which has matured into a CSF-filled cavity with the same diffusion characteristics as the adjacent ventricle.

This is why DWI must be interpreted alongside a quantitative diffusion map. The most commonly used apparent diffusion coefficient (ADC) map is calculated from the diffusion scans and quantitatively assesses the magnitude of tissue diffusivity. Areas of diffusion restriction will demonstrate a *lower* signal (and thus appear darker) on the ADC map compared to normal tissue (Fig. 7.6(c)). Therefore, once an area of high signal has been identified on the DWI sequence, a corresponding low signal must be present on the ADC map to confirm true diffusion restriction. It should also be noted that DWI hyperintensity and diffusion restriction are physical properties rather than being disease specific, and are not exclusively seen in stroke patients—abscesses and hypercellular brain tumours also cause diffusion restriction.

Evolution of ADC changes in subacute infarction

The described DWI hyperintense/ADC hypointense changes seen in acute infarction persist for around a week. After this, there is a steady increase in ADC signal, thought to be due to a combination of tissue necrosis and increased extracellular oedema, allowing greater diffusion of water molecules. When the ADC value rises to that of normal brain tissue, it is termed 'pseudonormalization'. After around 2 weeks, the ADC value will rise above that of normal tissue. The ADC map therefore has potential for estimating the age of an infarct. This can be useful in patients with multiple infarcts of varying ages, indexing an embolic source. DWI is not as helpful, as DWI signal remains high for the first few weeks, influenced by T2 shine-through effects.[7]

Advanced MR modalities

Contrast-enhanced MR perfusion is largely equivalent to CT perfusion in the quantification of haemodynamic parameters. In patients with impaired renal function, a contrast-free technique called arterial spin labelling can be used to derive absolute CBF maps.

MR spectroscopy offers non-invasive information of the metabolite composition of brain regions. Two metabolites are of particular interest in stroke; lactate, indexing anaerobic glycolysis, and N-acetyl-aspartate (NAA), a marker of neuronal viability. Lactate and NAA have prognostic value but are not routinely used in diagnostic work-up of strokes.[8,9] The specificity of MR spectroscopy allowing confirmation, exclusion, or even quantification of lactic acidosis can be diagnostically useful in challenging clinical scenarios including vasculitis, metabolic strokes, or global hypoxia.

Subacute imaging findings

Haemorrhagic transformation

Haemorrhagic transformation is usually seen in the first few days following infarction, and is thought to result from collateral perfusion, or reperfusion, of infarcted tissue with compromised vessel integrity. There are two distinct types of haemorrhagic transformation: petechial haemorrhage, and parenchymal haematoma (Fig. 7.7). The CT appearances of petechial haemorrhage are of punctate or patchy hyperdensities, which typically involve the margins of the infarct, but may also be seen within the infarct itself. Parenchymal haematomas are larger confluent areas of haemorrhage, which may extend outside the infarct area, affect remote areas, extend into the extraparenchymal spaces, and cause mass effect. Parenchymal haematomas, particularly the large ones, are associated with adverse clinical outcomes, unlike petechial haemorrhage, therefore it is important to differentiate the two when seen on imaging.[10]

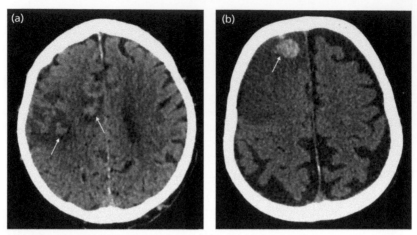

Fig. 7.7 (a) Petechial haemorrhages within a right frontal lobe infarct (arrows). (b) A different patient with small volume parenchymal haemorrhage within a right frontal lobe infarct (arrow).

Haemorrhagic transformation may occur spontaneously, but is also one of the most feared complications of reperfusion therapy and can be excluded by repeat CT in acute clinical deterioration after thrombolysis.

Fogging effect

The fogging effect is a well-described phenomenon which typically occurs in the second or third week after infarction. Infarcted areas of the brain which were initially hypodense transiently appear isodense to normal brain, masking or 'fogging' the area of abnormality (Fig. 7.8). This is thought to be due to influx of lipid-laden macrophages, proliferation of capillaries, and reduction of oedema.[11,12] It is important to be aware of this phenomenon, as it may cause diagnostic confusion when imaging patients in the subacute stage. The infarcted brain will later become hypodense once more as necrosis progresses.

Although fogging is more widely recognized on CT, a similar process has been described on T2-weighted MRI.[13]

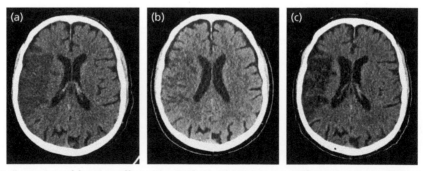

Fig. 7.8 Illustration of fogging effect. (a) Unenhanced CT imaging performed at time of symptom onset demonstrates MCA territory infarction. (b) Changes are less evident on the CT performed 1 week later, due to fogging effect. (c) A further CT performed 2 months later demonstrates an established infarct.

Contrast enhancement

Parenchymal enhancement of infarcted brain tissue may be patchy, ring-like, or gyral (serpiginous) in appearance, and is thought to be secondary to breakdown of the blood–brain barrier. It is typically present on CT in the second or third week after stroke, but may be seen earlier on MRI.[14,15] Delayed postcontrast imaging is not usually performed in the stroke setting; however, if the diagnosis is unclear and it is carried out, it has the potential to cause confusion, as enhancement of infarcted tissue may be mistaken for a neoplastic or infectious process. It is therefore important to consider infarction in the differential for an enhancing intra-axial lesion.

Vascular imaging

Determination of the most likely aetiology and decisions regarding management of stroke often require dedicated vascular assessment, in both acute and non-acute settings.

Guidelines regarding carotid intervention are predominantly based on the grade of carotid stenosis, based on historic randomized controlled trials using conventional angiography.[1,16] Patients with TIA or non-disabling stroke should undergo dedicated carotid imaging within 24 hours in order to identify severe carotid stenosis, potentially treatable with carotid endarterectomy or endovascular intervention.[1]

There are a variety of vascular imaging modalities available, which each have their own benefits and limitations.

CT angiography

Contrast-enhanced CT angiography (CTA) requires intravenous (IV) injection of iodinated contrast media, but is quick and easy to perform, and can be used to evaluate both intracranial and extracranial arteries. Vascular calcification is demonstrated particularly well but may obscure accurate assessment of the degree of stenosis.

In the acute stroke setting, CTA is used to localize the site of arterial occlusion (Fig. 7.9), and may demonstrate arterial dissection as a potential cause of infarction. Following the introduction of intra-arterial thrombectomy as a first-line treatment for stroke, the use of CTA has gained an important role in the selection of patients for neurointervention. Patients with ischaemic stroke who

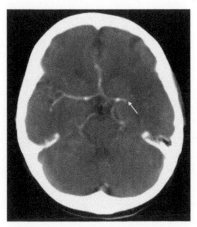

Fig. 7.9 CT angiogram in a patient with acute left MCA territory infarction demonstrating abrupt cut off of contrast within the left MCA (arrow), in keeping with vessel occlusion.

are eligible for endovascular therapy should have a CT angiogram from aortic arch to skull vertex. This is used to confirm the presence of large vessel occlusion, a prerequisite for thrombectomy, and to demonstrate the quality of collateral circulation, a further important consideration.[1,17]

CTA may also be used when posterior circulation infarction is suspected, as evaluation of the posterior fossa is limited on unenhanced CT. Vertebrobasilar thrombus can be readily identified on CTA; however, brainstem infarcts are best seen on MRI.

MR angiography

MR angiography (MRA) is also used to evaluate both intracranial and extracranial arteries. There are two main MRA techniques used in daily practice: time-of-flight (TOF) MRA and contrast-enhanced MRA (CE-MRA) (Fig. 7.10). Time-of-flight imaging uses the principle of flow-based contrast, and does not require injection of a contrast medium, but is limited at lower magnetic field strengths (1.5 T). Contrast-enhanced MRA requires IV injection of a gadolinium-based contrast agent; however, it provides greater resolution and is less susceptible to artefact than the flow-based techniques. CE-MRA is usually the sequence of choice for the neck vessels, unless the patient has any contraindication to IV contrast. MRA can be performed as an addition to the standard sequences in a TIA MRI protocol.

Direct plaque imaging

Patients with thromboembolic events from the carotid artery (amaurosis fugax, TIA, or stroke) are at increased risk of stroke despite best medical treatment. There is increasing evidence that improved risk prediction can be afforded by MRI detection of intraplaque haemorrhage, one of the key histological plaque features defining a vulnerable plaque with increased thromboembolic risk. Carotid plaque haemorrhage can be easily visualized on unenhanced fat and blood-flow nulled T1-weighted MRI scans. Presence of plaque haemorrhage (Fig. 7.11) is associated with around a fivefold increase in stroke risk. Direct plaque imaging may therefore offer risk stratification in clinically uncertain cases.[18]

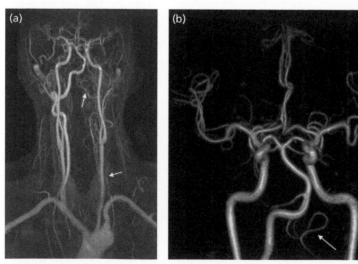

Fig. 7.10 Contrast-enhanced MRA of the neck vessels and 3D reconstruction of a TOF MRA of the circle of Willis in the same patient performed on a 3 T MRI. Note the hypoplastic left vertebral artery (arrowed) with dominant right vertebral artery, a normal variant.

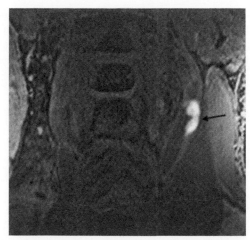

Fig. 7.11 Unenhanced fat-suppressed, black-blood T1-weighted MR image. Bright signal can be seen within a plaque in the wall of the left common carotid artery (arrow). This represents intraplaque haemorrhage.

Doppler ultrasound

Doppler ultrasound imaging is frequently used for carotid assessment, as it is cost-effective, non-invasive, and easily accessible. It can provide detailed anatomical information, such as plaque location and morphology, as well as physiological information about vessel flow. The disadvantage of ultrasound is that it is a highly operator dependent technique, and may be susceptible to artefact and misinterpretation. It is also only useful for evaluation of the extracranial arteries. Ultrasound may be limited by anatomical factors such as a short neck, high bifurcation, or tortuous vessels, or by other factors such as bandages, central lines, or a patient's inability to cooperate.

Colour Doppler is used to provide an overall assessment of flow within a vessel. A colour map is superimposed onto the greyscale ultrasound image, with the colours red and blue representing blood flow either towards, or away from, the probe (Fig. 7.12). Pulsed-wave Doppler is used to analyse flow at specific sites within the vessel, and produces a spectral wave form from which the peak systolic velocity (PSV) and end diastolic velocity (EDV) are calculated. The common carotid (CCA), internal carotid (ICA), external carotid (ECA), and vertebral arteries should be separately interrogated.[19–21]

The degree of ICA stenosis should be graded using the North American Symptomatic Carotid Endarterectomy Trial (NASCET) method.[1] This uses angiographic measurements of luminal diameter for the calculation of carotid stenosis,[16] and has been widely adopted and applied to ultrasound. With this method, the narrowest luminal diameter at the site of stenosis (B) and the luminal diameter of the normal ICA beyond the carotid bulb (A) are measured. Percentage diameter stenosis is calculated using the formula A–B/A.

Stenosis can also be graded using velocity criteria. Absolute velocity measurements were originally used to grade carotid stenosis, but these are subject to many variables and are not as reliable as velocity ratios. PSV ratio (the ratio of PSV in the ICA to PSV in the CCA) and St Mary's ratio (the ratio of PSV in the ICA to EDV in the CCA) are most commonly measured, and are used to stratify the degree of stenosis. It is important that carotid imaging reports clearly state which criteria are used when measuring and grading carotid stenosis, in order to avoid confusion.[21]

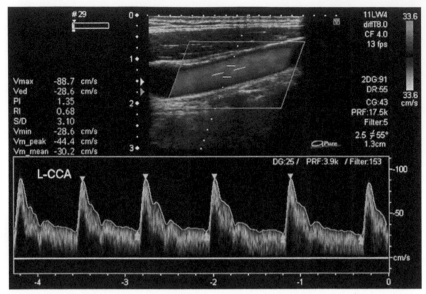

Fig. 7.12 Colour Doppler imaging of the common carotid artery (top) with pulsed-wave Doppler demonstrating a normal spectral wave form (bottom).

Ultrasound is a very useful screening tool, but as discussed, does have its limitations. It may be necessary to perform further imaging studies such as CT or MRA for definitive diagnosis.[21]

Conclusion

Imaging is an integral part of stroke medicine. Due to the time-critical nature of treatment in stroke, it is important that imaging is readily accessible. With the many different imaging modalities and studies available, it is important that clinicians have sufficient knowledge to be able to select the most appropriate test for the patient, and to be aware of potential limitations and diagnostic pitfalls.

References

1. **Intercollegiate Stroke Working Party**. *National Clinical Guideline for Stroke*, 5th edition. London, UK: Royal College of Physicians, 2016.

2. **Latchaw RE, Alberts MJ, Lev MH**, et al. Recommendations for imaging of acute ischaemic stroke. *Stroke* 2009;**40**:3646–78.

3. **Marco de Lucas E, Sánchez E, Gutiérrez A**, et al. CT protocol for acute stroke: tips and tricks for general radiologists. *RadioGraphics* 2008;**28**(6):1673–87.

4. **Warwick Pexman JH, Barber PA, Hill MD**, et al. Use of the Alberta Stroke Program Early CT Score (ASPECTS) for assessing CT scans in patients with acute stroke. *AJNR Am J Neuroradiol* 2001;**22**:1534–42.

5. **Fiebach JB, Schellinger PD, Jansen O**, et al. CT and diffusion-weighted MR imaging in randomized order: diffusion-weighted imaging results in higher accuracy and lower interrater variability in the diagnosis of hyperacute ischemic stroke. *Stroke* 2002;**33**:2206–10.

6. **Wardlaw J, Brazzelli M, Miranda H,** et al. An assessment of the cost-effectiveness of magnetic resonance, including diffusion-weighted imaging, in patients with transient ischaemic attack and minor stroke: a systematic review, meta-analysis and economic evaluation. *Health Technol Assess* 2014;**18**:1–6.

7. **Lansberg MG, Tijs VN, O'Brien MW,** et al. Evolution of apparent diffusion coefficient, diffusion-weighted, and T2-weighted signal intensity of acute stroke. *AJNR Am J Neuroradiol* 2001;**22**:637–44.

8. **Pereira AC, Saunders DE, Doyle VL,** et al. Measurement of initial *N*-Acetyl aspartate concentration by magnetic resonance spectroscopy and initial infarct volume by MRI predicts outcome in patients with middle cerebral artery territory infarction. *Stroke* 1999;**30**:1577–82.

9. **Parsons MW, Li T, Barber PA,** et al. Combined 1H MR spectroscopy and diffusion-weighted MRI improves the prediction of stroke outcome. *Neurology* 2000;**55**(4):498–506.

10. **Berger C, Fiorelli M, Steiner T,** et al. Hemorrhagic transformation of ischemic brain tissue. *Stroke* 2001;**32**:1330–5.

11. **Skriver EB & Olsen TS.** Transient disappearance of cerebral infarcts on CT scan, the so-called fogging effect. *Neuroradiology* 1981;**22**(2):61–5.

12. **Becker H, Desch H, Hacker H, & Pencz A.** CT fogging effect with ischemic cerebral infarcts. *Neuroradiology* 1979;**18**(4):185–92.

13. **O'Brien P, Sellar RJ, & Wardlaw JM.** Fogging on T2-weighted MR after acute ischaemic stroke: how often might this occur and what are the implications? *Neuroradiology* 2004;**46**:635–41.

14. **Hornig CR, Busse O, Buettner T, Dorndorf W, Agnoli A, & Akengin Z.** CT contrast enhancement on brain scans and blood-CSF barrier disturbances in cerebral ischemic infarction. *Stroke* 1985;**16**:268–73.

15. **Karonen JO, Kaarina Partanen PL, Vanninen RL, Vainio PA, & Aronen HJ.** Evolution of MR contrast enhancement patterns during the first week after acute ischemic stroke. *AJNR Am J Neuroradiol* 2001;**22**:103–11.

16. **North American Symptomatic Carotid Endarterectomy Trial.** Methods, patient characteristics, and progress. *Stroke* 1991;**22**:711–20.

17. **White PM, Bhalla A, Binsmore J, James M,** et al. Standards for providing safe acute ischaemic stroke thrombectomy services (September 2015). *Clin Radiol* 2017;**72**(2):175.e1–9.

18. **Hosseini AA, Kandiyil N, Altaf N, MacSweeney S, & Auer DP.** MRI plaque hemorrhage strongly predicts recurrent cerebrovascular events. *Ann Neurol* 2013;**73**(6):774–84.

19. **Tahmasebpour HR, Buckley AR, Cooperberg PL, & Fix CH.** Sonographic examination of the carotid arteries. *RadioGraphics* 2005;**25**(6):1561–75.

20. **von Reutern GM, Goertler MW, Bornstein NM,** et al. Grading carotid stenosis using ultrasonic methods. *Stroke* 2012;**43**:916–21.

21. **Oates CP, Naylor AR, Hartshorne T,** et al. Joint recommendations for reporting carotid ultrasound investigations in the United Kingdom. *Eur J Vasc Endovasc Surg* 2009;**37**:251–61.

Chapter 8

Atrial fibrillation and stroke in the older person

David Mangion

Introduction

Atrial fibrillation (AF) is the commonest sustained cardiac arrhythmia encountered in clinical practice.[1] In 2010, the number of individuals with diagnosed AF globally was estimated to be 33.5 million.[2] People with AF have an increased risk of death, stroke, and non-stroke cardiovascular disease.[3,4] Additionally, AF is associated with increased risk of kidney dysfunction, dementia, physical disability, and poor subjective health.[3,4] Costs and hospitalizations attributable to AF have increased over recent decades and are expected to increase further.[5] Thus, AF constitutes a significant public health problem.[2,4]

Stroke as the second most common cause of death and the third most common cause of disability worldwide, with the burden greater in developing countries.[6] Atrial fibrillation accounts for between one in three to four of ischaemic strokes[7-9] and around 80% of cardioembolic strokes.[10] A robust evidence base for the prevention of AF-related stroke exists.[10]

AF is predominantly a disease of older people.[11-13] However, the application of guideline recommendations to older people can be difficult[14,15] and adherence often suboptimal.[16] This review provides an update on the contribution of AF to stroke in the older person.

Epidemiology

Incidence and prevalence

Both the incidence and prevalence increase with age.[12,13,17,18] The incidence of new onset of AF doubles with each decade of age, independent of the increasing prevalence of known predisposing conditions.[19] In the Rotterdam study, the overall incidence was 9.9/1000 person-years, rising from 1.1/1000 person-years in age group 55–59 years to 20.7/1000 person-years in the age group 80–84 years and stabilized in those aged 85 years and above.[12] Overall prevalence of AF was 5.5%, rising from 0.7% in the age group 55–59 years to 17.8% in those aged 85 years and above.[12] Incidence and prevalence were higher in men. Although rates differ by population, these age-related trends are similar in other studies.[2,17,18,20,21] Approximately 70% of individuals with AF are between 65 and 85 years of age.[20] The lifetime risk for development of AF is around 1 in 4 for men and women.[12,22] Permanent AF occurs in approximately 50% of patients, and paroxysmal and persistent AF in 25% each.[18] Since AF is commonly asymptomatic, prevalence rates are likely to be an underestimate in the absence of screening. The prevalence of AF has increased recently and is predicted to more than double over the next two to three decades, reflecting an ageing population and increased prevalence of risk factors.[13,23-25]

Risk factors for AF in older people

Multiple factors contribute to the increased frequency of AF with age. Ageing is associated with an atrial cardiopathy, secondary to electrical and structural remodelling, that promotes AF.[26–28] Cardiovascular diseases predispose to AF[26,29] and their prevalence increase with age.[4] Traditional cardiovascular risk factors including obesity,[30] diabetes,[31] and hypertension[4] are commoner in older people, as are chronic kidney disease[11,32] and sleep-related breathing disorders.[11,33] Age-related androgen deficiency[34,35] predicts incident AF. Physical inactivity accounted for 26% of all new AF cases in older people.[36] Improved treatment of cardiovascular disease and risk factors has increased the numbers of older survivors who remain at risk of developing AF.[26] Traditional risk factors predict the development of AF only partially. Biomarkers, such as B-type natriuretic peptide, and genetics may be important determinants of risk in old age.[27,37]

Secular changes in lifestyle have increased the contribution of diabetes[29] and obesity[29,38] to risk. While the risk associated with hypertension has declined,[29,38] blood pressure combined with antihypertensive treatment and body mass index continue to constitute the greatest population-attributable risks.[29,38] Better management of these modifiable risk factors may reduce the burden of AF.[39]

Stroke in AF

Stroke risk in AF

AF increases the risk of stroke two- to fivefold. [3,21,40] The risk of stroke increases with age both in men and women with AF.[41] Being aged 65 years or older was associated with a threefold increased risk of stroke.[42] However, stroke risk is a continuum rather than a dichotomous variable.[41,43] The risk of stroke increases 1.4-fold per decade of age.[41] In the Framingham Study, the attributable risk for stroke associated with AF increased from 1.5% at ages 50–59 to 23.5% at ages 80–89.[40] Most strokes occur in the very elderly. In the Oxford Vascular Study,[44] around 60% of AF-related ischaemic strokes occurred in people ≥80 years old.

Atrial fibrillation, previously known or newly diagnosed, was found in 18–33% of those admitted with ischaemic stroke.[7,8,45–48] In these, the prevalence of AF increased with advancing age, from around 2% in those aged 40 years or younger[48] to around 50% in those older than 90 years.[7,8,48] In those admitted with stroke, the CHA_2DS_2-VASc score was directly related to the prevalence of AF. In those aged ≥75 years with heart failure, around 70% had underlying AF.[7]

The incidence of ischaemic stroke has declined in those aged more than 65 years, perhaps reflecting better management of stroke and risk factors.[9,49] However, the frequency of AF-related stroke has increased[7,44,47] probably reflecting an increasing prevalence of AF due to demographic changes and lack of anticoagulation before stroke.[7,8,44,47] The numbers of AF-related ischaemic strokes at age ≥80 years increased nearly threefold from 1981–1986 to 2002–2012.[44] Based on demographic change alone, at current incidence rates the absolute number of AF-related strokes in those aged ≥80 years are projected to treble again by 2050 without better preventative measures.[44]

Stroke severity

Prognosis is worse in AF-related stroke. Those with AF-related strokes have an increased risk of mortality[46,48,50–52] and recurrence[48,51,52] after stroke. Age and sex adjusted 1-year mortality after stroke is increased 1.2- to 1.7- fold. [48,51] In-hospital mortality is around 20–25%[46,53] while 1-year mortality is around 40–50%.[50,51,54] In people with AF, ischaemic stroke triples long-term mortality with median survival of only 1.8 years after stroke.[54] Survivors are more likely to be chronically disabled, bedridden, and to require constant nursing care and institutionalization, particularly if very elderly.[44,48,52] Older age[46,48] and increased stroke severity[46,48,54] largely account for the poorer outcomes of AF-related ischaemic stroke. Costs are higher for AF-related stroke care.[55] Potentially preventable AF-related events in the United Kingdom were estimated to cost £467 million in 2010, of which £374 million were attributable to care for those aged ≥80 years.[44] By 2050, estimated cost attributable to stroke alone for those aged ≥80 years, is £1.4 billion, with more than 50% of costs (£720 million) attributable to long-term institutionalization.[44]

Stroke prevention

Mechanism of stroke in AF

AF-related strokes are due to embolization of fibrin rich thrombi originating from the left atrial appendage.[56,57] Blood stasis due to AF itself is a plausible mechanism for thrombus formation.[56] However, the pathogenesis of thromboembolism in AF is complex. It involves not only abnormal flow within the left atrial appendage but also endothelial dysfunction, the presence of a procoagulant environment, inflammation, neurohumoral factors, and structural changes within the atrial myocardium, primarily atrial fibrosis.[27,57] Thus, AF may be related to but separate from thromboembolism, both effects of an atrial cardiopathy that may be the actual cause of stroke.[58] However, it is also estimated that around a quarter of strokes in people with AF are due to atherothrombotic mechanisms, reflecting the atherosclerotic risk factors embodied in CHADS$_2$ and CHA$_2$DS$_2$-VASc scores.[59]

Antithrombotic treatment in AF

Stroke prevention is central to the management of AF, irrespective of symptoms, rhythm management, or pattern of AF since risk is largely independent of these.[60] Anticoagulation with vitamin K antagonists (VKA) effectively reduces the risk of stroke by 64% compared to placebo and by 39% compared to antiplatelet treatment.[61] Anticoagulation has other benefits. Therapeutic anticoagulation at the time of stroke was associated with lower odds of moderate or severe stroke and in-hospital mortality,[62] and better functional recovery and survival[63] after stroke. After ischaemic stroke, anticoagulation reduces recurrence[64] and mortality.[65] Commencing anticoagulants 4–14 days after ischaemic stroke seems optimal after balancing the risks of stroke recurrence and bleeding.[60,66] A residual risk of stroke remains after anticoagulation[61,64,67] arguing for coexisting non-cardioembolic mechanisms.[10] In very elderly (≥85 years) people, this risk varied from 3.9%/year[68] to 1%/year.[69]

Antiplatelet treatment provides a stroke risk reduction of 22% in AF, possibly due to its effect on non-cardioembolic mechanisms.[61] Although often perceived as a viable alternative to anticoagulation, aspirin is neither safe nor effective.[70] In very elderly people warfarin was superior to preventing stroke without excess bleeding risk.[71,72] In elderly people (≥75 years), apixaban was superior to aspirin in reducing thromboembolic events.[69] In patients ≥85 years, rates of major bleeding were similar but intracranial bleeding less frequent on apixaban compared to aspirin.[69]

Aspirin is itself associated with an increased bleeding risk compared to no treatment in trial[73] and real-world settings.[74] In community settings, the relative risk of intracranial bleeding is doubled with VKA compared to no treatment or aspirin but the absolute risk is small (0.46 vs. 0.23 per 100 person-years).[75] In people aged more than 65 years, a systematic review found that the risk of intracranial bleeding is increased with anticoagulants but antiplatelet drugs carry a risk of major bleeding which appears to be equal or very close to that of oral anticoagulants, translating into an estimated excess absolute risk of major bleeding events of only 1 to 2/100 patients/year with anticoagulants.[76] Stroke risk increases with age while the protective effect of aspirin declines with age, unlike warfarin[77] or apixaban.[69] Therefore, older people have substantially greater benefits from anticoagulation.[69,77,78] Where anticoagulant treatment is not feasible no treatment may be safer, and preferable, to antiplatelet treatment[60,70,79] although North American guidelines continue to support a role for aspirin.[80]

Well-managed warfarin therapy is effective and associated with a low risk of complications.[60,80–83] However, many factors, including medication and diet, can affect VKA control.[84] A 'time within therapeutic range' (TTR) of at least 70% is regarded as ideal.[82,83] This is difficult to achieve.[85,86] Those at highest risks for stroke and bleeding are least likely to be in therapeutic range.[85] Younger age is a predictor of good control.[87] Age-related predictors of poor control include frailty[85] and dementia.[86] Where TTR remains poor (<65%) a direct oral anticoagulants (DOAC) could be considered.[88] The SAME-TT$_2$R$_2$ >2[87] can help identify those likely to experience complications related to poor VKA control[89] and to benefit from a DOAC from the outset (Fig. 8.1).[90]

Compared to VKA, DOACs offer significant reductions in stroke and mortality.[67] Major bleeding events were similar but DOACs were associated with a 50% reduction in the risk of intracranial haemorrhage (ICH).[67] While observational studies do not offer direct comparison, postmarketing studies broadly confirm results of these trials[91–93] although differences between these agents may exist.[92,93] This may allow individualization of anticoagulant therapy.[94] VKAs remain the currently recommended treatment for AF patients with rheumatic mitral valve disease and/or a mechanical heart valve prosthesis.[60,80]

In those aged ≥75 years, DOACs were at least as effective as VKA in preventing stroke and systemic embolization.[67,95,96] Compared to VKA, a significant reduction in the risk of intracranial

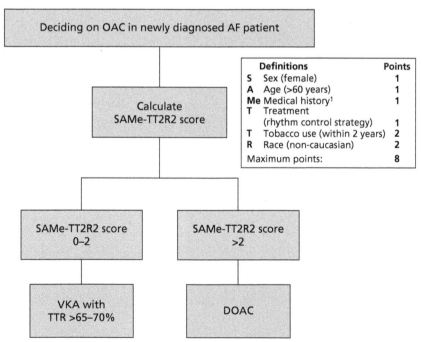

Fig. 8.1 Possible strategy for choosing oral anticoagulation in patients with non-valvular AF.[1] Medical history defined as more than two of the following: hypertension, diabetes, coronary artery disease/myocardial infarction, peripheral arterial disease, congestive heart failure, previous stroke, pulmonary disease, hepatic or renal disease. DOAC, non-VKA oral anticoagulant; VKA, vitamin K antagonists.

bleeding was observed with dabigatran and apixaban and for clinically relevant bleeding with apixaban.[95] Gastrointestinal bleeding was increased with dabigatran but little data exists for other DOACs.[95] Indirect comparison suggests that the risk of major or clinically relevant non-major bleeding appears least with apixaban compared to rivaroxaban and dabigatran.[96] This may make apixaban the preferred agent in elderly individuals.[94] Low-dose regimes may appear attractive in terms of safety. However, these are often associated with higher risk of stroke and bleeding although this may reflect the less favourable risk profiles of patients who received lower doses.[91] Major bleeding rates were low (1.37 per 100 person-years) in very old individuals ($\geq$75) on DOACs but deterioration of renal function was associated with these events.[97] Given the ease of deterioration of renal function in older individuals, regular monitoring is necessary.[98]

Risk stratification and net clinical benefit

Individual assessments of the competing risks of stroke and bleeding empower patients to make informed decisions about their treatment.[60,80,88,99,100] Prediction tools can guide decision-making.[60,80,100] The risk of stroke is similar in those with paroxysmal, persistent, or permanent AF.[10,60,80,88]

Commonly used stroke risk prediction tools are the CHADS2 and CHA$_2$DS$_2$-VASc tools (Table 8.1).[100] Compared to the CHADS$_2$ score, the CHA$_2$DS$_2$-VASc score is better at identifying truly 'low-risk' individuals and is as good at identifying 'high risk' individuals.[100,101] Even one risk factor increases thromboembolic risk.[102] Better, safer control of VKA therapy and the advent of safer and effective anticoagulants has allowed a paradigm shift away from identifying high risk individuals likely to benefit from VKA therapy to identifying those at truly low risk and who are unlikely to benefit from anticoagulation.[10,60,88,102] While VKA may have a positive net benefit with a stroke rate more than 1.7% per year, use of DOACs allows lowering of the threshold for anticoagulation to a stroke rate of 0.9% per year.[103] This favours use of DOACs.[102] Stroke risk prediction systems provide useful thresholds to inform decision-making regarding anticoagulation

Table 8.1 CHA$_2$DS$_2$-vasc score

CHA$_2$DS$_2$-vasc risk factor	Points
Signs/symptoms of heart failure or objective evidence of reduced left ventricular ejection fraction	1
Hypertension Resting BP >140/90 on at least two occasions or currently taking antihypertensive medication	1
Age 75 years or older	2
Previous stroke, transient ischaemic attack, or thromboembolism	
Diabetes mellitus Fasting glucose >125 mg/dl (7 mmol/litre) or treatment with oral hypoglycaemic agent and/or insulin	1
Vascular disease Previous myocardial infarction, peripheral artery disease, or aortic plaque	1
Age 65–74 years	1
Sex category (female)	1

rather than provide exact assessment of stroke risk[104] since not all risk factors carry the same weight.[105]

Age is a major risk factor for AF-related stroke[41,105] although this is modified by other variables.[41] Age ≥75 years is recognized as a strong risk factor.[41] However, since the lifetime AF-related stroke incidence sharply increases during the sixth decade of life, individuals reach the threshold for anticoagulation at 65 years of age even in the absence of other risk factors.[41,60,88,106] Approximately 50% of patients with only one risk factor had age as the only risk factor (≥65 years), and 90% had either age or hypertension as the risk factor.[106] In East Asians, an increased thromboembolic risk is evident at lower age (≥50 years).[107] Female sex accentuates risk in those 65 years and older or with at least one other risk factor.[10]

The HAS-BLED score predicts major bleeding in people on anticoagulants, antiplatelet therapy alone, or no antithrombotic treatment (Table 8.2).[108] It performs better than other clinically based prediction tools.[100] A score of ≥3 requires caution and identification and addressing of correctable risk but should not, on its own, preclude anticoagulation.[60] Bleeding risk is similar for international normalized ratios less than 2.0 compared to 2–3 but increases further with increasing intensity of anticoagulation.[81]

Neither the CHA_2DS_2-VASc score nor the HAS-BLED score show perfect discrimination and decision-making can be difficult in those at borderline risk.[101,103] Imaging and biological markers may refine prediction where risk is indeterminate or low.[101] Systems that incorporate biomarkers show potential to improve prediction both for stroke[109] and bleeding risk.[110] Age is a major clinical risk factor in both systems.[109,110]

Assessments of the competing risks of stroke and bleeding allow determination of net clinical benefit of anticoagulation.[78] Stroke risk and bleeding risk stratification systems share many of the same risk factors and those at high risk of bleeding are also at high risk of stroke.[100] This situation in common in older people.[41] The risk of ICH increases with age, with or without anticoagulant therapy.[69,77,78,81,111] However, the higher the bleeding risk, the greater is the risk of stroke and hence the wider the gap between stroke and bleeding risks.[69,79,112,113] Consequently, in older people the net clinical benefit favours anticoagulation.[69,77,78,113] This is highest in the very old.[69,78]

Table 8.2 HAS-BLED score

Clinical factor	Points
Hypertension (uncontrolled, >160 mmHg systolic)	1
Abnormal renal (dialysis, transplant, Cr >2.26 mg/dl or >200 µmol/litre) and (liver function Cirrhosis or bilirubin >2× normal with AST/ALT/AP >3× normal) (1 point each)	1 or 2
Stroke previous history, particularly lacunar	1
Bleeding bleeding history or predisposition (anaemia)	1
Labile INRs	1
Elderly	1
Drugs (antiplatelet agents, non-steroidal anti-inflammatory drugs); or alcohol (≥8 drinks/week) (1 point each)	1 or 2

Any beneficial effect of aspirin is lost with advancing age.[77,79] The net benefit may be greater with apixaban compared to VKA.[79]

Anticoagulant treatment in older people

Despite the efficacy of anticoagulation in preventing stroke, treatment often does not conform with current guidelines.[10,16] Consequently, opportunities for stroke prevention are lost.

Around a third of people who present with ischaemic stroke have atrial fibrillation.[7,47] Most people suffering ischaemic AF-related strokes are not on anticoagulants at the time of onset of the stroke.[7,45,47,53,114] In those with known AF prior to stroke, 13%[45] to 44%[47] were taking anticoagulants at the time of stroke. However, only 10%[53] to 25%[47] were therapeutically anticoagulated. Individuals in these studies (mean age >70 years) were predominantly elderly.[7,45,53,114] The chance of being anticoagulated was reduced by 4% per year of increasing age.[114]

Anticoagulation reduces stroke recurrence and mortality in elderly stroke survivors.[114] Only 35–44% of survivors of AF-related stroke received warfarin after discharge.[7,114] Anticoagulant use after stroke was inversely related to CHA_2DS_2-VASc score[7] and age.[115] In very elderly individuals (>90 years old), only 6.6% of patients received warfarin after discharge.[7]

In the United Kingdom, around 80% of people with AF are aged ≥65 years, with one-quarter aged ≥85 years.[68] In community settings, around 80–90% of individuals with AF are eligible for anticoagulants[116,117] but a treatment gap is commonly evident. Around 40% of those with CHA_2DS_2-VASc score of ≥2 were not receiving anticoagulants in the absence of contraindications or refusal.[117] About a quarter of patients at high risk of stroke received antiplatelet monotherapy.[117] Similar patterns of under treatment exist elsewhere.[113,118–120] Conversely, approximately 1 in 4 individuals with the lowest thrombotic risk were treated with oral anticoagulation.[120] The use of anticoagulants declined while that of aspirin increased with age.[68] In the very elderly (>85 years), only 36% received anticoagulation compared with 57% in the 75–84 year age group.[68] Almost half aged ≥85 years received aspirin monotherapy.[68]

While increased use of DOACS may have improved adherence to guidelines, regional differences in anticoagulation practices exist.[118] Significant proportion of individuals with AF remain without anticoagulation, particularly in Asia and North America.[118] Indeed, in the Veterans Health Administration system, initiation of anticoagulant in individuals with newly diagnosed AF (60% older than 70 years), and who also had additional risk factors for stroke, fell from 51.3% in 2002 to 43.1% in 2011.[121,122]

Recorded perceived contraindications and declines were highest in the very elderly[68,123] but these only accounted partially for the lower use of anticoagulants in these individuals.[123] Frailty[123,124] and measures of poor health and functional status[125] are predictors of non-use of anticoagulants. However, age was the strongest predictor of non-use of anticoagulants in people ≥80 years old, independent of frailty, dementia, or bleeding risk.[122] In institutionalized people, rates of anticoagulation ranged from 17% to 57%, even among residents with high stroke risk and low bleeding risk.[126,127] Optimizing the use of anticoagulants remains key to reducing the burden of preventable stroke in older people.

Screening for AF

A goal of secondary prevention is the detection and treatment of occult AF after stroke.[60,79,128] About 25% of ischaemic strokes remain without a readily identifiable cause despite investigation.[129] Embolic sources, including undiagnosed paroxysmal AF, may be the cause of stroke in many of these cryptogenic strokes, perhaps better defined as embolic stroke of undetermined source.[129]

Since AF is often paroxysmal and absent at the time of stroke, current guidelines recommend between 12[79] and 72 hours[60] of initial post-stroke electrocardiographic monitoring to detect occult AF. Such monitoring is recommended for all stroke survivors without an established diagnosis of AF[60,80,128] since AF can also be detected in strokes of presumed atherosclerotic aetiology.[59,130] Prolonged use of internal[130] or external[131] cardiac monitoring devices increases detection of AF and may be necessary.[60,88] In stroke survivors, sequential use of cardiac monitoring strategies has an overall yield of 24% of newly detected AF.[132,133] Since about 20% of people with ischaemic stroke are already know to have AF, this means that AF can be detected in around 40% of strokes.[100] Late diagnosis of AF (>7 days post-stroke) is associated with an increased risk of stroke recurrence.[134] About 50% of episodes of AF detected after stroke are shorter than 30 seconds.[133,135] The clinical significance of such short episodes of AF is uncertain.[60,129,135] Increasing age is a consistent predictor of incident AF detected after stroke.[135–137] However, ambulatory monitoring is used infrequently in stroke survivors, with lost opportunities for stroke prevention.[134,138]

Previously undiagnosed AF is found in around quarter of AF-related strokes.[7,45] Community-based screening has the potential to reduce the burden of AF-related stroke.[16,139] Systematic screening detected new AF in 1.5–3% of elderly populations screened.[140–142] In people aged 75–76 years, prolonged monitoring with a hand-held electrocardiogram (ECG) device allowed detection of paroxysmal AF in 7.4% of those with ≥2 risk factors for stroke.[143] In primary care, opportunistic pulse taking with follow-up electrocardiography was as effective as systematic screening in people aged more than 65 years and allowed detection of an additional third of cases of AF.[144]

Guidelines recommend opportunistic screening in high risk individuals, including those aged ≥65 years.[60,88] This is a reasonable strategy since nearly all will be eligible for anticoagulation.[10,140–143] However, experience from British primary care shows striking variation in rates of detected AF (range 0.1–16.7%), suggesting differences in the efficiency of case finding.[16] Also, initiation of anticoagulation after detection of AF remains variable, ranging from 17%[140] to over 90%.[142]

Non-pharmacological treatment

Since 90% of thrombi in AF originate in the left atrial appendage (LAA), occlusion of the LAA may be a viable treatment option, particularly in those where anticoagulants are unsuitable.[145] LAA occlusion resulted in less intracranial bleeding but more ischaemic stroke compared to VKA.[146] When periprocedural events were excluded, the difference in ischaemic stroke rate was not significant. Almost half of individuals in the pooled analysis were aged ≥75 years. The procedure is currently reserved for those with contraindications to anticoagulation.[60,145]

Barriers to anticoagulation

The failure to use anticoagulants reflects choices made by physicians or patients.[147] Patients' decisions are influenced by individual perceptions of the balance between risk and benefit of anticoagulation.[148] Professionals often consider management of anticoagulation in older people to be more challenging. Difficulties in achieving adequate control, ensuring adequate monitoring and the increased risk of bleeding among them are issues of concern.[149–151] However, the underuse of anticoagulants in older people is not readily explained by assessments of stroke or bleeding risk or by indicators of frailty.[116,121,151,152]

Age itself is often given a reason for failure to use anticoagulants.[114,152] Each advancing decade of life is associated with a 14% reduction in warfarin use.[153] Warfarin was discontinued within 1 year of initiation in 26% of individuals ≥80 years of age, the majority (81%) due to safety concerns.[154]

Older patients often have increased sensitivity to warfarin and generally require lower initiation and maintenance dosage.[155] Age-related physiological changes affect the pharmacokinetics of anticoagulants.[156] However, interaction with other medications and diet, as well as the effect of other comorbidities and disease, have the potential to increase the risk of bleeding.[14,155,156] Cerebral pathologies, including amyloid angiopathy and cerebral microbleeds, may contribute to increased bleeding risk.[155,156] Reasons commonly given by physicians to withhold anticoagulants in older people include risk of bleeding and falls, comorbidities, disability, poor prognosis, and ability to comply with treatment.[114,152,157] However, physicians are reluctant to prescribe warfarin to individuals older than 80 years even if otherwise healthy.[152] Risks of falls and bleeding are commonly overestimated and appear to be disproportionate barriers to anticoagulation.[152] Older age *per se* is not a contraindication to anticoagulation but lower doses and tighter monitoring may be required and DOACs may be preferred.[155]

The risk of bleeding related to aspirin[81] or anticoagulants[69,81] increases with age. In frail, older people, the prescription of anticoagulants is influenced more by bleeding risk than by the risk of stroke.[158] Medications predisposing to bleeding, including antiplatelet therapy, are sometimes used together with anticoagulants in elderly people.[156,159] Intercurrent illness and resultant changes in medication and diet have the potential to affect VKA control.[159] Drug–drug interactions are less common with DOACs but remain possible.[160] Chronic kidney disease, common in older people, increases the risk of stroke and VKA-related bleeding, although net benefit favours anticoagulation.[14,161] In older people, renal insufficiency is easily aggravated by the effects of intercurrent illness, dehydration, medication, and radiocontrast media.[14,155] This can affect the clearance of drugs primarily dependent on renal excretion, such as dabigatran.[155] However, warfarin is minimally dependent on renal excretion.[60] Only about 9% of people with AF who suffer intracerebral bleed restart anticoagulants, reflecting physicians' justifiable concerns with the possibility of recurrent bleeding.[162] Concern with the risk of bleeding should prompt a review of possible modifiable factors that may contribute to bleeding risk rather than withholding of anticoagulants.[60,100]

Disability and frailty, although separate constructs, are related.[163] Frailty is a syndrome commonly, though not exclusively, found in older subjects. It represents a state of increased vulnerability to health stressors resulting from reduced reserve across multiple physiological systems.[164] It is associated with reduced survival, increased risk of hospitalization, and poor quality of life.[165] Frailty is akin to biological age and may be a better indicator than chronological age on which to base treatment decisions for older persons.[165]

Physicians are particularly reluctant to prescribe anticoagulants to older patients with poor health and functional status, and short life expectancy.[15] Even when adherence to guidelines is good, those with higher risk of bleeding and higher frailty status were less likely to receive anticoagulants.[166] The suboptimal use of anticoagulants in older people, particularly the very elderly, may reflect a misunderstanding of the concept of frailty and its associated risk, with physicians equating chronological with biological age.[165] Frail people have an increased risk of stroke as well as bleeding, so measures of frailty may have limited utility in evaluating risk.[155] However, an anticoagulation-focused frailty assessment additional to standard bleeding and stroke risk assessments may allow for better awareness and correction of risk in frail elderly people.[165,167] Older people also have a high risk of non-stroke death. Accounting for this competing risk attenuates the protective effect of warfarin.[168] Decisions regarding anticoagulation should also consider the patient's risk of non-stroke death and not only the risk of stroke.[169]

The estimated risk of falling in elderly people is commonly based on physicians' perceptions rather than objective assessment.[170,171] However, the risks of falls and falls-related bleeding are common reasons why physicians fail to use anticoagulants in older people.[114,152,157] In elderly people who have fallen, mortality after a first fall, as well as eventual death due to head injury, were increased in those on anticoagulants.[172] In people with head injury, preinjury warfarin increased the odds of ICH by 40% and doubled the risk of 30-day in-hospital mortality.[173] Elderly people, assessed as being at high risk of falls, had more falls-related bone fractures, major bleeding, life-threatening bleeding, and all-cause death on anticoagulants, even after adjusting for frailty.[171] A history of prior fall was a predictor of ischaemic stroke/thromboembolism, major bleeding, and mortality but not anticoagulant-related haemorrhagic stroke.[174] The increased risk of stroke/thromboembolism and mortality in those with a prior history of falling may reflect increased comorbidities and higher stroke risk scores.[173] In individuals perceived at high risk of falling, the risk of traumatic ICH was increased but prescription of warfarin or aspirin at baseline did not significantly affect risk of ICH.[175] People at high risk of falls also have a high risk of stroke.[175,176] Therefore, such individuals appear to benefit from anticoagulation.[174] In people taking anticoagulants, falls-related bleeds are uncommon.[177] For individuals at an average risk of falling, warfarin increases quality adjusted life years compared to aspirin or no treatment.[178] Where a significant falls risk is identified, interventions to reduce this may allow safer use of anticoagulants[170] while consideration could be given to withholding anticoagulation for those at low risk of stroke.[172] It is unclear whether DOACs are safer than VKA in minimizing the risk of falls-related bleeding.[171,176]

While initiation of warfarin declined with age, persistence with treatment was better in those aged ≥65 years.[179] Half of those who discontinue warfarin have questionable reasons for doing so and most of these do not receive other thromboprohylaxis.[180] Although persistence with DOAC treatment was better than with VKA, up to half of individuals discontinued DOAC treatment.[181] Non-adherence with anticoagulation increases the risk of stroke but this risk may be more important in individuals with CHA_2DS_2-VASc score ≥2.[181] The shorter duration of action of DOACs makes adherence to a regular schedule particularly important and this may be an issue in older people.[14]

Contraindications to anticoagulant therapy, while common, are often subjective.[182] Many individuals with AF continue to receive anticoagulants despite reported contraindications, suggesting that the perceived benefit outweighed the potential harm posed by the relative contraindication.[183] Physicians may consider that older people have valid reasons to avoid anticoagulation.[154,157] However, few individuals have absolute contraindications and most are eligible for either VKA or DOACs.[184] Nonetheless, many frail individuals may not be optimal candidates for warfarin despite a high stroke risk.[15,157] While North American practice allows for antiplatelets as an alternative in these individuals,[80,150] this does not reflect other guidance.[60,88]

Many older people have limited health literacy, the degree to which individuals can obtain, process, and understand the information and services necessary to make appropriate decisions involving their health and knowledge.[185] Low health literacy is associated with poor disease-related knowledge regarding stroke risk and anticoagulation.[186] This may contribute to difficulty in evaluating the risks and benefits of anticoagulation.[99,187] Low health literacy contributes to non-adherence to medication, as does impaired cognition.[188,189] Education may improve disease-related knowledge.[99]

Cognitive abilities significantly influence medication adherence.[189] Cognitive impairment affects approximately 30% of individuals between 80 and 89 years old[190] and is associated with poor control of VKA.[191] Anticoagulants were used in only 46% of individuals with dementia although this may be a relative rather than absolute contraindication.[184] Elderly individuals may find difficulty coping with complexities of medication regimens, drug formulations, and monitoring needs.[189] The support of caregivers may allow better coordination of care and encourage adherence.[14,189]

Shared decision-making

Patient may prefer to not use anticoagulants.[99,192] This reflects their understanding of stroke risk, anticoagulation, and their consequences.[9,193] Patients place a high importance on reducing stroke risk and limiting the risk of major bleeding.[194] About half of the patients perceive major ischaemic stroke and ICH to be worse than death.[195] However, generally, patients tend to accept many serious bleeds to avoid one stroke.[196] They are often willing to accept a higher risk of bleeding than professionals for an associated reduction in the risk of stroke.[192,197] However, a significant number of patients would refuse anticoagulants even when told that benefits were high and risks low.[196] Patients' experiences of anticoagulants influence their decisions regarding anticoagulation.[187] With regard to choice of treatment, patients preferred attributes that describe DOAC treatment[192] although they were also sensitive to cost pressures.[196]

Physicians show significant interindividual variation when evaluating the risks of stroke against bleeding.[190] Patients also show similar differences.[194,196,197] Many patients view bleeding and stroke risk differently from both physicians and clinical guidelines.[192] Indeed, based solely on patients' preferences, fewer patients would receive anticoagulation treatment than recommended by guidelines.[198] Practitioners should balance the recommendations of guidelines with patients' preferences and prioritize patient involvement for true shared decision-making.[60,188]

Most patients with AF significantly overestimate the perceived risks of both stroke and bleeding,[199] making informed discussion central to proper shared decision-making. Particularly in elderly individuals, good communication and appropriate framing of expected risks and benefits of anticoagulation may better inform patients and improve of uptake of treatment.[99,200] However, such interventions are often inadequate.[187]

Conclusion

Stroke due to AF is a devastating illness that mainly affects older people. Despite improvement in VKA control and the recent introduction of effective and safer anticoagulants, a significant proportion of older people do not receive appropriate stroke prophylaxis. Without improvements in stroke prevention, the problem of AF-related stroke will only increase. For professionals, this requires better understanding of guidelines. It also requires appreciation of the particular characteristics and challenges of treating older people. Ultimately, improved communication with patients promises a better partnership and more informed shared decision-making.

References

1. **Morin DP, Bernard ML, Madias C, Rogers PA, Thihalolipavan, S, & Estes III NNM**. The state of the art: atrial fibrillation epidemiology, prevention, and treat. *Mayo Clin Proc* 2016;**91**(12):1778–810.
2. **Chugh SS, Havmoeller R, Narayanan K**, et al. Worldwide epidemiology of atrial fibrillation: a global burden of disease 2010 study. *Circulation* 2013;**129**(8):837–47.
3. **Odutayo A, Wong CX, Hsiao AJ, Hopewell S, Altman DG, & Emdin CA**. Atrial fibrillation and risks of cardiovascular disease, renal disease, and death: systematic review and meta-analysis. *BMJ* 2016;**354**:i4482.
4. **Mozaffarian D, Benjamin EJ, Go AS**, et al. Heart disease and stroke statistics—2016 update. *Circulation* 2015;**133**(4):e38–360.
5. **Wolowacz SE, Samuel M, Brennan VK, Jasso-Mosqueda J- G, & Gelder ICV**. The cost of illness of atrial fibrillation: a systematic review of the recent literature. *Europace* 2011;**13**(10):1375–85.
6. **Feigin VL, Forouzanfar MH, Krishnamurthi R**, et al. Global and regional burden of stroke during 1990–2010: findings from the Global Burden of Disease Study 2010. *Lancet* 2014;**383**(9913):245–55.

7. Friberg L, Rosenqvist M, Lindgren A, Terént A, Norrving B, & Asplund K. High prevalence of atrial fibrillation among patients with ischemic stroke. *Stroke* 2014;**45**(9):2599–605.

8. Bjorck S, Palaszewski B, Friberg L, & Bergfeldt L. Atrial fibrillation, stroke risk, and warfarin therapy revisited: a population-based study. *Stroke* 2013;**44**(11):3103–8.

9. Pistoia F, Sacco S, Tiseo C, Degan D, Ornello R, & Carolei A. The epidemiology of atrial fibrillation and stroke. *Cardiology Clinics* 2016;**34**(2):255–68.

10. Freedman B, Potpara TS, & Lip GYH. Stroke prevention in atrial fibrillation. *Lancet* 2016;**388**(10046):806–17.

11. Ball J, Carrington MJ, McMurray JJ, & Stewart S. Atrial fibrillation: profile and burden of an evolving epidemic in the 21st century. *Int J Cardiol* 2013;**167**(5):1807–24.

12. Heeringa J. van der Kuip DA, Hofman A, et al. Prevalence, incidence and lifetime risk of atrial fibrillation: the Rotterdam study. *Eur Heart J* 2006;**27**(8):949–53.

13. Go AS, Hylek EM, Phillips KA, et al. Prevalence of diagnosed atrial fibrillation in adults. *JAMA* 2001;**285**(18):2370.

14. Foody J. Reducing the risk of stroke in elderly patients with non-valvular atrial fibrillation: a practical guide for clinicians. *Clin Interv Aging* 2017;**12**:175–87.

15. Bo M, Grisoglio E, Brunetti E, Falcone Y, & Marchionni N. Oral anticoagulant therapy for older patients with atrial fibrillation: a review of current evidence. *Eur J Intern Med* 2017;**41**:18–27.

16. Kearney M, Fay M, & Fitzmaurice DA. Stroke prevention in atrial fibrillation: we can do better. *Br J Gen Pract* 2016;**66**(643):62–3.

17. Murphy NF, Simpson CR, Jhund PS, et al. A national survey of the prevalence, incidence, primary care burden and treatment of atrial fibrillation in Scotland. *Heart* 2007;**93**(5):606–12.

18. Zoni-Berisso M, Lercari F, Carazza T, & Domenicucci S. Epidemiology of atrial fibrillation: European perspective. *Clin Epidemiol* 2014;**6**:213–20.

19. Kannel W, Wolf P, Benjamin E, & Levy D. Prevalence, incidence, prognosis, and predisposing conditions for atrial fibrillation: population-based estimates. *Am J Cardiol* 1998;**82**(8A):2N–9N.

20. Feinberg WM, Blackshear JL, Laupacis A, Kronmal R, & Hart RG. Prevalence, age distribution, and gender of patients with atrial fibrillation. Analysis and implications. *Arch Int Med* 1995; **155**(5):469–73.

21. Krahn AD, Manfreda J, Tate RB, Mathewson FA, & Cuddy TE. The natural history of atrial fibrillation: incidence, risk factors, and prognosis in the Manitoba follow-up study. *Am J Med* 1995;**98**(5):476–84.

22. Lloyd-Jones DM, Wang TJ, Leip EP, et al. Lifetime risk for development of atrial fibrillation: the Framingham Heart Study. *Circulation* 2004;**110**(9):1042–6.

23. Miyasaka Y1, Barnes ME, Gersh BJ, et al. Secular trends in incidence of atrial fibrillation in Olmsted County, Minnesota, 1980 to 2000, and implications on the projections for future prevalence. *Circulation* 2006;**114**(2):119–25.

24. Colilla S, Crow A, Petkun W, Singer DE, Simon T, & Liu X. Estimates of current and future incidence and prevalence of atrial fibrillation in the U.S. adult population. *Am J Cardiol* 2013;**112**(8):1142–7.

25. Krijthe BP, Kunst A, Benjamin EJ, et al. Projections on the number of individuals with atrial fibrillation in the European Union, from 2000 to 2060. *Eur Heart J* 2013;**34**(35):2746–51.

26. Kannel WB & Benjamin EJ. Current perceptions of the epidemiology of atrial fibrillation. *Cardiol Clini* 2009;**27**(1):13–24.

27. Hirsh BJ, Copeland-Halperin RS, & Halperin JL. Fibrotic atrial cardiomyopathy, atrial fibrillation, and thromboembolism. *J Am Coll Cardiol* 2015;**65**(20):2239–51.

28. Calenda BW, Fuster V, Halperin JL, & Granger CB. Stroke risk assessment in atrial fibrillation: risk factors and markers of atrial myopathy. *Nat Rev Cardiol* 2016;**13**(9):549–59.

29. Vermond RA, Geelhoed B, Verweij N, et al. Incidence of atrial fibrillation and relationship with cardiovascular events, heart failure, and mortality. *J Am Coll Cardiol* 2015;**66**(9):1000–7.

30. **Mathus-Vliegen EM, Basdevant A, Finer N,** et al. Prevalence, pathophysiology, health consequences and treatment options of obesity in the elderly: a guideline. *Obesity Facts* 2012;**5**(3):460–83.

31. **Wild S, Roglic G, Green A, Sicree R, & King H.** Global prevalence of diabetes: estimates for the year 2000 and projections for 2030. *Diabetes Care* 2004;**27**(5):1047–53.

32. **Anderson S, Halter JB, Hazzard WR,** et al. Prediction, progression, and outcomes of chronic kidney disease in older adults. *J Am Soc Nephrol* 2009;**20**(6):1199–209.

33. **Senaratna CV, Perret JL, Lodge CJ,** et al. Prevalence of obstructive sleep apnea in the general population: a systematic review. *Sleep Med Rev* 2016;**34**:70–81.

34. **Krijthe BP, Jong FHD, Hofman A,** et al. Dehydroepiandrosterone sulfate levels and risk of atrial fibrillation: the Rotterdam study. *Eur J Prev Cardiol* 2014;**21**(3):291–8.

35. **Magnani JW, Moser CB, Murabito JM,** et al. Association of sex hormones, aging, and atrial fibrillation in men: the Framingham Heart Study. *Circ Arrhythm Electrophysiol* 2014;**7**(2):307–12.

36. **Mozaffarian D, Furberg CD, Psaty BM, & Siscovick D.** Physical activity and incidence of atrial fibrillation in older adults: the Cardiovascular Health Study. *Circulation* 2008;**118**(8):800–7.

37. **Rienstra M, Mcmanus DD, & Benjamin EJ.** Novel risk factors for atrial fibrillation: useful for risk prediction and clinical decision making? *Circulation* 2012;**125**(20):e941–6.

38. **Schnabel RB, Yin X, Gona P,** et al. 50-year trends in atrial fibrillation prevalence, incidence, risk factors, and mortality in the Framingham Heart Study: a cohort study. *Lancet* 2015;**386**(9989):154–62.

39. **Wagoner DRV, Piccini JP, Albert CM,** et al. Progress toward the prevention and treatment of atrial fibrillation: a summary of the Heart Rhythm Society Research Forum on the Treatment and Prevention of Atrial Fibrillation, Washington, DC, December 9–10, 2013. *Heart Rhythm* 2015;**12**(1):e5–e29.

40. **Wolf PA, Abbott RD, & Kannel WB.** Atrial fibrillation as an independent risk factor for stroke: the Framingham Study. *Stroke* 1991;**22**(8):983–8.

41. **Marinigh R, Lip GY, Fiotti N, Giansante C, & Lane DA.** Age as a risk factor for stroke in atrial fibrillation patients. *J Am Coll Cardiol* 2010;**56**(11):827–37.

42. **Moulton AW, Singer DE, & Haas JS.** Risk factors for stroke in patients with nonrheumatic atrial fibrillation: a case-control study. *Am J Med* 1991;**91**(2):156–61.

43. **Lip GY, Nieuwlaat R, Pisters R, Lane DA, & Crijns HJ.** Refining clinical risk stratification for predicting stroke and thromboembolism in atrial fibrillation using a novel risk factor-based approach. *Chest* 2010;**137**(2):263–72.

44. **Yiin GS, Howard DP, Paul NL,** et al. Age-specific incidence, outcome, cost, and projected future burden of atrial fibrillation–related embolic vascular events. *Circulation* 2014;**130**(15):1236–44.

45. **Paciaroni M, Agnelli G, Caso V,** et al. Atrial fibrillation in patients with first-ever stroke: frequency, antithrombotic treatment before the event and effect on clinical outcome. *J Thromb Haemost* 2005;**3**(6):1218–23.

46. **Steger C, Pratter A, Martinekbregel M,** et al. Stroke patients with atrial fibrillation have a worse prognosis than patients without: data from the Austrian Stroke registry. *Eur Heart J* 2004;**25**(19):1734–40.

47. **Leyden JM, Kleinig TJ, Newbury J,** et al. Adelaide Stroke Incidence Study: declining stroke rates but many preventable cardioembolic strokes. *Stroke* 2013;**44**(5):1226–31.

48. **Mcgrath ER, Kapral MK, Fang J,** et al. Association of atrial fibrillation with mortality and disability after ischemic stroke. *Neurology* 2013;**81**(9):825–32.

49. **Koton S, Schneider ALC, Rosamond WD,** et al. Stroke incidence and mortality trends in US communities, 1987 to 2011. *JAMA* 2014;**312**(3); 259–68.

50. **Marini C, Santis FD, Sacco S,** et al. Contribution of atrial fibrillation to incidence and outcome of ischemic stroke: results from a population-based study. *Stroke* 2005;**36**(6):1115–19.

51. **Kaarisalo MM, Immonen-Räihä P, Marttila RJ,** et al. Atrial fibrillation in older stroke patients: association with recurrence and mortality after first ischemic stroke. *J Am Geriatr Soc* 1997;**45**(11):1297–301.

52. **Lin H-J, Wolf PA, Kelly-Hayes M,** et al. Stroke severity in atrial fibrillation: the Framingham Study. *Stroke* 1996;**27**(10):1760–4.

53. **Gladstone DJ, Bui E, Fang J,** et al. Potentially preventable strokes in high-risk patients with atrial fibrillation who are not adequately anticoagulated. *Stroke* 2008;**40**(1):235–40.

54. **Fang MC, Go AS, Chang Y,** et al. Long-term survival after ischemic stroke in patients with atrial fibrillation. *Neurology* 2014;**82**(12):1033–7.

55. **Miller PS, Andersson FL, & Kalra L.** Are cost benefits of anticoagulation for stroke prevention in atrial fibrillation underestimated? *Stroke* 2005;**36**(2):360–6.

56. **Blackshear JL & Odell JA.** Appendage obliteration to reduce stroke in cardiac surgical patients with atrial fibrillation. *Ann Thorac Surg*1996;**61**(2):755–9.

57. **Watson T, Shantsila E, & Lip GY.** Mechanisms of thrombogenesis in atrial fibrillation: Virchow's triad revisited. *Lancet* 2009;**373**(9658):155–66.

58. **Kamel H, Okin PM, Elkind MS, & Iadecola C.** Atrial fibrillation and mechanisms of stroke. *Stroke* 2016;**47**:895–900.

59. **Cha M-J, Kim YD, Nam HS, Kim J, Lee DH, & Heo JH.** Stroke mechanism in patients with non-valvular atrial fibrillation according to the CHADS2 and CHA2DS2-VASc scores. *Eur J Neurol* 2012;**19**(3):473–9.

60. **Kirchhof P, Benussi S, Kotecha D,** et al. 2016 ESC Guidelines for the management of atrial fibrillation developed in collaboration with EACTS. *Eur Heart J* 2016;**37**(38):2893–962.

61. **Hart RG, Pearce LA, & Aguilar MI.** Meta-analysis: antithrombotic therapy to prevent stroke in patients who have nonvalvular atrial fibrillation. *Ann Int Med* 2007;**146**(12):857–67.

62. **Xian Y, O'Brien EC, Liang L,** et al. Association of preceding antithrombotic treatment with acute ischemic stroke severity and in-hospital outcomes among patients with atrial fibrillation. *JAMA* 2017;**317**(10):1057–67.

63. **Hannon N, Arsava EM, Audebert HJ,** et al. Antithrombotic treatment at onset of stroke with atrial fibrillation, functional outcome, and fatality: a systematic review and meta-analysis. *Int J Stroke* 2015;**10**(6):808–14.

64. **EAFT (European Atrial Fibrillation Trial) Study Group.** Secondary prevention in non-rheumatic atrial fibrillation after transient ischaemic attack or minor stroke. *Lancet* 1993;**342**(8882):1255–62.

65. **Andersen KK & Olsen TS.** Reduced poststroke mortality in patients with stroke and atrial fibrillation treated with anticoagulants: results from a danish quality-control registry of 22 179 patients with ischemic stroke. *Stroke* 2006;**38**(2):259–63.

66. **Paciaroni M, Agnelli G, Ageno W, & Caso V.** Timing of anticoagulation therapy in patients with acute ischaemic stroke and atrial fibrillation. *Thromb Haemost* 2016;**116**(3):410–16.

67. **Ruff CT, Giugliano RP, Braunwald E,** et al. Comparison of the efficacy and safety of new oral anticoagulants with warfarin in patients with atrial fibrillation: a meta-analysis of randomised trials. *Lancet* 2014;**383**(9921):955–62.

68. **Wolff A, Shantsila E, Lip GYH, & Lane DA.** Impact of advanced age on management and prognosis in atrial fibrillation: insights from a population-based study in general practice. *Age Ageing* 2015;**44**(5):874–8.

69. **Ng KH, Shestakovska O, Connolly SJ,** et al. Efficacy and safety of apixaban compared with aspirin in the elderly: a subgroup analysis from the AVERROES trial. *Age Ageing* 2015;**45**(1):77–83.

70. **Freedman SB, Gersh BJ, & Lip GYH.** Misperceptions of aspirin efficacy and safety may perpetuate anticoagulant underutilization in atrial fibrillation. *Eur Heart J* 2014;**36**(11):653–6.

71. **Mant J, Hobbs FR, Fletcher K,** et al. Warfarin versus aspirin for stroke prevention in an elderly community population with atrial fibrillation (the Birmingham Atrial Fibrillation Treatment of the Aged Study, BAFTA): a randomised controlled trial. *Lancet* 2007;**370**(9586):493–503.

72. **Rash A, Downes T, Portner R, Yeo WW, Morgan N, & Channer KS.** A randomised controlled trial of warfarin versus aspirin for stroke prevention in octogenarians with atrial fibrillation (WASPO). *Age Ageing* 2007;**36**(2):151–6.

73. Baigent C, Blackwell L, Collins R, et al. Aspirin in the primary and secondary prevention of vascular disease: collaborative meta-analysis of individual participant data from randomised trials. *Lancet* 2009;**373**(9678):1849–60.

74. Garcia Rodríguez LA, Martín-Pérez M, Hennekens CH, Rothwell PM, & Lanas A. Bleeding risk with long-term low-dose aspirin: a systematic review of observational studies. *Plos One* 2016;**11**(8):e0160046.

75. Go AS, Hylek EM, Chang Y, et al. Anticoagulation therapy for stroke prevention in atrial fibrillation: how well do randomized trials translate into clinical practice? *JAMA* 2003;**290**(20): 2685–92.

76. Melkonian M, Jarzebowski W, Pautas E, Siguret V, Belmin J, & Lafuente-Lafuente C. Bleeding risk of antiplatelet drugs compared with oral anticoagulants in older patients with atrial fibrillation: a systematic review and meta-analysis. *J Thromb Haemost* 2017;**15**(7):1500–10.

77. van Walraven C, Hart RG, Connolly S, et al. Effect of age on stroke prevention therapy in patients with atrial fibrillation. The Atrial Fibrillation Investigators. *Stroke* 2009;**40**:1410–16.

78. Singer DE. The Net Clinical Benefit of Warfarin Anticoagulation in Atrial Fibrillation. *Ann Int Med* 2009;**151**(5):297–305.

79. Stroke Guidelines. RCP London. 2017. Available from: https://www.rcplondon.ac.uk/guidelines-policy/stroke-guidelines [Accessed: 20 April 2017].

80. January CT, Wann LS, Alpert JS, et al. 2014 AHA/ACC/HRS guideline for the management of patients with atrial fibrillation: executive summary: a report of the American College of Cardiology/American Heart Association Task Force on practice guidelines and the Heart Rhythm Society. *Circulation* 2014;**130**(23):2071–104.

81. Fang MC, Chang Y, Hylek EM, et al. Advanced age, anticoagulation intensity, and risk for intracranial hemorrhage among patients taking warfarin for atrial fibrillation. *Ann Int Med* 2004;**141**(10):745–52.

82. Björck F, Renlund H, Lip GYH, Wester P, Svensson PJ, & Själander A. Outcomes in a warfarin-treated population with atrial fibrillation. *JAMA Cardiol* 2016;**1**(2):172–80.

83. Lehto M, Niiranen J, Korhonen P, et al. Quality of warfarin therapy and risk of stroke, bleeding, and mortality among patients with atrial fibrillation: results from the nationwide FinWAF Registry. *Pharmacoepidemiol Drug Saf* 2017;**26**(6):657–65.

84. De Caterina R, Husted S, Wallentin L, et al. Vitamin K antagonists in heart disease: current status and perspectives (Section III). *Thromb Haemost* 2013;**110**(6):1087–107.

85. Pokorney SD, Simon DN, Thomas L, et al. Patients' time in therapeutic range on warfarin among US patients with atrial fibrillation: results from ORBIT-AF registry. *Am Heart J* 2015;**170**(1):141–8.

86. Razouki Z, Ozonoff A, Zhao S, & Rose AJ. Pathways to poor anticoagulation control. *J Thromb Haemost* 2014;**12**(5):628–34.

87. Apostolakis S, Sullivan RM, Olshansky B, & Lip GY. Factors affecting quality of anticoagulation control among patients with atrial fibrillation on warfarin: the SAMe-TT(2)R(2) score. *Chest* 2013;**144**:1555–63.

88. National Clinical Guideline Centre (UK). *Atrial Fibrillation: The Management of Atrial Fibrillation*. London, UK: National Institute for Health and Care Excellence (UK), 2014.

89. Lip GY, Haguenoer K, Saint-Etienne C, & Fauchier L. Relationship of the SAMe-TT2R2 score to poor-quality anticoagulation, stroke, clinically relevant bleeding, and mortality in patients with atrial fibrillation. *Chest* 2014;**146**:719–26.

90. Fauchier L, Angoulvant D, & Lip GYH. The SAMe-TT2R2 score and quality of anticoagulation in atrial fibrillation: a simple aid to decision-making on who is suitable (or not) for vitamin K antagonists. *Europace* 2015;**17**(5):671–3.

91. Potpara TS & Lip GYH. Post approval observational studies of non–vitamin K antagonist oral anticoagulants in atrial fibrillation. *JAMA* 2017;**317**(11):1115.

92. Larsen TB, Skjøth F, Nielsen PB, Kjældgaard JN, & Lip GYH. Comparative effectiveness and safety of non-vitamin K antagonist oral anticoagulants and warfarin in patients with atrial fibrillation: propensity weighted nationwide cohort study. *BMJ* 2016;**353**:i3189.

93. Nielsen PBCB, Skjøth F, Søgaard M, Kjældgaard JN, Lip GYH, & Larsen TB. Effectiveness and safety of reduced dose non-vitamin K antagonist oral anticoagulants and warfarin in patients with atrial fibrillation: propensity weighted nationwide cohort study. *BMJ* 2017;**356**:j510.

94. Diener H-C, Aisenberg J, Ansell J, et al. Choosing a particular oral anticoagulant and dose for stroke prevention in individual patients with non-valvular atrial fibrillation: part 2. *Eur Heart J* 2017;**38**(12):860–8.

95. Sharma M, Cornelius VR, Patel JP, Davies JG, & Molokhia M. Efficacy and harms of direct oral anticoagulants in the elderly for stroke prevention in atrial fibrillation and secondary prevention of venous thromboembolism. *Circulation* 2015;**132**(3):194–204.

96. Sadlon AH & Tsakiris DA. Direct oral anticoagulants in the elderly: systematic review and meta-analysis of evidence, current and future directions. *Swiss Medical Weekly* 2016;**146**:w14356.

97. Khan F, Huang H, & Datta YH. Direct oral anticoagulant use and the incidence of bleeding in the very elderly with atrial fibrillation. *J Thromb Thrombolysis* 2016;**42**(4):573–8.

98. Hart RG, Eikelboom JW, Brimble KS, McMurtry MS, & Ingram AJ. Stroke prevention in atrial fibrillation patients with chronic kidney disease. *Canad J Cardiol* 2013;**29**(7 Suppl):S71–8.

99. Cerasuolo JO, Montero-Odasso M, Ibañez A, Doocy S, Lip GY, & Sposato LA. Decision-making interventions to stop the global atrial fibrillation-related stroke tsunami. *Int J Stroke* 2017;**12**(3):222–8.

100. Dzeshka S & Lip GYH. Stroke and bleeding risk assessment: where are we now? *J Atrial Fibrillation* 2014;**6**(6):1042.

101. Chen JY, Zhang AD, Lu HY, Guo J, Wang FF, & Li ZC. CHADS$_2$ versus CHA$_2$DS$_2$-VASc score in assessing the stroke and thromboembolism risk stratification in patients with atrial fibrillation: a systematic review and meta-analysis. *J Geriatr Cardiol* 2013;**10**(3):258–66.

102. Potpara TS, Dagres N, Mujović N, et al. Decision-making in clinical practice: oral anticoagulant therapy in patients with non-valvular atrial fibrillation and a single additional stroke risk factor. *Adv Ther* 2017;**34**(2):357–77.

103. Eckman MH, Singer DE, Rosand J, & Greenberg SM. Moving the tipping point: the decision to anticoagulate patients with atrial fibrillation. *Circ Cardiovasc Qual Outcomes* 2010;**4**(1):14–21.

104. Lip GY, Nielsen PB. Should Patients with atrial fibrillation and 1 stroke risk factor (CHA$_2$DS$_2$-VASc score 1 in men, 2 in women) be anticoagulated?. *Circulation* 2016;**133**(15):1498–503.

105. Huang D, Anguo L, Yue W-S, Yin L, Tse H-F, & Siu C-W. Refinement of ischemic stroke risk in patients with atrial fibrillation and CHA$_2$DS$_2$-VASc score of 1. *Pacing Clin Electrophysiol* 2014;**37**(11):1442–7.

106. Lip GY, Skjøth F, Rasmussen LH, & Larsen TB. Oral anticoagulation, aspirin, or no therapy in patients with nonvalvular AF with 0 or 1 stroke risk factor based on the CHA$_2$DS$_2$-VASc score. *J Am Coll Cardiol* 2015;**65**(14):1385–94.

107. Chao T-F, Wang K-L, Liu C-J, et al. Age threshold for increased stroke risk among patients with atrial fibrillation. *J Am Coll Cardiol* 2015;**66**(12):1339–47.

108. Pisters R, Lane DA, Nieuwlaat R, Vos CBD, Crijns HJ, & Lip GY. A novel user-friendly score (HAS-BLED) to assess 1-year risk of major bleeding in patients with atrial fibrillation. *Chest.* 2010;**138**(5):1093–1100.

109. Hijazi Z, Lindbäck J, Alexander JH, al. The ABC (age, biomarkers, clinical history) stroke risk score: a biomarker-based risk score for predicting stroke in atrial fibrillation. *Eur Heart J* 2016;**37**(20):1582–90.

110. Hijazi Z, Oldgren J, Lindbäck J, et al. The novel biomarker-based ABC (age, biomarkers, clinical history)-bleeding risk score for patients with atrial fibrillation: a derivation and validation study. *Lancet* 2016;**387**(10035):2302–11.

111. Angelozzi A, Renda G, Mercuri M, & De Caterina R. *The Risk of Intracranial Hemorrhage with Anticoagulation in the Elderly—Estimates of Prevalence and Therapeutic Strategies.* Available from: http://www.acc.org/latest-in-cardiology/articles/2015/12/21/12/59/the-risk-of-intracranial-hemorrhage-with-anticoagulation-in-the-elderly [Accessed: 20 April 2017].

112. **Friberg L, Rosenqvist M, & Lip GYH.** Net clinical benefit of warfarin in patients with atrial fibrillation: a report from the Swedish Atrial Fibrillation Cohort Study. *Circulation* 2012;**125**(19):2298–307.

113. **Lip GYH, Clementy N, Pericart L, Banerjee A, & Fauchier L.** Stroke and major bleeding risk in elderly patients aged >=75 years with atrial fibrillation: the Loire Valley Atrial Fibrillation Project. *Stroke* 2014;**46**(1):143–50.

114. **Lamassa M, Di Carlo A, Pracucci G, et al.** Characteristics, outcome, and care of stroke associated with atrial fibrillation in Europe: data from a multicenter multinational hospital-based registry (The European Community Stroke Project). *Stroke* 2001;**32**:392–8.

115. **Mcgrath ER, Go AS, Chang Y, et al.** Use of oral anticoagulant therapy in older adults with atrial fibrillation after acute ischemic stroke. *J Am Geriatr Soc* 2016;**65**(2):241–8.

116. **Holt TA, Hunter TD, Gunnarsson C, Khan N, Cload P, & Lip GY.** Risk of stroke and oral anticoagulant use in atrial fibrillation: a cross-sectional survey. *Br J Gen Pract* 2012;**62**(603):710–17.

117. **Shantsila E, Wolff A, Lip GYH, Lane DA.** Optimising stroke prevention in patients with atrial fibrillation: application of the GRASP-AF audit tool in a UK general practice cohort. *Br J Gen Pract* 2015;**65**(630):e16–23.

118. **Huisman MV, Rothman KJ, Paquette M, et al.;** GLORIA-AF investigators the changing landscape for stroke prevention in AF: findings from the GLORIA-AF registry phase 2. *J Am Coll Cardiol* 2017;**69**(7):777–85.

119. **Kakkar AK, Mueller I, Bassand J-P, et al.** Risk profiles and antithrombotic treatment of patients newly diagnosed with atrial fibrillation at risk of stroke: perspectives from the international, observational, prospective GARFIELD registry. *PLoS One* 2013;**8**(5):e63479.

120. **Hsu JC, Maddox TM, Kennedy K, et al.** Aspirin instead of oral anticoagulant prescription in atrial fibrillation patients at risk for stroke. *J Am Coll Cardiol* 2016;**67**(25):2913–23.

121. **Buck J, Kaboli P, Gage BF, Cram P, & Sarrazin MSV.** Trends in antithrombotic therapy for atrial fibrillation: data from the Veterans Health Administration Health System. *Am Heart J* 2016;**179**:186–91.

122. **Scowcroft ACE, Lee S, & Mant J.** Thromboprophylaxis of elderly patients with AF in the UK: an analysis using the General Practice Research Database (GPRD) 2000–2009. *Heart* 2012;**99**(2):127–32.

123. **Cowan C, Healicon R, Robson I, et al.** The use of anticoagulants in the management of atrial fibrillation among general practices in England. *Heart* 2013;**99**(16):1166–72.

124. **Induruwa I, Evans NR, Aziz A, Reddy S, Khadjooi K, & Romero-Ortuno R.** Clinical frailty is independently associated with non-prescription of anticoagulants in older patients with atrial fibrillation. *Geriatr Gerontol Int* 2017;**17**(11):2178–83.

125. **Pilotto A, Gallina P, Copetti M, et al.** Warfarin treatment and all-cause mortality in community-dwelling older adults with atrial fibrillation: a retrospective observational study. *J Am Geriatr Soc* 2016;**64**(7):1416–24.

126. **O'Caoimh R, Igras E, Ramesh A, Power B, O'Connor K, & Liston R.** Assessing the appropriateness of oral anticoagulation for atrial fibrillation in advanced frailty: use of stroke and bleeding risk-prediction models. *J Frailty Ageing* 2017;**6**(1):46–52.

127. **Neidecker M, Patel AA, Nelson WW, & Reardon G.** Use of warfarin in long-term care: a systematic review. *BMC Geriatr* 2012;**12**:14.

128. **Kernan WN, Ovbiagele B, Black HR, et al.** Guidelines for the prevention of stroke in patients with stroke and transient ischemic attack: a guideline for healthcare professionals from the American Heart Association/American Stroke Association. *Stroke* 2014;**45**(7):2160–236.

129. **Hart RG, Diener HC, Coutts SB, et al.; Cryptogenic Stroke/ESUS International Working Group.** Embolic strokes of undetermined source: the case for a new clinical construct. *Lancet Neurol* 2014;**13**:429–38.

130. **Demeestere J, Fieuws S, Lansberg MG, & Lemmens R.** Detection of atrial fibrillation among patients with stroke due to large or small vessel disease: a meta-analysis. *J Am Heart Assoc* 2016;**5**(9):pii: e004151.

131. **Brachmann J, Morillo CA, Sanna T, et al.** Uncovering atrial fibrillation beyond short-term monitoring in cryptogenic stroke patients: three-year results from the cryptogenic stroke and underlying atrial fibrillation trial. *Circ Arrhythm Electrophysiol* 2016;**9**(1):e003333.

132. **Gladstone DJ, Spring M, Dorian P, et al.** Atrial fibrillation in patients with cryptogenic stroke. *N Engl J Med* 2014;**370**(26):2467–77.

133. **Sposato LA, Cipriano LE, Saposnik G, Vargas ER, Riccio PM, & Hachinski V.** Diagnosis of atrial fibrillation after stroke and transient ischaemic attack: a systematic review and meta-analysis. *Lancet Neurol* 2015;**14**(4):377–87.

134. **Lip GYH, Hunter TD, Quiroz ME, Ziegler PD, & Turakhia MP.** Atrial fibrillation diagnosis timing, ambulatory ECG monitoring utilization, and risk of recurrent stroke. *Circ Cardiovasc Qual Outcomes* 2017;**10**(1):e002864.

135. **Cerasuolo JO, Cipriano LE, & Sposato LA.** The complexity of atrial fibrillation newly diagnosed after ischemic stroke and transient ischemic attack. *Curr Opin Neurol* 2017;**30**(1):28–37.

136. **Fauchier L, Clementy N, Pelade C, Collignon C, Nicolle E, & Lip GY.** Patients with ischemic stroke and incident atrial fibrillation. *Stroke* 2015;**46**(9):2432–7.

137. **Favilla CG, Ingala E, Jara J, et al.** Predictors of finding occult atrial fibrillation after cryptogenic stroke. *Stroke* 2015;**46**(5):1210–15.

138. **Edwards JD, Kapral MK, Fang J, Saposnik G, & Gladstone DJ.** Underutilization of ambulatory ECG monitoring after stroke and transient ischemic attack. *Stroke* 2016;**47**(8):1982–9.

139. **Healey JS & Sandhu RK.** Are we ready for mass screening to detect atrial fibrillation? *Circulation* 2015;**131**(25):2167–8.

140. **Sandhu RK, Dolovich L, Deif B, et al.** High prevalence of modifiable stroke risk factors identified in a pharmacy-based screening programme. *Open Heart* 2016;**3**(2):e000515.

141. **Lowres N, Neubeck L, Salkeld G, et al.** Feasibility and cost-effectiveness of stroke prevention through community screening for atrial fibrillation using iPhone ECG in pharmacies: the SEARCH-AF study. *Thromb Haemost* 2014;**111**:1167–76.

142. **Svennberg E, Engdahl J, Al-Khalili F, Friberg L, Frykman V, & Rosenqvist M.** Mass screening for untreated atrial fibrillation: the STROKESTOP study. *Circulation* 2015;**131**:2176.

143. **Engdahl J, Andersson L, Mirskaya M, & Rosenqvist M.** Stepwise screening of atrial fibrillation in a 75-year-old population: implications for stroke prevention. *Circulation* 2013;**127**(8):930–7.

144. **Fitzmaurice DA, Hobbs FDR, Jowett S, et al.** Screening versus routine practice in detection of atrial fibrillation in patients aged 65 or over: cluster randomised controlled trial. *BMJ* 2007;**335**(7616):383.

145. **Holmes DR & Reddy VY.** Left atrial appendage and closure: who, when, and how: cardiovascular interventions. *Circ Cardiovasc Interv* 2016;**9**(5):e002942.

146. **Holmes DR, Doshi SK, Kar S, et al.** Left atrial appendage closure as an alternative to warfarin for stroke prevention in atrial fibrillation. *J Am Coll Cardiol* 2015;**65**(24):2614–23.

147. **Lane DA & Lip GYH.** Atrial fibrillation: stroke prevention in atrial fibrillation: can we do better? *Nat Rev Cardiol* 2016;**13**(9):511–12.

148. **Lane DA & Lip GYH.** Patient's values and preferences for stroke prevention in atrial fibrillation: balancing stroke and bleeding risk with oral anticoagulation. *Thromb Haemost* 2014;**111**(3):381–3.

149. **Jacobs LG.** Warfarin pharmacology, clinical management, and evaluation of hemorrhagic risk for the elderly. *Cardiol Clin* 2008;**26**(2):157–67.

150. **Desai Y, El-Chami MF, Leon AR, & Merchant FM.** Management of atrial fibrillation in elderly adults. *J Am Geriatr Soc* 2017;**65**(1):185–93.

151. Maes F, Dalleur O, Henrard S, et al. Risk scores and geriatric profile: can they really help us in anticoagulation decision making among older patients suffering from atrial fibrillation? *Clin Interv Aging* 2014;9;1091–9.

152. Pugh D, Pugh J, & Mead GE. Attitudes of physicians regarding anticoagulation for atrial fibrillation: a systematic review. *Age Ageing* 2011;40(6):675–83.

153. Brophy MT, Snyder KE, Gaehde S, Ives C, Gagnon D, & Fiore LD. Anticoagulant use for atrial fibrillation in the elderly. *J Am Geriatr Soc* 2004;52(7):1151–6.

154. Hylek EM, Evans-Molina C, Shea C, Henault LE, & Regan S. Major hemorrhage and tolerability of warfarin in the first year of therapy among elderly patients with atrial fibrillation. *Circulation* 2007;115(21):2689–96.

155. Sebastian JL & Tresch DD. Use of oral anticoagulants in older patients. *Drugs Aging* 2000;16(6):409–35.

156. Andreotti F, Rocca B, Husted S, et al. Antithrombotic therapy in the elderly: expert position paper of the European Society of Cardiology Working Group on Thrombosis. *Eur Heart J* 2015; 36(46):3238–49.

157. Hylek EM, D'Antonio J, Evans-Molina C, Shea C, Henault LE, & Regan S. Translating the results of randomized trials into clinical practice: the challenge of warfarin candidacy among hospitalized elderly patients with atrial fibrillation. *Stroke* 2006;37(4):1075–80.

158. Frain B, Castelino R, & Bereznicki LR. The utilization of antithrombotic therapy in older patients in aged care facilities with atrial fibrillation. *Clin Appl Thromb Hemost* 2018:24(3):519–24.

159. Zarraga IGE & Kron J. Oral anticoagulation in elderly adults with atrial fibrillation: integrating new options with old concepts. *J Am Geriatr Soc* 2013;61(1):143–50.

160. Fitzgerald JL & Howes I.G. Drug interactions of direct-acting oral anticoagulants. *Drug Safety* 2016;39(9):841–5.

161. Olesen JB, Lip GY, Kamper AL, et al. Stroke and bleeding in atrial fibrillation with chronic kidney disease. *N Engl J Med* 2012;367():625–35.

162. Pennlert J, Overholser R, Asplund K, et al. Optimal timing of anticoagulant treatment after intracerebral hemorrhage in patients with atrial fibrillation. *Stroke* 2016;48(2):314–20.

163. Blodgett J, Theou O, Kirkland S, Andreou P, & Rockwood K. Frailty in NHANES: comparing the frailty index and phenotype. *Arch Gerontol Geriatr* 2015;60(3):464–70.

164. Bergman H, Ferrucci L, Guralnik J, et al. Frailty: an emerging research and clinical paradigm—issues and controversies. *J Gerontol Series A Biol Sci Med Sci* 2007;62(7):731–7.

165. Heckman GA & Braceland B. Integrating frailty assessment into cardiovascular decision making. *Canad J Cardiol* 2016;32(2):139–41.

166. Lefebvre M-CD, St-Onge M, Glazer-Cavanagh M, et al. The effect of bleeding risk and frailty status on anticoagulation patterns in octogenarians with atrial fibrillation: the FRAIL-AF study. *Canad J Cardiol* 2016;32(2):169–76.

167. Granziera S, Cohen AT, Nante G, Manzato E, & Sergi G. Thromboembolic prevention in frail elderly patients with atrial fibrillation: a practical algorithm. *J Am Med Dir Assoc* 2015;16(5):358–64.

168. Ashburner JM, Go AS, Chang Y, et al. Influence of competing risks on estimating the expected benefit of warfarin in individuals with atrial fibrillation not currently taking anticoagulants: the anticoagulation and risk factors in atrial fibrillation study. *J Am Geriatr Soc* 2017;65(1):35–41.

169. Murphy TE & Chaudhry SI. Benefit of warfarin in older persons with atrial fibrillation. *J Am Geriatr Soc* 2017;65(1):25–6.

170. Sellers MB & Newby LK. Atrial fibrillation, anticoagulation, fall risk, and outcomes in elderly patients. *Am Heart J* 2011;161(2):241–6.

171. Steffel J, Giugliano RP, Braunwald E, et al. Edoxaban versus warfarin in atrial fibrillation patients at risk of falling. *J Am Coll Cardiol* 2016;68(11):1169–78.

172. Inui TS, Parina R, Chang DC, Inui TS, & Coimbra R. Mortality after ground-level fall in the elderly patient taking oral anticoagulation for atrial fibrillation/flutter: a long-term analysis of risk versus benefit. *J Trauma Acute Care Surg* 2014;**76**(3):642–9.

173. Collins CE, Witkowski ER, Flahive JM, Anderson FA, & Santry HP. Effect of preinjury warfarin use on outcomes after head trauma in Medicare beneficiaries. *Am J Surg* 2014;**208**(4).

174. Banerjee A, Clementy N, Haguenoer K, Fauchier L, & Lip GY. Prior history of falls and risk of outcomes in atrial fibrillation: the Loire Valley Atrial Fibrillation Project. *Am J Med* 2014;**127**(10):972–8.

175. Gage BF, Birman-Deych E, Kerzner R, Radford MJ, Nilasena DS, & Rich MW. Incidence of intracranial hemorrhage in patients with atrial fibrillation who are prone to fall. *Am J Med* 2005;**118**(6):612–17.

176. Hylek EM & Ko D. Atrial fibrillation and fall risk. *J Am Coll Cardiol* 2016;**68**(11):1179–80.

177. Donzé J, Clair C, Hug B, et al. Risk of falls and major bleeds in patients on oral anticoagulation therapy. *Am J Med* 2012;**125**(8):773–8.

178. Man-Son-Hing M, Nichol G, Lau A, et al. Choosing antithrombotic therapy for elderly patients with atrial fibrillation who are at risk for falls. *Arch Intern Med* 1999;**159**:677–85.

179. Gallagher AM, Rietbrock S, Plumb J, & Staa TPV. Initiation and persistence of warfarin or aspirin in patients with chronic atrial fibrillation in general practice: do the appropriate patients receive stroke prophylaxis? *J Thromb Haemost* 2008;**6**(9):1500–6.

180. Björck F, Ek A, Johansson L, & Själander A. Warfarin persistence among atrial fibrillation patients—why is treatment ended? *Cardiovasc Ther* 2016;**34**(6):468–74.

181. Yao X, Abraham NS, Alexander GC, et al. Effect of adherence to oral anticoagulants on risk of stroke and major bleeding among patients with atrial fibrillation. *J Am Heart Assoc* 2016;**5**(2);pii: e003074.

182. Spivey CA, Liu X, Qiao Y, et al. Stroke associated with discontinuation of warfarin therapy for atrial fibrillation. *Curr Med Res Opin* 2015;**31**(11):2021–9.

183. O'Brien EC, Holmes DN, Ansell JE, et al. Physician practices regarding contraindications to oral anticoagulation in atrial fibrillation: findings from the outcomes registry for better informed treatment of atrial fibrillation (ORBIT-AF) registry. *Am Heart J* 2014;**167**(4);601–9.

184. Steinberg BA, Greiner MA, Hammill BG, et al. Contraindications to anticoagulation therapy and eligibility for novel anticoagulants in older patients with atrial fibrillation. *Cardiovasc Ther* 2015;**33**(4):177–83.

185. Paasche-Orlow MK, Parker RM, Gazmararian JA, Nielsen-Bohlman LT, & Rudd RR. The prevalence of limited health literacy. *J Gen Int Med* 2005: **20**(2):175–84.

186. Fang MC, Machtinger EL, Wang F, & Schillinger D. Health literacy and anticoagulation-related outcomes among patients taking warfarin. *J Gen Int Med* 2006;**21**(8):841–6.

187. Borg Xuereb C, Shaw RL, & Lane DA. Patients' and health professionals' views and experiences of atrial fibrillation and oral-anticoagulant therapy: a qualitative meta-synthesis. *Patient Educ Couns* 2012;**88**(2):330–7.

188. Gellad WF, Grenard JL, & Marcum ZA. A systematic review of barriers to medication adherence in the elderly: looking beyond cost and regimen complexity. *Am J Geriatr Pharmacother* 2011;**9**(1):11–23.

189. Yap AF, Thirumoorthy T, & Kwan YH. Systematic review of the barriers affecting medication adherence in older adults. *Geriatr Gerontol Int* 2015;**16**(10):1093–101.

190. Plassman BL, Langa KM, Fisher GG, et al. Prevalence of dementia in the United States: the aging, demographics, and memory study. *Neuroepidemiology* 2007;**29**:125–32.

191. Deelen BA, Van Den Bemt PM, Egberts TC, Van 't Hoff A, & Maas HA. Cognitive impairment as determinant for sub-optimal control of oral anticoagulation treatment in elderly patients with atrial fibrillation. *Drugs Aging* 2005;**22**(4):353–60.

192. Wilke T, Bauer S, Mueller S, Kohlmann T, & Bauersachs R. Patient preferences for oral anticoagulation therapy in atrial fibrillation: a systematic literature review. *Patient* 2016;**10**(1):17–37.

193. **Lip G, Agnelli G, Thach A, Knight E, Rost D, & Tangelder M.** Oral anticoagulation in atrial fibrillation: a pan-European patient survey. *Eur J Int Med* 2007;**18**(3):202–8.

194. **Edwards NT, Greanya ED, Kuo IF, Loewen PS, & Culley CL.** Patient preferences regarding atrial fibrillation stroke prophylaxis in patients at potential risk of atrial fibrillation. *Int J Clin Pharmacy* 2017;**39**(2):468–72.

195. **Wang Y, Xie F, Kong MC, Lee LH, Ng HJ, & Ko Y.** Patient-reported health preferences of anticoagulant-related outcomes. *J Thromb Thrombolysis* 2015;**40**(3):268–73.

196. **Loewen PS, Ji AT, Kapanen A, & Mcclean A.** Patient values and preferences for antithrombotic therapy in atrial fibrillation. *Thromb Haemost* 2017;**117**(6):1007–22.

197. **Alonso-Coello P, Montori VM, Díaz MG, et al.** Values and preferences for oral antithrombotic therapy in patients with atrial fibrillation: physician and patient perspectives. *Health Expect* 2014;**18**(6):2318–27.

198. **Man-Son-Hing M.** Preference-based antithrombotic therapy in atrial fibrillation: implications for clinical decision making. *Med Decis Making* 2005;**25**(5):548–59.

199. **Hijazi M, Aljohani S, Alqahtani F, et al.** Perception of the risk of stroke and the risks and benefits of oral anticoagulation for stroke prevention in patients with atrial fibrillation: a cross-sectional study. *Mayo Clin Proc* 2019;**94**(6):1015–23.

200. **Lane D.** Anti-thrombotic therapy for atrial fibrillation and patients' preferences for treatment. *Age Ageing* 2005;**34**(1):1–3.

Chapter 9

Early management of acute ischaemic stroke

Paul Guyler

Introduction

What is an acute ischaemic stroke?

An ischaemic stroke is a stroke that occurs when a blood clot (or rarely a piece of other debris, such as fat) narrows or blocks a blood vessel so that the blood cannot reach a particular area of the brain. This clot may form inside the blood vessel itself (thrombosis) or may form in the heart or on a damaged carotid artery and travel from its origin via the blood stream (embolus) until it is forced into a smaller artery, thus obstructing blood flow (see example in Fig. 9.1). Brain cells which normally receive blood by the way of this blocked blood vessel are starved of the oxygen and glucose that they require for cellular metabolism and unless the blood flow is restored, they permanently die. The signs and symptoms of a stroke vary from person to person, depending on which part of the brain is affected and the extent of damage. A stroke is said to be 'acute' if the symptoms appear very suddenly, as opposed to 'chronic' symptoms which last or progress over a long period of time.

Sometimes the artery will unblock (recanalize) spontaneously if the clot breaks up or dissolves, but this is uncertain and does not always occur, or occur before permanent damage has been done. There are two main techniques that can be used to unblock the obstructed artery: intra-venous thrombolysis and endovascular mechanical thrombectomy. The aim of both of these techniques is to break down or remove the blockage and to re-establish the blood flow before the lack of oxygen irreversibly damages the brain neurones. The clinical results of such interventions are that people may make a better physical recovery from their stroke. The effect of treatment is time-dependent; earlier treatment may reopen an occluded vessel more quickly and save more brain, and hence increases the probability of a favourable outcome (a patient being 'cured' of his symptoms or reducing the disability caused by the stroke).

Fig. 9.2 endeavours to explain this further. A clot has blocked an artery in our patient and the ischaemic area in light blue (the 'penumbra') is at threat. If the artery were able to be unblocked after 1 minute, all of the penumbral area would be saved with no injury, and our patient would suffer no disabling symptoms. However, over time, more and more of this penumbra is irrevers-ibly damaged (the 'core' infarct), and even if blood flow is restored at this point, the core area of brain will not be saved and its function permanently lost.

Ischaemic brain will produce symptoms but if treated quickly this brain can be salvaged (before progressing to permanent brain damage) although *infarcted* brain is dead and cannot be saved.

Typically, 1.9 million neurons are lost for each minute that brain remains ischaemic. Therefore, for either intravenous thrombolysis or endovascular mechanical thrombectomy, rapid treatment is essential. In reducing time to treatment, we are literally saving brain.

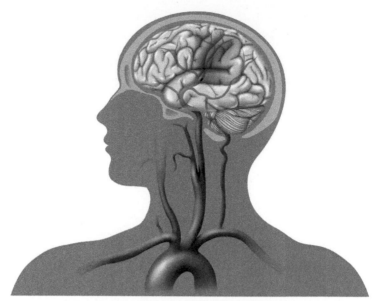

Fig. 9.1 Acute ischaemic stroke: a clot from atheromatous carotid artery in the neck has embolized into a cerebral artery and occluded the blood vessel. The area of brain shaded in blue is starved of oxygen and will die unless blood flow can be restored, causing major permanent brain damage.
JACOPIN/BSIP/age fotostock.

The most commonly used method to unblock (revascularize) the blood vessel is treatment with a clot-dissolving drug to break down the blood clot (thrombus). This intravenous treatment is commonly known as 'thrombolysis'. The administration of thrombolysis can happen very quickly, but thrombolysis is less effective on large clots and may have no effect at all in debris of occluding the vessel which is made up of non-clot material. Thrombolytic drugs can also cause serious

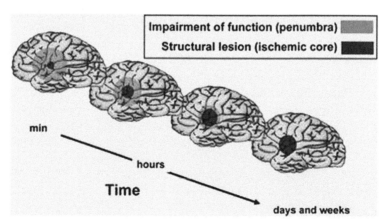

Fig. 9.2 Ischaemic core and penumbra.

Reproduced from Mergenthaler P, Dirnagl U, Kunz A, Ischemic Stroke: Basic Pathophysiology and Clinical Implication. In: Pfaff DW [ed], *Neuroscience in the 21st Century*, pp. 2543–63, Copyright (2013), with permission from Springer Science Business Media, LLC.

bleeding in the brain (intracranial haemorrhage), which can be fatal. Before thrombolysis can be administered, urgent brain imaging (usually a computed tomography (CT) scan) is required to exclude a haemorrhagic stroke (a stroke caused by a bleed rather than a clot), as it is not possible to do this by clinical examination alone. Thrombolysis given to a person with a stroke caused by haemorrhage rather than a clot would likely have fatal results.

Endovascular mechanical thrombectomy requires an interventional specialist to pass a special wire and catheter up inside the arteries to the clot, and use a device to remove the clot. A stent retriever can trap the clot or other material and physically remove this out from the body, or an aspiration catheter can 'suck' out the clot similar to a vacuum cleaner. This requires the patient to remain very still and often necessitates the patient to be sedated or have a general anaesthetic. Usually the arterial system is accessed via the femoral artery in the groin and the wire passed up the aorta, into the carotid or vertebral arteries in the neck and then to the clot in the cerebral arteries. This procedure is more difficult to organize, requiring the patient to be in a specialized catheter laboratory with a consultant interventional radiologist and anaesthetist, so it takes longer to happen than intravenous thrombolysis. However, it is more effective on removing larger clots, or other debris, which thrombolysis would not break down. Also, it can be performed if, for whatever reason, intravenous thrombolysis is contraindicated (such as if the patient has recently had an operation, or has a problem with active bleeding).

Stroke medicine is swiftly evolving with new evidence from specialist research

Over the last 20 years, there have been major evidence-based changes in the immediate hyperacute treatment of acute ischaemic stroke.

Stroke medicine changed for ever with clinical trials of thrombolytic agents and subsequent licensing of the fibrinolytic drug named Alteplase—Recombinant Tissue Plasminogen Activator (rt-PA). Alteplase is produced by a recombinant DNA technique using a Chinese hamster ovary cell-line. Intravenous thrombolysis was slow to be introduced as a mainstream stroke treatment in the United Kingdom; in 2006 fewer than 1% of patients with acute ischaemic stroke received treatment with clot-busting drugs.

As a result, in 2007, a national stroke strategy was developed by the Department of Health[1] which required major reconfiguration of stroke services. Patients were to be transferred to the closest specialist hyperacute stroke centre to receive rapid brain imaging, and, where indicated, urgent interventions such as intravenous thrombolytic therapy. However, when alteplase was licensed for use in acute ischaemic stroke in April 2003 in the United Kingdom, this licence listed any patient over the age of 80 years as a contraindication to treatment. By definition, this contraindication inevitably ensured that many elderly patients were not treated with rt-PA, although in many experienced stroke centres elderly patients were treated with alteplase regardless of this.

In the years since intravenous thrombolysis was implemented, there have been many discussions regarding its risks and benefits, particularly with concerns in relation to patient age. These debates have taken place between medical professionals in scientific journals, and within regulatory authorities at both national and international levels.

A major concern of treating patients with thrombolysis is the possible development of intracranial haemorrhage (bleeding into the brain), which can be fatal. Treatment decisions have to be made very quickly with delays being minimized as speed of treatment is related to a better neurological outcome. However, this process also requires a clinician to balance treatment efficacy and risk with many other clinical parameters and variables, as well as the patient's perspective of how their symptoms will affect their life. Understandably, this is not a simple task. Stroke specialists had often to decide whether or not to treat patients outside the available evidence and medication licence, especially in older patients. In our society, the proportion of older people is rising. In the United Kingdom, the population aged over 80 has doubled since 1982 and life expectancy is increasing in the rest of Europe and in other countries. As a result, the percentage of patients undergoing thrombolysis will decline in the future if patients aged over 80 are not treated. It is therefore understandable why opinions on the overall balance of benefits and risks have varied substantially.

More recently, endovascular thrombectomy (intra-arterial clot retrieval procedures) for patients with a proximal intracranial arterial occlusion has been shown to improve neurological outcome and functional independence in patients with acute ischaemic stroke. The debate about how we provide such treatments to all such patients and, indeed, which patients should have such procedures has also started.

Intravenous thrombolysis in older people—the journey and controversy

Until the publication of the results of the Third International Stroke Trial, IST3[2] in 2012, there had been very little randomized controlled trial data specifically regarding elderly patients over the age of 80 years. Major trials had compared intravenous alteplase against control (no treatment)— examples include NINDS,[3] ECASS,[4] ECASS II,[5] ATLANTIS,[6] ECASS 3,[7] and EPITHET.[8] The fact that only very small number of older patients were enrolled despite multiple trials can be put down to either there being only small numbers of patients in this age category presenting within the appropriate trial time window from the onset of their symptoms, or the trial excluding older patients purely on the basis of their chronological age, or both. Initially, patients over the age of 80 were excluded from the NINDS trial. This age criterion was subsequently removed after part A of the trial had enrolled 188 patients, but after this only 25 patients were randomised in the treatment thrombolysis trial arm and 19 in the placebo arm of the trial. Patients aged over 80 years old were excluded from all of the ECASS trials.

The problem at this time for stroke physicians treating older patients was—what to do for such patients presenting within 4.5 hours with an acute ischaemic stroke? In 2012, the National Institute for Health and Care Excellence (NICE), in its technology appraisal guidance,[9] had no definitive recommendation for the use of alteplase for treating ischaemic stroke in elderly people, but acknowledged that 'patients outside the licensed indication for alteplase (under 18 years and over 80 years of age) . . . may have the potential to benefit from treatment with the technology'.

It was generally agreed that although less favourable outcomes with thrombolytic treatment may be expected when treating elderly patients (mostly because of other coexisting comorbidities), effective treatments should not be withheld in the absence of convincing data suggesting either a proven lack of benefit or an unacceptable risk. The concerns for withholding thrombolytic treatment in clinical practice were mainly due to fears that advancing age would be associated with a higher risk for haemorrhagic complications, poorer outcomes with increased levels of disability, and increased risk of dying in hospital.[10–12]

One particular fear primarily relating to older patients is whether the presence of a burden of leukoaraiosis (cerebral white matter changes or periventricular white matter disease which is seen on brain imaging) is associated with the development of symptomatic intracerebral haemorrhage when thrombolytic therapy is administered. In trials this happens in around 2.5–5% of patients treated with intravenous alteplase (depending on the specific trial definition of symptomatic intracerebral haemorrhage which was used). Leukoaraiosis can be seen on brain imaging— such as the standard baseline CT scan of the brain carried out in acute stroke patients which is required before thrombolysis can be administered—and is an indication of chronic ischaemic damage of the cerebral microcirculation. It has been hypothesized that acute ischaemia may worsen this microcirculatory cerebral damage at the blood–brain barrier and hence thrombolytic treatment may then increase the risk of intracranial haemorrhage (clinically causing worsening disability or death). Several studies[13,14] have indicated that in patients with severe leukoaraiosis and multiple lacunes (small cerebrospinal fluid-filled cavities in the basal ganglia or cerebral white matter) which are observed coincidentally on imaging in older people, and there may be a rate of symptomatic intracerebral haemorrhage of around 10%. The presence of moderate to severe leukoaraiosis in the deep white matter should be considered as an independent risk factor and could be included cautiously as one of several factors to be considered in the decision-making process of a clinician when weighing up the risks and benefits of thrombolytic treatment (others include examples such as time from symptom onset or very high blood pressure).

As a result of the lack of data and medication licence, there were multiple publications in scientific literature endeavouring to aid decision-making in whether to treat older patients outside of the alteplase licence. In 2006, a meta-analysis of pooled thrombolysis data concluded that despite less favourable clinical disability outcomes, the risk of symptomatic intracerebral haemorrhage did not increase in elderly patients treated with intravenous thrombolysis.[15] Similarly in 2011, an updated review concluded that patients aged over 80 years receiving thrombolysis for their acute ischaemic stroke may have worse functional recovery rates and higher mortality than younger patients, but appeared not to have increased rates of symptomatic cerebral haemorrhage.[16] However, such reviews do have limitations, such as potential selection biases in the primary studies, and the authors in their discussions concurred that such conclusions required cautious interpretation.

A comparison between patients who had received thrombolysis as part of routine clinical practice and who had been entered into SITS-ISTR (Safe Implementation of Treatments in Stroke International Stroke Thrombolysis Registry) and a different group of patients who had not received thrombolysis (who acted as controls) from VISTA (Virtual International Stroke Trials Archive) added further information for those centres treating older patients.[17] Some 29 228 patients in these databases were analysed and adjusted for age and stroke baseline severity; of these, 3472 patients were aged over 80. A major strength of this approach was that as the real-life treated patients were compared against controls from the rigorously conducted neuroprotection trials, any bias in quality of care should have favoured the non-treated control group. Despite this, the patients who were treated with intravenous alteplase had better clinical outcomes than untreated patients and this effect was not dependent on age. Patients aged over 80 years derived similar benefits from thrombolytic treatment as younger patients. There was also no difference in the rates of symptomatic intracerebral haemorrhage among patients aged over 80 years old as compared with the younger group.

The weight of evidence seemed to be moving towards clinicians being cautious and performing individual assessments of older patients but with an increasing tendency to give thrombolytic treatment in view of this having a likely potential for benefitting the patients. Increasing age was associated with poorer outcome than in younger patients but the association between thrombolysis treatment and improved outcome was maintained in very elderly people. It seemed that age alone should not be a barrier to treatment. Treatment of patients aged over 80 years increased after the publication of data from SITS, but what was needed was randomized controlled trial data, and results of the Third International Stroke trial[2] were eagerly awaited. IST-3 was purposely designed to include patients who were considered to be outside of the licence for rt-PA—especially elderly patients—and to therefore determine the balance of benefits and harms of thrombolytic therapy with rt-PA for this group. It is still the best resource of data for such patients; 3035 patients were enrolled, of whom 53% (1617) were older than 80 years of age.

Not only was a significant difference found in the adjusted effect of treatment between patients older than 80 years and in patients aged 80 years or younger, against expectations this in fact suggested a greater benefit in those older than 80 years of age. Thrombolytic treatment appeared at least as effective in the older age group as in younger patients. In recruiting older patients and patients who did not strictly meet prevailing licence criteria for thrombolytic therapy, it had been anticipated that there would be a higher risk of symptomatic intracranial haemorrhage than in previous trials. The IST-3 trial patient information leaflet stated that rt-PA treatment might be associated with an increased risk of fatal intracranial haemorrhage of 4%, which turned out to be the rate that the trial indeed registered.

IST-3 afforded confidence that mortality was not increased by thrombolysis, but also estimates on the benefits and harms of such treatment outside the current licence.

Clinicians now had randomized controlled trial data in addition to registry comparisons and meta-analyses, and a new Cochrane review of intravenous thrombolysis was published[18] containing 40% more data than the previous update from 2009. This new review included 27 trials, involving 10 187 participants; in the previous review only 0.5% patients were aged over 80 years but in this update 16% of participants were over 80 years of age.

The conclusions were that:

(i) Treatment within 3 hours of stroke with thrombolysis was more effective in reducing death or dependency without any increase in death than no treatment.

(ii) Thrombolysis could reduce the risk of long-term dependency on others for daily activities, in spite of an increased risk of bleeding in the brain, which also increased the risk of early death. Once that this early bleeding risk had passed, at 3 or 6 months after stroke, people treated with clot-dissolving drugs were more likely to have recovered from their stroke and to be independent, especially if they had been treated within the first three hours after stroke.

These are illustrated in Fig. 9.3.

(iii) Thrombolytic therapy administered up to 6 hours after ischaemic stroke also significantly reduced the proportion of participants who were dead or dependent at 3–6 months after stroke. Treatment could reduce the risk of long-term dependency on others for daily activities (illustrated in Figs. 9.4 and 9.5).

Importantly, participants aged over 80 years benefited equally to those aged less than 80 years. Older people benefited as much as younger people.

Despite all of this, there have remained concerns among healthcare professionals about thrombolytic treatment of acute ischaemic stroke.[19] On a population basis, taking the previous evidence into account, it would seem that treatment would benefit more patients than cause harm. However, given that such treatment can and does cause fatal intracerebral haemorrhage, the question remained if the potential reduction in disability justified this risk. Advocates for thrombolysis[20] pointed out other hazards that patients may be more likely to encounter in untreated stroke that receive a smaller degree of attention, such as impaired mobility causing venous thromboembolism or impaired swallowing increasing the risk of aspiration pneumonia, or a high death rate from complications in the brain such as malignant ischaemic swelling. It is likely that the reason that patients are likely to overall make a better recovery if treated with rt-PA is that by 3–6 months after stroke, the total deaths in the control group (from such complications) and in alteplase-treated patients (from early treatment-associated intracerebral haemorrhage) have balanced out.

Review: Thrombolysis for acute ischaemic stroke
Comparison: 1 Any thrombolytic agent versus control
Outcome: 32 Death or dependency (mRS 3 to 6) by the end of follow-up, participants treated within 3 hours aged ≤ 80 years versus > 80 years

Study or subgroup	Thrombolysis n/N	Control n/N	Peto Odds Ratio Peto, Fixed, 95 CI	Weight	Peto Odds Ratio Peto, Fixed, 95 CI
1 Participants aged ≤ 80 years					
ECASS 1995	28/49	25/38		5.3%	0.70 [0.29, 1.66]
NINDS 1995	127/273	170/283		35.6%	0.58 [0.42, 0.81]
ECASS II 1998	39/81	44/77		10.2%	0.70 [0.37, 1.30]
ATLANTIS B 1999	3/13	12/26		2.2%	0.39 [0.10, 1.49]
ATLANTIS A 2000	7/10	7/12		1.4%	1.62 [0.29, 8.90]
IST3 2012	54/87	57/90		10.7%	0.95 [0.52, 1.74]
Subtotal (95% CI)	**513**	**526**		**65.3%**	**0.66 [0.52, 0.85]**

Total events: 258 (Thrombolysis), 315 (Control)
Heterogeneity: Chi² = 3.64, df = 5 (P = 0.60); I² = 0.0%
Test for overall effect: Z = 3.28 (P = 0.0010)

Study or subgroup	Thrombolysis n/N	Control n/N	Peto Odds Ratio Peto, Fixed, 95 CI	Weight	Peto Odds Ratio Peto, Fixed, 95 CI
2 Participants aged > 80 years					
NINDS 1995	13/25	22/29		3.2%	0.36 [0.12, 1.09]
IST3 2012	245/344	266/328		31.5%	0.58 [0.41, 0.83]
Subtotal (95% CI)	**369**	**357**		**34.7%**	**0.56 [0.40, 0.78]**

Total events: 258 (Thrombolysis), 288 (Control)
Heterogeneity: Chi² = 0.67, df = 1 (P = 0.41); I² = 0.0%
Test for overall effect: Z = 3.41 (P = 0.00066)

Study or subgroup	Thrombolysis n/N	Control n/N	Peto Odds Ratio Peto, Fixed, 95 CI	Weight	Peto Odds Ratio Peto, Fixed, 95 CI
Total (95% CI)	**882**	**8883**		**100.0%**	**0.62 [0.51, 0.76]**

Total events: 516 (Thrombolysis), 603 (Control)
Heterogeneity: Chi² = 4.98, df = 7 (P = 0.66); I² = 0.0%
Test for overall effect: Z = 4.66 (P < 0.00001)
Test for subgroup differences: Chi² = 0.67, df = 1 (P = 0.41), I² = 0.0%

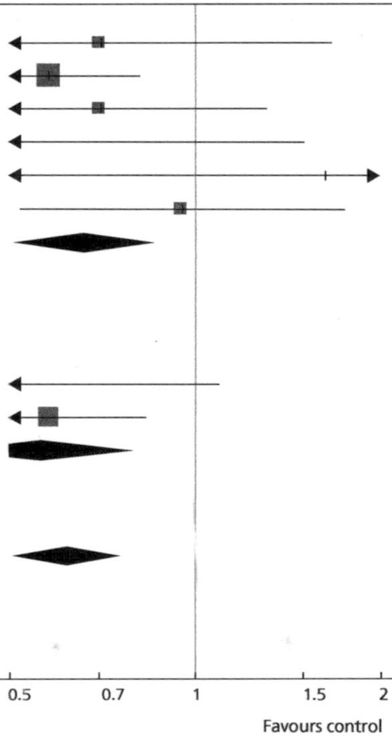

Scale: 0.5 0.7 1 1.5 2 — Favours thrombolysis / Favours control

Fig. 9.3 Review of thrombolysis trials of acute ischaemic stroke.

This specifically focuses on the outcome of death or dependency (mRS 3–6) by the end of the trial follow-up period, for trial participants treated within 3 hours, aged <=80 versus >80 years; all ages have favourable results with thrombolytic treatment instead of control treatment.

Reproduced with permission from Wardlaw JM, et al. Thrombolysis for acute ischaemic stroke. *Cochrane Database of Systematic Reviews*, Issue 7, Art. No.: CD000213. Copyright © 2016 The Cochrane Collaboration. Published by John Wiley & Sons, Ltd. doi:10.1002/14651858.CD000213.pub3.

Review: Thrombolysis for acute ischaemic stroke
Comparison: 1 Any thrombolytic agent versus control
Outcome: 31 Death or dependency (m RS 3 to 6) by the end of follow-up; participants treated up to 6 hours ≤ 80 years versus > 80 years

Study or subgroup	Thrombolysis n/N	Control n/N	Peto Odds Ratio Peto, Fixed, 95% CI	Weight	Peto Odds Ratio Peto, Fixed, 95% CI
1 Participants age ≤ 80 years					
Mori 1992	11/19	10/12		0.4%	0.32 [0.07, 1.48]
NINDS 1995	127/273	170/283		8.8%	0.58 [0.42, 0.81]
ECASS 1995	171/313	185/307		9.7%	0.79 [0.58, 1.09]
ECASS II 1998	187/409	211/391		12.8%	0.72 [0.55, 0.95]
ATLANTS B 1999	141/307	135/306		9.7%	1.08 [0.78, 1.48]
ATLANTS A 2000	64/71	56/71		1.2%	2.35 [0.95, 5.82]
Wang 2003	14/67	11/33		1.1%	0.52 [0.20, 1.35]
EPITHET 2008	18/38	18/36		1.2%	0.90 [0.36, 2.23]
ECASS 3 2008	140/418	155/403		12.1%	0.81 [0.61, 1.07]
IST3 2012	367/698	374/720		22.6%	1.03 [0.83, 1.26]
Subtotal (95% CI)	**2613**	**2562**		**79.4%**	**0.85 [0.76, 0.95]**
Total events: 1240 (Thrombolysis), 1325 (Control)					
Heterogeneity: Chi² = 19.38, df = 9 (P = 0.02); I² = 54%					
Test for overall effect: Z = 2.85 (P = 0.0044)					
2 Participants aged > 80 years					
NINDS 1995	13/25	22/29		0.8%	0.36 [0.12, 1.09]
EPITHET 2008	11/13	10/12		0.2%	1.10 [0.13, 8.92]
IST3 2012	594/817	612/800		19.5%	0.82 [0.65, 1.02]
Subtotal (95% CI)	**855**	**841**		**20.6%**	**0.80 [0.64, 0.99]**
Total events: 618 (Thrombolysis), 644 (Control)					
Heterogeneity: Chi² = 2.14, df = 2 (P = 0.34); I² = 7%					
Test for overall effect: Z = 2.06 (P = 0.040)					
Total (95% CI)	**3468**	**3403**		**100.0%**	**0.84 [0.76, 0.93]**
Total events: 1858 (Thrombolysis), 1969 (Control)					
Heterogeneity: Chi² = 21.82, df = 12 (P = 0.04); I² = 45%					
Test for overall effect: Z = 3.47 (P = 0.00052)					
Test for subgroup differences: Chi² = 0.29, df = 1 (P = 0.59); I² = 0.0%					

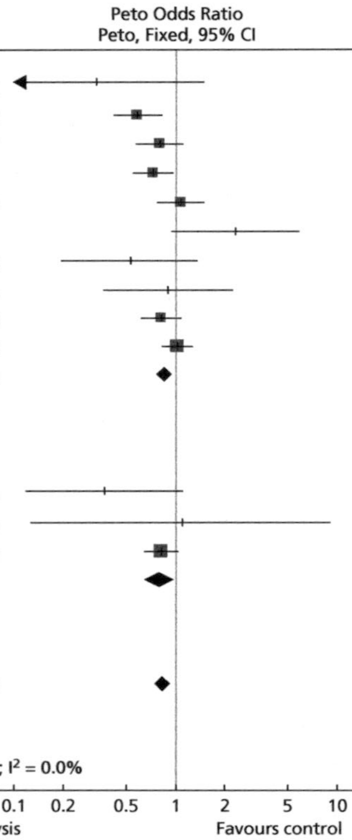

0.1 0.2 0.5 1 2 5 10
Favours thrombolysis   Favours control

Fig. 9.4 Review of thrombolysis trials of acute ischaemic stroke. This specifically focuses on the outcome of death or dependency (mRS 3–6) by the end of the trial follow-up period, for trial participants treated within 6 hours, aged <=80 versus >80 years; all ages have favourable results with thrombolytic treatment instead of control treatment.

Reproduced with permission from Wardlaw JM, et al. Thrombolysis for acute ischaemic stroke. *Cochrane Database of Systematic Reviews*, Issue 7, Art. No.: CD000213. Copyright © 2016 The Cochrane Collaboration. Published by John Wiley & Sons, Ltd. doi:10.1002/14651858.CD000213.pub3.

Review: Thrombolysis for acute ischaemic stroke
Comparison: 1 Any thrombolytic agent versus control
Outcome: 33 Alive and independent (m RS 0 to 2) at end of follow up, treaged up to 6 hours aged ≤ 80 years versus > 80 years

Study or subgroup	Thrombolysis n/N	Control n/N	Peto Odds Ratio Peto, Fixed, 95% CI	Weight	Peto Odds Ratio Peto, Fixed, 95% CI
1 Participants age ≤ 80 years					
Mori 1992	8/19	10/12		0.4%	3.09 [0.67, 14.12]
NINDS 1995	145/272	113/283		8.8%	1.71 [1.23, 2.39]
ECASS 1995	142/312	122/307		9.7%	1.26 [0.92, 1.73]
ECASS II 1998	222/409	180/391		12.7%	1.39 [1.05, 1.83]
ATLANTS B 1999	166/307	171/306		9.7%	0.93 [0.68, 1.28]
ATLANTS A 2000	7/71	15/71		1.2%	0.43 [0.17, 1.05]
Wang 2003	53/67	22/33		1.1%	1.93 [0.74, 5.03]
EPITHET 2008	20/38	18/36		1.2%	1.11 [0.45, 2.74]
ECASS 3 2008	278/418	248/403		12.0%	1.24 [0.93, 1.65]
IST3 2012	331/698	346/720		22.5%	0.97 [0.79, 1.20]
Subtotal (95% CI)	2612	2562		79.4%	1.17 [1.05, 1.31]
Total events: 1372 (Thrombolysis), 1237 (Control)					
Heterogeneity: Chi² = 19.20, df = 9 (P = 0.02); I² = 53%					
Test for overall effect: Z = 2.83 (P = 0.0046)					
2 Participants aged > 80 years or over					
NINDS 1995	12/40	7/29		0.9%	1.34 [0.46, 3.86]
EPITHET 2008	2/13	2/12		0.2%	0.91 [0.11, 7.43]
IST3 2012	223/817	188/800		19.5%	1.22 [0.98, 1.53]
Subtotal (95% CI)	870	841		20.6%	1.22 [0.98, 1.52]
Total events: 237 (Thrombolysis), 197 (Control)					
Heterogeneity: Chi² = 0.10, df = 2 (P = 0.95); I² = 0.0%					
Test for overall effect: Z = 1.81 (P = 0.071)					
Total (95% CI)	3482	3403		100.0%	1.18 [1.07, 1.31]
Total events: 1609 (Thrombolysis), 1434 (Control)					
Heterogeneity: Chi² = 19.40, df = 12 (P = 0.08); I² = 38%					
Test for overall effect: Z = 3.35 (P = 0.00082)					
Test for subgroup differences: Chi² = 0.10, df = 1 (P = 0.75); I² = 0.0%					

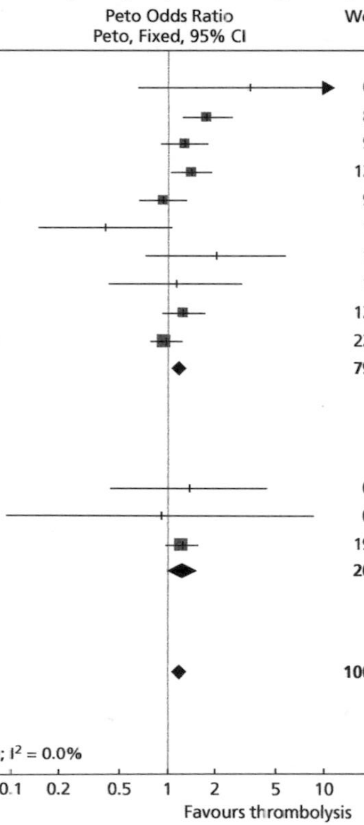

0.1 0.2 0.5 1 2 5 10
Favours control   Favours thrombolysis

Fig. 9.5 Review of thrombolysis trials of acute ischaemic stroke.

This specifically focusses on the outcome of alive and independent (mRS 0–2) by the end of the trial follow-up period, for trial participants treated within 6 hours, aged <=80 versus >80 years; all ages have favourable results with thrombolytic treatment instead of control treatment.

After these questions and other concerns regarding the evidence base for treatment, it was announced in August 2014 that there would be an in-depth independent expert review of intravenous alteplase use in acute ischaemic stroke.[21]

This working group of the United Kingdom's Commission on Human Medicines had expertise in statistics, epidemiology, emergency medicine, neurology, and also patient representation. A thorough scientific assessment was conducted by staff who had not previously been involved in the licensing of alteplase. Its report[22] rigorously reviewed and discussed all available data, including a new meta-analysis of intravenous thrombolysis (the most current summary of all clinical data available on rt-PA use in acute ischaemic stroke).[23] It unanimously concluded that alteplase remained safe and effective for use in the treatment of acute ischaemic stroke up to 4.5 hours after the onset of symptoms. It reiterated that the earlier that treatment is given the greater the chance of a more favourable outcome for patients.

A few points are worth noting from this review. There had been questions raised about the differing outcomes between the IST-3 and ECASS III trials. IST-3 had aimed to establish the balance of benefits and harms of thrombolytic therapy with rt-PA in patients who did not meet the licence criteria (especially elderly patients), whereas in contrast, trials such as ECASS III were managed according to the specifics of the treatment licence. As a result of these differences, it was not surprising that the ECASS III trial results were unlike from the IST-3 results. Importantly, the benefits and risks of rt-PA treatment in elderly patients (over 80 years of age) were discussed and the available data suggested that the benefits of rt-PA were not age-related. Information from IST-3,[2] a new meta-analysis which highlighted that faster treatment with alteplase improved disability outcomes within 4.5 hours and showed bigger benefits with earlier treatment[23] and other observational sources, did not raise concern about the off-label use of rt-PA in patients over 80 years old.

Hopefully, this review has now addressed concerns and clarified the role of intravenous alteplase as a standard treatment in acute ischaemic stroke for now—at least until new treatments or other agents are developed in the future with the potential to either be more efficacious or to have a lower risk of haemorrhagic side effects.

The current fourth edition of the National Clinical Guideline for Stroke in the UK[24] recommends:

(i) Any patient, regardless of age or stroke severity, where treatment can be started within 3 hours of known symptom onset and who has been shown not to have an intracerebral haemorrhage or other contraindications should be considered for treatment using alteplase.

(ii) Between 3 and 4.5 hours of known stroke symptom onset, patients under 80 years who have been shown not to have an intracerebral haemorrhage or other contraindication, should be considered for treatment with alteplase.

(iii) Between 3 and 6 hours of known stroke symptom onset, patients should be considered for treatment with alteplase on an individual basis, recognizing that the benefits of treatment are likely to be smaller than those treated earlier, but that the risks of a worse outcome, including death, will on average not be increased.

Further work is continuing on the use of intravenous alteplase in acute ischaemic stroke for patients who could not live alone without help of another person before this stroke (dependent patients). This group of patients (who are often elderly) are frequently denied thrombolysis due to similar concerns discussed earlier regarding efficacy and haemorrhagic complications. However, a recent trial[25] concluded that although these dependent patients carry a higher risk of dying from their stroke when compared with a group of previously independent patients, the risk of symptomatic intracranial haemorrhage and the likelihood of poor outcome were not independently influenced by previous dependency. It seems that assuming that the patient survives their stroke, they are likely to avoid a poor outcome at least as successfully as independent patients would and therefore withholding intravenous thrombolysis in this dependent group may not be justified.

Endovascular mechanical thrombectomy

For many years, mechanical thrombectomy has been performed to open an occluded cerebral vessel in an acute stroke, using different devices to improve the vessel recanalization rate and patient outcome.[26–41] The advantages of using a mechanical device is that patients with contraindications to intravenous thrombolysis can receive treatment as occluded vessels can be directly opened without the haemorrhagic risks of intravenous thrombolysis. Intravenous thrombolysis can also be administered in suitable patients in addition to an endovascular approach; the recanalization rates of large artery occlusions are also much higher than with intravenous thrombolysis alone. The interventional procedure can be performed under conscious sedation or general anaesthesia. Currently, expert consensus[42] is that general anaesthesia is recommended for patients who are comatose with a Glasgow Coma Scale score of less than 8, those who are severely agitated and in whom an intervention could not be performed safely under sedation, or either respiratory or airway compromise (which may be related to the stroke itself or complications such as seizures or vomiting). Conscious sedation for endovascular treatment is preferred by some stroke centres. A subanalysis of the MR CLEAN study[35] suggested an association with better patient neurological outcomes and lower mortality when compared with general anaesthesia but biases such as quicker procedural treatment and differences in patient selection may well have influenced these results (e.g. patients presenting with more severe strokes will require a general anaesthetic and may be more likely to subsequently have a worse neurological outcome). More research is ongoing in this area.

In the early days, catheter-based treatments were performed by positioning microcatheters up into the intracranial arteries to deliver thrombolysis—such as in the PROACT Trial.[26] In this study intra-arterial thrombolysis with a pro-urokinase infusion was used in patients aged less than 85 years old to attempt to dissolve the occluding thrombus. However, during this trial, the interventional neuroradiologists performing the procedure noted that the lytic process may be enhanced by using the wire to manipulate the thrombus.

Following this, microcatheter- and wire-based mechanical devices were developed with some promising results. One of the so-called older-generation devices is the MERCI retrieval device.

On deploying the device, it adopted a corkscrew-shape (demonstrated in Fig. 9.6(a)) which endeavoured to pierce the clot (Fig. 9.6(b), parts 1 and 2) and then remove it (Fig. 9.6(b), part 3). This device underwent subsequent modifications in attempting to better anchor the clot and prevent it being released while being retracted.[27] Suction aspiration catheters were next developed; these utilized either large catheters to suck up and remove occluded thrombi in the larger proximal cerebral vessels, or smaller catheters to gain access to smaller blood vessels and retrieve clots which had passed more distally. The Penumbra Pivotal trial in 2009 reported 25% of patients experienced a good clinical outcome.[28] In 2013, three endovascular treatment trials—IMS III, MR RESCUE, and SYNTHESIS EXPANSION, reported neutral results with respect to clinical outcomes. This was a setback to developing interventional thrombectomy services and pathways. There were limitations of these studies that could have influenced the results, such as the use of wire manipulation instead of thrombectomy devices leading to lower than desired vessel recanalization rates, and long delays between onset of stroke symptoms and thrombectomy treatment. In IMS III only four patients were treated with the 'new-generation' stent retrievers and

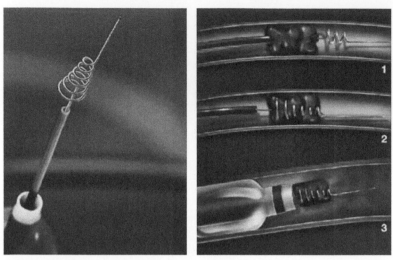

Fig. 9.6 The MERCI clot retrieval device.

Reproduced with permission from Smith WS, et al. Technology Insight: recanalization with drugs and devices during acute ischemic stroke. *Nature Reviews Neurology*, 3, 45–53. Copyright © 1969, Springer Nature. https://doi.org/10.1038/ncpneuro0372.

often occlusion of a vessel was not confirmed.[39] The SYNTHESIS EXPANSION trial also used very few stent retrievers,[40] with the MR RESCUE[41] using previous generation MERCI or penumbra devices and achieving a good vessel recanalization in only two-thirds of patients.

More recently, 'new-generation' stent retrievers have been developed, which currently produced the most favourable clinical outcomes in trials; an example is shown in Fig. 9.7.

A microcatheter is pushed across the thrombus, followed by the stent retriever. The microcatheter is then withdrawn and the stent retriever is deployed, ideally covering the entire length of the occlusion. Sometimes crushing the thrombus against the vessel wall will restore some cerebral blood

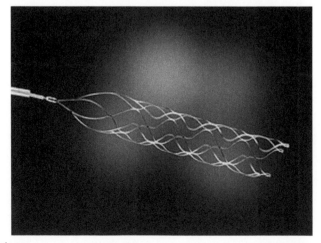

Fig. 9.7 Stent retriever.

Reproduced with permission of Medtronic, Inc.

flow but the main aim is to capture the thrombus within the stent mesh. This process is demonstrated in Fig. 9.8.

The stent retriever is then slowly and carefully retrieved along with the clot. If necessary, this can be repeated multiple times to achieve complete clot removal.

In order to gain US Food and Drug Administration approval, two new stent retrievers were mandated to be tested against the older-generation MERCI device in two randomized controlled trials, SWIFT and TREVO-2, in 2012. The SWIFT trial[43] was halted prematurely by the steering committee after only 113 patients had been randomized because the new Solitaire stent retriever showed a significant improvement in recanalizing the occluded cerebral artery vessel; this in turn led to better clinical outcomes for patients with reduced disability 3 months after the stroke. TREVO-2[44] also displayed more frequent vessel reperfusion as compared to the MERCI device and better patient—3-month clinical outcomes. In 2014, an analysis of 9300 patients from the United States,[45] of whom 18% were over 80 years of age, suggested that the death rate of older patients who received endovascular thrombectomy was double that of younger patients. This caused concern, but as the time period related to 2008–2010 and the types of device used were not stated, it was not clear how this would relate to treatment with stent retrievers (nor was there any age-matched control group to compare with).

In 2015, multiple large randomized controlled trials reported evidence for endovascular stroke treatment. The first was MR CLEAN from the Netherlands; this trial had no age limit with patients ranging between 23 and 96 years old.[29] Some 16% were 80 years or older. Patients within 6 hours of symptom onset who had a proven large artery occlusion that would be amenable to endovascular thrombectomy treatment were randomised either to usual care (which included intravenous thrombolysis where indicated) or intraarterial treatment plus usual care. 89.0% patients received treatment with intravenous alteplase before randomization. The results showed that the intra-arterial treatment was safe (with no significant difference in symptomatic intracranial haemorrhage between the two trial arms) and effective—33% patients in the interventional group had very good outcomes in their neurological functioning in daily life compared to only 19% in the usual care group. These treatment outcomes were observed irrespective of age, the

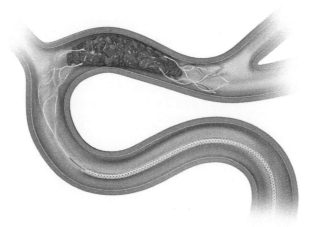

Fig. 9.8 A deployed stent retriever.

Courtesy of Stryker.

treatment effect was positive in this older age group and there was no difference between patients aged less than or older than 80 years old.

As a result of the results from MR CLEAN, other ongoing randomized trials were halted prematurely. ESCAPE[30]—the randomized assessment of rapid endovascular treatment of ischaemic stroke—had no defined upper age limit, with the oldest person enrolled in the trial being 93 years of age. CT imaging was undertaken to confirm patients had an intracranial proximal arterial occlusion of the anterior circulation. The infarct volume had to be small with an Alberta Stroke Program Early CT Score (ASPECTS) score of more than 5, aiming for patients with good collateral blood supply and a large penumbra with only small core infarct. ASPECTS stands for 'Alberta Stroke Program Early CT Score', a score based on 10 specific areas of the brain which are affected first by ischaemia in the middle cerebral artery territory; a score of 10 is normal with no evidence of brain damage and 0 represents complete brain infarction in these areas.

All patients received intravenous thrombolysis when clinically indicated. This trial confirmed the MR CLEAN findings, with the interventional group being less likely to die from their stroke and achieving better clinical outcomes—regardless of age. In EXTEND-IA,[31] patients were randomized if they were functionally independent prior to the stroke occurring and could receive intravenous alteplase within 4.5 hours after stroke onset; plus they had to have a favourable penumbra on CT perfusion imaging as well as an occluded anterior circulation artery occlusion on CT angiography. This trial had no older age limits.

With the addition of thrombectomy to standard care within 8 hours of stroke onset, the results suggest that compared to the use of alteplase alone, only 3.2 patients require endovascular treatment with endovascular therapy to ensure another patient becoming independent from this severe stroke. SWIFT PRIME[32] treated patients aged 18–85 years of age, as did REVASCAT.[33] These also showed positive outcomes from endovascular treatment.

After these positive trials, several new meta-analyses were published. One of these evaluating endovascular treatments of thrombectomy using Solitaire stent retrievers in the anterior circulation was completed in 2016.[34] This analysed 787 patients: 401 treated using endovascular thrombectomy against 386 being treated with intravenous thrombolysis/standard stroke treatments only. There was no difference in intracranial haemorrhage or death when comparing the two groups, but patients treated using stent retrievers were less likely to be disabled and more likely to return to independent living. The authors concluded that age alone should not prevent patients from receiving endovascular stroke treatment; there was no evidence of treatment being less effective in older patients who were previously in good health; furthermore, there was a clinically and statistically significant 20% absolute reduction in mortality in patients aged 80 years or over.

The Hermes collaboration[46] used individual patient data from five trials' databases, and therefore was able to conduct a meta-analysis to clarify whether endovascular treatments were efficacious in different subgroups of patients. Of particular note, clinical outcomes after endovascular thrombectomy were significantly better than the control groups in patients aged 80 years or older. Also, from a safety point of view, there was no difference between groups with respect to the risk of symptomatic intracranial haemorrhage.

When analysing patient-level data pooled from trials in which the Solitaire device was the only or the predominant device (SWIFT PRIME, ESCAPE, EXTEND-IA, REVASCAT), a meta-analysis showed that mechanical thrombectomy has a favourable effect over standard care in patients ≥80 years old.[47] However, the number of patients in these trials who were 90 years of age or older was very small, and the benefit of mechanical thrombectomy over standard care in patients who are 90 years of age or older is still not absolutely clear.

In February 2016, NICE produced new guidance for mechanical clot retrieval in the treatment of acute ischaemic stroke.[36] This concludes that the current evidence on the safety and efficacy of mechanical clot retrieval for treating acute ischaemic stroke is adequate to support the use of this procedure. There are no exclusions defined on the basis of an older age.

Single-centre published experience backs up the trial data in very elderly patients (age ≥80 years) and aged patients (60–79 years). Patients older than 80 years of age undergoing mechanical thrombectomy for acute infarction were more difficult to recanalize due to inaccessible occlusion sites, but mortality and other complications were similar to those in younger patients.[48] Another centre[49] evaluated patients having thrombectomy aged more than 80 years old and ≤80 years old; 43.4% of patients in the younger group and 25.7% of patients in the older group achieved an 'excellent outcome'. A 'good outcome' was achieved in 65.1% of patients in the younger group, and 60% of patients in the older group. There was no significant difference seen between these groups after adjusting for gender, NIHSS score at admission, ASPECTS, and thrombolysis. Although age may be a prognostic factor, patients should not be excluded based on age criteria alone. Others[50] found that being aged 80 years or older was not significant, with complete recanalization being more important when predicting outcome in older people.

More recently, randomized controlled trials have used more complex imaging to further select patients for thrombectomy treatment but who are over 6 hours from their symptom onset.

The DAWN trial[51] randomized patients who had both large anterior circulation vessel occlusion and clinical imaging mismatch (a combination of NIHSS score and imaging findings on CT perfusion imaging or diffusion-weighted MRI imaging) between 6 and 24 hours from last known normal to treatment with either mechanical thrombectomy or standard care. The mismatch imaging attempted to look for patients who had disproportionately severe clinical symptoms relative to the volume of their stroke core infarct. The mismatch criteria were defined according to age (<80 years or ≥80 years). Only 12% of patients had strokes of witnessed onset. Patients receiving thrombectomy had better functional outcomes at 90 days (49% in the thrombectomy group as compared with 13% in the control group).

The DEFUSE 3 trial[52] used imaging to select patients with remaining ischaemic brain tissue that was not yet infarcted who also had large anterior circulation occlusion 6–16 hours after they were last known to be well. Again, endovascular therapy (thrombectomy) showed better functional outcome at 90 days than standard medical therapy (44.6% vs. 16.7%) and benefit was independently demonstrated for the subgroup of patients who met DAWN eligibility criteria and also for the subgroup who did not.

In conclusion, the current evidence suggests that endovascular thrombectomy, particularly using new-generation stent retrievers, is beneficial to most patients with acute ischaemic stroke caused by a large artery occlusion of the cerebral anterior circulation, regardless of their age. As with any treatment decision in an elderly patient, consideration of comorbidities and risks should factor into the decision-making for mechanical thrombectomy. This will require reconfiguration of stroke services on a global basis to provide interventional endovascular treatment to individuals that require it for their acute ischaemic stroke.

Multidisciplinary stroke care

Not every patient with acute ischaemic stroke will be eligible to receive intravenous thrombolysis (currently the national average is 11% of patients)[53] or have a mechanical thrombectomy—for example, patients with a delayed presentation of their stroke. Nevertheless, all can still benefit from coordinated specialist services that a multidisciplinary approach on a dedicated ward-based acute stroke unit can offer.

There is overwhelming evidence that treating all patients with acute ischaemic stroke on stroke units reduces their risk of dying and increases their chances of returning home and looking after themselves independently.[37] The latest Cochrane review from 2013[38] evaluated 5855 patients and 28 trials and confirmed that these benefits occur regardless of age.

Why do patients benefit? It is likely to be a combination of multiple small gains, aiming for excellence in all areas of care.

An acute stroke unit delivers this high-dependency care. Patients treated by stroke specialist multidisciplinary staff are more likely to have faster and more accurate investigations, diagnoses, and personalized management plans. A patient receives neurological and physiological monitoring on a specialist unit to maintain homeostasis in the early acute phase of their stroke, combined with regular standardized assessments to treat acute stroke and prevent complications (such as venous thromboembolism and aspiration pneumonia). Measures are taken to optimize nutrition, hydration, swallowing, and plans made for any disturbance of bladder and bowel control. Positioning of the patients and early rehabilitation targeting specific patient goals, with early discharge planning into specialist early supported discharge stroke services, helps optimize the best functional outcome for an individual patient. The team facilitate communication and personal treatment plans with patients and their carers. Finally, palliative care for dying patients is also of huge importance; the only possible exception for stroke unit care would be symptom control for patients dying of stroke in their own home and those having end-stage comorbidities such as advanced dementia. Guidelines for such best management are regularly updated by the Royal College of Physicians.[24]

After all of this, what should an older person who suffers an acute stroke now do?

The treatment approach for acute ischaemic stroke in an older person is unambiguous: re-establish cerebral blood flow as quickly, completely, and safely as possible.

If any patient, younger or older, feels that they have any symptoms (particularly 'FAST' symptoms: the Face Arm and Speech Test) that suggest that they may be suffering a stroke, then they should immediately call for emergency assistance and get to hospital or specialist stroke centre as quickly as possible. They should not hesitate by thinking that they will be 'too old' for treatment.

On arrival, they will be assessed by a stroke doctor and undergo urgent brain imaging. Intravenous thrombolytic treatment should be considered (weighing up different individual risks against the benefits) to be given as quickly as possible, as this is very effective if started within 3 hours of stroke and definitely improves outcome if given up to 4.5 hours after stroke.

Mechanical thrombectomy may be considered for patients with large artery occlusions up to 6 hours after symptom onset, but should not prevent treatment with intravenous thrombolysis where this is indicated; similarly, intravenous thrombolysis should not delay mechanical thrombectomy. If intravenous thrombolysis is contraindicated, then mechanical thrombectomy should be considered as a first-line treatment in large vessel occlusions. Selected acute stroke patients (with evidence of a large vessel occlusion in the anterior circulation and a region of tissue that is ischaemic but not yet infarcted on favourable perfusion imaging) within 6–24 hours of last known normal may also be candidates for endovascular thrombectomy.

All patients with stroke benefit from a multidisciplinary approach and stroke unit care, and all stroke patients (regardless of age) should be moved swiftly to a stroke unit for monitoring, acute treatments, and rehabilitation in order to achieve the best possible recovery from their stroke.

References

1. **Department of Health.** *National Stroke Strategy.* December 2007. Available from: https://webarchive. nationalarchives.gov.uk/20130104224925/http://www.dh.gov.uk/prod_consum_dh/groups/dh_ digitalassets/documents/digitalasset/dh_081059.pdf [Accessed: 24 July 2019].

2. IST-3 2012. The IST-3 collaborative group. The benefits and harms of intravenous thrombolysis with recombinant tissue plasminogen activator within 6 hours of acute ischaemic stroke (the third international stroke trial (IST-3)): a randomised controlled trial. *Lancet* 2012;**379**:2364–72.

3. **The National Institute of Neurological Disorders and Stroke rt-PA Stroke Study Group.** Tissue plasminogen activator for acute ischemic stroke. *N Engl J Med* 1995;**333**:1581–7.

4. **Hacke W, Kaste M, Fieschi C,** et al. Intravenous thrombolysis with recombinant tissue plasminogen activator for acute hemispheric stroke: the European Cooperative Acute Stroke Study (ECASS). *JAMA* 1995; **274**: 1017–25.

5. **Hacke W, Kaste M, Fieschi C,** et al. Randomised double-blind placebo-controlled trial of thrombolytic therapy with intravenous alteplase in acute ischaemic stroke (ECASS II). *Lancet* 1998;**352**:1245–51.

6. **Clark WM, Albers GW, Madden KP, & Hamilton S.** The rtPA (alteplase) 0- to 6-hour acute stroke trial, part A (A0276g): results of a double-blind, placebo-controlled, multicenter study: thrombolytic therapy in Acute Ischemic Stroke Study investigators. *Stroke* 2000;**31**:811–16

7. **Hacke W, Kaste M, Bluhmki E,** et al. **for the European Cooperative Acute Stroke Study (ECASS) investigators.** Alteplase compared with placebo within 3 to 4·5 hours for acute ischemic stroke. *N Engl J Med* 2008;**359**:1317–29.

8. **Davis SM, Donnan GA, Parsons MW,** et al. and **for the EPITHET investigators.** Effects of alteplase beyond 3 h after stroke in the Echoplanar Imaging Thrombolytic Evaluation Trial (EPITHET): a placebo-controlled randomised trial. *Lancet Neurol* 2008;**7**:299–309.

9. **NICE.** *Alteplase for Treating Ischaemic Stroke. NICE Technology Appraisal Guidance (TA264).* Available from: http://www.nice.org.uk/guidance/ta264/chapter/4-Consideration-of-the-evidence [Accessed: 24 July 2019].

10. **Heuschmann PU, Kolominsky-Rabas PL, Roether J,** et al. Predictors of in-hospital mortality in patients with acute ischemic stroke treated with thrombolytic therapy. *JAMA* 2004;**292**:1831–8.

11. **Bateman BT, Schumacher HC, Boden-Albala B,** et al. Factors associated with in-hospital mortality after administration of thrombolysis in acute ischemic stroke patients: an analysis of the nationwide inpatient sample 1999 to 2002. *Stroke* 2006;**37**:440–6.

12. **Hacke W, Donnan G, Fieschi C,** et al. Association of outcome with early stroke treatment: pooled analysis of ATLANTIS, ECASS, and NINDS rt-PA stroke trials. *Lancet* 2004;**363**:768–74.

13. **Tobias Neumann-Haefelin T, Hoelig S, Berkefeld J,** et al., **for the MR Stroke Group.** Leukoaraiosis is a risk factor for symptomatic intracerebral hemorrhage after thrombolysis for acute stroke. *Stroke* 2006;**37**:2463–6.

14. **B Palumbo V, Boulanger JM, Hill MD,** et al. Leukoaraiosis and intracerebral hemorrhage after thrombolysis in acute stroke. *Neurology* 2007;**68**:1020–4.

15. **Engelter ST, Bonati LH, & Lyrer PA.** Intravenous thrombolysis in stroke patients of > or = 80 versus < 80 years of age—a systematic review across cohort studies. *Age Ageing* 2006;**35**:572–80.

16. **Bhatnagar P, Sinha D, Parker RA, Guyler P, & O'Brien A.** Intravenous thrombolysis in acute ischaemic stroke: a systematic review and meta-analysis to aid decision making in patients over 80 years of age. *J Neurol Neurosurg Psychiatry* 2011;**82**:712–17.

17. **Mishra NK, Ahmed N, Andersen G,** et al. for the VISTA and SITS collaborators. Thrombolysis in very elderly people: controlled comparison of SITS International Stroke Thrombolysis Registry and Virtual International Stroke Trials Archive. *BMJ* 2010;**341**:c6046.

18. **Wardlaw JM, Murray V, Berge E, & del Zoppo GJ.** Thrombolysis for acute ischaemic stroke. *Cochrane Database Syst Rev* 2014;**7**:CD000213.

19. **Shinton R.** Questions about authorisation of alteplase for ischaemic stroke. *Lancet* 2014;**384**:659–60.

20. **Sandercock P, Lindley R, Wardlaw JM, Murray V, Whiteley W, & Cohen G.** Alteplase for ischaemic stroke—responses. *Lancet* 2014;**384**:661–2.

21. BBC News. *Safety Review into Stroke Clot-Buster Drug Alteplase.* 22 August 2014. Available from: http://www.bbc.co.uk/news/health-28900824 [Accessed: 24 July 2019].

22. **Gov.uk.** *Alteplase for Treatment of Acute Ischaemic Stroke: Independent Review.* 2015. Available from: https://www.gov.uk/government/publications/alteplase-for-treatment-of-acute-ischaemic-stroke-independent-review [Accessed: 24 July 2019].

23. **Emberson J, Lees KR, Lyden P, et al.** Effect of treatment delay, age, and stroke severity on the effects of intravenous thrombolysis with alteplase for acute ischaemic stroke: a meta-analysis of individual patient data from randomised trials. *Lancet* 2014;**384**:1929–35.

24. **Intercollegiate Stroke Working Party.** *National Clinical Guideline for Stroke,* 5th edition. London, UK: Royal College of Physicians, 2016.

25. **Gensicke H, Strbian D, Zinkstok S, et al.** Intravenous thrombolysis in patients dependent on the daily help of others before stroke. *Stroke* 2016;**47**:450–6.

26. **PROACT Investigators.** PROACT: a phase II randomized trial of recombinant prourokinase by direct arterial delivery in acute middle cerebral artery stroke. Prolyse in acute thromboembolism. *Stroke* 1998;**29**:4–11.

27. **Smith WS, Sung G, Saver J, et al.** Mechanical thrombectomy for acute ischemic stroke: final results of the MULTIMERCI trial. *Stroke* 2008;**39**:1205–12.

28. **The Penumbra Pivotal Stroke Trial Investigators.** The Penumbra pivotal stroke trial: safety and effectiveness of a new generation of mechanical devices for clot removal in intracranial large vessel occlusive disease. *Stroke* 2009;**40**:2761–8.

29. **Berkhemer OA, Fransen PS, Beumer D, et al.** MR CLEAN Investigators. A randomized trial of intraarterial treatment for acute ischemic stroke. *N Engl J Med* 2015;**372**:11–20.

30. **Goyal M, Demchuk AM, Menon BK, et al.** ESCAPE Trial Investigators. Randomized assessment of rapid endovascular treatment of ischemic stroke. *N Engl J Med* 2015;**372**:1019–30.

31. **Campbell BC, Mitchell PJ, Kleinig TJ, et al.** EXTEND-IA Investigators. Endovascular therapy for ischemic stroke with perfusion-imaging selection. *N Engl J Med* 2015;**372**:1009–18.

32. **Saver JL, Goyal M, Bonafe A, et al.** SWIFT PRIME Investigators. Stent-retriever thrombectomy after intravenous t-PA vs. t-PA alone in stroke. *N Engl J Med* 2015;**372**:2285–95.

33. **Jovin TG, Chamorro A, Cobo E, et al.** REVASCAT Trial Investigators. Thrombectomy within 8 hours after symptom onset in ischemic stroke. *N Engl J Med* 2015;**372**:2296–306.

34. **Campbell B, Hill M, Rubiera M, et al.** Safety and efficacy of solitaire stent thrombectomy. individual patient data meta-analysis of randomized trials. *Stroke* 2016;**47**:798–806.

35. **Van den Berg LA, Koelman D, Berkhemer OA, et al.** Type of anesthesia and differences in clinical outcome after intra-arterial treatment for ischemic stroke. *Stroke* 2015;**46**:1257–62.

36. **NICE.** *Mechanical Clot Retrieval for Treating Acute Ischaemic Stroke.* NICE interventional procedure guidance [IPG548]. 2016. Available from: http://www.nice.org.uk/guidance/ipg548 [Accessed: 24 July 2019].

37. **Stroke Unit Trialists' Collaboration.** Collaborative systematic review of the randomised trials of organised in-patient (stroke unit) care after stroke. *BMJ* 1997;**314**:1151–9.

38. **Stroke Unit Trialists' Collaboration.** Organised inpatient (stroke unit) care for stroke. *Cochrane Database Syst Rev* 2013;(9):CD000197.

39. **Broderick JP, Palesch YY, Demchuk AM, et al.** Endovascular therapy after intravenous t-pa versus t-pa alone for stroke. *N Engl J Med* 2013;**368**:893–903.

40. **Ciccone A, Valvassori L, Nichelatti M, et al.** Endovascular treatment for acute ischemic stroke. *N Engl J Med* 2013;**368**:904–13.

41. **Kidwell CS, Jahan R, & Saver JL.** Endovascular treatment for acute ischemic stroke. *N Engl J Med* 2013;**368**:2434–5.

42. **Talke PO, Sharma D, Heyer EJ, Bergese SD, Blackham KA, & Stevens RD.** Society for neuroscience in anaesthesiology and critical care expert consensus statement: anaesthetic management of endovascular treatment for acute ischemic stroke. *Stroke* 2014;**45**:138–50.

43. **Saver JL, Jahan R, Levy E, et al.** Solitaire flow restoration device versus the Merci retriever in patients with acute ischaemic stroke (swift): a randomised, parallel-group, non-inferiority trial. *Lancet* 2012;**380**:1241–9.

44. **Nogueira RG, Lutsep HL, Gupta R, et al.** Trevo versus Merci retrievers for thrombectomy revascularisation of large vessel occlusions in acute ischaemic stroke (trevo 2): a randomised trial. *Lancet* 2012;**380**:1231–40.

45. **Villwock MR, Singla A, Padalino DJ, et al.** Acute ischaemic stroke outcomes following mechanical thrombectomy in the elderly versus their younger counterpart: a retrospective cohort study. *BMJ Open* 2014;**4**:e004480.

46. **Goyal M, Menon K, van Zwam WH et al., for the HERMES collaborators.** Endovascular thrombectomy after large-vessel ischaemic stroke: a meta-analysis of individual patient data from five randomised trials. *Lancet* 2016;**387**(10029):1723–31.

47. **Campbell BC, Hill MD, Rubiera M, et al.** Safety and efficacy of solitaire stent thrombectomy: individual patient data meta-analysis of randomized trials. *Stroke* 2016;**47**:798–806.

48. **Kim DH, Kim SU, Sung JH, Lee DH, Yi HJ, & Lee SW.** Significances and outcomes of mechanical thrombectomy for acute infarction in very elderly patients: a single center experience. *J Korean Neurosurg Soc* 2017;**60**(6):654–60.

49. **Figueiredo S, Carvalho A, Rodrigues M, et al.** Endovascular stroke treatment of patients over 80 years old: cumulative evidence from the "real world". *J Stroke Cerebrovasc Dis* 2017;**26**(12):2949–53.

50. **Imahori T, Tanaka K, Arai A, et al.** Mechanical thrombectomy for acute ischemic stroke patients aged 80 years or older. *J Stroke Cerebrovasc Dis* 2017;**26**(12):2793–9.

51. **Nogueira RG, Jadhav AP, Haussen DC, et al. for the DAWN Trial Investigators.** Thrombectomy 6 to 24 hours after stroke with a mismatch between deficit and infarct. *N Engl J Med* 2018; **378**:11–21.

52. **Albers GW, Marks MP, Kemp S, et al. for the DEFUSE 3 Investigators.** Thrombectomy for stroke at 6 to 16 hours with selection by perfusion imaging. *N Engl J Med* 2018;**378**:708–18.

53. **Dunnell K.** Ageing and mortality in the UK—national statistician's annual article on the population. *Population Trends* 2008;**134**:6–23.

Chapter 10

Intracerebral haemorrhage in older people

Zhe Kang Law and Nikola Sprigg

A brief overview of cerebral haemorrhage

Intracranial haemorrhage refers to any accumulation of blood within the cranial vault.[1] Intracranial haemorrhage comprises intracerebral haemorrhage, subarachnoid haemorrhage, subdural haemorrhage, and extradural haemorrhage.[2,3] Intracerebral haemorrhage refers to bleeding within brain parenchyma and may occur with or without intraventricular extension.[4] Subdural haemorrhage or haematoma refers to accumulation of blood within the subdural space (between the dura and arachnoid layers of meninges). Extradural or epidural haemorrhage refers to accumulation of blood in the extradural space (i.e. between the dura mater and skull).[2] Subarachnoid haemorrhage refers to bleeding in the subarachnoid space (i.e. between the arachnoid and pia mater).[2] The subarachnoid space is where the circle of Willis and major intracranial arteries lie.

Intracerebral haemorrhage (ICH) and subarachnoid haemorrhage (SAH) are two types of haemorrhagic strokes as they are of presumed vascular aetiology. On the other hand, subdural and extradural haemorrhages are almost always secondary to head trauma. This chapter will focus mainly on intracerebral haemorrhage.

Intracerebral haemorrhage

Introduction

Intracerebral haemorrhage is a common and devastating medical emergency. Approximately 10–15% of all strokes are intracerebral haemorrhage.[5] The 30-day median mortality rate in ICH is 40%.[6] Increasing age is associated with increasing incidence of intracerebral haemorrhage. The incidence ratio of spontaneous ICH is nearly 10 times greater in people ≥85 years compared to people <55 years.[6] In addition, an older age is an independent poor prognostic factor in ICH. The risk of death or dependency 90 days post-ICH was four times higher in people ≥75 years compared to those <52 years.[7] Prompt diagnosis and optimal management of ICH is highly relevant for older people.

Risk factors

Hypertension is the most important risk factor for ICH, increasing the risk by three to five times.[8] Other risk factors include older age, male sex, alcohol excess, and smoking.[8] These risk factors lead to degenerative changes in cerebral blood vessels, with consequent weakening and rupture. Anticoagulation and antiplatelet therapy increases the risk of ICH; with anticoagulation carrying the higher risk. With an increasing prevalence of cardiovascular diseases with age, more elderly people are taking antithrombotic agents.[9] Furthermore, the risk of antithrombotic-related ICH is higher in older people, in part due to the higher prevalence of cerebrovascular diseases including cerebral amyloid angiopathy and cerebral small vessel disease.[10] Diabetes is a minor risk factor for ICH, if at all. The role of hypercholesterolaemia in ICH is controversial, with various studies reporting no association, increased and reduced risk of ICH with hypercholesterolaemia.[11-14] Similarly the risk of ICH with statin therapy is uncertain. The Stroke Prevention by Aggressive Reduction in Cholesterol Levels (SPARCL) trial reported a slight increase in risk of ICH with statins.[15] However, a meta-analysis of 31 randomized controlled trials reported no significant increase in ICH with statin therapy.[16]

Causes of intracerebral haemorrhage

The two most common causes of ICH are hypertension and cerebral amyloid angiopathy (CAA), accounting for approximately 70–80% of ICH.[17] Other less common causes (Table 10.1) are important to identify, as there are specific treatment options.

Hypertensive ICH

Long-standing poorly controlled hypertension can result in degenerative changes in the cerebral arterial wall: fibrinoid necrosis, lipohyalinosis, and formation of Charcot-Bouchard microaneuryms.[18] Rupture of penetrating arteries or arterioles affected by hypertensive vascular changes causes ICH in deep-seated locations such as basal ganglia, thalamus, cerebellum, and brainstem, though lobar haemorrhage may occur as well.[19] However, hypertension is not the only cause of deep-seated ICH. Only 50–70% of patients with deep-seated ICH were hypertensive.[14,20,21] On the other hand, acute hypertensive response occurs in approximately 60% of ICH in the first 24 hours and may be a result of raised intracranial pressure, dysregulated autonomic system, and stress response.[22] Hence, the finding of elevated blood pressure during acute phase of ICH may not indicate hypertension as the cause of ICH. In summary, most deep-seated ICHs are hypertensive related, though alternative causes should be considered.

Cerebral amyloid angiopathy

Sporadic CAA is predominantly a disease of older people. It affects 33% of people aged 60–70 years with increasing prevalence of up to 75% in those more than 90 years old.[23] It rarely affects people below the age of 55 years. In addition, APOE ε4 and ε2 alleles are risk factors for development of CAA and CAA-related ICH.[24]

Sporadic CAA is characterized by deposition of β-amyloid (Aβ) in the media and adventitia of small and medium blood vessels in the cortex and leptomeninges.[25] A varying degree of CAA is recognized from pathological studies. Mild CAA appeared as Congo red staining of the smooth muscles in tunica media; moderate CAA results in progressive wall thickening and amyloid infiltration of tunica media, while severe CAA results in double barrelling of the vessel wall, development of microaneurysms, and fibrinoid necrosis.[26] Spontaneous ICH occurs when the vessels weakened by CAA rupture. CAA often coexists with chronic hypertension. Though hypertension is not a risk factor for CAA, elevated blood pressure may increase the risk of CAA-related ICH.[26] A subgroup analysis of the PROGRESS trial showed that lowering BP by 9/4 mmHg with perindopril and indapamide in patients with CAA-related ICH reduced the risk of recurrence by 77%.[27]

In addition, CAA may result in small vessel ischaemia resulting from vasculopathic occlusion, thus increasing the risk of ischaemic stroke. Other clinical spectrums of CAA include cognitive impairment, transient neurological symptoms, seizures, and acute inflammatory encephalopathy.[26]

Diagnosing CAA is important as CAA-related ICH has a high recurrence rate of between 10% and 22% per year.[28, 29] Furthermore, CAA may increase the risk of anticoagulation-related ICH

Table 10.1 Causes of intracerebral haemorrhage

Causes	Characteristics	Specific treatment
Common in older people		
Hypertensive arteriopathy	Deep-seated haematoma in basal ganglia, thalamus, and brainstem. Presence of cerebral microbleeds in the same region, white matter lesion, old lacunes, and long-standing uncontrolled hypertension are supportive.	Secondary prevention with optimal blood pressure control.
Cerebral amyloid angiopathy	Multiple lobar haematomas in cortical/subcortical areas. Presence of cerebral microbleeds in cortical/subcortical areas, cortical superficial siderosis, leukoaraiosis and absence of hypertension are supportive (Fig. 10.1).	Optimizing blood pressure control if hypertension is comorbidity. Avoidance of anticoagulation therapy is controversial and should be individualized (see 'Restarting antithrombotics after intracerebral haemorrhage').
Cerebral small vessel disease	White matter lesion, lacunar infarction, lacunes, perivascular spaces, cerebral microbleeds and atrophy are radiological features of cerebral small vessel disease.	Optimizing blood pressure and glycaemic control, smoking cessation, and moderation of alcohol intake.
Anticoagulation related	History of anticoagulant intake and abnormal coagulation profile. DOACs may not cause abnormality on coagulation profile. Heterogeneous density or fluid level within the haematoma is suggestive.	Reversal of anticoagulation effects with four-factor prothrombin complex concentrates and specific antidotes (idarucizumab for dabigatran).
Haemorrhagic transformation of cerebral infarctions	History of recent large ischaemic infarction. May occur after intravenous thrombolysis or endovascular therapy.	Avoidance of antiplatelet therapy or anticoagulant for a specific timeframe, depending on size of infarction.
Uncommon in older people		
Haemorrhagic brain metastasis	Multiple brain lesions and history of prior/current malignancy.	Treatment options include radiotherapy, surgical excision, chemotherapy, and high-dose corticosteroids depending on type of primary malignancy.
Cerebral venous thrombosis	Bilateral midline haemorrhage with infarction is suggestive. Contrast-enhanced CT shows empty delta sign. Flow void on CTV or MRV.	Anticoagulation therapy should be started despite ICH for 3 to 6 months at least. Intrasinus thrombolysis or mechanical thrombectomy may be considered if thrombus progresses despite anticoagulation.

(*continued*)

Table 10.1 Continued

Causes	Characteristics	Specific treatment
Arteriovenous malformation	ICH commonly occurs between 20 and 40 years old. Consist of a tangle of abnormal arteries and veins, known as nidus with early venous drainage and occasional intranidal feeding artery or venous aneurysm. Typically described as 'bag of worms' appearance on MRI. DSA is the gold standard for diagnosis and assessment of AVM architecture.	Surgical resection, endovascular embolization, and radiosurgery are three treatment options. Unruptured AVMs are best treated conservatively.
Cavernous malformation	Commonly presents at 40–60 years old. 'Popcorn'-like appearance on MRI—consisting of a mixed signal core indicating haemorrhage of different ages and T2 hypointense haemosiderin rim. Blooming effect on T2 GRE or SWI.	Treated with surgical resection.
Dural arteriovenous fistula	Commonly present at 50–60 years old. May present with pulsatile tinnitus, cranial neuropathies, and proptosis. CT or MRI shows dilated cortical veins manifesting as multiple flow void tubular structures along cortical sulci.	Treated with endovascular interventions, surgical resection, or stereotactic radiosurgery.
Intracranial aneurysm	May have concurrent subarachnoid haemorrhage as well. DSA is gold standard in diagnosing aneurysm— appear as outpouching of an arterial wall segment.	Endovascular coiling or surgical clipping of aneurysm. Oral nimodipine should be used to prevent vasospasms.
Septic or mycotic embolism	Fever, raised leukocytes, and other signs of septicaemia. Echocardiogram may reveal vegetation, diagnostic of subacute bacterial endocarditis.	Prolonged course of intravenous antibiotics.

AVM, arteriovenous malformation; CTV, computed tomography venography; DSA, digital subtraction angiography; DOAC, Direct oral anti-coagulant; GRE, gradient-recalled echo; MRI, magnetic resonance imaging; MRV, magnetic resonance venography; SWI, susceptibility-weighted imaging.

and post-thrombolysis haemorrhagic transformation.[30] This has important bearing when considering anticoagulation, antiplatelet therapy, and thrombolysis in older people.

Superficial lobar haemorrhage, multiple or recurrent haemorrhage, and the presence of convexity subarachnoid haemorrhage are supportive of the diagnosis of CAA. CAA-related ICH most commonly affects occipital and temporal lobes, followed by frontal and parietal lobes. CAA may also cause cerebellar haemorrhage, but most brainstem haemorrhages are not CAA related.[31,32]

Magnetic resonance imaging (MRI) is a useful tool for diagnosis of CAA. In particular, susceptibility-weighted imaging (SWI) or T2*gradient-recalled echo (GRE) is highly sensitive in demonstrating haemosiderin deposition from previous haemorrhage. Cerebral microbleeds in the cortical–subcortical junction and cortical superficial siderosis demonstrated on SWI or GRE MRI are two characteristic signs of CAA (Fig. 10.1).[33] However, these signs are not pathognomonic. Cerebral microbleeds are also found in hypertensive arteriopathy, though their locations are mostly in the deep-seated areas (basal ganglia, thalamus, brainstem). Cavernous malformation

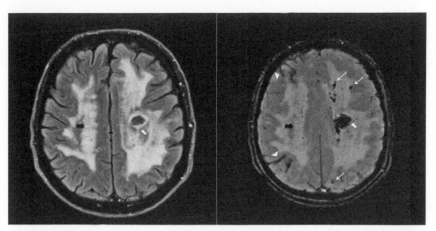

Fig. 10.1 MRI FLAIR image (left panel) showing left cortical superficial haematoma (thick white arrow) and extensive white matter disease (black arrow). Susceptibility-weighted imaging (right panel) showing numerous cerebral microbleeds (thin white arrow) and cortical superficial siderosis (white arrowheads).

Department of Medicine, National University of Malaysia, Kuala Lumpur, Malaysia.

is also associated with cerebral microhaemorrhage. Cortical superficial siderosis is indicative of previous subarachnoid haemorrhage and support the diagnosis of CAA if present in the cortical convexity. Patients with cortical superficial siderosis may present with recurrent amyloid 'spells' (see 'Clinical features').[34] Apart from diagnostic significance, a greater number of cerebral microbleeds and the presence of cortical superficial siderosis are prognostic markers for recurrent ICH. CAA may also cause small vessel disease manifesting as leukoaraiosis on MRI or computed tomography (CT). The Boston diagnostic criteria for CAA are widely accepted (Box 10.1).[35] In addition, the Edinburgh CT and genetic diagnostic criteria used three criteria: finger-like projections, subarachnoid haemorrhage on CT, and APOE ε4 possession on genetic testing to diagnose CAA in lobar haemorrhage (Fig. 10.2).[36] The presence of at least two of the three criteria indicates a high probability of moderate to severe CAA with a high rule-in specificity of 96%.[36]

Cerebral small vessel disease

Cerebral small vessel disease refers to disorders affecting small arteries, arterioles, and rarely veins of cerebral circulation. This is often diagnosed radiologically as lacunar infarction, lacunes, white matter lesions, perivascular spaces, cerebral microbleeds, and atrophy.[37] There is considerable overlap between cerebral small vessel disease with hypertensive arteriopathy and cerebral amyloid angiopathy, as both hypertension and CAA are causes of cerebral small vessel disease. However, cerebral small vessel disease may occur in older people as a result of age-related arteriolosclerosis without coexisting hypertension or CAA. Other causes of cerebral small vessel disease include genetic (cerebral autosomal-dominant arteriopathy with subcortical infarcts and leukoencephalopathy—CADASIL), immune-mediated, and venous collagenosis, which are all uncommon in older people.[38] The clinical manifestations of cerebral small vessel disease include ischaemic stroke, ICH, cognitive impairment, dementia, mood disturbance, and gait disorder.[38] Identification of this neurological entity is important, as it is an independent predictor of poor outcome after ICH.[39] In addition, the presence of cerebral small vessel disease on CT scan correlates strongly with normal vasculature on digital subtraction angiography.[40] Hence, invasive imaging for vascular abnormalities is not necessary in older people with cerebral small vessel disease.

Box 10.1 Boston criteria for diagnosis of cerebral amyloid angiopathy

Criteria for diagnosis of CAA

Definite CAA:

Full post-mortem examination reveals lobar, cortical, or cortical/subcortical haemorrhage and pathological evidence of severe cerebral amyloid angiopathy

Probable CAA with supporting pathological evidence:

Clinical data and pathological tissue from evacuated haematoma or cortical biopsy demonstrate an ICH in typical location and some degree of vascular amyloid deposition

Probable CAA:

Pathological confirmation not required
Age ≥ 55 years
Appropriate clinical history
MRI findings reveal multiple haemorrhages of varying sizes/ages with no other explanation

Possible CAA:

Age ≥ 55 years
Appropriate clinical history
MRI findings reveal a single lobar, cortical, or cortical/subcortical haemorrhage without another cause, multiple ICH with a possible but not a definite cause, or ICH in an atypical location

Reproduced with permission from Knudsen KA, et al. Clinical diagnosis of cerebral amyloid angiopathy: validation of the Boston criteria. *Neurology*, 56(4), 537–539. Copyright © 2001, American Academy of Neurology. doi:https://doi.org/10.1212/WNL.56.4.537

Anticoagulant-related ICH

Anticoagulant drugs are an increasingly important cause of ICH in older people due to their increasing use. As conditions such as atrial fibrillation, for which anticoagulation is indicated, increase with older age, so does the risk for anticoagulation-related bleeding. Older age and comorbidities associated with advancing age are predictors of bleeding complications. Anticoagulation-related ICH is associated with prolonged haematoma expansion leading to worse outcome.[41,42] In warfarin-related ICH, a supratherapeutic international normalized ratio (INR) of more than 4.0 increases the risk of ICH, though most cases of warfarin-related ICH have therapeutic range INR.[43] Direct oral anticoagulants (DOACs) are being increasingly used in place of warfarin due to their relatively lower risk of ICH and other significant bleeding.

ICH secondary to brain metastasis

Haemorrhagic brain metastasis should be considered as a cause of ICH in older people due to higher incidence of malignancy at this age. Multiple brain lesions or a previous history of malignancy should raise suspicion of brain metastasis. Malignant melanoma, renal cell carcinoma, thyroid carcinoma, breast carcinoma, and bronchogenic carcinoma (mnemonic 'MR-TB') are commonly associated with ICH.[44]

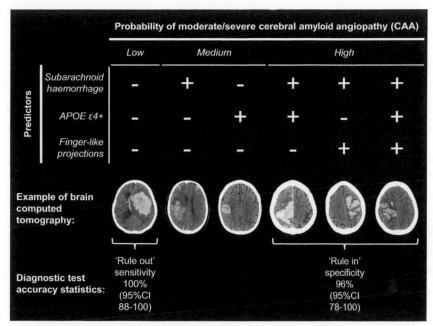

Fig. 10.2 Summary of the Edinburgh diagnostic criteria for lobar ICH associated with CAA, illustrative cases, and the diagnostic test accuracy of two cut-points.

Reproduced from Salman, Rustam Al-Shahi; Rodrigues, Mark. (2017). The Edinburgh diagnostic criteria for lobar intracerebral haemorrhage associated with moderate/severe cerebral amyloid angiopathy, 2010–2016 University of Edinburgh. Centre for Clinical Brain Sciences. Reproduced under the Creative Commons Attribution CC BY 4.0 License (https://creativecommons.org/licenses/by/4.0/).

Uncommon causes of ICH in older people

Other uncommon causes of ICH are listed in Table 10.1. In general, vascular malformations have a genetic predisposition, thus manifesting in early adult life. Despite that fact, these should still be excluded in older people as they may be amenable to endovascular or surgical treatment.

There may be more than one cause of ICH in a patient. For example, a patient with anticoagulant-related ICH may have underlying hypertensive arteriopathy or CAA, which increases the risk of ICH despite therapeutic range INR.

Clinical features

The onset of ICH is often gradual with progression over minutes or hours, as opposed to sub-arachnoid haemorrhage or cardioembolic cerebral infarction, which present with relatively sudden deterioration. The neurological deficits resulting from ICH depends on the location of the haematoma. The common locations of haematoma include basal ganglia (40–60%), thalamus (~30%), lobar/cortical (~20%), brainstem, or cerebellum (<10%).[45,46] Symptoms are the results of direct damage to the involved region and compression of surrounding tissues. Putaminal haematoma presents as hemiparesis, facial weakness, dysarthria, hemisensory loss, gaze palsy, and homonymous hemianopia. Thalamic haematoma causes hemisensory loss, while expansion of haematoma to midbrain inferiorly causes gaze palsy, cranial nerves palsy, and reduced conscious level. Cortical haematoma causes hemiparesis, hemisensory loss, dysarthria, dysphasia, homonymous hemianopia, and other cortical signs depending on cortical area involved. Cerebellar haematoma manifests as ataxia, clumsiness, and vertigo. Brainstem haematoma often rapidly leads to coma. In addition, quadriparesis, cranial nerve palsies, and gaze palsy may occur with brainstem haematoma. Haematoma at any location can lead to reduced level of consciousness and coma if it causes raised intracranial pressure, hydrocephalus, or cerebral oedema or disrupts the reticular activating system, the pathway responsible for consciousness. Older patients with ICH may also present with delirium and agitation, particularly those with a temporal lobe lesion.

Bleeding into the brain parenchyma *per se* does not cause headache, as brain parenchyma is devoid of pain receptors. However, headache occurs in half of patients with ICH due to stretching of meningeal pain fibres or irritation caused by blood in the cerebrospinal fluid and ventricles. Headache occurs more commonly with large lobar or cerebellar ICH and less commonly in older people, possibly because the presence of cerebral atrophy allows more space for haematoma expansion to occur.[47] Vomiting commonly occurs together with headache and may signify raised intracranial pressure. Neck stiffness is uncommon unless there is concurrent subarachnoid haemorrhage or extensive intraventricular haemorrhage (IVH). Seizures are more common in lobar/cortical haemorrhage and occur in 4–11% of patients with acute ICH.[48–53] In addition, acute hypertensive response occurs in 60% of patients in the first 24 hours.[22,54]

Small ICHs may present with rapidly resolving neurological symptoms resembling a transient ischaemic attack, hence the importance of neuroimaging in patients with clinically diagnosed transient ischaemic attack.[55] CAA may present with transient focal neurological episodes, also known as amyloid 'spells'. There may be positive symptoms: recurrent paraesthesia that spread from fingers to arm and then to face lasting several minutes; or negative: weakness and dysphasia. An MRI may not show any haematoma but instead reveal cortical superficial siderosis in up to half of patients with transient focal neurological episodes.[34] Approximately one-quarter of these patients may have a symptomatic lobar ICH in the following 2 months, hence the importance of recognizing and diagnosing CAA.[34]

Differential diagnosis

Ischaemic stroke

Clinical features of ischaemic stroke are similar to spontaneous ICH. Thrombotic infarction may have a stepwise progression while cardioembolic infarction presents with maximal severity at onset (unless recurrent). Several scoring systems have been designed to distinguish supratentorial ICH from ischaemic stroke clinically, including the Siriraj stroke score and Guy's hospital score.[56, 57] However, clinical scores are unreliable in the diagnosis of ICH making neuroimaging mandatory.[58]

Subarachnoid haemorrhage (SAH)

SAH typically presents with thunderclap headache, described as 'the worst headache ever' evolving to maximum severity over seconds.[59] The suddenness of onset is a better diagnostic feature than severity.[60] Other presentations include focal neurological deficits, impaired consciousness, meningism (neck stiffness, positive Kernig's and Brudzinski's signs), low-grade fever, and seizures.[61–63] About 30–50% of patients have a history of 'sentinel' headache: a sudden and severe headache that precedes more debilitating headache with neurological deficits by 6–20 days, probably a result of minor haemorrhage that stopped.[64] A non-contrast CT brain has a sensitivity of nearly 100% if performed within 6 hours and 97% if done within 3 days.[65] In cases of clinically suspected SAH with negative non-contrast CT, lumbar puncture should be considered to look for xanthochromia.[66] A ruptured intracranial aneurysm may rarely present with intracerebral haemorrhage without subarachnoid haemorrhage.

Subdural haematoma

Subdural haematoma results from tearing of cortical veins that drain into dural sinuses, usually caused by trauma such as falls, although this may be very minor or undetected.[67] Older people are at higher risk of subdural haematoma due to presence of cerebral atrophy and hence the stretching of cortical veins within the subdural space. Rarely, subdural haemorrhage may complicate intracerebral haemorrhage or subarachnoid haemorrhage. Anticoagulant and antiplatelet therapy may increase the risk of subdural haemorrhage.[68]

The typical presentation of acute subdural haematoma is of rapid decline in consciousness and neurological deficits. Although typically described in epidural haematoma, lucid interval occurs in about 12–38% of people with acute subdural haematoma, when the patient appears relatively well for a few hours before having progressive neurological deterioration.[69] Posterior fossa subdural haematoma may present with rapid decline in consciousness, headache, vomiting, cranial nerve palsies, and meningism, similar to the presentation of a posterior fossa ICH. On the other hand, chronic subdural haematoma presents more insidiously with headache, falls, focal neurological deficits, cognitive impairment, dizziness, reduced consciousness level, and seizures.[70]

Other space occupying lesions

Brain tumours and metastasis may present with focal neurological deficits, although the onset is often gradual. Other causes of space occupying lesion include extradural haematoma and brain abscess. Extradural haematoma is uncommon in people older than 50 to 60 years.

Hemiplegic migraine

Hemiplegic migraine is characterized by episodes of typical migraine with aura and accompanying motor aura (hemiparesis). The patients may have severe headache, visual, sensory, and aphasic aura as well.[71] Rarely, severe attacks of hemiplegic migraine may cause encephalopathy and coma.[72]

Todd's paralysis

Todd's paralysis is transient postictal hemiparesis that last less than 24 hours. Patients with structural lesion as well as older people have a higher risk of Todd's paralysis. Todd's paralysis typically presents with weakness of an upper limb, lower limb, or both that occurs after a focal seizure involving that limb in patients with pre-existing epilepsy.[73] The occurrence of postictal headache may raise the possibility of ICH. Neuroimaging would not show any new lesions in patients with Todd's paralysis.

Investigations

Neuroimaging

CT is usually the first-line neuroimaging in diagnosing spontaneous ICH. Acute haematoma appears hyperdense (40–60 Hounsfield units) on CT scan before the evolution to isodense then hypodense over few days to weeks.[74] In addition, MRI is equally accurate in diagnosing ICH, although the appearance of haematoma on MRI depends on the sequence and timing of scan (Table 10.2).[74]

Apart from diagnosis of ICH, neuroimaging is important for the detection of complications of ICH in the acute stage. Haematoma expansion, hydrocephalus, intraventricular extension of haemorrhage, perihaematomal oedema, midline shift, and herniation are common complications of spontaneous ICH that result in neurological deterioration after spontaneous ICH (Fig. 10.3).

Table 10.2 Appearance and evolution of haematoma on MRI

Stage	Time	T1	T2-	DWI	T2*GRE/ SWI
Hyperacute	<24 hours	Hypointense	Hyperintense	Hyperintense	Hypointense
Acute	1–3 days	Isointense/ hypointense	Hypointense	Hypointense	Hypointense
Early subacute	> 3 days	Hyperintense	Hypointense	Hypointense	Hypointense
Late Subacute	> 7 days	Hyperintense	Hyperintense	Hyperintense	Hypointense
Chronic	>14 days	Isointense/ hypointense	Hypointense	Hypointense	Hypointense

DWI, diffusion-weighted imaging; GRE, gradient-recalled echo; SWI, susceptibility-weighted imaging.

CT scan is the best modality to diagnose these complications, as the patients may be medically unstable or too restless to undergo MRI.

Neuroimaging is crucial to explore the underlying aetiologies for spontaneous ICH (Table 10.3). As vascular/structural causes of ICH are rare in older people, should we include vascular/structural neuroimaging as part of the routine investigations? One study suggested that even among older, hypertensive patients with deep-seated haemorrhage, a vascular anomaly is picked up in up to 20% of patients.[75] In patients with ICH who are otherwise medically well, a non-invasive vascular (computed tomography angiography (CTA) and/or magnetic resonance angiography (MRA)) and structural (MRI) neuroimaging should be considered. CTA and MRA are highly sensitive in detecting vascular anomalies. On the other hand, invasive procedures such as digital subtraction angiography should be reserved for those with particular high risk of vascular abnormality in whom intervention is anticipated.

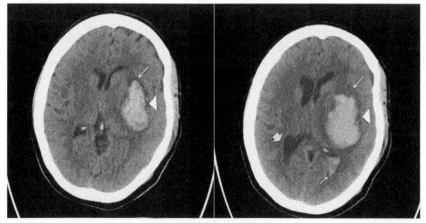

Fig. 10.3 Non-contrast CT scan (left panel) showing left basal ganglia haematoma (white arrowhead) with perihaematomal oedema (thin white arrow) and mass effect. A repeat CT scan 24 hours later (right panel) showed haematoma expansion (white arrowhead), worsening perihaematomal oedema (hypodense area, thin white arrow), mass effect, intraventricular extension of haemorrhage (yellow thin arrow), and hydrocephalus (yellow thick arrow).

Department of Medicine, National University of Malaysia, Kuala Lumpur, Malaysia.

Table 10.3 Investigation of patients with ICH

Investigations	Indication/justification	Comment
Neuroimaging CT, CTA, MRI, and MRA	For diagnosis of ICH and detection of complications Investigation for aetiology of ICH	Mandatory unless moribund at presentation
DSA	Investigation for aetiology of ICH (intracranial aneurysm and vascular anomalies)	Selected patients
Full blood count	Thrombocytopenia increases the risk of haematoma expansion. Raised white cell count and anaemia associated with poorer outcome	Mandatory
C-Reactive protein	Raised C-Reactive protein is a predictor of poorer outcome	Optional
Renal profile	The risk of haematoma expansion is greater in patients with renal failure. Hyponatraemia secondary to SIADH or cerebral salt wasting syndrome is a complication of ICH, and may lead to neurological deterioration	Mandatory
Coagulation profile	Coagulopathy leads to haematoma expansion and needs to be corrected	Mandatory
Anti-Xa, ECT, dTT	Specific test to detect anticoagulant activity in patients on DOACs	Selected patients
Troponin I/T	Raised troponin levels is a negative prognostic factor	Optional
Serum glucose	Higher glucose level is associated with worse outcome. Hypoglycaemia is a stroke mimic	Mandatory
Liver function test	Chronic liver disease may lead to coagulopathy and cause ICH	Mandatory
Electrocardiography	Detection of left ventricular hypertrophy is supportive of chronic hypertension	Optional

CT, computed tomography; CTA, computed tomography angiography; ECT, ecarin clotting time; DSA, digital subtraction angiography; dTT, diluted thrombin time; MRA, magnetic resonance angiography; MRI, magnetic resonance imaging; DOAC, direct oral anticoagulant; SIADH, syndrome of inappropriate antidiuretic hormone secretion.

Management of intracerebral haemorrhage

Acute stroke unit/intensive care unit

The benefit of organized stroke care for stroke patients is established. A systematic review pooling data from 5855 patients concluded that admission to an acute stroke unit improves outcome in terms of death and dependency (OR 0.79, 95% CI 0.68–0.90; $P = 0.0007$).[75] Patients with ICH showed similar reduction in death and dependency compared to patients with ischaemic stroke (Table 10.4).[76,77] In addition, a subgroup analysis comparing those <75 years and ≥75 years showed similar benefits on functional outcome in older people as well.[76] A meta-analysis that included ischaemic stroke and ICH suggested that better care planning in stroke units including prevention of aspiration, avoidance of urinary catheters, use of oxygen for hypoxia and paracetamol for fever, may have led to better outcome.[78] In addition, continuous monitoring of physiological parameters blood pressure, heart rate, oxygen saturation, temperature, and electrocardiogram (ECG) carried out in a stroke unit ensure early detection and treatment of complications.[79]

Table 10.4 General medical management in intracerebral haemorrhage

Management	Comments
Acute stroke unit	All patients should be admitted to acute stroke unit with close monitoring of vital signs and neurological status (GCS and neurological deficits).
DNAR order	DNAR order should be made with caution in the first few days so it would not affect active medical or surgical care.
Blood pressure reduction	Blood pressure should be lowered to SBP <140 mmHg in patients presenting within 6 hours of onset. However, excessive reduction of SBP to ~120 mmHg should be avoided.
Correcting coagulopathy	Four-factor PCC should be given as soon as possible to warfarin-related ICH targeting normalization of INR. Idaricizumab should be given to dabigatran-related ICH. Andexanet may be given for anti-Xa related ICH if available locally.
Thromboprophylaxis	Intermittent pneumatic compression should be used for thromboprophylaxis. Graduated compression stockings should be avoided. The role of low-molecular-weight heparin (LMWH) is unclear and cannot be recommended.
Dysphagia screening	All patients should have formal swallowing assessment prior to commencement of oral feeding.
Antiepileptic agents	Patients with clinical seizures should be treated with antiepileptic agents.
Fever and infection	Temperature of >38°C should be lowered. Empirical antibiotics should be started for suspected infection.
Glycaemic control	Avoidance of hypo- or hyperglycaemia (aiming for blood glucose level of 5–15 mmol/litre).
Hydration	Dehydration and overhydration should be avoided. Dextrose containing fluid should be avoided.
Bowel care	Constipation should be prevented by stool softener/laxative.
Neurosurgery	Hydrocephalus should be treated with EVD insertion. Posterior decompression should be performed for cerebellar haemorrhage >3 cm and those with obstructive hydrocephalus. Certain patients with supratentorial haematoma may benefit from craniotomy (see text).

EVD, external ventricular drain; GCS, Glasgow Coma Scale; PCC, Prothrombin Complex Concentrate; DNACPR, Do not attempt cardiopulmonary resuscitation.

Blood pressure reduction in acute ICH

Elevated blood pressure is deleterious in ICH, leading to worse functional outcome, death, and haematoma expansion.[80,81] Elevated arterial blood pressure may elevate the hydrostatic pressure within the haematoma, increasing the extravasation of blood, resulting in haematoma expansion and oedema formation.[80] At the same time, the mass effect of the haematoma is thought to impede blood supply to perihaematomal tissues, causing perihaematomal ischaemia, and excessive lowering of blood pressure may exacerbate this effect. This is a particular concern in older people where cerebral autoregulation may be impaired.[82] However, empirical evidence suggests that this is untrue. A zone of perihaematomal hypoperfusion without ischaemia was demonstrated in a positron emission tomography (PET) imaging study.[83] A study of diffusion-weighted MRI and proton magnetic resonance spectroscopy concluded there was no perihaematomal ischaemia.[84]

In several large clinical trials, intensive blood pressure reduction was shown to be safe and may be effective in improving outcome. In the INTERACT trial (n = 404) intensive blood pressure reduction to systolic blood pressure (SBP) of less than 140 mmHg significantly reduced haematoma expansion (mean haematoma volume difference of 3.15 ml at 24 hours, $P = 0.004$).[85] Similarly, the INTERACT-2, ATACH, and ATACH-2 trials reported non-significant reduction in haematoma expansion with intensive blood pressure reduction.[86–88] In the INTERACT-2 trial, intensive blood pressure reduction showed a trend towards improvement of functional outcome based on secondary analysis of ordinal shift of modified Rankin scale scores (OR 0.87; 95% CI, 0.77–1.00; $P = 0.04$).[86] In the ATACH-2 trial, the intensive blood pressure reduction arm achieved a mean minimum blood pressure of 129 mmHg compared to 141 mmHg in standard blood pressure control, but showed no beneficial effect.

Intensive blood pressure reduction to SBP of <140 mmHg is probably safe and may be effective and should be started within 6 hours of ICH. Excessive lowering to SBP to 110–120 is not necessary and may be harmful. However, a question remains whether the results of these trials apply to older people? In general, patients in the INTERACT, INTERACT-2 and ATACH-2 trial were in the 'young-old' age group with a mean/median age of 62 to 64 years. In addition, subgroup analysis of the INTERACT and INTERACT-2 showed no difference in the ≥65 years group compared to <65 years. Hence, there is no evidence that blood pressure treatment in older people with acute ICH should be different. However, long-term blood pressure control may need to be individualized (see 'Prevention of recurrent ICH').

Reversal of anticoagulation

In vitamin K antagonist-related ICH, intravenous vitamin K, prothrombin complex concentrate (PCC) and fresh frozen plasma (FFP) are effective haemostatic agents. PCC is more effective than FFP in reversal of anticoagulation. The INR Normalization in Coumadin Associated Intracerebral Haemorrhage (INCH) trial found that four-factor PCC reversed INR to less than 1.2 within 3 hours in 67% (18 of 27 patients) compared to FFP (9%, 2 of 23 patients) in sICH.[89] Protocols should be in place to reduce delay in giving PCC, including implementing point-of-care INR measurement and storage of PCC in emergency departments or hyperacute stroke units.[90]

ICH secondary to direct oral anticoagulants (DOACs-dabigatran, rivaroxaban, apixaban, and edoxaban) may be treated similarly with PCC and FFP. In addition, a specific reversal agent, idarucizumab, is available for dabigatran.[91] Idarucizumab normalizes diluted thrombin time and ecarin thrombin time within minutes in 88–98% of patients.[92] Andexanet alfa, a reversal agent for direct and indirect factor Xa inhibitor, was found to reverse the anti-Xa activities of rivaroxaban and apixaban within minutes of administration.[92,93] It was tested in a single-arm study among 352 patients who had intracranial and other major bleeding secondary to rivaroxaban, apixaban, edoxaban, and enoxaparin. Good or excellent haemostasis was achieved in 82% of the patients within 12 hours.[93,94] Andexanet alfa was approved as an antidote in May 2018.[95] The role of an antifibrinolytic agent, tranexamic acid in DOAC-related ICH, is being examined.[96]

Surgery

Selected patients may benefit from neurosurgery in ICH, depending on haematoma location, presence of complications, severity of ICH, and overall prognosis.

Infratentorial haematoma Posterior decompression is life-saving in large cerebellar haematoma (>3 cm) and those that resulted in obstructive hydrocephalus.[97] In addition, external ventricular drainage (EVD) reduces intracranial pressure and drains cerebrospinal fluid in patients with hydrocephalus. Conversely, brainstem haemorrhages are treated conservatively.

Supratentorial haematoma The role of craniotomy and evacuation of clot for supratentorial haematomas is less clear. The International Surgical Trial in Intracerebral Haemorrhage (STICH) trial was a prospective trial that randomized 1033 patients with ICH to early surgical haematoma evacuation or initial conservative treatment. There was no significant difference in outcome between the two groups.[98] However, a subgroup analysis of the trial showed that patients with superficial haematoma (<1 cm from surface) benefited from early surgery. The trial also found that patients with poor initial Glasgow Coma Scale (GCS) of less than 8 and IVH had poor outcome despite surgery.[98]

The subsequent STICH II trial randomized 601 patients with superficial lobar haematoma, with haematoma volume of 10–100 ml and without intraventricular extension to undergo early surgery or initial conservative management. There was a small absolute reduction in mortality of 6% and increase in favourable outcomes of 4% in the early surgery arm, although the difference was not statistically significant.[99] One reason that may explain this result is that the trial recruited patients who were conscious or mildly confused who might not benefit from surgery, and excluded those in whom chances of successful surgery were greatest. Patients with GCS of between 9 and 12 benefited from early surgery.[99] A meta-analysis including STICH II and 14 other trials (3366 patients) concluded overall benefit for early surgery (OR 0.74; 95% CI 0.64–0.86).[99] However, the meta-analysis should be interpreted cautiously as there was significant heterogeneity in the trials. It is unclear whether surgical intervention might benefit certain subgroups of patients. Subgroup analysis of STICH and STICH II showed no differences in outcome between patients ≥65 years and <65 years. The current European Stroke Organisation (ESO) guideline does not recommend routine surgery for supratentorial haematoma, though early surgery may be considered in patients with GCS of 9–12.[100] Similarly, the American Heart Association/American Stroke Association (AHA/ASA) guideline does not recommend routine surgery for supratentorial haematoma except in patients who are deteriorating.[101]

Minimally invasive surgery for clot evacuation was evaluated in the Minimally Invasive Surgery and rt-PA in ICH Evacuation phase II (MISTIE II) trial. The trial found that minimal invasive surgery, whether alone or with intraclot recombinant tissue-type plasminogen activator (rt-PA), results in greater removal of haematoma and significant reduction in perihaematomal oedema.[102] However, MISTIE II did not include patients ≥75 years. MISTIE III, a phase III randomized controlled trial, found that clot removal with intraclot rt-PA via image-guided catheter did not improve functional outcome in patients with large intracerebral haemorrhage (>30 ml) despite significant reduction in mortality on secondary analysis.[103] In view of these results, minimally invasive surgery cannot be routinely recommended.

Presence of complications In patients with hydrocephalus and IVH, EVD reduces and monitors intracranial pressure.[104] Decompressive craniectomy may be life-saving in patients with rapid deterioration secondary to mass effects.[105] Intraventricular recombinant tissue plasminogen activator (rt-PA) is a promising treatment for IVH. The Clot Lysis: Evaluating Accelerated Resolution of Intraventricular Hemorrhage Phase III (CLEAR III) trial showed no improvement in functional outcome in patients treated with intraventricular rt-PA compared to placebo (relative risk (RR) 1.06, 95% confidence interval (CI) 0.88–1.28; $P = 0.554$) though there was a 50% reduction in odds of death (adjusted OR 0.50, 95% CI 0.31–0.80; $P = 0.004$).[106] A secondary analysis showed that greater volume of IVH removal results in significantly better outcomes (mRS ≤3; adjusted OR 0·96, 95% CI 0.94–0.97; $P < 0.0001$).[106] However, the effects of intraventricular rt-PA in very elderly people could not be ascertained as the trial recruited relatively young patients (mean 59 years) with age ≥80 years as an exclusion criterion.

Severity of ICH and overall prognosis Patients with an initial GCS of ≤8, haematoma volume of ≥60 ml, and IVH have poor prognosis.[107] In addition, age of more than 80 years is associated with worse prognosis.[107] The benefits of intensive care in patients older than 80 years, especially those with medical or unplanned surgical admission are unclear, given the overall poor prognosis of this group of patients.[108] When considering age, frailty should be considered as well. However, although several preoperative frailty assessments are available, evidence of their use in decision-making for emergency neurosurgery in ICH is scant.[109] In summary, the expected benefit of surgery and intensive care, premorbid condition, ICH-specific prognostic factors, and patient's/family's wishes should come into consideration when making individualized decision on active surgical treatment. Patients should not be denied active surgical treatment solely on the basis of being 'too old'.

Prevention of recurrent ICH

Long-term blood pressure control is the most important secondary prevention after ICH. The Perindopril Protection Against Recurrent Stroke Study (PROGRESS; 6105 patients) found that reducing blood pressure by 12/5 mmHg decreased the risk of first and recurrent ICH by 56% and 63%, respectively.[110] The risk reduction is greatest in patients who achieved the lowest follow up blood pressure (median 112/72 mmHg). The effect of blood pressure reduction on preventing recurrence is significant in both hypertensive ICH and CAA-related ICH.[27] In addition, the Secondary Prevention of Small Subcortical Strokes (SPS3) trial showed that in patients with small vessel disease, lowering of blood pressure to <130/80 mmHg reduced the risk of recurrent ICH by up to 60%.[111] Given these results, long-term blood pressure target should be less than 130/80 mmHg in patients with ICH and intervention to reduce blood pressure can be started immediately post-ICH.[101] On the other hand, orthostatic hypotension is a common adverse effect when treating older people with antihypertensive agents. Orthostatic hypotension may increase the risk of cognitive impairment, delirium, and falls in older people.[112–114] In fact, orthostatic hypotension, cognitive impairment, delirium, falls, and intolerance to antihypertensive agents are all markers of frailty.[115] Treating hypertension too aggressively may be harmful. Therefore, blood pressure targets should be individualized according the patient's tolerance to antihypertensive agents.

Other measures for secondary ICH prevention include smoking cessation, moderation of alcohol intake, weight reduction for obese patients, diabetic control, and optimal management of antithrombotics.[101,116] In terms of glycaemic control, treatment targets should be individualized, as avoiding hypoglycaemia is an equally high priority. In frail older people, an HbA1c of ≥8% may be acceptable.[117]

Restarting antithrombotics after intracerebral haemorrhage

Anticoagulants and antiplatelet therapy should be stopped in the first 24 hours after ICH, as the risk of haematoma expansion is the greatest during this interval. Thereafter, it is unclear whether and when antithrombotic should be restarted in patients with clear indication. This clinical dilemma is particularly common in older people as conditions such as prosthetic heart valves or atrial fibrillation becomes increasingly common in the ageing population. The treatment decision should be individualized, weighing the risks and benefits of antithrombotics.

The risk of recurrent ICH is higher in patients with lobar haemorrhage, CAA, and cerebral microbleeds.[29,118,119] A higher number of cerebral microbleeds predicts higher risk of haemorrhage as well. Other risk factors for recurrent ICH include labile INR, advanced age (>65 years), poorly controlled hypertension, and vascular abnormality such as arteriovenous malformation (AVM).[120–122]

On the other hand, older age is an independent risk factor for thromboembolism, for example, in atrial fibrillation. The CHA_2DS_2-VASc score (Congestive cardiac failure-1, Hypertension-1, Age ≥75 years-2, Diabetes mellitus-1, Stroke-2, Vascular disease-1, Age 65 to 74 years-1, and sex category (female)-1) is widely used to predict the risk of thromboembolism in non-valvular atrial fibrillation. The score ranges from 0 to 9 with a risk of nearly 0 when the score is 0 but nearly 15% when the score is 9.[123] In addition, the HASBLED score (Hypertension, Abnormal renal/liver function, Stroke, Bleeding history or predisposition, Labile INR, Elderly (> 65 years), Drugs/alcohol concomitantly) predicts the risk of significant bleeding with anticoagulation.[124] Older age is a risk factor for both thromboembolism and significant bleeding. As a result, it is often a very difficult decision whether to start anticoagulants in older people after ICH, particularly if the risk of both thromboembolism and bleeding is deemed high.

While it is intuitive to avoid anticoagulation after ICH, there are emerging evidences that the benefit of anticoagulation may outweigh the risk in selected patients. A recent individual patient data meta-analysis found that resuming oral anticoagulant after anticoagulant-related ICH was associated with reduced mortality (hazard ratio (HR) = 0.25, 95% CI 0.17 to 0.38; P <0.0001) and favourable outcome (HR = 4.89, 95% CI = 3.25–7.36; P <0.0001) in lobar haemorrhage as well as non-lobar haemorrhage (mortality: HR = 0.22, 95% CI 0.16–0.30; P <0.0001 and improved outcome: HR = 5.12, 95% CI = 3.86–6.80; P <0.0001).[125] Similarly, another meta-analysis found that resumption of oral anticoagulation after ICH in patients with atrial fibrillation reduced the risk of ischaemic stroke (pooled RR 0.47, 95% CI = 0.29–0.77, P = 0.002) without increasing the risk of recurrent ICH (pooled RR 0.93, 95% CI = 0.45–1.90, P = 0.84).[126] However, these meta-analyses are based on data from observational studies. There is currently no established evidence based on randomized controlled trials to guide treatment decision in this respect. A general approach would be avoiding anticoagulant therapy in patients with high risk of recurrent ICH (CAA, presence of microbleeds, lobar haemorrhage, uncontrolled hypertension) with low risk of thromboembolic events.[127] Conversely, in patients with high risk of thromboembolism (prosthetic heart valves, high risk atrial fibrillation, high risk coronary artery disease, intracardiac thrombus) and low risk of recurrent ICH (deep-seated haemorrhage, well-controlled blood pressure) antithrombotic therapy may be considered. Left atrial appendage occlusion is an alternative for stroke prevention in atrial fibrillation when anticoagulation is deemed too high risk.[128] Anticoagulation should be withheld for at least 1–2 weeks after ICH based on observational data.[129]

Considering ageing and frailty in ICH

The physiological effects of ageing influence multiple systems including central nervous system, cardiovascular, renal, endocrine, and immunological systems. The reduced physiological reserves in compensating after an insult contribute to higher systemic complications, less chance for meaningful recovery and poorer functional outcome. This decline in physiological reserves results in frailty. Frailty is defined as a state of increased vulnerability to poor outcomes in the face of a stressor.[130] A frail older person may not recover to previous baseline function even after resolution of a 'minor' stress such as upper respiratory tract infection or falls. The effect of intracerebral haemorrhage on the frail person is even greater, given that it is by no means a 'minor' event. Frailty affects approximately 25–50% of people older than 85 years and is a prognostic factor for poor outcome.[130,131] This leads to frail older people being treated more conservatively in conditions such as diabetes mellitus or cancer. However, using frailty score to guide treatment decisions in intracerebral haemorrhage had not been well studied.

While advanced age is an independent prognostic factor for poor outcome, a higher rate of do-not-attempt-resuscitation (DNAR) order among older people may be a self-fulfilling prophecy.

Early withdrawal of medical care in patients with ICH is an independent factor for poor out-come.[132-134] While a DNAR order means that there should be no attempt for cardiopulmonary resuscitation in case of cardiopulmonary arrest, it should not mean withdrawal of all active medical and surgical care. One study showed that an increase in age of 10 years reduced the odds of transfer to neurosurgical care by 60%, even when active surgical treatment could have improved outcome.[135] While DNAR may be appropriate in some patients, the decision should be made with caution. An early DNAR order could result in suboptimal medical care and poor outcome.[101]

Key messages

♦ CAA should be considered as a cause of intracerebral haemorrhage in older people apart from hypertension.

♦ Transient focal neurological episodes or amyloid 'spells' may be a harbinger of CAA-related haemorrhage.

♦ The decision to restart anticoagulation or antiplatelet therapy should be individualized, taking into account risks and benefits.

♦ Most patients with ICH should be investigated with non-invasive imaging (CTA/MRA/MRI) for underlying causes. Vascular anomalies may be present in 20% of patients with ICH.

♦ All patients with ICH should be managed in acute stroke unit with close monitoring of vital signs and neurological status with protocol to prevent complications. Intermittent pneumatic compression should be used for thromboprophylaxis. Routine swallowing assessment should be done before oral feeding.

♦ Blood pressure should be lowered to SBP of less than 140 mmHg in patients presenting within 6 hours of onset. Long-term blood pressure reduction to a level of less than 130/80 mmHg reduces recurrence. Treatment targets may be individualized in frail or very elderly patients.

♦ Reversal of anticoagulation should be done as soon as possible using four-factor PCC in patients with warfarin-related ICH, idarucizumab for dabigatran-related ICH, and andexanet alfa for anti-Xa related ICH.

♦ Insertion of EVD in patients with hydrocephalus and posterior decompression in patients with cerebellar haematoma is life-saving. Neurosurgery may be beneficial for patients with superficial lobar haemorrhage with intermediate GCS (9–12) or when deteriorating.

♦ Active treatment leads to better outcome. An early DNAR order should be made with caution, even in older people.

References

1. **Caceres JA & Goldstein JN.** Intracranial hemorrhage. *Emerg Med Clin North Am* 2012;30:771–94.
2. **Kidwell CS & Wintermark M.** Imaging of intracranial haemorrhage. *Lancet Neurol* 2008;7:256–67.
3. **Al-Shahi Salman R, Labovitz DL, & Stapf C.** Spontaneous intracerebral haemorrhage. *BMJ* 2009;339:b2586.
4. **Aguilar MI & Brott TG.** Update in intracerebral hemorrhage. *Neurohospitalist* 2011;1:148–59.
5. **Feigin VL, Lawes CM, Bennett DA, Barker-Collo SL, & Parag V.** Worldwide stroke incidence and early case fatality reported in 56 population-based studies: a systematic review. *Lancet Neurol* 2009;8:355–69.
6. **van Asch CJ, Luitse MJ, Rinkel GJ, et al.** Incidence, case fatality, and functional outcome of intracerebral haemorrhage over time, according to age, sex, and ethnic origin: a systematic review and meta-analysis. *Lancet Neurol* 2010;9:167–76.

7. **Radholm K, Arima H, Lindley RI**, et al. Older age is a strong predictor for poor outcome in intracerebral haemorrhage: the INTERACT2 study. *Age Ageing* 2015;**44**:422–7.

8. **Ariesen MJ, Claus SP, Rinkel GJ, & Algra A.** Risk factors for intracerebral hemorrhage in the general population: a systematic review. *Stroke* 2003;**34**:2060–5.

9. **Go AS, Hylek EM, Phillips KA**, et al. Prevalence of diagnosed atrial fibrillation in adults: national implications for rhythm management and stroke prevention: the AnTicoagulation and Risk Factors in Atrial Fibrillation (ATRIA) Study. *JAMA* 2001;**285**:2370–5.

10. **Fang MC, Chang Y, Hylek EM**, et al. Advanced age, anticoagulation intensity, and risk for intracranial hemorrhage among patients taking warfarin for atrial fibrillation. *Ann Intern Med* 2004;**141**:745–52.

11. **Martini SR, Flaherty ML, Brown WM**, et al. Risk factors for intracerebral hemorrhage differ according to hemorrhage location. *Neurology* 2012;**79**:2275–82.

12. **Leppala JM, Virtamo J, Fogelholm R, Albanes D, & Heinonen OP.** Different risk factors for different stroke subtypes: association of blood pressure, cholesterol, and antioxidants. *Stroke* 1999; **30**:2535–40.

13. **Giroud M, Creisson E, Fayolle H**, et al. Risk factors for primary cerebral hemorrhage: a population-based study—the Stroke Registry of Dijon. *Neuroepidemiology* 1995;**14**:20–6.

14. **Thrift AG, McNeil JJ, Forbes A, & Donnan GA.** Three important subgroups of hypertensive persons at greater risk of intracerebral hemorrhage. Melbourne Risk Factor Study Group. *Hypertension* 1998;**31**:1223–9.

15. **Amarenco P, Bogousslavsky J, Callahan A**, 3rd, et al. High-dose atorvastatin after stroke or transient ischemic attack. *N Engl J Med* 2006;**355**:549–59.

16. **McKinney JS & Kostis WJ.** Statin therapy and the risk of intracerebral hemorrhage: a meta-analysis of 31 randomized controlled trials. *Stroke* 2012;**43**:2149–56.

17. **Foulkes MA, Wolf PA, Price TR, Mohr JP, & Hier DB.** The Stroke Data Bank: design, methods, and baseline characteristics. *Stroke* 1988;**19**:547–54.

18. **Fisher CM.** Cerebral miliary aneurysms in hypertension. *Am J Pathol* 1972;**66**:313–30.

19. **Zia E, Hedblad B, Pessah-Rasmussen H**, et al. Blood pressure in relation to the incidence of cerebral infarction and intracerebral hemorrhage. Hypertensive hemorrhage: debated nomenclature is still relevant. *Stroke* 2007;**38**:2681–5.

20. **Saloheimo P, Juvela S, & Hillbom M.** Use of aspirin, epistaxis, and untreated hypertension as risk factors for primary intracerebral hemorrhage in middle-aged and elderly people. *Stroke* 2001;**32**:399–404.

21. **Juvela S, Hillbom M, & Palomaki H.** Risk factors for spontaneous intracerebral hemorrhage. *Stroke* 1995;**26**:1558–64.

22. **Qureshi AI, Ezzeddine MA, Nasar A**, et al. Prevalence of elevated blood pressure in 563,704 adult patients with stroke presenting to the ED in the United States. *Am J Emerg Med* 2007;**25**:32–8.

23. **Yamada M, Tsukagoshi H, Otomo E, & Hayakawa M.** Cerebral amyloid angiopathy in the aged. *J Neurol* 1987;**234**:371–6.

24. **O'Donnell HC, Rosand J, Knudsen KA**, et al. Apolipoprotein E genotype and the risk of recurrent lobar intracerebral hemorrhage. *N Engl J Med* 2000;**342**:240–5.

25. **Attems J, Jellinger K, Thal DR, & Van Nostrand W.** Review: sporadic cerebral amyloid angiopathy. *Neuropathol Appl Neurobiol* 2011;**37**:75–93.

26. **Charidimou A, Gang Q, & Werring DJ.** Sporadic cerebral amyloid angiopathy revisited: recent insights into pathophysiology and clinical spectrum. *J Neurol Neurosurg Psychiatry* 2012;**83**:124–37.

27. **Arima H, Tzourio C, Anderson C**, et al. Effects of perindopril-based lowering of blood pressure on intracerebral hemorrhage related to amyloid angiopathy: the PROGRESS trial. *Stroke* 2010;**41**:394–6.

28. **Vinters HV.** Cerebral amyloid angiopathy. A critical review. *Stroke* 1987;**18**:311–24.

29. **Viswanathan A, Rakich SM, Engel C**, et al. Antiplatelet use after intracerebral hemorrhage. *Neurology* 2006;**66**:206–9.

30. **McCarron MO & Nicoll JA.** Cerebral amyloid angiopathy and thrombolysis-related intracerebral haemorrhage. *Lancet Neurol* 2004;**3**:484–92.

31. **Itoh Y, Yamada M, Hayakawa M, Otomo E, & Miyatake T.** Cerebral amyloid angiopathy: a significant cause of cerebellar as well as lobar cerebral hemorrhage in the elderly. *J Neurol Sci* 1993;**116**:135–41.

32. **Rosand J, Muzikansky A, Kumar A,** et al. Spatial clustering of hemorrhages in probable cerebral amyloid angiopathy. *Ann Neurol* 2005;**58**:459–62.

33. **Linn J, Herms J, Dichgans M,** et al. Subarachnoid hemosiderosis and superficial cortical hemosiderosis in cerebral amyloid angiopathy. *AJNR Am J Neuroradiol* 2008;**29**:184–6.

34. **Charidimou A, Peeters A, Fox Z,** et al. Spectrum of transient focal neurological episodes in cerebral amyloid angiopathy: multicentre magnetic resonance imaging cohort study and meta-analysis. *Stroke* 2012;**43**:2324–30.

35. **Knudsen KA, Rosand J, Karluk D, & Greenberg SM.** Clinical diagnosis of cerebral amyloid angiopathy: validation of the Boston criteria. *Neurology* 2001;**56**:537–9.

36. **Rodrigues MA, Samarasekera N, Lerpiniere C,** et al. The Edinburgh CT and genetic diagnostic criteria for lobar intracerebral haemorrhage associated with cerebral amyloid angiopathy: model development and diagnostic test accuracy study. *Lancet Neurol* 2018;**17**(3):232–40.

37. **Wardlaw JM, Smith EE, Biessels GJ,** et al. Neuroimaging standards for research into small vessel disease and its contribution to ageing and neurodegeneration. *Lancet Neurol* 2013;**12**:822–38.

38. **Pantoni L.** Cerebral small vessel disease: from pathogenesis and clinical characteristics to therapeutic challenges. *Lancet Neurol* 2010;**9**:689–701.

39. **Sato S, Delcourt C, Heeley E,** et al. Significance of cerebral small-vessel disease in acute intracerebral hemorrhage. *Stroke* 2016;**47**:701–7.

40. **Wilson D, Adams ME, Robertson F, Murphy M, & Werring DJ.** Investigating intracerebral haemorrhage. *BMJ* 2015;**350**:h2484.

41. **Flibotte JJ, Hagan N, O'Donnell J, Greenberg SM, & Rosand J.** Warfarin, hematoma expansion, and outcome of intracerebral hemorrhage. *Neurology* 2004;**63**:1059–64.

42. **Lee SB, Manno EM, Layton KF, & Wijdicks EF.** Progression of warfarin-associated intracerebral hemorrhage after INR normalization with FFP. *Neurology* 2006;**67**:1272–4.

43. **Rosand J, Hylek EM, O'Donnell HC, & Greenberg SM.** Warfarin-associated hemorrhage and cerebral amyloid angiopathy: a genetic and pathologic study. *Neurology* 2000;**55**:947–51.

44. **Kondziolka D, Bernstein M, Resch L,** et al. Significance of hemorrhage into brain tumors: clinicopathological study. *J Neurosurg* 1987;**67**:852–7.

45. **Mayer SA, Brun NC, Begtrup K,** et al. Recombinant activated factor VII for acute intracerebral hemorrhage. *N Engl J Med* 2005;**352**:777–85.

46. **Steiner T, Kaste M, Forsting M,** et al. Recommendations for the management of intracranial haemorrhage—part I: spontaneous intracerebral haemorrhage. The European Stroke Initiative Writing Committee and the Writing Committee for the EUSI Executive Committee. *Cerebrovasc Dis* 2006;**22**:294–316.

47. **Melo TP, Pinto AN, & Ferro JM.** Headache in intracerebral hematomas. *Neurology* 1996;**47**:494–500.

48. **Woo KM, Yang SY, & Cho KT.** Seizures after spontaneous intracerebral hemorrhage. *J Korean Neurosurg Soc* 2012;**52**:312–19.

49. **de Greef BT, Schreuder FH, Vlooswijk MC,** et al. Early seizures after intracerebral hemorrhage predict drug-resistant epilepsy. *J Neurol* 2015;**262**:541–6.

50. **Sung CY & Chu NS.** Epileptic seizures in intracerebral haemorrhage. *J Neurol Neurosurg Psychiatry* 1989;**52**:1273–6.

51. **Passero S, Rocchi R, Rossi S, Ulivelli M, & Vatti G.** Seizures after spontaneous supratentorial intracerebral hemorrhage. *Epilepsia* 2002;**43**:1175–80.

52. **Bladin CF, Alexandrov AV, Bellavance A,** et al. Seizures after stroke: a prospective multicenter study. *Arch Neurol* 2000;**57**:1617–22.

53. **Kilpatrick CJ, Davis SM, Tress BM**, et al. Epileptic seizures in acute stroke. *Arch Neurol* 1990;**47**:157–60.

54. **Willmot M, Leonardi-Bee J, & Bath PM.** High blood pressure in acute stroke and subsequent outcome: a systematic review. *Hypertension* 2004;**43**:18–24.

55. **Kumar S, Selim M, Marchina S, & Caplan LR.** Transient neurological symptoms in patients with intracerebral hemorrhage. *JAMA Neurol* 2016;**73**:316–20.

56. **Poungvarin N, Viriyavejakul A, & Komontri C.** Siriraj stroke score and validation study to distinguish supratentorial intracerebral haemorrhage from infarction. *BMJ* 1991;**302**:1565–7.

57. **Sandercock PA, Allen CM, Corston RN, Harrison MJ, & Warlow CP.** Clinical diagnosis of intracranial haemorrhage using Guy's Hospital score. *Br Med J (Clin Res Ed)* 1985;**291**:1675–7.

58. **Weir CJ, Murray GD, Adams FG**, et al. Poor accuracy of stroke scoring systems for differential clinical diagnosis of intracranial haemorrhage and infarction. *Lancet* 1994;**344**:999–1002.

59. **Ducros A & Bousser MG.** Thunderclap headache. *BMJ* 2013;**346**:e8557.

60. **Perry JJ, Stiell IG, Sivilotti ML**, et al. Clinical decision rules to rule out subarachnoid hemorrhage for acute headache. *JAMA* 2013;**310**:1248–55.

61. **Macdonald RL & Schweizer TA.** Spontaneous subarachnoid haemorrhage. *Lancet* 2017;**389**(10069):655–66.

62. **van Gijn J, Kerr RS, & Rinkel GJ.** Subarachnoid haemorrhage. *Lancet* 2007;**369**:306–18.

63. **Butzkueven H, Evans AH, Pitman A**, et al. Onset seizures independently predict poor outcome after subarachnoid hemorrhage. *Neurology* 2000;**55**:1315–20.

64. **Gorelick PB, Hier DB, Caplan LR, & Langenberg P.** Headache in acute cerebrovascular disease. *Neurology* 1986;**36**:1445–50.

65. **Perry JJ, Stiell IG, Sivilotti ML**, et al. Sensitivity of computed tomography performed within six hours of onset of headache for diagnosis of subarachnoid haemorrhage: prospective cohort study. *BMJ* 2011;**343**:d4277.

66. **Steiner T, Juvela S, Unterberg A**, et al. European Stroke Organization guidelines for the management of intracranial aneurysms and subarachnoid haemorrhage. *Cerebrovasc Dis* 2013;**35**:93–112.

67. **Howard MA, 3rd, Gross AS, Dacey RG, Jr., & Winn HR.** Acute subdural hematomas: an age-dependent clinical entity. *J Neurosurg* 1989;**71**:858–63.

68. **Hylek EM & Singer DE.** Risk factors for intracranial hemorrhage in outpatients taking warfarin. *Ann Intern Med* 1994;**120**:897–902.

69. **Bullock MR, Chesnut R, Ghajar J**, et al. Surgical management of acute subdural hematomas. *Neurosurgery* 2006;**58**:S16–24; discussion Si–iv.

70. **Adhiyaman V, Asghar M, Ganeshram KN, & Bhowmick BK.** Chronic subdural haematoma in the elderly. *Postgrad Med J* 2002;**78**:71–5.

71. **Thomsen LL & Olesen J.** Sporadic hemiplegic migraine. *Cephalalgia* 2004;**24**:1016–23.

72. **Russell MB & Ducros A.** Sporadic and familial hemiplegic migraine: pathophysiological mechanisms, clinical characteristics, diagnosis, and management. *Lancet Neurol* 2011;**10**:457–70.

73. **Binder DK.** A history of Todd and his paralysis. *Neurosurgery* 2004;**54**:480–6; discussion 486–7.

74. **Smith EE, Rosand J, & Greenberg SM.** Imaging of hemorrhagic stroke. *Magn Reson Imaging Clin N Am* 2006;**14**:127–40, v.

75. **Cordonnier C, Klijn CJ, van Beijnum J, & Al-Shahi Salman R.** Radiological investigation of spontaneous intracerebral hemorrhage: systematic review and trinational survey. *Stroke* 2010;**41**:685–90.

76. **Stroke Unit Trialists' Collaboration.** Organised inpatient (stroke unit) care for stroke. *Cochrane Database Syst Rev* 2013;**9**:CD000197.

77. **Langhorne P, Fearon P, Ronning OM**, et al. Stroke unit care benefits patients with intracerebral hemorrhage: systematic review and meta-analysis. *Stroke* 2013;**44**:3044–9.

78. **Govan L, Langhorne P, & Weir CJ.** Does the prevention of complications explain the survival benefit of organized inpatient (stroke unit) care?: further analysis of a systematic review. *Stroke* 2007;**38**:2536–40.

79. **Ciccone A, Celani MG, Chiaramonte R, Rossi C, & Righetti E.** Continuous versus intermittent physiological monitoring for acute stroke. *Cochrane Database Syst Rev* 2013;(5):CD008444.

80. **Ohwaki K, Yano E, Nagashima H,** et al. Blood pressure management in acute intracerebral hemorrhage: relationship between elevated blood pressure and hematoma enlargement. *Stroke* 2004;**35**:1364–7.

81. **Qureshi AI.** Acute hypertensive response in patients with stroke: pathophysiology and management. *Circulation* 2008;**118**:176–87.

82. **Matsuda H, Maeda T, Yamada M,** et al. Age-matched normal values and topographic maps for regional cerebral blood flow measurements by Xe-133 inhalation. *Stroke* 1984;**15**:336–342.

83. **Zazulia AR, Diringer MN, Videen TO,** et al. Hypoperfusion without ischemia surrounding acute intracerebral hemorrhage. *J Cereb Blood Flow Metab* 2001;**21**:804–10.

84. **Carhuapoma JR, Wang PY, Beauchamp NJ,** et al. Diffusion-weighted MRI and proton MR spectroscopic imaging in the study of secondary neuronal injury after intracerebral hemorrhage. *Stroke* 2000;**31**:726–32.

85. **Anderson CS, Huang Y, Arima H,** et al. Effects of early intensive blood pressure-lowering treatment on the growth of hematoma and perihematomal edema in acute intracerebral hemorrhage: the Intensive Blood Pressure Reduction in Acute Cerebral Haemorrhage Trial (INTERACT). *Stroke* 2010;**41**:307–12.

86. **Anderson CS, Heeley E, Huang Y,** et al. Rapid blood-pressure lowering in patients with acute intracerebral hemorrhage. *N Engl J Med* 2013;**368**:2355–65.

87. **Qureshi AI, Palesch YY, Martin R,** et al. Effect of systolic blood pressure reduction on hematoma expansion, perihematomal edema, and 3-month outcome among patients with intracerebral hemorrhage: results from the antihypertensive treatment of acute cerebral hemorrhage study. *Arch Neurol* 2010;**67**:570–6.

88. **Qureshi AI, Palesch YY, Barsan WG,** et al. Intensive blood-pressure lowering in patients with acute cerebral hemorrhage. *N Engl J Med* 2016;**375**:1033–43.

89. **Steiner T, Poli S, Griebe M,** et al. Fresh frozen plasma versus prothrombin complex concentrate in patients with intracranial haemorrhage related to vitamin K antagonists (INCH): a randomised trial. *Lancet Neurol* 2016;**15**:566–73.

90. **Parry-Jones A.** Cutting delays in reversing anticoagulation after intraccrebral haemorrhage: three key changes at a UK comprehensive stroke centre. *BMJ Qual Improv Rep* 2015;**4**:u208763.w3521.

91. **Pollack CV, Jr., Reilly PA, Eikelboom J,** et al. Idarucizumab for dabigatran reversal. *N Engl J Med* 2015;**373**:511–20.

92. **Siegal DM, Curnutte JT, Connolly SJ,** et al. Andexanet alfa for the reversal of factor Xa inhibitor activity. *N Engl J Med* 2015;**373**:2413–24.

93. **Connolly SJ, Crowther M, Eikelboom JW,** et al. Full study report of andexanet alfa for bleeding associated with factor Xa inhibitors. *N Engl J Med* 2019;**380**(14):1326–35.

94. **Connolly SJ, Milling TJJ, Eikelboom JW,** et al. Andexanet alfa for acute major bleeding associated with factor Xa inhibitors. *N Engl J Med* 2016;**375**:1131–41.

95. **Heo YA.** Andexanet alfa: first global approval. *Drugs* 2018;**78**(10):1049–55.

96. **Seiffge D, Peters N, Sprigg N,** et al. Treatment of intracerebral hemorrhage in patients on direct oral anticoagulants with tranexamic acid-TICH-DOAC. *Int J Stroke* 2015;**10**:76.

97. **van Loon J, Van Calenbergh F, Goffin J, & Plets C.** Controversies in the management of spontaneous cerebellar haemorrhage. A consecutive series of 49 cases and review of the literature. *Acta Neurochir (Wien)* 1993;**122**:187–93.

98. **Mendelow AD, Gregson BA, Fernandes HM,** et al. Early surgery versus initial conservative treatment in patients with spontaneous supratentorial intracerebral haematomas in the International Surgical Trial in Intracerebral Haemorrhage (STICH): a randomised trial. *Lancet* 2005;**365**:387–97.

99. Mendelow AD, Gregson BA, Rowan EN, et al. Early surgery versus initial conservative treatment in patients with spontaneous supratentorial lobar intracerebral haematomas (STICH II): a randomised trial. *Lancet* 2013;**382**:397–408.

100. Steiner T, Al-Shahi Salman R, Beer R, et al. European Stroke Organisation (ESO) guidelines for the management of spontaneous intracerebral hemorrhage. *Int J Stroke* 2014;**9**:840–55.

101. Hemphill JC, 3rd, Greenberg SM, Anderson CS, et al. Guidelines for the management of spontaneous intracerebral hemorrhage: a guideline for healthcare professionals from the American Heart Association/American Stroke Association. *Stroke* 2015;**46**:2032–60.

102. Mould WA, Carhuapoma JR, Muschelli J, et al. Minimally invasive surgery plus recombinant tissue-type plasminogen activator for intracerebral hemorrhage evacuation decreases perihematomal edema. *Stroke* 2013;**44**:627–34.

103. Hanley DF, Thompson RE, Rosenblum M, et al. Efficacy and safety of minimally invasive surgery with thrombolysis in intracerebral haemorrhage evacuation (MISTIE III): a randomised, controlled, open-label, blinded endpoint phase 3 trial. *Lancet* 2019;**393**(10175):1021–32.

104. Adams RE & Diringer MN. Response to external ventricular drainage in spontaneous intracerebral hemorrhage with hydrocephalus. *Neurology* 1998;**50**:519–23.

105. Takeuchi S, Wada K, Nagatani K, Otani N, & Mori K. Decompressive hemicraniectomy for spontaneous intracerebral hemorrhage. *Neurosurg Focus* 2013;**34**:E5.

106. Hanley DF, Lane K, McBee N, et al. Thrombolytic removal of intraventricular haemorrhage in treatment of severe stroke: results of the randomised, multicentre, multiregion, placebo-controlled CLEAR III trial. *Lancet* 2017;**389**:603–11.

107. Hemphill JC, 3rd, Bonovich DC, Besmertis L, Manley GT, & Johnston SC. The ICH score: a simple, reliable grading scale for intracerebral hemorrhage. *Stroke* 2001;**32**:891–7.

108. Nguyen YL, Angus DC, Boumendil A, & Guidet B. The challenge of admitting the very elderly to intensive care. *Ann Intensive Care* 2011;**1**:29.

109. Amrock LG & Deiner S. The implication of frailty on preoperative risk assessment. *Curr Opin Anaesthesiol* 2014;**27**:330–5.

110. Arima H, Tzourio C, Butcher K, et al. Prior events predict cerebrovascular and coronary outcomes in the PROGRESS trial. *Stroke* 2006;**37**:1497–502.

111. White CL, Pergola PE, Szychowski JM, et al. Blood pressure after recent stroke: baseline findings from the secondary prevention of small subcortical strokes trial. *Am J Hypertens* 2013;**26**:1114–22.

112. Ooi WL, Hossain M, & Lipsitz LA. The association between orthostatic hypotension and recurrent falls in nursing home residents. *Am J Med* 2000;**108**:106–11.

113. Wolters FJ, Mattace-Raso FU, Koudstaal PJ, Hofman A, & Ikram MA. Orthostatic hypotension and the long-term risk of dementia: a population-based study. *PLoS Med* 2016;**13**:e1002143.

114. Fong TG, Tulebaev SR, & Inouye SK. Delirium in elderly adults: diagnosis, prevention and treatment. *Nat Rev Neurol* 2009;**5**:210–20.

115. Joosten E, Demuynck M, Detroyer E, & Milisen K. Prevalence of frailty and its ability to predict in hospital delirium, falls, and 6-month mortality in hospitalized older patients. *BMC Geriatr* 2014;**14**:1.

116. Kase CS, Kurth T. Prevention of intracerebral hemorrhage recurrence. *Continuum (Minneap Minn)* 2011;**17**:1304–17.

117. Mallery LH, Ransom T, Steeves B, et al. Evidence-informed guidelines for treating frail older adults with type 2 diabetes: from the Diabetes Care Program of Nova Scotia (DCPNS) and the Palliative and Therapeutic Harmonization (PATH) program. *J Am Med Dir Assoc* 2013;**14**:801–8.

118. Poon MT, Fonville AF, & Al-Shahi Salman R. Long-term prognosis after intracerebral haemorrhage: systematic review and meta-analysis. *J Neurol Neurosurg Psychiatry* 2014;**85**:660–7.

119. Charidimou A, Kakar P, Fox Z, & Werring DJ. Cerebral microbleeds and recurrent stroke risk: systematic review and meta-analysis of prospective ischemic stroke and transient ischemic attack cohorts. *Stroke* 2013;**44**:995–1001.

120. **Biffi A, Anderson CD, Battey TW,** et al. Association between blood pressure control and risk of recurrent intracerebral hemorrhage. *JAMA* 2015;**314**:904–12.

121. **Al-Shahi R & Warlow C.** A systematic review of the frequency and prognosis of arteriovenous malformations of the brain in adults. *Brain* 2001;**124**:1900–26.

122. **Vermeer SE, Algra A, Franke CL, Koudstaal PJ, & Rinkel GJ.** Long-term prognosis after recovery from primary intracerebral hemorrhage. *Neurology* 2002;**59**:205–9.

123. **Lip GY, Nieuwlaat R, Pisters R, Lane DA, & Crijns HJ.** Refining clinical risk stratification for predicting stroke and thromboembolism in atrial fibrillation using a novel risk factor-based approach: the euro heart survey on atrial fibrillation. *Chest* 2010;**137**:263–72.

124. **Pisters R, Lane DA, Nieuwlaat R,** et al. A novel user-friendly score (HAS-BLED) to assess 1-year risk of major bleeding in patients with atrial fibrillation: the Euro Heart Survey. *Chest* 2010;**138**:1093–100.

125. **Biffi A, Kuramatsu J, Leasure A,** et al. Resumption of Oral Anticoagulation after intracerebral hemorrhage is associated with decreased mortality and favorable functional outcome (CCI.003). *Neurology* 2017;**88**.

126. **E Korompoki, F Filippidis, P Nielsen,** et al. Long-term antithrombotic treatment in intracranial hemorrhage survivors with atrial fibrillation: a systematic review and meta-analysis. *Eur Stroke J* 2017;**2**:477–95.

127. **Law ZK, Appleton JP, Bath PM, & Sprigg N.** Management of acute intracerebral haemorrhage—an update. *Clin Med (Lond)* 2017;**17**:166–72.

128. **Reddy VY, Doshi SK, Sievert H,** et al. Percutaneous left atrial appendage closure for stroke prophylaxis in patients with atrial fibrillation: 2.3-Year follow-up of the PROTECT AF (Watchman Left Atrial Appendage System for Embolic Protection in Patients with Atrial Fibrillation) Trial. *Circulation* 2013;**127**:720–9.

129. **Phan TG, Koh M, & Wijdicks EF.** Safety of discontinuation of anticoagulation in patients with intracranial hemorrhage at high thromboembolic risk. *Arch Neurol* 2000;**57**:1710–13.

130. **Fried LP, Tangen CM, Walston J,** et al. Frailty in older adults: evidence for a phenotype. *J Gerontol A Biol Sci Med Sci* 2001;**56**:M146–56.

131. **Clegg A, Young J, Iliffe S, Rikkert MO, & Rockwood K.** Frailty in elderly people. *Lancet* 2013;**381**:752–62.

132. **Zahuranec DB, Brown DL, Lisabeth LD,** et al. Early care limitations independently predict mortality after intracerebral hemorrhage. *Neurology* 2007;**68**:1651–7.

133. **Becker KJ, Baxter AB, Cohen WA,** et al. Withdrawal of support in intracerebral hemorrhage may lead to self-fulfilling prophecies. *Neurology* 2001;**56**:766–72.

134. **Hemphill JC, 3rd, Newman J, Zhao S, & Johnston SC.** Hospital usage of early do-not-resuscitate orders and outcome after intracerebral hemorrhage. *Stroke* 2004;**35**:1130–4.

135. **Abid KA, Vail A, Patel HC,** et al. Which factors influence decisions to transfer and treat patients with acute intracerebral haemorrhage and which are associated with prognosis? A retrospective cohort study. *BMJ Open* 2013;**3**:e003684.

Chapter 11

Cerebral small vessel disease: Potential interventions for prevention and treatment

Gordon Blair, Jason P. Appleton, Joanna M. Wardlaw, and Philip M. Bath

Introduction

Cerebral small vessel disease (SVD) is the underlying cause of most (85–90%) lacunar ischaemic strokes, which make up a quarter of all ischaemic strokes. As well as causing clinically evident lacunar ischaemic stroke, SVD can present clinically as vascular cognitive impairment and vascular dementia, intracerebral haemorrhage, late onset depression, or as gait or bladder dysfunction.[1] Its incidence increases with age such that some radiological features of SVD are present in around 10% of people in their sixties rising to 90% of people in their eighties.[2] In the United Kingdom, SVD is responsible for about 35 000 incident lacunar strokes per year[3] and about 350 000 cases of dementia. While usually being the cause of lacunar stroke, patients with other ischaemic stroke subtypes also frequently have some features of SVD present on their brain imaging.[4] It is thus an increasingly important condition to consider when treating the older stroke patient.

SVD is characterized by damage to deep grey and white matter structures of the brain and is thought to result from damage to perforating arterioles and capillaries; however, the contribution of venular damage to the disease process remains underinvestigated.[5] Radiologically, SVD is most commonly diagnosed based on the appearance of hypoattenuated areas in the periventricular and deep white matter, lacunes ('lakes' of cerebrospinal fluid (CSF) attenuation) in the deep grey or white matter, and global atrophy on computed tomography (CT) scans (Fig. 11.1). Magnetic resonance imaging (MRI) allows the full range of background SVD lesions to be seen as well as clearly distinguishing acute from old lacunar infarcts using diffusion imaging, for example, in patients presenting with a recent lacunar stroke syndrome and occasionally identifying asymptomatic acute lacunar infarcts[6] (Fig. 11.2). These background features include white matter hyperintensities (WMH) in the periventricular and deep white and grey matter structures, lacunes ('lakes' of signal similar to cerebrospinal fluid), old small haemorrhages, microbleeds, superficial siderosis and visible perivascular spaces (previously called Virchow–Robin spaces) (Fig. 11.1). The reason why such damage can accumulate in the brain without discrete symptoms seems to be related mainly to whether the lesions are sited in primary motor or sensory pathways where a small lesion may be more likely to be noticed than one in the frontal white matter, for example.[7]

Histologically, and depending on the population studied, SVD is seen to diffusely affect arterioles measuring 40–200 micrometres in size. The abnormalities of the arterioles are described as 'arteriolosclerosis', 'lipohyalinosis', and 'fibrinoid necrosis' (Fig. 11.3).[1] Plasma components and inflammatory cells are seen to infiltrate the arteriole walls and pass into perivascular tissue

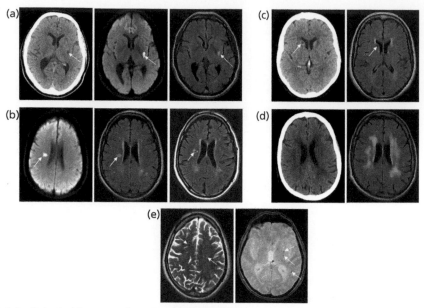

Fig. 11.1 Radiological features of small vessel disease.

(a) CT scan, DWI MRI scan, and FLAIR MRI scan showing acute lacunar infarction in the left posterior lentiform nucleus.

(b) DWI MRI scan, FLAIR MRI scan, and further follow-up FLAIR MRI scan showing acute lacunar infarction in the right centrum semiovale and subsequent cavitation into a chronic lacune.

(c) CT scan and FLAIR MRI scan showing a chronic lacune in the right caudate head.

(d) CT scan showing characteristic periventricular hypoattenuation and FLAIR MRI scan in same patient showing characteristic periventricular hyperintense lesions that are the radiological hallmarks of small vessel disease.

(e) T2-Weighted MRI scan showing enlarged perivascular spaces in the centrum semiovale and GRE MRI scan showing microbleeds (arrows).

Images courtesy of the Brain Research Imaging Centre, University of Edinburgh and NHS Lothian and obtained during the Mild Stroke Study II (funded by Wellcome Trust) and CVR Lacunar Stroke Study (funded by Chief Scientist Office).

resulting in damage to these structures. The precise pathological correlates of the radiological lesions are currently under investigation.

Causes of SVD

Despite being such a common condition with devastating consequences, SVD remains a very poorly understood disorder. Recently, evidence has grown to show that SVD is not simply due to atherosclerosis of the small blood vessels.[1]

For example, while patients with lacunar stroke share certain risk factors with those having other (e.g. cortical) stroke subtypes such as hypertension, diabetes-raised cholesterol, and smoking, there is little association with other traditional stroke risk factors such as atrial fibrillation, ipsilateral carotid artery stenosis, and ischaemic heart disease.[1] While vascular risk factors explain about 70% of the variance in large artery atheromatous disease, they explain less than 2% of the variance in WMH in community-dwelling older subjects and 0.1% in patients with recent minor ischaemic stroke.[8] Indeed, patients who have recent lacunar ischaemic stroke have the same chance as having significant carotid stenosis on the contralateral (asymptomatic) side of the neck as on their symptomatic (ipsilateral) side,[9] and WMH are almost always distributed

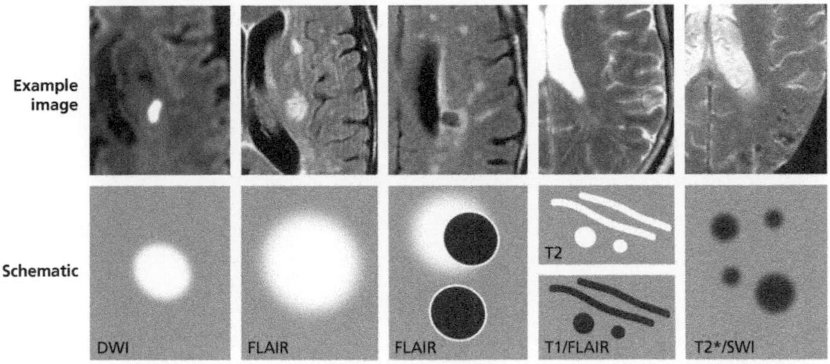

	Recent small subcortical infarct	White matter hyperintensity	Lacune	Perivascular space	Cerebral microbleed
Example image					
Schematic	DWI	FLAIR	FLAIR	T2 / T1/FLAIR	T2*/SWI
Usual diameter	≤20 mm	Variable	3–15 mm	≤2 mm	≤10 mm
Comment	Best identified on DWI	Located in white matter	Usually have hyperintense rim	Most linear without hyperintense rim	Detected on GRE seq., round or ovoid, blooming
DWI	↑	↔	↔/(↓)	↔	↔
FLAIR	↑	↑	↓	↓	↔
T2	↑	↑	↑	↑	↔
T1	↓	↔/(↓)	↓	↓	↔
T2*-weighted GRE	↔	↑	↔/(↓ if haemorrhage)	↔	↓↓

↑ Increased signal ↓ Decreased signal ↔ Iso-intense signal

Fig. 11.2 MRI appearances of the individual radiological features of SVD. Up arrows indicate hyperintense signal, down arrows indicate hypointense signal, sideways arrows indicate no difference in signal compared to normal appearing brain. DWI, diffusion weighted imaging; FLAIR, fluid attenuated inversion recovery; GRE, gradient echo.

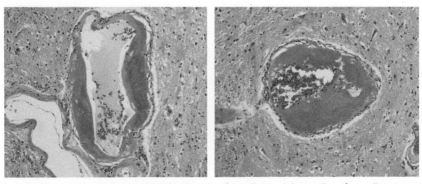

Fig. 11.3 Pathology sections showing lipohyalinosis of small arteriolar wall. Left, earlier stage; right, advanced lipohyalinosis/fibrinoid necrosis.

Images courtesy of Prof Colin Smith, University of Edinburgh.

Box 11.1 Summary for SVD

- SVD is common in older people and particularly in older stroke patients
- It is the underlying cause of 25% of ischaemic strokes
- It is the major contributor to vascular cognitive impairment
- Is a common cause of haemorrhagic stroke in older people
- Lacunar stroke correlates poorly with cardio- or atherothromboembolic risk factors such as AF and carotid artery stenosis
- SVD is not 'atherosclerosis of the small blood vessel'. Instead it is more likely a consequence of microvascular endothelial dysfunction
- Lacunar ischaemic stroke and other SVD presentations will likely require different treatments to other stroke subtypes

symmetrically in the two cerebral hemispheres regardless of the presence of a unilateral internal carotid artery stenosis.[9,10] Overall, cardioembolic or large artery atheromatous embolic sources were found in only around 10% of patients with a recent lacunar ischaemic stroke in the basal ganglia and in only around 3% of patients when the recent lacunar ischaemic stroke was in the centrum semiovale.[11] These findings strongly suggest lacunar stroke and SVD are separate from atherosclerotic vascular disease.

While the exact cause of SVD remains unclear, certain factors are known to play a key role. Damage to the endothelial cells lining the arterioles appears as an important early step.[11] This results in blood–brain barrier breakdown, which has been demonstrated in humans with both gadolinium-enhanced MRI scan and analysis of cerebrospinal fluid albumin levels (Box 11.1 and Fig. 11.4).[12] Inflammation is also involved in this process with a systematic review of pathology specimens in lacunar stroke showing perivascular inflammation to be a common feature.[13] Further evidence for the role of inflammation comes from elevated levels of blood markers of inflammation and endothelial activation,[14] although the extent to which this represents risk factor exposure is unclear. However, patients with systemic sources of inflammation such as rheumatoid arthritis or systemic lupus erythematosis have both increased risk of stroke[15] and of having WMH, lacunes, and prominent perivascular spaces on neuroimaging.[15] Hence, endothelial dysfunction and inflammation appear to result in thickening of the arteriolar wall, which becomes less able to vasodilate when required.[11] Risk factor exposures (hypertension, diabetes, smoking) make this worse. As well as increased interstitial fluid having adverse effects on the function of multiple cells in the brain, the tissue supplied by these thickened and stiff arterioles may then be at risk of ischaemia and the vessel wall itself more liable to precipitate secondary thrombosis.[11]

Given this differing disease process, most lacunar ischaemic strokes and other clinical SVD presentations are likely to require a different set of therapies to that used routinely in other stroke subtypes.

Acute treatment

The current acute treatment of ischaemic stroke comprises thrombolysis, aspirin, mechanical thrombectomy,[16] and hemicraniectomy.[17] While the latter two are not usually relevant to the acute presentation of SVD, aspirin and thrombolysis are discussed as follows.

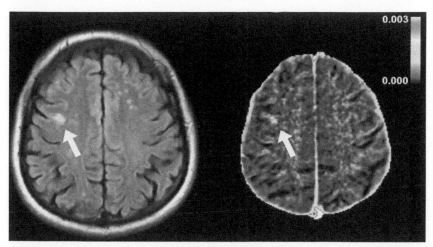

Fig. 11.4 Image showing a FLAIR MRI scan demonstrating a centrum semiovale white matter hyperintensity (arrow) and a dynamic contrast enhanced MRI showing increased blood brain barrier permeability in the lesion.

Image courtesy of Anna Heye and the Brain Research Imaging Centre. Image taken as part of the Mild Stroke Study II funded by Wellcome Trust(16).

Thrombolysis and SVD

Thrombolysis in lacunar stroke

The benefits of intravenous thrombolysis in patients presenting with lacunar ischaemic stroke have been debated throughout the history of stroke thrombolysis. No clinical trial has yet been powered for subgroup analysis by stroke type and most trials excluded patients with lacunar stroke.

Of the two trials of alteplase that did include lacunar stroke, the National Institute of Neurological Disorders and Stroke (NINDS) trial of intravenous alteplase up to 3 hours after onset of acute ischaemic stroke included 51/624 patients with small vessel occlusive stroke and found no evidence of an interaction between alteplase effect and stroke subtype, the benefit of thrombolysis being seen across all stroke subtypes.[18] The third International Stroke Trial (IST-3) of alteplase given up to 6 hours after onset of acute ischaemic stroke included 300/3032 patients with lacunar ischaemic stroke and also found no evidence of an alteplase stroke-subtype interaction.[19,20] On closer analysis, the odds ratio (OR) for good functional outcome at 6 months in lacunar stroke patients allocated alteplase vs. control was 1.17 (95% CI 0.7–1.94, P = ns) but the sample was underpowered: 5/168 patients allocated alteplase (3%) died within 7 days versus 1/164 (1%) allocated control; 8/168 (5%) patients allocated alteplase had a symptomatic intracerebral haemorrhage (ICH) (sICH) versus 0/164 allocated control.[20]

Observational data on 1630 lacunar stroke patients thrombolysed in the Canadian Stroke Register showed a relative risk for good functional outcome of 1.84 (1.59–2.13), for discharge home of 1.38 (1.19–1.60) and for death of 0.89 (0.54–1.47) for those with lacunar stroke receiving thrombolysis compared to those not receiving thrombolysis.[21]

The WAKE-UP trial showed the benefit of alteplase in patients with stroke of unknown onset time with MRI evidence of diffusion-weighted imaging (DWI)/FLAIR mismatch (implying ischaemic but not yet infarcted tissue). A recent secondary analysis explored differences between the treatment effect in patients with MRI confirmed lacunar infarct and those with non-lacunar infarcts. In 105 lacunar patients OR for favourable outcome (mRS0-1) with alteplase treatment was 1.68 (95% CI, 0.76–3.69) and in 385 non-lacunar patients OR for favourable outcome was 1.62 (95% CI, 1.04–2.01), implying no difference in treatment effect by stroke type. However, the trial was not powered for this non-specified secondary analysis and had not recruited its target 800 patients after being stopped early due to withdrawal of funding.[22]

Thrombolysis in mild stroke (i.e. National Institutes of Health Stroke Scale (NIHSS) ≤5)

Lacunar strokes are generally milder than other stroke types, typical NIHSS scores being lower than 5. Thrombolysis in mild stroke remains a matter of debate; previous views on the benefits of thrombolysis being small in this group while risks are poorly defined, are increasingly challenged given our improving awareness of the longer-term cognitive and functional consequences of even the mildest strokes.

IST-3 showed patients thrombolysed with an NIHSS score of <5 had an OR of 1.14 (0.79–1.65) for good 6-month functional outcome compared to those receiving standard post-stroke care. As with thrombolysis in any stroke, death within 7 days and sICH were increased with thrombolysis (death: 7/304 patients (2%) vs. 3/308 (1%); sICH: 9/304 (3%) vs. 0/308).[20] Meta-analysis of individual patient data from nine thrombolysis trials show that for patients with NIHSS of 0–4 thrombolysis has an OR of 1.48 (1.07–2.06) for an outcome of modified Rankin score 0–1[23] compared to standard care. This equates to an absolute increase in excellent outcome of 8%, with an absolute excess of haemorrhage with alteplase of 1.5% (95% CI 0.8–2.6%).[24] Observational data from the Austrian Stroke Register of 890 thrombolysed mild stroke patients showed an OR of improved functional outcome at 3 months of 1.49 (95% CI 1.17–1.89) compared to those with mild stroke who were not thrombolysed.[25]

These data in lacunar stroke and in mild stroke are in line with the overall effects of alteplase and the samples are too small to determine if the benefits or risks of alteplase are significantly different in lacunar or mild stroke. Hence two trials of thrombolysis in patients with mild stroke (NIHSS ≤5) are ongoing in North America, PRISMS (alteplase, Khatri, ClinicalTrials.gov: NCT02072226), and TEMPO-2 (tenecteplase, Coutts, ClinicalTrials.gov: NCT02398656).

Thrombolysis for stroke in the presence of SVD on imaging

Another important aspect to consider is whether the presence of SVD features on neuroimaging at presentation with acute ischaemic stroke should influence the decision to give intravenous thrombolysis. Some imaging features of SVD seen on MRI are not discernible on CT (e.g. cerebral microbleeds [CMBs]),[6] which is important given that CT is more widely available than MRI.

The most reliable data on the outcome after thrombolysis for acute ischaemic stroke in patients with SVD who receive intravenous alteplase comes from randomized trials. IST-3 was the only trial that included large numbers of older people, there being only about 100 patients aged over 80 in all prior alteplase trials combined. IST-3 (n = 3017),[26] examined three CT visible components of SVD and found that leukoaraiosis, presence of cerebral atrophy and having a prior infarct (many of which were lacunes) were each independently associated with a reduction (total when all three present = 50% reduction, each feature individually contributing a third of the 50%) in the chances of favourable outcome at 6 months after stroke, with no evidence of an interaction with alteplase. Neither leukoaraiosis nor atrophy independently predicted sICH individually after correcting for age, NIHSS, and time after stroke, but having an old infarct plus a hyperattenuated artery (visible acute arterial thrombus) increased the absolute risk of sICH with (versus without) alteplase to 13.8%, versus 3.2% when both signs were absent.

Most other studies assessed effects of individual rather than combined SVD features on outcome after thrombolysis, and many were observational studies rather than randomized controlled trials (RCTs). In a systematic review of 55 studies to assess risk factors for intracerebral haemorrhage (ICH) following intravenous alteplase,[27] presence of leukoaraiosis (akin to WMH on MRI)(6) (6/55 studies) was associated independently with an increased risk of ICH (OR 2.45, 95% CI 1.64–3.66).[27] A recent retrospective observational study (n = 311) found that patients with leukoaraiosis had an increased risk of sICH and haemorrhagic transformation post-thrombolysis.[28]

In a Finnish retrospective cohort (n = 2485), leukoaraiosis was independently associated with worse functional outcome (modified Rankin Scale (mRS)) 3 months post-thrombolysis.[29] An updated retrospective analysis of the Canadian Alteplase for Stroke Effectiveness Study (CASES) assessed SVD as presence of leukoaraiosis and lacunes on baseline CT in 820 patients and found that severe SVD in those aged less than 80 years was associated with an increased risk of sICH and less favourable functional outcome (mRS) at 3 months compared with absent or moderate SVD.[30] However, these associations were not seen in those aged more than 80 years, which could represent selection bias; clinicians may have been more likely to administer thrombolysis to octogenarians with less comorbidity, thus creating a cohort not representative of older people eligible for thrombolysis.

Two systematic reviews and meta-analyses of the same five observational studies (n = 790) demonstrated a non-significant increased risk of sICH post-thrombolysis in patients with CMBs on pretreatment MRI.[31,32] Despite the use of different meta-analytical methods the results were similar: relative risk (RR) of 1.90 (95% CI 0.92–3.93)[31] and OR 1.98 (95% CI 0.90–4.35).[32] Shoamanesh et al.[32] also noted an association between CMB burden and ICH; a finding replicated in a retrospective report (n = 326) in which higher numbers of CMBs were associated with increased rates of sICH.[33] In observational studies in patients without thrombolysis, having large numbers of CMBs is a risk factor for sporadic ICH, therefore use of alteplase should be very carefully weighed in patients known to have many CMBs.

In summary, for the present, intravenous thrombolysis should not routinely be withheld in those known to have leukoaraiosis or lacunes on CT or MRI (or CMBs on pretreatment MRI) but may be taken into account after clinical factors, particularly age, stroke severity, and time after stroke have been considered. In some situations where the decision based on clinical findings is marginal, the presence of the imaging SVD findings may be useful to tip the decision in one way or the other. Meanwhile, prospective research is required to establish in which patients with imaging evidence of SVD do the risks of ICH outweigh the benefits of thrombolysis or are the benefits of alteplase so low that the treatment is unlikely to be helpful. In the meantime, evidence of severe SVD on baseline imaging should be taken into consideration as part of the decision to give intravenous thrombolysis in patients with acute ischaemic stroke of any subtype.

The challenges regarding thrombolysis in SVD and lacunar stroke are also discussed in Chapter 9, 'Early management of acute ischaemic stroke'.

Preventing SVD

Given the slow progression of SVD and its chronic nature, treatment will likely require long-term therapies in a similar way to current vascular secondary prevention. The very high prevalence of SVD suggests treatments will have to be affordable and easy to administer. Given SVD's association with age and the increasing numbers of medications older people are now taking, any treatment will also have to be safe, simple, and have only limited interactions with other common drugs. To achieve these goals, older people and specifically patients over the age of 80 will need to be included in future trials.[34] Patients with concurrent severe ipsilateral carotid stenosis and/or atrial fibrillation will need these treated as normal.

Drugs previously tested in SVD

Next we summarize the evidence for various therapies that have been tested in lacunar ischaemic stroke or other presentations of SVD, or may be beneficial. The information comes from searches of several electronic databases including the Cochrane Library, WHO meta-register for trials, Internet Stroke Center, MEDLINE, and EMBASE as well as the authors' own reference databases (years 1990–2016) and prior publications.[34] The searches sought articles describing clinical trials in patients with lacunar stroke or other presentations of SVD, or who were at risk of developing the disease.

Anticoagulation

Emboli from cardiac sources are an uncommon cause of lacunar ischaemic stroke (<10%) but in patients found to have a cardioembolic source, secondary prevention, in the form of oral anticoagulation, should be considered. The beneficial role of oral anticoagulation in secondary stroke prevention in patients with atrial fibrillation (AF) is well known.[35] Warfarin reduces any stroke recurrence by two-thirds while the direct oral anticoagulants—dabigatran, apixaban, edoxaban, and rivaroxaban—are as effective as warfarin at preventing both initial and recurrent strokes.[36]

   Data focusing on the effects of oral anticoagulation in patients with acute lacunar ischaemic stroke or neuroimaging signs of SVD are lacking; none of the direct oral anticoagulant trials or subsequent meta-analysis reported outcomes in patients with SVD as a subgroup, or of the effect of treatment on SVD or cognition as outcomes.[36] In addition, these trials included relatively young participants (median age 72 years)[36] with probably less SVD or comorbidity raising the question of risk of ICH in the context of SVD, AF, oral anticoagulation, and the older person. The Stroke Prevention in Reversible Ischaemia Trial (SPIRIT) (n = 1316) found that patients with a previous ischaemic stroke who were in sinus rhythm treated with high dose warfarin, international normalized ratio (INR) of 3–4.5, had an increased risk of ICH compared to aspirin. This risk was higher in those with multiple WMH detected on CT (HR 7.5 (3.4–16)) but did not assess bleeding risk with other imaging features of SVD.[37] To help answer this question, the observational Clinical Relevance of Microbleeds in Stroke study (CROMIS-2)[38] has two main aims: to identify factors associated with increased ICH risk following oral anticoagulation for secondary prevention following ischaemic stroke with concomitant AF; and to determine clinical, genetic, and imaging biomarkers associated with anticoagulation-associated ICH. Such research may potentially be used to predict the risk of oral anticoagulation-associated ICH in patients with SVD in future.

Antidementia drugs

Five medications are licensed to treat Alzheimer's disease. Four of these drugs are acetyl-cholinesterase inhibitors (donepezil, galantamine, rivastigmine, tacrine) and the fifth is a non-competitive antagonist of the N-methyl-D-aspartate (NMDA) receptor (memantine). The acetyl-cholinesterase inhibitors prevent the breakdown of the neurotransmitter acetylcholine[39] and memantine helps prevent excitotoxicity which can damage neurons.[40] From a pathophysio-logical point of view, acetyl-cholinesterase inhibitors would appear unlikely to improve vascular dementia; however, the high prevalence of SVD features in patients with Alzheimer's disease[41] suggests there may be some benefit, albeit the effects of these agents on Alzheimer's disease are modest at best. However, many trials of these drugs only involved patients with Alzheimer's disease, with far fewer studies including participants with vascular or mixed dementias.[42]

Some trials to date of donepezil (two studies, 1219 patients[43,44]), memantine (two studies, 900 patients[45,46]), and galantamine (two studies, 1378 patients[47,48]) in vascular cognitive impairment and dementia have shown modest beneficial effects on cognitive function and activities of daily living, although results from all trials are mixed and none specifically commented on inclusion of patents with vascular risk factors or imaging SVD features or used small vessel disease as an outcome measure.[39,40,49] The clinical significance of these effects is questionable as the improvement in cognitive scores was generally less than is considered clinically relevant and many of the outcome measures were obtained on scales designed for use in Alzheimer's disease rather than vascular cognitive impairment; specifically, the Alzheimer's disease cognitive scale does not measure executive function which is particularly affected by vascular cognitive impairment.

All the trials were short duration treatment studies in patients with cognitive impairment or dementia and no trials have attempted to prevent vascular cognitive impairment using these drugs.

Antiplatelet treatments

The antiplatelet drugs aspirin, cilostazol, clopidogrel, dipyridamole, and triflusal are commonly administered following ischaemic stroke, though use varies by world region. Of these cilostazol, dipyridamole, and triflusal have weak antiplatelet effects, while aspirin and clopidogrel have moderately potent effects on platelets. Cilostazol, dipyridamole, and triflusal also have effects on smooth muscle activity, white cells,[50] blood brain barrier integrity, and inflammatory markers[51] in addition to their antiplatelet properties.[52–55] Although all have been shown to be efficacious at preventing recurrence following ischaemic stroke of all types, there is limited specific data on patients with lacunar infarcts.

The role of dual antiplatelet agents has been assessed in both the acute and chronic setting following ischaemic stroke.[56–60] Short-term use of dual antiplatelets (i.e. a few weeks) reduces stroke recurrence without increasing major bleeding.[56,57] The effect of chronic use of dual antiplatelet agents post-stroke depends on the combination: aspirin and dipyridamole are superior to each drug in isolation,[61,62] while aspirin and clopidogrel increase major bleeding risk, outweighing the potential benefit of reduced stroke recurrence.[63,64] This imbalance is greater in lacunar stroke.[65] Chronic triple therapy with aspirin, clopidogrel, and dipyridamole in a population (n = 17) where the majority (71%) had lacunar stroke, also resulted in increased bleeding risk when compared with aspirin alone.[66]

The aforementioned data are from a mixed population of lacunar and non-lacunar strokes without deep phenotyping at baseline. In contrast, the Secondary Prevention of Small Subcortical Stroke (SPS3) trial randomized 3020 patients with a symptomatic lacunar stroke, as demonstrated on MRI, to chronic aspirin and clopidogrel versus aspirin alone.[65] The study was stopped early when dual antiplatelet therapy was associated with more bleeding and death than aspirin. Excess haemorrhage was also seen in a subgroup of patients with previous stroke (47% lacunar) from the Thrombin Receptor Antagonist in Secondary Prevention of Atherothrombotic Ischaemic Events (TRA 2P)-Thrombolysis in Myocardial Infarction (TIMI) 50 trial of vorapaxar and existing antiplatelet therapy (dual antiplatelet) versus existing antiplatelet therapy only (monotherapy).[67]

In rat models, cilostazol reduces infarct size and improves motor and cognitive function compared to aspirin,[68] and improves recovery of ischaemic white matter lesions.[69] The ECLIPse trial[70] evaluated cilostazol in patients with acute lacunar infarction and found that compared to placebo, cilostazol reduced transcranial Doppler pulsatility index at day 90 from baseline. The authors proposed that pleiotropic effects of cilostazol beyond antiplatelet activity may explain their findings. In acute lenticulostriate artery territory infarction (n = 100), cilostazol was not superior to ozagrel in preventing neurological deterioration at 30 days.[71] Cilostazol has been assessed in both the acute and chronic post-stroke setting in trials from Asia Pacific countries (China, Korea, Japan).[72–75] A meta-analysis of 5491 patients (55–75% lacunar strokes) found that in the acute phase following stroke cilostazol had no significant effect on stroke recurrence, haemorrhagic events, functional outcome, or death as compared to aspirin or placebo, although the data were from small studies. In the chronic setting, cilostazol reduced recurrent stroke (RR 0.53, 95% CI 0.34–0.81) when compared to placebo, while it reduced haemorrhagic strokes (RR 0.29, 95% CI 0.15–0.56) but had no effect on stroke recurrence or death compared to aspirin.[75] More recently, the prevention of cardiovascular events in Asian patients with ischaemic stroke at high risk of cerebral haemorrhage (PICASSO) trial recruited 1534 patients with recent ischaemic stroke and a history or imaging findings of ICH or two or more microbleeds. Patients were randomized to cilostazol, aspirin, cilostazol plus probucol, or aspirin plus probucol. Cilostazol was non-inferior to aspirin at preventing cardiovascular events (including stroke) over 2 years of follow-up.[76] Despite having a high proportion of lacunar strokes at baseline, these trials involved young people (59–67 years) and therefore their relevance to older persons from different ethnic backgrounds and geographical regions is not known.

The effect of cilostazol on cognition is not clear. One unpublished report, the Cilostazol versus Aspirin for Vascular Dementia in post-stroke patients with white matter lesions (CAVAD) study, randomly assigned 52 patients to cilostazol 200 mg/day or aspirin 100 mg/day for 12 months.[77] The cilostazol group had improved cognitive function at 6 and 12 months with fewer bleeding events compared to those taking aspirin. Recent UK data from the LACI-1 trial has demonstrated that 9 weeks of cilostazol, in isolation or combination with isosorbide mononitrate, was well-tolerated in 57 patients with recent lacunar ischaemic stroke.[78] Further larger studies assessing cilostazol's effects on stroke recurrence and imaging outcomes including older people's cognition are awaited (CASID: NCT01409564, Efficacy Study of Cilostazol and Aspirin on Cerebral Small Vessel Disease: NCT01932203, LACI-2: EUDRACT 2016-002277-35, Taiwan Registry Data).

The lack of efficacy of drugs primarily acting as antiplatelet agents in trials involving patients with lacunar events provides more evidence for a non-atheromatous aetiology for lacunar strokes. Of note, the effects of antiplatelet agents on WMH, lacunes, and microbleeds have not yet been reported.

Blood pressure (BP) lowering

Hypertension is an important modifiable vascular risk factor for both SVD and stroke.[79] It is prevalent, especially in those aged over 60 years, affecting 1 billion people worldwide.[80] Treating high BP reduces the risk of first stroke. In the Systolic Hypertension in the Elderly Program (SHEP) antihypertensives reduced rates of ischaemic stroke and lacunar events.[81] Secondary prevention with BP management reduces stroke recurrence but there is limited data on stroke categories at baseline and as outcomes.[82]

As well as assessing dual versus single antiplatelet agents in lacunar stroke, the SPS3 trial assessed, in a multifactorial design, intensity of BP lowering and found no difference in stroke recurrence between the lower-target (<130 mmHg) and higher-target (130–149 mmHg) groups.[83] In addition, a post-hoc analysis found there was no improvement in long-term cognition in the intensive BP arm.[84] A large BP intensity trial (Systolic blood PRessure INtervention Trial (SPRINT))[85] found that intensive BP control (<120 mmHg) in 9361 patients (mean age 68 years) at high risk of cardiovascular events without diabetes or previous stroke resulted in fewer major cardiovascular events and death, and a non-significant 11% lower incidence of stroke (subtypes not specified). Intensive BP lowering was not associated with a reduced risk of probable dementia, but did reduce the risk of mild cognitive impairment (HR 0.81, 95% CI 0.69–0.95) and when combined with probable dementia (HR 0.95, 95% CI 0.74–0.97).[86] Further data on the effects on imaging findings of SVD have yet to be published. The UK-based Prevention Of Decline in Cognition After Stroke Trial (PODCAST) stopped early due to under-recruitment and failed to demonstrate an effect of intensive BP lowering on cognitive outcomes after stroke.[87] There are on-going studies examining intensive BP management in SVD and its potential impact on cognition, such as PRESERVE (ISRCTN37694103).

The effect of antihypertensives on WMH progression has been assessed in the substudies of two RCTs.[88,89] In the perindopril protection against recurrent stroke study (PROGRESS) MRI substudy, there was a non-significant reduction in the risk of new WMH and a significant re-duction in the mean total volume of new WMH in the treatment group compared to placebo.[88] However, in the PRoFESS MRI substudy there was no difference in WMH progression in the group receiving telmisartan compared to placebo.[89]

It is worth noting that the effect of excessive lowering of BP in certain groups of individuals, especially the very elderly, remains unclear. Systolic BP levels of <120 mmHg, 140–150 mmHg, or >150 mmHg during follow-up after ischaemic stroke were associated with stroke recurrence in one study, suggesting a 'J-shaped curve'.[90] In a Dutch population-based study of 513 people aged 85 years, high systolic BP in those with impaired physical or cognitive functioning was associated with a reduced stroke risk, while those with unimpaired functioning who had higher diastolic BP and mean arterial pressure had a higher risk of stroke.[91] Despite being observational, this study suggests that lowering of BP in the frail elderly patient may be detrimental. Of note, another observational study found that increasing BP was continuously related to the risk of developing vascular dementia when aged ≤70 years and that BP was a strong risk factor for vascular dementia following stroke or transient ischaemic attack (TIA).[92] However, as age increased, the strength of these associations reduced but did not reverse, implying that the effect of BP on the risk of developing vascular dementia reduces over the age of 70 years. This data should be interpreted with caution, however, given its observational nature.

Other haemodynamic measures influenced by antihypertensive agents such as BP variability, heart rate, peak pressure, pulse pressure, and rate pressure product are important considerations in stroke, cognitive impairment, and vascular dementia.[93,94] Equally, the diverse mechanisms of action of antihypertensive medications are likely to have differing effects on these outcomes and warrant further investigation.

Endothelin

Endothelin-1 is a potent vasoconstrictor and physiological NO antagonist that is released from endothelium. It has, therefore, been used to induce ischaemic stroke in experimental models. Endothelin receptor antagonists have been trialled in patients in the management of vasospasm in subarachnoid haemorrhage, and in both pulmonary and systemic hypertension.[95,96] Unfortunately there is no current evidence available regarding their use or effects in people with SVD.[97]

Lipid lowering

Statins (HMG-CoA reductase inhibitors) are most commonly used to prevent first and recurrent vascular events,[98,99] through their effect on lowering low density lipoprotein cholesterol (LDL-c) in patients at high risk of stroke or large artery atheromatous disease. However, they have pleio-tropic actions which include antiplatelet, anti-inflammatory, and endothelial stabilizing actions.[34]

No trial has looked at statin use exclusively in lacunar stroke. However, in the SPARCL trial, stroke recurrence was shown to be reduced by atorvastatin to a similar degree in both subgroups of patients with large artery atheromatous stroke and patients with SVD lacunar stroke (hazard ratios [HR] 0.70 and 0.85, respectively).[100,101]

Trials assessing the effect of statins on other endpoints relevant to SVD have had more mixed results. The Heart Protection Study (n = 20 536) assessed simvastatin's effects on cognitive decline and showed no effect with treatment.[102] The PROSPER study assessed the effects of pravastatin (less potent than either simvastatin or atorvastatin at lipid lowering) on cognitive function (n = 5804) and WMH progression (n = 535),[103,104] while the ROCAS study looked at the effects of simvastatin on WMH progression (n = 227).[105] Both showed neutral effects. Atorvastatin has been shown to increase cerebrovascular reactivity and endothelial function in one small study.[106] Intensive lipid lowering in the PODCAST trial (n = 83) was associated with improvements in some secondary cognitive outcomes over 2 years of follow-up, but this may represent chance due to the small sample size.[87]

Anti-inflammatory drugs

Increasing evidence of a role for inflammation in the pathogenesis of SVD raises the possibility of using anti-inflammatory agents to treat SVD. Both steroids and non-steroidal anti-inflammatory drugs are likely to be unsuitable due to long-term side effects and increased cardiovascular risk. However, many other drugs have anti-inflammatory properties—these include statins, phospho-diesterase inhibitors, prostacyclin, and nitric oxide donors.[34]

Blood–brain barrier (BBB) modulation

Subtle increased BBB permeability occurs in normal ageing but is accelerated in SVD including in patients with more severe WMH and in those with lacunar stroke versus non-lacunar stroke.[12,107,108] Some currently licensed drugs are suggested to improve BBB function. These include antivascular endothelial growth hormone antibodies, cyclic guanylate mono-phosphate (cGMP) modulators (e.g. dipyridamole), cyclic adenylate mono-phosphate (cAMP) modulators (e.g. cilostazol, pentoxifylline), fasudil (a rho-kinase inhibitor, discussed next), and topiramate (an antiepileptic finding increasing use in many other neurological disorders).[34] However, the effects of these on SVD remain unknown and are being evaluated in ongoing trials (LACI-2: EUDRACT 2016-002277-35).[78]

Neurotrophins

Neurotrophins are proteins that control the development and growth of neurones. Cerebrolysin is a neurotrophic peptide with putative neurotrophic and neuroprotective effects; it is administered as a once daily intravenous injection. Six small studies (total n = 597) have suggested that cerebrolysin may be effective in treating vascular dementia.[109] Further trials are required and if found to be effective, an alternative route of delivery would be needed. Cerebrolysin's effects on features of SVD are unknown at present.

Nitric oxide/cyclic GMP/PDE5 system

Nitric oxide (NO) has antiplatelet, antivascular smooth muscle cell, anti-inflammatory, antileukocyte, pro-endothelial, and blood–brain barrier integrity actions, as well as being neuroprotective, modulating cerebral autoregulation, and inhibiting apoptosis.[110–114] It is therefore a potential therapeutic target for prevention and management of SVD. NO is synthesized by NO synthase from L-arginine, and from reduction of nitrate and nitrite. Downstream signalling occurs via the second messenger cGMP, which is broken down by phosphodiesterase (PDE). Therefore, this pathway can be upregulated using a variety of approaches: increase L-arginine and levels; increase NO synthase activity; administer NO donors; or inhibit PDE activity.[111,114]

NO donors can be split into organic nitrates (e.g. glyceryl trinitrate [GTN], isosorbide mononitrate), which have no antiplatelet effects and inorganic nitrates (e.g. sodium nitroprusside), which inhibit platelet activity.[115,116] Endogenous NO levels are low in acute,[117] chronic,[118] and probably in lacunar stroke.[119] Supplementation of vascular NO levels by NO donors may therefore improve vascular compliance[120,121] but there are limited data to support this at present. In preclinical studies of acute large artery cerebral ischaemia, NO donors reduce infarct volume, increase penumbral blood flow, and improve functional outcome.[122] In acute stroke of ischaemic and haemorrhagic type (though very few with lacunar stroke), transdermal GTN administered within 6 hours of onset, and continued for up to 7 days improved functional outcome and cognition at 90 days.[123] GTN's efficacy is currently being assessed within 4 hours of stroke ictus in patients stratified by imaging burden of SVD on baseline imaging presenting with any type of ischaemic or haemorrhagic stroke requiring hospital admission. Secondary outcome measures include cognition (RIGHT-2: ISRCTN26986053). Of note, although isosorbide mononitrate is extensively used in the chronic management of ischaemic heart disease, there are no data on its use in stroke of any type, including SVD. The aforementioned completed LACI-1 and ongoing LACI-2 trials assess isosorbide mononitrate, in isolation and combination with cilostazol, in patients with recent lacunar ischaemic stroke.

PDE inhibitors are either non-selective—such as methylxanthines (pentoxifylline, theophylline)—or selective (dipyridamole (PDE5 inhibitor), cilostazol (PDE3 inhibitor)). As alluded to previously, dipyridamole is a weak antiplatelet but also has an inhibitory effect on adenosine reuptake with resultant effects on endothelial, smooth muscle, and white cells similar to the effects of NO.[52–54] It is licensed for stroke secondary prevention either as monotherapy or in combination with aspirin, but there are no specific data on SVD.[124] See 'antiplatelet treatments' section for summary of cilostazol.

Peroxisome proliferator-activated receptor (PPAR)-gamma agonists

Peroxisome proliferator-activated receptor-gamma agonists (e.g. pioglitazone) licensed for glycaemic control in diabetes mellitus have effects that could be potentially beneficial in patients with SVD. Such attributes include antifibrinolysis, anti-inflammation, antihypertensive, antismooth muscle cell proliferation, lipid metabolism regulation, and pro-endothelial activity. The prospective pioglitazone clinical trial in macrovascular events (PROactive) randomized 5238 patients with type 2 diabetes to pioglitazone or placebo.[125] In those without prior stroke, pioglitazone did not prevent first stroke, while in a subgroup analysis of 984 patients with previous stroke, pioglitazone reduced stroke recurrence, and major adverse cardiovascular events. Pioglitazone given for an average of 4.8 years in patients with recent ischaemic stroke or TIA and insulin resistance, but not diabetes, in the Insulin Resistance Intervention after Stroke (IRIS) trial (n = 3876) resulted in less fatal or non-fatal stroke or myocardial infarction compared with placebo.[126] However, neither of these trials stratified by stroke type at baseline or outcome, or provide data on differential effects in patients with imaging evidence of SVD.

Of note, adverse effects such as weight gain, fluid retention, risk of heart failure, fractures, and possibly bladder cancer have raised concern.[127] Future development of selective PPAR-gamma modulators may hold promise by retaining the beneficial properties while avoiding unwanted effects.[128]

Prostacyclin/cyclic AMP/PDE3 system

Prostacyclin, its prostaglandin derivatives (e.g. PGE2) and mimetics (e.g. beraprost) have similar effects to those seen with the NO and cGMP pathway but are mediated via the second messenger cAMP, which is degraded by PDE. Several small studies of intravenous prostacyclin in acute stroke have been performed.[129] However, as no oral preparations are available it is not suitable for chronic administration in a condition such as SVD.

The prostaglandin-cAMP pathway can be chronically stimulated by using an oral PDE3 inhibitor such as cilostazol, pentoxifylline, or triflusal. Pentoxifylline, like cilostazol, is licensed for the management of peripheral vascular disease. There have been several trials in acute ischaemic stroke and dementia prevention involving pentoxifylline or related methylxanthines but unfortunately they were small and had flawed designs.[130,131] Triflusal is licensed for use in high-risk individuals to prevent recurrent vascular events.[132] As well as its antiplatelet and PDE3 inhibiting properties, it promotes release of NO from white cells. Data on cilostazol is discussed in the 'antiplatelet treatments' section.

To date, none of the PDE-inhibitor trials in stroke have focused on lacunar stroke or SVD, though some are now ongoing (LACI-2: EUDRACT 2016-002277-35).

Rho-kinase antagonists

Rho-kinase is a kinase involved in regulating the cytoskeleton. Fasudil is a selective rho-kinase inhibitor, which reduces smooth muscle cell proliferation and increases blood brain barrier integrity. In one study of 160 patients it improved early neurological deficit in acute ischaemic stroke of any subtype.[133] SVD is associated with chronic blood–brain barrier dysfunction, which may be due to a different process than the dysfunction seen in acute ischaemia, however.

Stimulants

The sympathomimetic, amphetamine, has been assessed in 329 patients in 11 trials to improve motor recovery following stroke but is associated with increased BP and mortality, and has not been assessed specifically in people with SVD.[134] Modafinil inhibits dopamine transport and is licensed for use in narcolepsy to reduce fatigue and improve cognition. A RCT of modafinil versus placebo in 41 patients assessing post-stroke fatigue found no difference in the multidimensional fatigue inventory-20 general fatigue domain at day 90 but there were significant improvements in other fatigue scoring scales (secondary outcomes) that could be explored further.[135] Again, this medication's use has not been reported in the context of SVD.

Vitamins

The vitamins most likely to improve SVD are those that affect homocysteine metabolism. These include vitamins B_6, B_{12}, and folate. Low levels of B_{12} have been associated with more severe WMH.[136] Trials have failed to show that administration of these vitamins reduces stroke recurrence,[137,138] but a small substudy from the VITATOPS trial suggested that patients with severe WMH had slower WMH progression when given B vitamins.[139] These findings remain to be replicated.

Xanthine oxidase inhibitors

Inhibition of xanthine oxidase lowers plasma uric acid levels, and allopurinol and febuxostat are used for this purpose for the treatment of gout. Allopurinol has multiple other effects including modulation of vascular function through increasing nitric oxide availability, reducing blood vessel stiffness, BP, and left ventricular hypertrophy, as well as anti-inflammatory effects[34] and may be beneficial in prevention of myocardial ischaemia. The effects on vascular function may simply be due to co-association with body mass index, however.[140] One small study of 50 patients with small subcortical stroke failed to show any effect of allopurinol on cerebral vasoreactivity, augmentation index (a marker of vessel stiffness), or soluble markers of inflammation.[141] A further trial in 80 patients with any type of ischaemic stroke (50% of participants had lacunar strokes) showed reduced central systolic BP, augmentation index, and carotid intimamedia thickness progression following 1 year of allopurinol therapy.[142] Larger trials, such as Xilo-FIST (ClinicalTrials. gov: NCT02122718), are ongoing.

Immunosuppressive agents

Immunosuppressive agents exhibit anti-inflammatory effects and might interfere with the inflammatory processes involved in the development of SVD.[34] Methotrexate and monoclonal antibodies may not be best suited to treating SVD due to the likely lifelong treatment required and toxicity of these agents. Monoclonal antibodies also have difficulty penetrating the brain. Other less expensive and toxic agents that might merit consideration include thalidomide, which has anti-TNF alpha and antiangiogenic effects and currently has a role in treating multiple myeloma.

Lifestyle interventions

A number of observational studies suggest that lifestyle measures may have a role in preventing SVD or slowing its progression. Whether lifestyle changes would specifically affect SVD pathogenesis or simply improve general health is unclear (Box 11.2).

Given the strong association of smoking with sporadic lacunar ischaemic stroke[143] as well as in patients with CADASIL,[144] smoking cessation should be strongly encouraged. Smoking has been demonstrated to have a dose-dependent effect on WMH progression that persists for at least 6 years after cessation of smoking.[145] In older community-based non-stroke subjects, smoking also thins the cerebral cortex in a dose-dependent manner, which requires on average 25 years after cessation for cortical thickness to equate to that seen in non-smokers.[146]

Exercise similarly may improve SVD. One cohort study has shown that higher levels of physical activity are associated with greater integrity of white matter tracts, greater grey and normal white matter volumes, and lower atrophy and WMH volume.[147] However, association is not causation and no intervention studies on the role of increasing exercise on WMH progression exist.

Other interventions include salt reduction. Higher self-reported salt intake has been associated with increased WMH.[148] Reducing dietary salt is known to lower BP, platelet activity, and oxidative stress.

Interventions to reduce emotional stress may also have a role, although these remain untested. Perceived stress has been associated with subclinical cerebral infarction.[149]

Box 11.2 Potential future SVD interventions for testing

♦ BP and lipid lowering: intensity (intensive versus guideline) or drug class comparison trials would be needed due to their standard usage in secondary prevention after ischaemic stroke.

♦ Polymechanistic agents: NO donors, statins, prostacyclin agonists, PDE3 inhibitors (cilostazol, pentoxifylline, triflusal) and PDE5 inhibitors (dipyridamole) each have multiple mechanisms of action that could be beneficial.

♦ Drug combinations that maximize the modulation of multiple potential mechanisms of action:

  • Unrelated but synergistic effects: assessment of two or more agents (e.g. xanthine oxidase inhibitor and PPAR-gamma agonist, intensive BP and lipid lowering, NO modulation and BP lowering).

  • Related effects: assessment of interventions with similar mechanisms (e.g. cAMP and cGMP modulation (cilostazol and dipyridamole,[54] cilostazol and pentoxifylline,[147] cilostazol and isosorbide mononitrate, or cilostazol dinitrate, a hybrid drug)).

♦ Potential RCT designs[34]:

  • Aim: prevention versus stabilization/reduction of existing disease.

  • Patients: pre- or post-stroke, cognitive impairment present or absent, imaging evidence of SVD present or absent.

  • Comparators: open label or placebo controlled.

  • Outcomes: functional (e.g. mRS), cognitive, imaging based, stroke prevention, SVD prevention.

  • Design: single-blinded blinded outcome, double-blinded placebo-controlled, open-label blinded outcome.

Conclusion

The stroke, cognitive, and imaging manifestations of SVD are common, especially in the ageing population, and therefore its incidence and prevalence are likely to increase. The pathophysiology of SVD is different to other stroke subtypes thus requiring singular interventions. Future trials in SVD will have to define their population more clearly in order to identify the beneficial effects on SVD.

Although there are currently no proven treatments for the prevention or treatment of SVD, there are several agents that in isolation or combination may be beneficial. Careful management of hypertension, avoidance of smoking, management of other vascular risk factors such as with statins and good glycaemic control in diabetics, and encouraging a healthy lifestyle are all sensible with some supporting evidence. Participation in the several ongoing randomized controlled trials (RCTs) is to be encouraged. The use of medications licensed in other areas, so-called drug repurposing, should be investigated. Ongoing and future research will aim to find specific biomarkers and tailored treatments for the management of this common, insidious, and disabling condition.

Acknowledgements

Bath is Stroke Association Professor of Stroke Medicine, is an NIHR Senior Investigator and receives funding from the British Heart Foundation (BHF, CS/14/4/30972, CS/15/5/31475), National Institute of Health Research (NIHR) Health Technology Assessment Programme (10/104/24) and the Alzheimer's Society Ref 252 (AS-PG-14-033). Appleton is funded on the British Heart Foundation (BHF, CS/14/4/30972) and National Institute of Health Research (NIHR) Health Technology Assessment Programme (10/104/24). Blair receives funding from the European Union Horizon 2020, PHC-03-15, project No 666881, 'SVDs@Target' grant, the Alzheimer Society Ref: 252 (AS-PG-14-033) and the Edinburgh and Lothians Health Foundation. Wardlaw receives funding from the Medical Research Council through the UK Dementia Research Institute at The University of Edinburgh, the Foundation Leducq Transatlantic Network of Excellence for the Study of Perivascular Spaces in Small Vessel Disease (16 CVD 05), the Chief Scientist Office (ETM/326), the Row Fogo Charitable Trust (BRO-D.FID3668413), the Wellcome Trust (WT088134/Z/09/A), the Alzheimer's Society Ref 252 (AS-PG-14-033), and British Heart Foundation (through grant CS/15/5/31475 and the British Heart Foundation Centre of Research Excellence).

References

1. **Wardlaw J, Smith C, & Dichgans M.** Mechanisms of sporadic cerebral small vessel disease: insights from neuroimaging. *Lancet Neurol* 2013;**12**(5):483–97.

2. **Debette S & Markus HS.** The clinical importance of white matter hyperintensities on brain magnetic resonance imaging: systematic review and meta-analysis. *BMJ* 2010;**341**:c3666.

3. **Warlow C, Sudlow C, Dennis M, Wardlaw J, & Sandercock P.** Stroke. *Lancet* 2003;**362**:1211–24.

4. **Rost NS, Rahman RM, Biffi A,** et al. White matter hyperintensity volume is increased in small vessel stroke subtypes. *Neurology* 2010;**75**(19):1670–7.

5. **Ostergaard L, Sondergaard T, Moreton F,** et al. Cerebral small vessel disease: capillary pathways to stroke and cognitive decline. *J Cereb Blood Flow Metab* 2016; **36**(2):302–25.

6. **Wardlaw JM, Smith EE, Biessels GJ,** et al. Neuroimaging standards for research into small vessel disease and its contribution to ageing and neurodegeneration. *Lancet Neurol* 2013;**12**(8):822–38.

7. **Valdes Hernandez MC, Maconick LC, Munoz Maniega S,** et al. A comparison of location of acute symptomatic versus 'silent' small vessel lesions. *Int J Stroke* 2015;**10**:1044–50.

8. **Wardlaw JM, Allerhand M, Doubal FN,** et al. Vascular risk factors, large-artery atheroma, and brain white matter hyperintensities. *Neurology* 2014;**82**(15):1331–8.

9. **Mead GE, Lewis SC, Wardlaw JM, Dennis MS, & Warlow CP.** Severe ipsilateral carotid stenosis and middle cerebral artery disease in lacunar ischaemic stroke: innocent bystanders? *J Neurol* 2002;**249**(3):266–71.

10. **Potter GM, Doubal FN, Jackson CA, Sudlow CL, Dennis MS, & Wardlaw JM.** Lack of association of white matter lesions with ipsilateral carotid artery stenosis. *Cerebrovasc Dis* 2012;**33**(4):378–84.

11. **Del Bene A, Makin SD, Doubal FN, & Wardlaw JM.** Do risk factors for lacunar ischaemic stroke vary with the location or appearance of the lacunar infarct? *Cerebrovasc Dis* 2012;**33**(1):21.

12. **Farrall AJ & Wardlaw JM.** Blood-brain barrier: ageing and microvascular disease - systematic review and meta-analysis. *Neurobiol Aging* 2009;**30**(3):337–52.

13. **Bailey EL, Smith C, Sudlow CL, & Wardlaw JM.** Pathology of lacunar ischemic stroke in humans—a systematic review. *Brain Pathol* 2012;**22**(5):583–91.

14. **Wiseman S, Marlborough F, Doubal F, Webb DJ, & Wardlaw J.** Blood markers of coagulation, fibrinolysis, endothelial dysfunction and inflammation in lacunar stroke versus non-lacunar stroke and non-stroke: systematic review and meta-analysis. *Cerebrovasc Dis* 2014;**37**:64–75.

15. **Wiseman SJ, Ralston SH, & Wardlaw JM.** Cerebrovascular disease in rheumatic diseases: a systematic review and meta-analysis. *Stroke* 2016;47(4):943–50.

16. **Goyal M, Menon BK, van Zwam WH,** et al. Endovascular thrombectomy after large-vessel ischaemic stroke: a meta-analysis of individual patient data from five randomised trials. *Lancet* 2016;397(10029):1723–31.

17. **Vahedi K, Hofmeijer J, Vacaut E,** et al. Early decompressive surgery in malignant infarction of the middle cerebral artery: a pooled analysis of three randomised controlled trials. *Lancet Neurol* 2007;6:215–22.

18. **The National Institute of Neurological Disorders and Stroke rt-PA Stroke Study Group.** Tissue plasminogen activator for acute stroke. *N Engl J Med* 1995;333:1581–7.

19. **Sandercock P, Wardlaw JM, Lindley RI,** et al. The benefits and harms of intravenous thrombolysis with recombinant tissue plasminogen activator within 6 h of acute ischaemic stroke (the third international stroke trial [IST-3]): a randomised controlled trial. *Lancet* 2012;379(9834):2352–63.

20. **Lindley RI, Wardlaw JM, Whiteley WN,** et al. Alteplase for acute ischemic stroke: outcomes by clinically important subgroups in the Third International Stroke Trial. *Stroke* 2015;46:746–56.

21. **Shobha N, Fang J, & Hill MD.** Do lacunar strokes benefit from thrombolysis? Evidence from the Registry of the Canadian Stroke Network. *Int J Stroke* 2013;8:45–9.

22. **Barow E, Boutitie F, Cheng B,** et al. Functional outcome of intravenous thrombolysis in patients with lacunar infarcts in the WAKE-UP Trial. *JAMA Neurol* 2019.

23. **Emberson J, Lees K, Lyden P,** et al. Effect of treatment delay, age and stroke severity on the effects of intravenous thrombolysis with alteplase for acute ischaemic stroke: a meta-analysis of individual patient data from randomised trials. *Lancet* 2014;384(9958):1929–35.

24. **Whiteley WN, Emberson J, Lees KR,** et al. Risk of intracerebral haemorrhage with alteplase after acute ischaemic stroke: a secondary analysis of an individual patient data meta-analysis. *Lancet Neurol* 2016;15:925–33.

25. **Greisenegger S, Seyfang L, Kiechi S, Lang W, Ferrari J, & Collaborators ASUR.** Thrombolysis in patients with mild stroke: results from the Austrian Stroke Unit Registry. *Stroke* 2014;45(3):765–9.

26. **group TI-c.** Association between brain imaging signs, early and late outcomes, and response to intravenous alteplase after ischaemic stroke in the third International Stroke Trial (IST-3): a secondary analysis of a randomised controlled trial. *Lancet Neurol* 2015;14(5):485–96.

27. **Whiteley WN, Bruins Slot K, Fernandes P, Sandercock P, & Wardlaw JM.** Risk factors for intracranial haemorrhage in acute ischemic stroke patients treated with recombinant tissue plasminogen activator: a systematic review and meta-analysis of 55 studies. *Stroke* 2012;43:2904–9.

28. **Willer L, Havsteen I, Ovesen C, Christensen AF, & Christensen H.** Computed tomography-verified leukoaraiosis is a risk factor for post-thrombolytic hemorrhage. *J Stroke Cerebrovasc Dis* 2015;24(6):1126–30.

29. **Curtze S, Melkas S, Sibolt G,** et al. Cerebral computed tomography-graded white matter lesions are associated with worse outcome after thrombolysis in patients with stroke. *Stroke* 2015;46:1554–60.

30. **Arba F, Palumbo V, Boulanger JM,** et al. Leukoaraiosis and lacunes are associated with poor clinical outcomes in ischemic stroke patients treated with intravenous thrombolysis. *Int J Stroke* 2016;11(1):62–7.

31. **Charidimou A, Kakar P, Fox Z, & Werring DJ.** Cerebral microbleeds and the risk of intracerebral haemorrhage after thrombolysis for acute ischaemic stroke: systematic review and meta-analysis. *J Neurol Neurosurg Psychiatry* 2013;84:277–80.

32. **Shoamanesh A, Kwok CS, Lim PA, & Benavente OR.** Postthrombolysis intracranial hemorrhage risk of cerebral microbleeds in acute stroke patients: a systematic review and meta-analysis. *Int J Stroke* 2012;8(5):348–56.

33. **Dannenberg S, Scheitz JF, Rozanski M,** et al. Number of cerebral microbleeds and risk of intracerebral hemorrhage after intravenous thrombolysis. *Stroke* 2014;45:2900–5.

34. **Bath PM & Wardlaw JM.** Pharmacological treatment and prevention of cerebral small vessel disease: a review of potential interventions. *Int J Stroke* 2015;**10**(4):469–78.

35. **Saxena R & Koudstaal P.** Anticoagulants for preventing stroke in patients with nonrheumatic atrial fibrillation and a history of stroke or transient ischaemic attack. Cochrane Database Syst Rev 2004(2):CD000185.

36. **Ruff CT, Giugliano RP, Braunwald E, et al.** Comparison of the efficacy and safety of new oral anticoagulants with warfarin in patients with atrial fibrillation: a meta-analysis of randomised trials. *Lancet* 2014;**383**(9921):955–62.

37. **SPIRIT Study Group.** A randomized trial of anticoagulants versus aspirin after cerebral ischemia of presumed arterial origin. The Stroke Prevention in Reversible Ischemia Trial (SPIRIT) Study Group. *Ann Neurol* 1997;**42**(6):857–65.

38. **Charidimou A, Wilson D, Shakeshaft C, et al.** The Clinical Relevance of Microbleeds in Stroke study (CROMIS-2): rationale, design and methods. *Int J Stroke* 2015;**10**:155–61.

39. **Malouf R & Birks J.** Donepezil for vascular cognitive impairment. *Cochrane Database Syst Rev* 2004(1):CD004395.

40. **McShane R, Areosa Sastre A, & Minakaran N.** Memantine for dementia. *Cochrane Database Syst Rev* 2006(2):CD003154.

41. **Snowdon DA, Greiner LH, Mortimer JA, Riley KP, Greiner PA, & Markesbery WR.** Brain infarction and the clinical expression of Alzheimer disease: the Nun Study. *JAMA* 1997;**277**(10):813–17.

42. **Qaseem A, Snow V, Cross JT, Jr., et al.** Current pharmacologic treatment of dementia: a clinical practice guideline from the American College of Physicians and the American Academy of Family Physicians. *Ann Intern Med* 2008;**148**(5):370–8.

43. **Black S, Roman GC, Geldmacher DS, et al.** Efficacy and tolerability of donepezil in vascular dementia: positive results of a 24-week, multicenter, international, randomized, placebo-controlled clinical trial. *Stroke* 2003;**34**(10):2323–30.

44. **Wilkinson D, Doody R, Helme R, et al.** Donepezil in vascular dementia: a randomized, placebo-controlled study. *Neurology* 2003;**61**(4):479–86.

45. **Orgogozo JM, Rigaud AS, Stoffler A, Mobius HJ, & Forette F.** Efficacy and safety of memantine in patients with mild to moderate vascular dementia: a randomized, placebo-controlled trial (MMM 300). *Stroke* 2002;**33**(7):1834–9.

46. **Wilcock G, Mobius HJ, Stoffler A, & MMM 500 group.** A double-blind, placebo-controlled multicentre study of memantine in mild to moderate vascular dementia (MMM500). *Int Clin Psychopharmacol* 2002;**17**(6):297–305.

47. **Erkinjuntti T, Kurz A, Gauthier S, Bullock R, Lilleneld S, & Damaraju CV.** Efficacy of galantamine in probable vascular dementia and Alzheimer's disease combined with cerebrovascular disease: a randomised trial. *Lancet* 2002;**359**(9314):1283–90.

48. **Auchus AP, Brashear HR, Salloway S, Korczyn AD, De Deyn PP, Gassmann-Mayer C, et al.** Galantamine treatment of vascular dementia: a randomized trial. *Neurology* 2007;**69**(5):448–58.

49. **Craig D & Birks J.** Galantamine for vascular cognitive impairment. *Cochrane Database Syst Rev* 2006;(1):CD004746.

50. **Zhao L, Fletcher S, Weaver C, et al.** Effects of aspirin, clopidogrel and dipyridamole administered singly and in combination on platelet and leucocyte function in normal volunteers and patients with prior ischaemic stroke. *Thromb Haemost* 2005;**93**(3):527–34.

51. **Zhao L, Gray LJ, Leonardi-Bee J, Weaver CS, Heptinstall S, & Bath PM.** Effect of aspirin, clopidogrel and dipyridamole on soluble markers of vascular function in normal volunteers and patients with prior ischaemic stroke. *Platelets* 2006;**17**(2):100–4.

52. **Liu S, Yu C, Yang F, Paganini-Hill A, & Fisher MJ.** Phosphodiesterase inhibitor modulation of brain microvascular endothelial cell barrier properties. *J Neurol Sci* 2012;**320**(1–2):45–51.

53. **Gresele P, Momi S, & Falcinelli E.** Anti-platelet therapy: phosphodiesterase inhibitors. *Br J Clin Pharmacol* 2011;**72**(4):634–46.

54. **Rondina MT & Weyrich AS.** Targeting phosphodiesterases in anti-platelet therapy. *Handb Exp Pharmacol* 2012(210):225–38.

55. **Pullamsetti SS, Savai R, Schaefer MB, et al.** cAMP phosphodiesterase inhibitors increases nitric oxide production by modulating dimethylarginine dimethylaminohydrolases. *Circulation* 2011;**123**(11):1194–204.

56. **Geeganage CM, Diener HC, Algra A, et al.** Dual or mono antiplatelet therapy for patients with acute ischemic stroke or transient ischemic attack: systematic review and meta-analysis of randomized controlled trials. *Stroke* 2012;**43**(4):1058–66.

57. **Wong KSL, Wang Y, Leng X, et al.** Early dual versus mono antiplatelet therapy for acute non-cardioembolic ischemic stroke or transient ischemic attack: an updated systematic review and meta-analysis. *Circulation* 2013;**128**(15):1656–66.

58. **Antithrombotic Trialists Collaboration.** Collaborative meta-analysis of randomised trials of antiplatelet therapy for prevention of death, myocardial infarction, and stroke in high risk patients. *BMJ* 2002;**324**(7329):71–86.

59. **Palacio S, Hart RG, Pearce LA, & Benavente OR.** Effect of addition of clopidogrel to aspirin on mortality: systematic review of randomized trials. *Stroke* 2012;**43**(8):2157–62.

60. **Squizzato A, Keller T, Romualdi E, & Middeldorp S.** Clopidogrel plus aspirin versus aspirin alone for preventing cardiovascular disease. Cochrane Database Syst Rev 2011(1):CD005158.

61. **Diener HC, Cunha L, Forbes C, Sivenius J, Smets P, & Lowenthal A.** European stroke prevention study 2. Dipyridamole and acetylsalicylic acid in the secondary prevention of stroke. *J Neurol Sci* 1996;**143**(1–2):1–13.

62. **The ESPRIT Study Group.** Aspirin plus dipyridamole versus aspirin alone after cerebral ischaemia of arterial origin (ESPRIT): randomised controlled trial. *Lancet* 2006;**367**:1665–73.

63. **Bhatt DL, Fox KAA, Hacke W, et al.** Clopidogrel and aspirin versus aspirin alone for the prevention of atherothrombotic events. N Engl J Med 2006;**354**(16):1706–17.

64. **Diener HC, Bogousslavsky J, Brass LM, et al.** Aspirin and clopidogrel compared with clopidogrel alone after recent ischaemic stroke or transient ischaemic attack in high-risk patients (MATCH): randomised, double-blind, placebo-controlled trial. *Lancet* 2004;**364**(9431):331–7.

65. **SPS3 Investigators BO, Hart RG, McClure LA, Szychowski JM, Coffey CS, & Pearce LA.** Effects of clopidogrel added to aspirin in patients with recent lacunar stroke. *N Engl J Med* 2012;**376**(9):817–25.

66. **Sprigg N, Gray LJ, England T, et al.** A randomised controlled trial of triple antiplatelet therapy (aspirin, clopidogrel and dipyridamole) in the secondary prevention of stroke: safety, tolerability and feasibility. *PLoS One* 2008;**3**(8):e2852.

67. **Morrow D, Braunwald M, Bonaca M, et al.** Vorapaxar in the secondary prevention of atherothrombotic events. *N Engl J Med* 2012;**366**:1404–13.

68. **Omote Y, Deguchi K, Tian F, et al.** Clinical and pathological improvement in stroke-prone spontaneous hypertensive rats related to the pleiotropic effect of cilostazol. *Stroke* 2012;**43**(6):1639–46.

69. **Miyamoto N, Tanaka R, Shimura H, et al.** Phosphodiesterase III inhibition promotes differentiation and survival of oligodendrocyte progenitors and enhances regeneration of ischemic white matter lesions in the adult mammalian brain. *J Cereb Blood Flow Metab* 2010;**30**(2):299–310.

70. **Han SW, Lee SS, Kim SH, et al.** Effect of cilostazol in acute lacunar infarction based on pulsatility index of transcranial Doppler (ECLIPse): a multicenter, randomized, double-blind, placebo-controlled trial. *Eur Neurol* 2013;**69**(1):33–40.

71. **Kondo R, Matsumoto Y, Furui E, et al.** Effect of cilostazol in the treatment of acute ischemic stroke in the lenticulostriate artery territory. *Eur Neurol* 2013;**69**(2):122–8.

72. **Uchiyama S, Demaerschalk BM, Goto S, et al.** Stroke prevention by cilostazol in patients with atherothrombosis: meta-analysis of placebo-controlled randomized trials. *J Stroke Cerebrovasc Dis* 2009;**18**(6):482–90.

73. **Kamal AK, Naqvi I, Husain MR, & Khealani BA.** Cilostazol versus aspirin for secondary prevention of vascular events after stroke of arterial origin. *Cochrane Database Syst Rev* 2011;(1):CD008076.

74. **Dinicolantonio JJ, Lavie CJ, Fares H,** et al. Meta-analysis of cilostazol versus aspirin for the secondary prevention of stroke. *Am J Cardiol* 2013;**112**:1230–4.

75. **Shi LG, Pu JL, Xu L, Malaguit J, & Zhang J.** The efficacy and safety of cilostazol for the secondary prevention of ischaemic stroke in acute and chronic phases in Asian population - an updated meta-analysis. *BMC Neurol* 2014;**14**:251.

76. **Kim BJ, Lee E-J, Kwon SU,** et al. Prevention of cardiovascular events in Asian patients with ischaemic stroke at high risk of cerebral haemorrhage (PICASSO): a multicentre, randomised controlled trial. *Lancet Neurol* 2018;**17**(6):509–18.

77. **Li W & Tai LW.** Cilostazol verse aspirin for vascular dementia in poststroke patients with white matter lesions (CAVAD)2012 05/02/2016.

78. **Blair GW, Appleton JP, Flaherty K,** et al. Tolerability, safety and intermediary pharmacological effects of cilostazol and isosorbide mononitrate, alone and combined, in patients with lacunar ischaemic stroke: the LACunar Intervention-1 (LACI-1) trial, a randomised clinical trial. *EClin Med* 2019;**11**:34–43.

79. **Jackson CA, Hutchison A, Dennis MS, Wardlaw JM, Lewis SC, & Sudlow CL.** Differences between ischemic stroke subtypes in vascular outcomes support a distinct lacunar ischemic stroke arteriopathy: a prospective, hospital-based study. *Stroke* 2009;**40**(12):3679–84.

80. **Kerney PM, Whelton M, Reynolds K, Muntner P, Whelton PK, & He J.** Global burden of hypertension: analysis of worldwide data. *Lancet* 2005;**365**:217–23.

81. **Perry HM, Jr., Davis BR, Price TR,** et al. Effect of treating isolated systolic hypertension on the risk of developing various types and subtypes of stroke: the Systolic Hypertension in the Elderly Program (SHEP). *JAMA* 2000;**284**(4):465–71.

82. **Rashid P, Leonardi-Bee J, & Bath P.** Blood pressure reduction and the secondary prevention of stroke and other vascular events: a systematic review. *Stroke* 2003;**34**:2741–9.

83. **Benavente OR, Coffey CS, Conwit R,** et al. Blood-pressure targets in patients with recent lacunar stroke: the SPS3 randomised trial. *Lancet* 2013;**382**(9891):507–15.

84. **Pearce L, McClure L, Anderson D,** et al. Effects of long-term blood pressure lowering and dual antiplatelet treatment on cognitive function in patients with recent lacunar stroke: a secondary analysis from the SPS3 randomised trial. *Lancet Neurol* 2014;**13**(12):1177–85.

85. **SPRINT Research Group, Wright JT Jr, Williamson JD,** et al. A randomized trial of intensive versus standard blood-pressure control. *N Engl J Med* 2015;**373**(22):2103–16.

86. **Group TSMIftSR.** Effect of intensive vs standard blood pressure control on probable dementia: a randomized clinical trial. *JAMA* 2019;**321**(6):553–61.

87. **Bath PM, Scutt P, Blackburn DJ,** et al. Intensive versus guideline blood pressure and lipid lowering in patients with previous stroke: main results from the pilot 'Prevention of Decline in Cognition after Stroke Trial' (PODCAST) Randomised Controlled Trial. *PLoS One* 2017;**12**(1):e0164608.

88. **Dufouil C, Chalmers J, Coskun O,** et al. Effects of blood pressure lowering on cerebral white matter hyperintensities in patients with stroke: the PROGRESS (Perindopril Protection Against Recurrent Stroke Study) Magnetic Resonance Imaging Substudy. *Circulation* 2005;**112**(11):1644–50.

89. **Weber R, Weimar C, Blatchford J,** et al. Telmisartan on top of antihypertensive treatment does not prevent progression of cerebral white matter lesions in the prevention regimen for effectively avoiding second strokes (PRoFESS) MRI substudy. *Stroke* 2012;**43**(9):2336–42.

90. **Ovbiagele B, Diener H-C, Yusuf S,** et al. Level of systolic blood pressure within the normal range and risk of recurrent stroke. *JAMA* 2011;**306**(19):2137–44.

91. **Sabayan B, van Vliet P, de Ruijter W, Gussekloo J, de Craen AJ, & Westendorp RG.** High blood pressure, physical and cognitive function, and risk of stroke in the oldest old: the Leiden 85-plus Study. *Stroke* 2013;**44**(1):15–20.

92. **Emdin CA, Rothwell PM, Salimi-Khorshidi G**, et al. Blood pressure and risk of vascular dementia: evidence from a primary care registry and a cohort study of transient ischemic attack and stroke. *Stroke* 2016;**47**:1429–35.

93. **Bohm M, Cotton D, Foster L**, et al. Impact of resting heart rate on mortality, disability and cognitive decline in patients after ischaemic stroke. *Eur Heart J* 2012;**33**(22):2804–12.

94. **Rothwell PM, Howard SC, Dolan E**, et al. Prognostic significance of visit-to-visit variability, maximum systolic blood pressure, and episodic hypertension. *Lancet* 2010;**375**(9718):895–905.

95. **Hainsworth AH & Markus HS.** Do in vivo experimental models reflect human cerebral small vessel disease? A systematic review. *J Cereb Blood Flow Metab* 2008;**28**(12):1877–91.

96. **Bailey EL, McCulloch J, Sudlow C, & Wardlaw JM.** Potential animal models of lacunar stroke: a systematic review. *Stroke* 2009;**40**(6):e451–8.

97. **Pedder H, Vesterinen HM, Macleod MR, & Wardlaw JM.** Systematic review and meta-analysis of interventions tested in animal models of lacunar stroke. *Stroke* 2014;**45**:563–70.

98. **Manktelow BN & Potter JF.** Interventions in the management of serum lipids for preventing stroke recurrence. *Cochrane Database Syst Rev* 2009;**8**(3):CD002091.

99. **Amarenco P, Labreuche J, Lavallee P, & Touboul P-J.** Statins in stroke prevention and carotid atherosclerosis: systematic review and up-to-date meta-analysis. *Stroke* 2004;**35**:2902–9.

100. **Amarenco P, Bogousslavsky J, Callahan A**, 3rd, et al. High-dose atorvastatin after stroke or transient ischemic attack. *N Engl J Med* 2006;**355**(6):549–59.

101. **Amarenco P, Benavente O, Goldstein LB**, et al. Results of the Stroke Prevention by Aggressive Reduction in Cholesterol Levels (SPARCL) trial by stroke subtypes. *Stroke* 2009;**40**(4):1405–9.

102. **Heart Protection Study Collaborative Group.** Effects of cholesterol-lowering with simvastatin on stroke and other major vascular events in 20536 people with cerebrovascular disease or other high-risk conditions. *Lancet* 2004;**363**(9411):757–67.

103. **Shepherd J, Blauw GJ, Murphy MB**, et al. Pravastatin in elderly individuals at risk of vascular disease (PROSPER): a randomised controlled trial. *Lancet* 2002;**360**:1623–30.

104. **ten Dam VH, van den Heuvel DM, van Buchem MA**, et al. Effect of pravastatin on cerebral infarcts and white matter lesions. *Neurology* 2005;**64**(10):1807–9.

105. **Mok VC, Lam WW, Fan YH**, et al. Effects of statins on the progression of cerebral white matter lesion: post hoc analysis of the ROCAS (Regression of Cerebral Artery Stenosis) study. *J Neurol* 2009;**256**(5):750–7.

106. **Lavallee PC, Labreuche J, Gongora-Rivera F**, et al. Placebo-controlled trial of high-dose atorvastatin in patients with severe cerebral small vessel disease. *Stroke* 2009;**40**(5):1721–8.

107. **Topakian R, Barrick TR, Howe FA, & Markus HS.** Blood-brain barrier permeability is increased in normal-appearing white matter in patients with lacunar stroke and leucoaraiosis. *J Neurol Neurosurg Psychiatry* 2010;**81**(2):192–7.

108. **Wardlaw JM, Doubal F, Armitage P**, et al. Lacunar stroke is associated with diffuse blood-brain barrier dysfunction. *Ann Neurol* 2009;**65**(2):194–202.

109. **Chen N, Yang M, Guo J, Zhou M, Zhu C, & He L.** Cerebrolysin for vascular dementia. *Cochrane Database Syst Rev* 2013;**1**:CD008900.

110. **Willmot MR & Bath PM.** The potential of nitric oxide therapeutics in stroke. *Expert Opin Investig Drugs* 2003;**12**(3):455–70.

111. **Radomski MW, Palmer RM, & Moncada S.** The role of nitric oxide and cGMP in platelet adhesion to vascular endothelium. *Biochem Biophys Res Commun* 1987;**148**(3):1482–9.

112. **Bath PMW, Hassall DG, Gladwin A-M, Palmer RMJ, & Martin JF.** Nitric oxide and prostacyclin. Divergence of inhibitory effects on monocyte chemotaxis and adhesion to endothelium in vitro. *Arterioscler Thromb* 1991;**11**:254–60.

113. **Vallance P, Collier J, & Moncada S.** Effects of endothelium-derived nitric oxide on peripheral arteriolar tone in man. *Lancet* 1989;**2**(8670):997–1000.

114. **Bath PMW.** The effect of nitric oxide-donating vasodilators on monocyte chemotaxis and intracellular cGMP concentrations in vitro. *Eur J Clin Pharmacol* 1993;**45**:53–8.

115. **Butterworth RJ, Cluckie A, Jackson SH, Buxton-Thomas M, & Bath PM.** Pathophysiological assessment of nitric oxide (given as sodium nitroprusside) in acute ischaemic stroke. *Cerebrovasc Dis* 1998;**8**(3):158–65.

116. **Bath PMW, Pathansali R, Iddenden R, & Bath FJ.** The effect of transdermal glyceryl trinitrate, a nitric oxide donor, on blood pressure and platelet function in acute stroke. *Cerebrovasc Dis* 2001;**11**:265–72.

117. **Rashid PA, Whitehurst A, Lawson N, & Bath PMW.** Plasma nitric oxide (nitrate/nitrite) levels in acute stroke and their relationship with severity and outcome. *J Stroke Cerebrovasc Dis* 2003;**12**(2):82–7.

118. **Ferlito S, Gallina M, Pitari GM, & Bianchi A.** Nitric oxide plasma levels in patients with chronic and acute cerebrovascular disorders. *Panminerva Med* 1998;**40**:51–4.

119. **Hassan A, Hunt BJ, O'Sullivan M, et al.** Markers of endothelial dysfunction in lacunar infarction and ischaemic leukoaraiosis. *Brain* 2003;**126**(Pt 2):424–32.

120. **Presley TD, Morgan AR, Bechtold E, et al.** Acute effect of a high nitrate diet on brain perfusion in older adults. *Nitric Oxide* 2011;**24**(1):34–42.

121. **Bath PM.** William M Feinberg award for excellence in clinical stroke: high explosive treatment for ultra-acute stroke: hype of hope. *Stroke* 2016;**47**:2423–6.

122. **Willmot M, Gray L, Gibson C, Murphy S, & Bath PMW.** A systematic review of nitric oxide donors and L-arginine in experimental stroke; effects on infarct size and cerebral blood flow. *Nitric Oxide* 2005;**12**(3):141–9.

123. **Bath P, Woodhouse L, Scutt P, et al.** Efficacy of nitric oxide, with or without continuing antihypertensive treatment, for management of high blood pressure in acute stroke (ENOS): a partial-factorial randomised controlled trial. *Lancet* 2015;**385**(9968):617–28.

124. **Leonardi-Bee J, Bath PM, Bousser MG, et al.** Dipyridamole for preventing recurrent ischemic stroke and other vascular events: a meta-analysis of individual patient data from randomized controlled trials. *Stroke* 2005;**36**(1):162–8.

125. **Wilcox R, Bousser M-G, Betteridge DJ, et al.** Effects of pioglitazone in patients with type 2 diabetes with or without previous stroke: results from PROactive (PROspective pioglitAzone Clinical Trial in macroVascular Events 04). *Stroke* 2007;**38**(3):865–73.

126. **Kernan WN, Viscoli CM, Furie KL, et al.** Pioglitazone after ischemic stroke or transient ischemic attack. *N Engl J Med* 2016;**374**(14):1321–31.

127. **Bath PM, Appleton JP, & Sprigg N.** The Insulin Resistance Intervention after Stroke trial: a perspective on future practice and research. *Int J Stroke* 2016;**11**(7):741–3.

128. **Ciudin A, Hernandez C, & Simo R.** Update on cardiovascular safety of PPARgamma agonists and relevance to medicinal chemistry and clinical pharmacology. *Curr Top Med Chem* 2012;**12**(6):585–604.

129. **Bath PMW.** Prostacyclin and analogues for acute ischaemic stroke. *Cochrane Database Syst Rev* 2004(3):CD000177.

130. **Bath PM, Bath-Hextall FJ.** Pentoxifylline, propentofylline and pentifylline for acute ischaemic stroke. *Cochrane Database Syst Rev* 2004(3):CD000162.

131. **Frampton M, Harvey RJ, & Kirchner V.** Propentofylline for dementia. *Cochrane Database Syst Rev* 2003(2):CD002853.

132. **Costa J, Ferro JM, Matias-Guiu J, Alvarez-Sabin J, & Torres F.** Triflusal for preventing serious vascular events in people at high risk. *Cochrane Database Syst Rev* 2005(3):CD004296.

133. **Shibuya M, Hirai S, Seto M, Satoh S, & Ohtomo E.** Effects of fasudil in acute ischemic stroke: results of a prospective placebo-controlled double-blind trial. *J Neurol Sci* 2005;**238**(1–2):31–9.

134. **Sprigg N & Bath PM.** Speeding stroke recovery? A systematic review of amphetamine after stroke. *J Neurol Sci* 2009;**285**(1–2):3–9.

135. **Poulsen MB, Damgaard B, Overgaard K, & Rasmussen RS.** Modafinil may alleviate poststroke fatigue: a randomized, placebo-controlled, double-blinded trial. *Stroke* 2015;**46**:3470–7.

136. **de Lau LM, Smith AD, Refsum H, Johnston C, & Breteler MM.** Plasma vitamin B12 status and cerebral white-matter lesions. *J Neurol Neurosurg Psychiatry* 2009;**80**(2):149–57.

137. **The VITATOPS Trial Study Group.** B vitamins in patients with recent transient ischaemic attack or stroke in the VITAmins TO Prevent Stroke (VITATOPS) trial: a randomised, double-blind, parallel, placebo-controlled trial. *Lancet Neurol* 2010;**9**:855–65.

138. **Toole JF, Malinow MR, Chambless LE, et al.** Lowering homocysteine in patients with ischemic stroke to prevent recurrent stroke, myocardial infarction, and death. *JAMA* 2004;**291**(5):565–75.

139. **Cavalieri M, Schmidt R, Chen C, et al.** B vitamins and magnetic resonance imaging-detected ischemic brain lesions in patients with recent transient ischemic attack or stroke: the VITAmins TO Prevent Stroke (VITATOPS) MRI-substudy. *Stroke* 2012;**43**(12):3266–70.

140. **Palmer TM, Nordestgaard BG, Benn M, et al.** Association of plasma uric acid with ischaemic heart disease and blood pressure: mendelian randomisation analysis of two large cohorts. *BMJ* 2013;**347**:f4262.

141. **Dawson J QT, Harrow C, Lees KR, & Walters MR.** The effect of allopurinol on the cerebral vasculature of patients with subcortical stroke; a randomized trial. *Br J Clin Pharmacol* 2009;**68**(5):662–8.

142. **Higgins P, Walters MR, Murray HM, et al.** Allopurinol reduces brachial and central blood pressure, and carotid intima-media thickness progression after ischaemic stroke and transient ischaemic attack: a randomised controlled trial. *Heart* 2014;**100**(14):1085–92.

143. **Staals J, Makin S, Doubal F, Dennis M, & Wardlaw J.** Stroke subtype, vascular risk factors, and total MRI brain small-vessel disease burden. *Neurology* 2014;**83**:1228–34.

144. **Chabriat H, Joutel A, Dichgans M, Tournier-Lasserve E, & Bousser MG.** Cadasil. *Lancet Neurol* 2009;**8**(7):643–53.

145. **Power MC, Deal JA, Sharrett AR, et al.** Smoking and white matter hyperintensity progression: the ARIC-MRI Study. *Neurology* 2015;**84**(8):841–8.

146. **Karama S, Ducharme S, Corley J, et al.** Cigarette smoking and thinning of the brain's cortex. *Mol Psychiatry* 2015;**20**:778–85.

147. **Gow AJ, Bastin ME, Munoz Maniega S, et al.** Neuroprotective lifestyles and the aging brain: activity, atrophy and white matter integrity. *Neurology* 2012;**79**:1802–8.

148. **Heye AK, Thrippleton MJ, Chappell FM, et al.** Blood pressure and sodium: association with MRI markers in cerebral small vessel disease. *J Cereb Blood Flow Metab* 2016;**36**:264–74.

149. **Aggarwal NT, Clark CJ, Beck TL, et al.** Perceived stress is associated with subclinical cerebrovascular disease in older adults. *Am J Geriatr Psychiatry* 2014;**22**(1):53–62.

Chapter 12

Nutrition, feeding, and dysphagia in the older patient with stroke

Jessica Beavan and Lisa Everton

Introduction

The management of dysphagia, nutrition, and hydration are an important part of care within the stroke pathway. Older patients with dysphagia may require enteral feeding and have higher rates of malnutrition, complications, institutionalization, and mortality.

Older people may have prior nutritional and swallowing problems. Both these and new impairments need to be considered when making decisions about interventions, the risks and benefits of each intervention, and how these might affect the recovery and quality of life following a stroke.

The evidence to guide us in the very old and frail is limited and generalizing evidence from available studies may be flawed. Some of the recommendations we make are, therefore, based on our experience rather than backed by substantial evidence. In this chapter we will describe the factors which may affect a person's nutritional status in their later years, the clear link in acute severe stroke with dysphagia, describe currently accepted management, emerging techniques, and suggest a framework which clinicians may find useful to approach these problems. Any clinical plan has to be based on a comprehensive geriatric assessment taking into account the stroke patient's wishes, with contributions from the multidisciplinary team (MDT) and the person's family, legal proxy, or other carers.

Nutrition problems in the older person and in stroke

Changes in the ageing gastrointestinal system as well as the development of physical frailty can lead to problems with nutrition (Table 12.1). A vicious cycle may develop where a system that is dependent on adequate nutrition is unable to function well enough to achieve this. This lack of physiological reserve is well-recognized in the development of frailty syndrome.

In addition to physiological changes specific to the gut, reduced mobility, falls, social isolation, and mental health problems can lead to a reduced dietary intake. Diseases of the gut are more common leading to nutritional deficiencies through lack of absorption or intolerance of certain foods. Body mass ratios change, with greater fat to muscle, as well as loss of stature.

Estimates of undernutrition in community dwelling elders are reported between 6 and 14%[1,2] varying between methods, residence, and country. The major contributors to undernutrition prevalence are dysphagia-related comorbidities[3] and poor dental status.[4]

Prevalence of undernutrition in patients admitted to stroke units is approximately 20%.[5] Markers linked with nutritional status deteriorate after stroke as many of the markers are affected by other processes, for example, loss of muscle mass due to disuse, mid arm circumference (MAC), weight (oedema, change in fat/muscle ratios), and albumin (acute phase responses), making definitions, and monitoring challenging, these being most severe in enterally fed patients. In the United Kingdom, the MUST (Malnutrition Universal Screening Tool) score is used to risk

Table 12.1 The ageing gastrointestinal system

Gastrointestinal unit	Ageing effects
Preparation/anticipation	Reduced appetite/taste/smell Difficulty in food preparation
Oral cavity Dentition	Partial or complete loss of teeth—inability to chew leading to an increasing soft diet Increased risk of oral cancers Increased prevalence of gingivitis and candidiasis Reduced taste Difficulty maintaining oral care
Oro-pharynx	Reduced swallowing times Sarcopaenia of swallow
Oesophagus	Incompetence of gastro-oesophageal junction Increased prevalence of hiatus hernia Early satiety Candidiasis Reduced peristalsis
Stomach	Gastric atrophy Reduced absorption—iron and B_{12} Drug side effects
Duodenum/Small intestine	Reduced absorption Reduced motility Reduced tolerance of different food types
Large bowel	Reduced motility Constipation Increased gastrointestinal malignancy
Ano-rectum	Haemorrhoids and prolapse common Reduction in sphincter control Faecal incontinence Constipation/Impaction

stratify patients.[6] In some patients, the MNA (Mini Nutritional Assessment) may be more useful in identifying factors affecting nutritional status and is well validated in older patients.[7]

Dysphagia in older people and acute stroke

Half of patients with acute stroke (the majority being total anterior circulation strokes) will experience dysphagia. Many will improve, some requiring short-term enteral feeding and a minority a gastrostomy. Older stroke patients are more likely to require interventional nutritional support and have greater complications. Even relatively minor strokes can decompensate an already compromised swallow and obtaining a prior history of problems may hint as to whether recovery is likely to occur.

Community prevalence studies of dysphagia report rates of 12–33% with up to 74% in high-risk cohorts (previous stroke, Parkinson's Disease, chronic obstructive pulmonary disease).[3,8,9] Swallow function changes with age, so swallowing parameters such as swallowing time increase. Generalized muscle loss and weakness (sarcopaenia) is recognized not just to affect girdle skeletal muscle but also swallowing muscles contributing to the frailty syndrome. Grip strength, general functional status, and mobility may be associated with swallow function and its ability to recover.[10] Cervical osteophytes, pharyngeal pouches, achalasia, hiatus hernia, oesophagitis, strictures, and malignancies can also lead to dysphagia.[11]

Dysphagia is a marker of a severe stroke and increases the risk of aspiration pneumonia sevenfold.[12,13] The physical impairments, in addition to aspiration and pneumonia, can lead to a downward spiral of failed feeding, recurrent infection, and deteriorating nutritional and physiological status with dwindling reserves and chance of survival.

Frailty, dysphagia, and stroke

Patients with stroke form a heterogeneous group, even more so as they become older and the concepts of frailty and biological vs. chronological age are useful in evaluating prognosis. Using the deficit model (Rockwood), demonstrating accumulation of problems, maybe more useful in this situation than the phenotype model (Fried).[14] Attention to detail early in admission may be key to preventing the downward feeding spiral, targeting rehabilitation interventions, managing expectations, and deciding when to take a predominantly palliative approach. Following standard treatment guidelines, modified to the individual situation will provide the best outcomes and should not be denied because of age.

Managing undernutrition in stroke

Managing nutrition and hydration requires a multidisciplinary approach to optimize intake considering seating, upper limb function, environmental enhancement, medication changes, and food preparation along with relevant goal setting. Improved nutritional status follows and leads to a good functional recovery.[15–18] Measuring changes of nutritional status post-stroke are difficult and there are currently no stroke specific tools. A generic risk assessment tool, for example, the MUST, along with measures of input, are helpful but are reliant on accurate documentation and interpretation.

Assessment

The MUST score identifies all patients with acute stroke and dysphagia as high risk. Rapid assessment of dysphagia allows clinicians to start early enteral feeding, modify medication, and advise dietary modification to reduce complications. For those with a clearly unsafe swallow and those who are only able to take limited modified diet (i.e. trials) supportive feeding is usually required within 24 hours of admission. Reassessment is best led by the dietitian and specialist nursing team.

Interventions

For many patients this will mean implementing a rehabilitation programme alongside nutritional support, which may be provided orally, enterally, or intravenously (Fig. 12.1).

Oral supplementation

Oral supplementation usually refers to commercial nutrient-dense supplements in addition to usual diet, but it may be more acceptable and sustainable long term to use energy-dense foods and add high calorie substances such as cream to usual foods. This can be a challenge in the hospital environment, and this is where nutrition assistants and family members can contribute and assist at mealtimes.

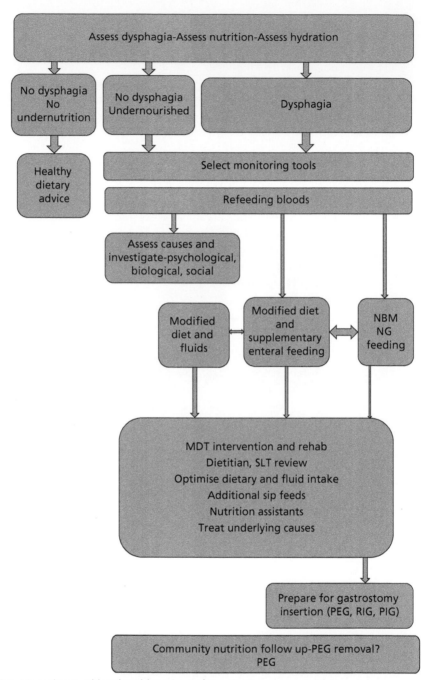

Fig. 12.1 Managing nutritional problems in stroke patients.

NBM, nil by mouth; SLT, speech and language therapist; PEG, percutaneous endoscopic gastrostomy; NG, nasogastric; MDT, multidisciplinary team; PIG, per oral image guided gastrostomy; RIG, radiologically inserted gastrostomy.

Evidence from the limited stroke trials in non-dysphagic patients[17–19] suggest supplementation is only of benefit in undernourished stroke patients, consistent with other trials in other disease groups.[19] Some will have problems of obesity, hypercholesterolaemia, and poor diabetic control, where supplementation may be detrimental and different dietary intervention is required.

Less is known about the optimum diet for rehabilitation. Vitamin supplementation may benefit some patients with inadequate intake and those at risk of refeeding syndrome (Fig. 12.2) will require high dose B vitamin[20] and electrolyte supplementation.

Patients on modified diets are at risk as diets offered may be high in salt, lack fibre, and be unbalanced.[21] Modified diets can form part of a therapeutic swallowing programme. Internationally agreed descriptors may lead to greater consistency in food textures and fluids patients receive (https://www.iddsi.org).

Dehydration is common in older patients with stroke, increasing the risks of infections, constipation, and venous thromboembolism. Ideal fluid intake can be difficult to estimate; most calculations are based on young people without comorbidities. For some patients most of their fluids come from the food they consume.[22] Those on thickened fluids may find them unpleasant and are less likely to be offered fluids as often, resulting in inadequate intake.[22] There is low quality evidence that free water protocols do not increase aspiration pneumonia risk in selected patients, may improve hydration status, and do appear to improve quality of life.[23] Fluid balance documentation and assistance by families, environmental optimization (e.g. seating, table positioning, and setup, red meal trays, e.g. to indicate need for help feeding) and nutrition assistants are helpful before resorting to intravenous fluids.

Enteral feeding

Enteral feeding rates vary between units and countries. Approximately half to two-thirds of dysphagic patients receive some form of nasogastric tube (NGT) feeding.[24] NGT feeding is the method of choice in the acute phase but is fraught with difficulties—securing the tube consistently and safely, delivering adequate feed, fluids, medication, and managing fluid balance and electrolyte abnormalities.[25–27] Gastrostomies improve nutritional indices and feed delivery but are associated with significant mortality and morbidity in stroke patients; therefore, careful selection is required to ensure complication rates are low.[25,28] The risks (Table 12.2) are higher in the acute phase and therefore it is important to optimize NGT feeding early. The use of a nasal bridle (looped NGT) improves the efficiency of feeding by reducing the numbers of NGTs required,[26] which may reduce the need for percutaneous endoscopic gastrostomy (PEG) insertion, but is associated with an increased risk of minor nasal trauma, sinusitis, and is not suitable when there is abnormal nasal anatomy. Forms of restraint such as mittens placed on the active or both hands may reduce the removal of tubes.[29] Their use should be time limited with agreement of family and MDT gained in patients who lack capacity, with a clear care plan (cannula and skin integrity checks, removal when undergoing therapy or relatives present).

The natural history of dysphagia in anterior circulation strokes is of improvement over the first 2–4 weeks,[30] however this is also the time period of greatest complications delaying recovery. Over time the risk of gastrostomy insertion reduces and a decision can be made in most patients by the end of week three whether a PEG insertion is likely to be required with a planned insertion in week four, allowing those with natural recovery to avoid insertion. The two most common methods of gastrostomy insertion are endoscopic (PEG) and radiological (RIG) although another technique; per oral image guided gastrostomy (PIG), is available.[31] There are no direct comparisons in stroke, but RIGs may have a lower complication rate around 1%[32] with PEG 3–10%,[29] although are less secure.[32,33] Surgical gastrostomies have the highest complication rates. The best indicator of likely need for a gastrostomy is stroke severity[34] and bilateral infarction.[35]

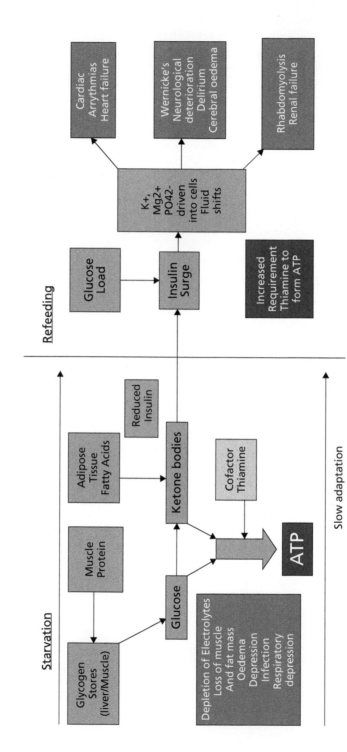

Fig. 12.2 Refeeding syndrome.

Table 12.2 Gastrostomy insertion risk (NPSA/NCEPOD)

Complication[37]	Frequency (approximate) if known* *Clinicians should be aware of their local PEG audit data to advise patients
Death	7 days 3% 1 month 10% 1 year 30–50%*
Local infection	10%
Leakage	58–78%
Blockage	16–31%
Pneumonia	Up to 50% stroke patients
Gastrointestinal bleeding	2.5%
Peritonitis	2.3%
Colonic perforation	2%
Buried bumper syndrome	Unreported
Tumour seeding, gastric volvulus, aorto-gastric fistula	Rare

In posterior circulation strokes, a decision to place an early gastrostomy maybe appropriate as prolonged enteral support is likely to be required.

In the long term, approximately 5–8% of patients will have a PEG,[35] but a significant number will have it removed and some (a third) will die of other stroke complications.

Reducing pneumonia risk with enteral feeding All patients requiring enteral feeding are at high risk of aspiration because of the severity of the stroke and dysphagia. There are a number of contributory factors to this: bacterial load of oral cavity, poor oral hygiene, and dental health, poor posture and trunk control, biofilms, gastric reflux, and reduced motility.[36]

Poor oral hygiene may be associated with stroke-associated pneumonia (SAP)[37,38] and causes pain and distress. Mouth care regimes help to reduce the incidence of SAP[37-40] and are important for both comfort and reducing bacterial load. Prepacked sets containing suction sponges, saliva replacement, adapted/suction toothbrushes, and high-fluoride, low taste, non-foaming toothpaste may be helpful. Staff should be trained in providing oral care (https://www.mouthcarematters. hee.nhs.uk). Oral care sponges have reported choking risks and are unavailable in some hospitals. Triple-headed or small-headed toothbrushes may be better tolerated and can be used as a hydration tool if disposable or cleaned thoroughly. Other tools (e.g. MouthEze) are also available. Chlorhexidine and antibacterial gel may reduce bacterial load.[41,42] Patients who are unable to control their saliva may be helped symptomatically by anticholinergics (atropine drops, hyoscine patches) but they should be used with caution due to anticholinergic side effects (many stroke patients have reduced saliva production). Artificial saliva preparations as sprays rather than gels may reduce accumulation if applied to a precleaned cavity. Ensuring oxygen is humidified and use of saline nebulizers will reduce oral drying.

A UK pilot cluster randomized controlled trial (RCT) (SOCLE-II) comparing an enhanced oral healthcare versus usual oral healthcare in stroke care settings has been completed and awaiting publication.[40]

Oral care may be difficult in severely impaired and confused people and desensitization techniques may be helpful in ensuring better delivery.

Timing, type of feeding regime, and whether bolus or continuous feeding is better is unknown. Titrating feed levels dependent on gastric residual volume (GRV) in stroke appear to reduce pneumonia,[43] a procedure commonly practised on intensive care units. Regular metoclopramide[44] in the first 10 days and jejunal tubes may reduce aspiration risk (but are more difficult to place on the ward).

PPI (Proton pump inhibitor) use may increase the risk of pneumonia[45] and therefore consideration should be given to cessation or converting to an H_2 antagonist. Statins and angiotensin-converting-enzyme (ACE) inhibitors are associated with less pneumonia.[46,47]

Prophylactic antibiotics reduce urinary, but not respiratory infections, and should only be given if there are clear signs of infection.[48,49] The ideal duration of antibiotic treatment is unclear—some patients will respond quickly, particularly if their functional status improves, whereas others may require prolonged treatment. In these patients, further imaging and respiratory specialist input may be helpful as there may be a combination of diagnoses (e.g. heart failure, pulmonary emboli, and aspiration).

Environmental assisted eating

Those with severe strokes are dependent on carers to maintain their nutrition and hydration. People who have access to their own fluids are more likely to drink sufficient amounts and be able to self-regulate, even though these homeostatic mechanisms are severely impaired in the sick. Appropriate seating, table set up, and limb support enhance the ability to do this. Use of nutrition assistants and priority 'red' trays can enhance patients' intake as well as provide psychological support.[50] Families should participate. Further technological advances such as robotic arm-assisted feeding and robotic chairs are subject to ongoing research.

Patients who are enterally fed become socially isolated and unable to benefit from some features of rehabilitation wards (e.g. attending dining rooms at mealtimes), so consideration should be made of how to ameliorate this (e.g. timetabling rehabilitation, open visiting times, and setting up of separate activities).

Special cases

Diabetes: People with poorly controlled diabetes are at risk of further deterioration in glycaemic control with enteral feeding.[51] It is important to ensure consistent feeding and using an early nasal bridle may help, as well as close liaison with nursing staff, dietitians, and diabetic teams to ensure an appropriate timed regime. Conversion to insulin therapy may be required.

Incarcerated hiatus hernia: these are relatively common and can cause difficulties with reflux and placement of tubes. Severe cases where the majority of the stomach is in the pulmonary cavity are high risk. Chest X-rays may be difficult to interpret, and it may be impossible to pass the NGT through to a position below the diaphragm. In these cases, consider ensuring feeding occurs upright, lower rates of feeding, accepting a longer feeding period, and using H_2-receptor antagonist drugs. Computed tomography (CT) scanning of the thorax and abdomen should be undertaken before a gastrostomy insertion is considered. In some cases a surgical PEG may be the only option, requiring careful counselling of patient and family.

Dementia: There is insufficient evidence to guide decisions here. In the acute phase, it is best to assume all severely dysphagic patients require nutritional support unless there is clear justification for withholding treatment. There is a wide range of dementia severity and gaining information about this is key to this decision-making. Those with dementia are less likely to make such a good recovery or to tolerate tube feeding well and their clinical status should be reassessed regularly. NGT feeding can be used short term and a separate decision made subsequently about PEG insertion. PEG feeding does not appear to change the prognosis in dementia, but may be appropriate in clear stroke-related dysphagia.[52]

Dysphagia incidence and identification after acute stroke

Incidence of dysphagia

The reported incidence of dysphagia after acute stroke is dependent on timing and method of assessment; ranging from 64% to 78% in studies using instrumental assessments and around 50% in studies utilizing bedside assessments.[53–55]

Clinical course of dysphagia

Cortical strokes (anterior circulation)

Cortical strokes contribute most to the burden of acute dysphagia (especially total anterior circulation strokes), however many of these will recover in the first two weeks with 50% incidence dropping to approximately 30% and then less than 20% at 4 weeks[53,56] and less than 10% at 6 months. Techniques such as transcranial magnetic stimulation (TMS) and functional magnetic resonance imaging have enhanced our understanding of the anatomical areas involved in swallowing and swallow recovery; demonstrating a dominant 'swallowing' hemisphere. If the lesion affects this area then initially both hemispheres show diffuse increased activity; the intact hemisphere can reorganize and take over swallowing function over time and greater localization of activity has been demonstrated over time in both hemispheres.[54,57] This change may be enhanced by rehabilitation techniques. There is insufficient evidence to prognosticate dysphagia recovery from imaging, however certain areas appear especially important: the cingulate gyrus, pre/post-central gyrus, the insular, operculum, and the inferior parietal (water swallowing) areas.[58,59]

Brainstem strokes

In brainstem stroke, the swallowing deficit can often be severe, even with a small volume lesion, necessitating a greater proportion of tube feeding over a longer period for some patients. However, recovery can still occur many months later. As these patients may have less severe physical and cognitive problems, they are able to actively participate in rehabilitation programmes, which require self-directed therapy or risk management (e.g. suctioning). Some patients may demonstrate 'pharyngeal mis-sequencing' which may occur in up to 50% of brainstem stroke patients due to abnormal pressure generation in the pharynx and may be particularly responsive to biofeedback.[60]

Identification of dysphagia

Swallow screening

All patients with a suspected diagnosis of stroke should have their swallow assessed within 4 hours of admission, using a validated swallow screening tool[61] administered by trained staff, usually nurses.[62] Some units have 'dysphagia trained nurses' who also assess with food and fluid modification as part of the swallow screen.

Effective swallow screening programmes are associated with a reduction in pneumonia rates,[63,64] with earlier swallow screens associated with lower rates of pneumonia.[65]

Table 12.3 Examples of different types of dysphagia outcome measures

Score	Components
Penetration-Aspiration Scale (PAS)[67]	Clinician rated scale of penetration and aspiration; based on videofluoroscopy (VFS) or fibreoptic endoscopic evaluation of swallowing (FEES); 8-point scale
Dysphagia Outcome Severity Scale (DOSS)[68]	Clinician rated scale of dysphagia severity based on VFS, makes recommendations for diet, supervision, and nutrition, 7-point scale
Therapy Outcome Measures for Rehabilitation Professionals (TOM)[69]	Updated version of original TOMs, has four domains: impairment, activity, participation, well-being/distress
American-Speech-Language-Hearing Association National Outcome Measurement System (ASHA NOMS)[70]	Clinician rated scale of oral intake, includes measures of compensation/strategies, levels 1–7
Royal Brisbane Hospital Outcome Measure for Swallowing (RBHOMS) [71]	Clinician rated scale of swallowing disability, four stages of oral intake with 10 levels at each stage
Dysphagia Severity Rating Scale (DSRS)[72]	Clinician rated scale of oral intake, 3 levels: fluids, diet, supervision, 12 items
Functional Oral Intake Scale (FOIS)[73]	Clinician rated scale of oral intake; 7-point scale, levels 4–7 score diet only
IDDSI Functional Diet Scale (FDS)[74]	Clinician rate scale of oral intake, based on IDDSI, 7 levels
Dysphagia Handicap Index (DHI)[75]	Patient-reported quality of life (QOL) measure; questionnaire plus visual analogue scale; 25 items
Swallowing Quality of Life Scale (SWAL-QOL)[76]	Patient-reported QOL measure, including general health indicators, questionnaire, 44 items plus extra questions
Eating Assessment Tool (EAT-10)[77]	Patient-reported outcome instrument, 10 items

Clinical bedside assessment

Further specialist assessment is conducted by a speech and language therapist (SLT) for patients who fail swallow screening. A recent large-scale study reported that earlier SLT assessments have been associated with a significantly lower risk of SAP in acute stroke.[65] SLT assessment involves examination of the oral cavity, cranial nerves, and observation of swallowing with different consistencies and compensatory measures (+/– use of pulse oximetry and cervical auscultation), to allow diagnosis of the dysphagia severity and type. The SLT will make recommendations regarding oral intake and/or advice regarding compensatory strategies or rehabilitation of the swallow mechanism, set goals and monitor outcomes (Table 12.3). Detection of silent aspiration (i.e. entry of food/fluids below the level of the vocal cords with no cough response) from a bedside assessment can be difficult and where this is suspected, or the clinical picture is unclear, further instrumental assessment is indicated. Cough reflex testing using citric acid may enhance the sensitivity of screening or bedside testing, however, further research is required. A recent large RCT resulted in a neutral outcome.[66]

Instrumental assessment

The two main forms of instrumental assessment are videofluoroscopy (VFS) and fibreoptic endoscopic evaluation of swallowing (FEES). Manometry (if available) may be useful if poor opening

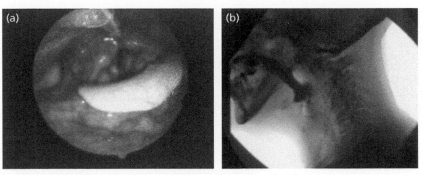

Fig. 12.3 FEES image post-swallow. Note presence of nasogastric tube.

of the upper oesophageal sphincter is suspected. Recent guidelines encourage the earlier and more widespread use of instrumental evaluation for guiding therapeutic decision-making.[62]

During VFS, patients are X-rayed swallowing a variety of barium-coated fluids and food in an upright position, resulting in a dynamic series of images depicting the whole swallowing process.

FEES involves passing a flexible endoscope transnasally to the level of the laryngopharynx (Fig. 12.3). The resulting image gives a view of the larynx and pharynx, while observing food and fluids being swallowed. Food dye can be used to enhance this visualization. Both methods examine for the presence of penetration or aspiration into the airway, the impact of modifying food and fluids or trialling strategies and postures. FEES does not allow visualization of the oral stage of swallowing, but can be repeated, delivered at the bedside and be used as part of active rehabilitation, including biofeedback.

VFS is limited by the need for patient stability and radiation exposure, and for this reason FEES may become more common on stroke units, but requires significant investment. Detection of aspiration[78–80] and risks are similar between both techniques.[81–83]

Interventions for dysphagia after acute stroke

Compensatory methods

Compensatory methods aim to manage risk and comprise mainly bolus modification, postural changes, and swallow strategies.

Bolus modification

The main form of bolus modification is thickening fluids and modifying food textures (e.g. to a pureed consistency) to enable easier swallowing. Thickened fluids are more cohesive, viscous, and move slower in the mouth, which generally allows dysphagic patients, who have poorly functioning oral musculature, greater control of the bolus in the oral cavity. Thickened fluids also slow down the speed at which the bolus enters the pharynx. Thickened fluids detected by touch and pressure mechanoreceptors[84] may provide greater sensory feedback.

Postural changes and swallow strategies

Postural changes include altering head positions (chin tuck or head turn) during swallowing. Swallow strategies include breath-hold techniques and swallow clearing techniques. These strategies are cheap, provide immediate reduction in aspiration risk (as demonstrated on VFS), and allow patients modified oral intake. These are thought to be compensatory rather than rehabilitative techniques and are not viable in those with severe cognitive or linguistic deficits.

When no compensatory strategy is effective, patients may be placed 'nil by mouth'. These patients experience a reduced quality of life and absence of swallowing practice may worsen outcome through the 'atrophy' of neural mechanisms linked to swallowing function,[85] which may be especially important in dementia.

Rehabilitative methods

Exercises

These treatments comprise muscle training and strengthening, such as tongue exercises (using pressure and resistance), the effortful swallow, the Mendelsohn's manoeuvre, and the Shaker exercise. These interventions require patients to learn and repeat these techniques and so precludes patients with severe cognitive or language impairments.

Inspiratory and expiratory muscle strength training (EMST) have also been explored for stroke patients,[86,87] but further research with greater numbers of participants and randomized controlled designs are required.

The McNeill Dysphagia Therapy Programme (MDTP), an exercise-based programme, has been combined with Neuromuscular Electrical Stimulation (NMES) in a placebo-controlled trial in dysphagia post-stroke—the full results are not yet published.[88]

Using biofeedback in swallowing therapy is also receiving increasing attention, but is limited by a lack of evidence.[89]

Peripheral sensory stimulation

Stimulation of local oropharyngeal structures to enhance swallowing has been explored with a number of stimuli in stroke patients. The most commonly investigated are chemical stimulation involving citric acid, Capsaicin, sour/cold-sour, black pepper oil,[90–93] as well as physical stimulation, which may activate more than one sensory pathway. Examples of the latter include air pulse therapy,[94] carbonated fluids,[95,96] and tactile and/or thermal stimulation to the posterior oropharynx with a swab, or a chilled laryngeal mirror or ice chips.[97–99]

Overall, studies show some improvement in swallowing parameters however most evidence is based on cohort studies in patients with chronic dysphagia with short-term outcomes.

Acupuncture

Acupuncture is a technique widely used in China. There are multiple different techniques and although some studies suggest benefit, there were many methodological problems and a 2008 Cochrane review showed no overall benefit.[100] A further systematic review in 2012 concluded that acupuncture requires further exploration in high-quality trials.[101]

Emerging methods

Neuro-stimulation methods

Many of these treatments (Table 12.4) are undergoing clinical trials and are not routinely available in many countries. They provide either a peripheral input to the muscles (internally or externally) or central sensory input (to the motor pharyngeal cortex) with the aim of improving swallowing by stimulating sensory drive to the brain and causing increased activity in the motor swallowing areas. These treatments have arisen as evidence from imaging studies with healthy subjects have demonstrated that a number of cortical- and subcortical regions of the brain are involved in

Table 12.4 Neurostimulation methods

Technique	Description	Evidence
Pharyngeal electrical stimulation (PES)	Electrical stimulus directly to pharyngeal muscles	Change in swallowing parameters—increases motor cortex excitability in healthy subjects and stroke patients consistent with improvement in swallowing function.[54,103,104,105] In one large multicentre randomized controlled trial in acute dysphagic stroke patients (N = 126) no benefit was shown.[106] However, a positive trial was reported in dysphagic stroke patients with tracheostomy[107]
Neuromuscular electrical stimulation (NMES)	External throat electrodes stimulating infra and suprahyoid muscles e.g. VitalStim AmpCare ES	Change in swallowing parameters. The most recent systematic review and meta-analysis into NMES examined eight studies and concluded that in the short-term, standard swallow treatment combined with NMES appeared to be more effective than standard swallow treatment alone[108]
Transcranial direct current stimulation (TCDS)	Application of direct current through the scalp	Change in swallowing parameters A number of studies have demonstrated that anodal TDCS at certain parameters resulted in increased cortical excitability in swallow related areas.[109,110] A further three RCTs using TDCS in stroke patients have also suggested improvements in swallowing parameters, up to 1–3 months' after intervention, but subject numbers are small[111]
Transcranial magnetic stimulation (TMS/rTMS)	Detection as well as delivery of magnetic field using circular coil over pharyngeal motor cortex. Provide stimulation to the pharyngeal motor cortex in the form of repetitive trains of magnetic pulses, i.e. repetitive TMS	Change in swallowing parameters Studies have involved healthy participants[112,113] and dysphagic participants. Five RCTs[111,114] involving stroke patients and rTMS showed some improvements in swallowing parameters
Paired associative stimulation (PAS)	Combination of PES and TMS	Change in swallowing parameters A recent study using PAS in stroke patients showed increased excitability in swallow related brain areas and a reduction in scores of penetration and aspiration[115] in 18 patients

volitional swallowing. In addition, a series of studies using TMS conducted by Hamdy et al.[54,57] demonstrated that recovery from dysphagia following stroke correlated with an increase in the size of the pharyngeal representation in the intact hemisphere. The broad aim of neurostimulation treatments, therefore, is to promote or enhance the speed of these changes.

Many of the earlier compensatory and exercise approaches have become part of routine clinical practice, and the SLT may choose to use a number of these depending on the patient. The most recent systematic review for swallowing therapy for post-stroke dysphagia, reported that swallowing therapy resulted in a number of positive outcomes.[102] However, the authors concluded that the results were based on variable quality evidence and that more high-quality trials were required to test the efficacy of specific interventions.[102] Stimulation therapies show promise and units should participate in trials to enhance understanding of this.

End-of-life care

Despite a number of advances in dysphagia rehabilitation, the prognosis for older stroke patients with dysphagia is poor. Decline in swallowing function often precedes the terminal phases of life as part of a general decline. Some patients will survive in a frail state with a high risk of further deterioration and this presents an opportunity for advanced care planning with the person and their family. Feeding tubes may form part of palliative care and a PEG may allow supportive hydration and limited medical intervention, thus minimizing the requirement for hospital admission or use of parenteral routes for drugs or feeding, if the risk of insertion is low, and following a fully informed shared decision-making process. People may feel relief when the pressure to eat and drink more is removed.

Quality of life is difficult to judge and decisions to withdraw feed and fluids provided medically need to be made carefully. These decisions are increasingly regulated and there needs to be clear documentation, collection of views and information before coming to a best interests decision, respecting the appropriate legal frameworks. Optimizing the person's ability to take part in the decision may require multiple sessions facilitated by SLTs. In the case of a person lacking mental capacity, a second opinion is required outside of the treating clinical team (physician or other healthcare professional).

Eating is a pleasure, which may be denied in dysphagia, and agreeing an 'at risk' feeding plan may be a more important goal than reducing aspiration. Dehydration can be distressing and a free water protocol may alleviate this. All people should be offered oral intake as wanted when the final days or hours of life are anticipated.

Framework for managing the older person with acute stroke and dysphagia

The future of dysphagia therapy

Although the consequences for someone with a severe stroke and dysphagia are bleak there is a growing number of potential treatments (Table 12.5). It is clear that as this area grows, there will be a need for consensus to deliver guidelines and maintain databases of outcomes in order to facilitate the transition from research to clinical practice.[116]

It is important that these interventions:

◆ continue to be tested rigorously, preferably in large RCTs
◆ have standardized outcome measures (return to oral intake, pneumonia, quality of life (QOL) measures, and control/sham groups)
◆ research should focus on establishing optimal treatment protocols and timing of interventions
◆ should make greater use of imaging technologies
◆ should investigate the use of combined stimulation and behavioural methods
◆ include research patient and public involvement
◆ evaluate cost effectiveness

Table 12.5 Framework for approach to person with acute stroke and dysphagia

Assessments	Actions
First 24 hours	
Swallow screening	Nurse led water swallow screen
	Institute oral care protocol for NBM and modified diet patients
	Access and assistance to toothbrushes for all
Nutritional risk and assessment	MUST or similar nutritional assessment
	Decision about mode of feeding
	Consider commencing metoclopramide
	Change PPI to H_2 antagonists unless active peptic ulcer disease
	Consider measuring gastric residual volume before increasing feed rates
	Ensure baseline electrolytes (U&E, Mg, Po4, Ca)
	Identify those at refeeding risk and monitor as per guidelines
Stroke severity and prognosis	NIHSS, OCSP classification
	Frailty assessment
	Comorbidity assessment
	Communication point
	Medication review and route
Research study eligibility	Offer opportunity for study participation, for all patients with dysphagia
First 7 Days	
Swallowing	Detailed SLT assessment for those patients who fail swallow screens (these can be repeated during first 18–24 hours if appropriate). If available Dysphagia-trained nurses (DTN) can assess with food and thickened fluids and liaise with SLT as appropriate
	SLT-led rehabilitation interventions
	Goal setting
	Oral care
	Denture and dental care
	Consider daytime feeding if respiratory problems and assistance with optimum positioning
	Instrumental evaluation—VFS or FEES if appropriate
	Consider/identify patients who might benefit from free water protocol
Nutrition	Nutrition assistant support
	Involve carers/families
	Consider use of adjuncts to improve NGT efficiency (Bridle)
	Dietitian subjective global assessment
	Optimize oral diet
	Refeeding bloods if required
	Review diuretic use

(continued)

Table 12.5 Continued

Assessments	Actions
Stroke recovery	Improving NIHSS suggests greater chance of recovery of swallow and less likely to need PEG-posterior circulation strokes behave differently and usually take longer to recover
	Communication point
Mental capacity assessments	Although will be assessed informally frequently this should be formalized if considering use of restraint device such as mittens to secure a feeding tube or if considering using or withdrawing tube feeding
First 14 days	
Swallowing	SLT reassessment and rehabilitation interventions
	Consider FEES or VFS
	Dental review if available
	Oral care—including antifungal treatments and saliva replacement if required.
	Positioning
Nutrition	If NG feeding still required at days 14–21, then likely to require PEG—begin preparation
	For patients not tolerating NG tubes, consider early PEG insertion
	Review feeding timing regime to optimize rehabilitation and pneumonia risk
	Feed/Fluid balance charts
	Monitor electrolytes
	Dietitian subjective global assessment
Stroke recovery	If recovery poor (no change, worsening NIHSS) or deterioration delay decisions about PEG insertion
	Communication point: counsel carers/family and patient about decisions
	Avoid clopidogrel until decision made about PEG insertion
Mental capacity assessments	Mental capacity assessments should be undertaken and best interests decisions to be made in patients lacking capacity and should be documented regarding PEG insertion
21–28 days	
Swallowing	SLT reassessment and rehabilitation interventions—start to transfer any interventions to patient-led for those with ability to do so
	Safest oral intake recommendations for palliative care situations
	Oral care—including antifungal treatments and saliva replacement if required
	Positioning
	Outcome assessments
Nutrition	PEG insertion for those with no or inadequate intake by other means if fit to undertake procedure.
	Teaching patient/family to manage PEG
	Feed/Fluid balance charts
	Dietary advice for rehabilitation (e.g. making meals with correct consistency, balanced diet)
	Optimize 'at risk' diet for those unable/fit for tube feeding
	Assess need for long-term multivitamins

Table 12.5 Continued

Assessments	Actions
Stroke recovery	Second opinions for patients with poor or uncertain prognosis
	Medical fitness for PEG procedure—rule out anatomical difficulties and optimize respiratory status. Some patients may benefit from bridging NIV
	Communication point—end-of-life care and prognosis
Mental capacity assessments	Mental capacity assessments should be undertaken for decision re PEG placement
	Best interests decisions to be made in patients lacking capacity and should be documented regarding PEG insertion and/or risks of oral intake
6 weeks, 3 months, 6 months	
Swallowing	Continued rehabilitation programme
	Repeat instrumental assessment for selected patients (esp. posterior circulation strokes)
	Community intervention
Nutrition	Community dietitian review
	PEG still required?
Stroke recovery	6-week and 3-month reviews
	Medication reviews
	NH telephone/visit or relative contact for those unable to attend OPC and/or lacking capacity
	Communication point-advanced care planning
	Planned removal of PEG
Mental capacity assessments	As appropriate depending on recovery and decisions
Other	

Abbreviations: PEG, percutaneous endoscopic gastrostomy; OPC, outpatient clinic; NBM, nil by mouth; NH, nursing home; NIV, non-invasive ventilation; SLT, speech and language therapist; NIHSS, National Institute of Health Stroke Scale; OCSP, Oxford Community Stroke Project.

Communication points—key times to update patients and next of kin and explain the next stages of decision-making.

The consequences of dysphagia, undernutrition, and pneumonia benefit from multiple combined interventions from all members of the MDT as part of stroke unit care. Oral care and providing nutrition and hydration are accepted to be good practice, but the best methods are unclear. This is a key area for quality improvement and audit strategies (e.g. implementing oral hygiene assessment tools, standardizing care protocols, training of staff, and appropriate equipment and products).

The rapid progress of technological innovations, such as therapy/education apps for tablets and telemedicine provides further opportunities to deliver patient-led rehabilitation.

Summary

The management of the older stroke patient with dysphagia requires active multidisciplinary interventions taking into account the person's physiological and prognostic status. Unlike other impairments it has huge emotional as well as physical impact because of its effect on nutritional intake which is not always felt to be wholly within a medical sphere. Careful reassessment, balancing risks and benefits, and discussions with patients and their families are required throughout the acute, subacute, and chronic phases to manage expectations and future care.

With further functional and other imaging techniques, we may be better able to prognosticate which patients are most likely to have enough neurobiological reserve to benefit from techniques that rely on neuroplasticity. It is likely that this degree of reserve will correlate with the person's measured frailty syndrome and overall prognosis. At this time, we do not know enough to do this accurately and we must rely on clinical judgement, optimize each individual's situation, ensure patient and family participation, be prepared to try new techniques, and involve all patients in research and audit.

References

1. **Kaiser MJ, Bauer JM, Ramsch C, et al.; Mini Nutritional Assessment International Group.** Frequency of malnutrition in older adults: a multinational perspective using the mini nutritional assessment. *J Am Geriatr Soc* 2010;**58** (9):1734–8.

2. **Iizika S, Tadaka E, & Sanada H.** Comprehensive assessment of nutritional status and associated factors in the healthy community dwelling elderly. *Geriatr Gerontol Int* 2008;**8** (1):24–31.

3. **Lindroos E, Saarela RK, Soini H, Muurinen S, Suominem MH, & Pitkala KH.** Care-giver reported swallowing difficulties, malnutrition and mortality in assisted living facilities. *J Nutr Health Aging* 2014;**18**(7):718–22.

4. **Semba RD, Blaum CS, Bartali B, et al.** Denture use, malnutrition, frailty and mortality among older women living in the community. *J Nutr Health Aging* 2006;**10** (2):161–7.

5. **Gariballa SE, Parker N, & Castleden M.** Nutritional status of hospitalised acute stroke patients. *Br J Nutr* 1998;**79**:481–7.

6. **BAPEN Malnutrition Advisory Group (2003/2010/2011).** *Malnutrition Universal Screening Tool (MUST).* Available from: https://www.bapen.org.uk/pdfs/must/must_full.pdf [Accessed: 26 July 2019].

7. **Guigoz Y.** The Mini Nutritional Assessment (MNA) review of the literature—what does it tell us? *J Nutr Health Aging* 2006;**10**(6):466–85; discussion 485–7.

8. **Yang EJ, Kim MH, Lim JY, & Paik NJ.** Oropharyngeal dysphagia in a community-based elderly cohort: the Korean longitudinal study on health and aging. *J Korean Med Sci* 2013;**28**(10):1534–9.

9. **Zhang J & Li J.** Investigation of swallowing function in the elderly (Chinese abstract). *J Clin Otorhinolaryngol Head Neck Surg* 2013;**27**(2):91–4.

10. **Maeshima S, Osawa A, Hayashi T, & Tanashi N.** Factors associated with prognosis and eating and swallowing disability after stroke: a study from a community based stroke system. *J Stroke Cerebrovasc Dis* 2013;**22**(7):926–30.e1.

11. **Kim Y, Park GY, Seo YJ, & Im S.** Effect of anterior cervical osteophyte in post stroke dysphagia: a case control study. *Arch Phys Med Rehabil* 2015;**96**(7):1269–76.

12. **Singh S & Hamdy S.** Dysphagia in Stroke Patients. *Postgrad Med J* 2006;**82**(968):383–91.

13. **Smithard DG, O' Neill PA, Parks C, & Morris J.** Complications and outcome after acute stroke. Does dysphagia matter? *Stroke* 1996;**27**(7):1200–4.

14. **Cesari M, Gambassi G, Abellan Van Kan G, & Vellas B.** The frailty phenotype and the frailty index: different instruments for different purposes. *Age Ageing* 2013;**0**:1–3.

15. **Nakayama E, Tohara H, Hino T, et al.** The effects of ADL on recovery of swallowing function in stroke patients after acute phase. *J Oral Rehabil* 2014;**41**(12):904–11.

16. **Rabadi MH, Coar PL, Lukin M, Lesser M, & Blass JP.** Intensive nutritional supplements can improve outcomes in stroke rehabilitation. *Neurology* 2008;**71**(23):1856–61.

17. **Gariballa SE, Parke SG, Taub N, & Castleden M.** A randomised, controlled, single blind trial of nutritional supplementation after acute stroke. *JPEN J Parenter Enteral Nutr* 1998;**22**(5):315–19.

18. **Ha l, Hauge T, & Iversen PI.** Body composition in older acute stroke patients after treatment with individualized, nutritional supplementation while in hospital. *BMC Geriatr* 2010;**10**:75.

19. **Milne AC, Avenell A, & Potter J.** Meta-analysis: protein and energy supplementation in older people. *Ann Int Med* 2006;**144**(1):37–48.

20. **BAPEN.** Refeeding Decision Tree 2012. Available from: http://www.bapen.org.uk/pdfs/decision-trees/refeeding-syndrome.pdf [Accessed: 26 July 2019].

21. **Wright L, Cotter D, Hickson M, & Frost G.** Comparison of energy and protein intakes of older people consuming a texture modified diet with a normal hospital diet. *J Hum Nutr Diet* 2005;**18**(3):213–19.

22. **McGrail A & Kelchner L.** Barriers to oral fluid intake: beyond thickened liquids. *J Neurosci Nurs* 2015;**47**(1):58–63.

23. **Gillman A, Winkler R, & Taylor N.** Implementing the free water protocol does not result in aspiration pneumonia in carefully selected patients with dysphagia: a systematic review. *Dysphagia* 2017;**32**:345–61.

24. **Hong J, Kim DK, & Seo KM.** Clinical factors of enteral tube feeding in acute ischaemic stroke patients. *Am J Phys Med Rehabil* 2015;**94**(8):595–601.

25. **Geeganage C, Beavan J, Ellender S, & Bath PM** Interventions for dysphagia and nutritional support in acute and subacute stroke. *Cochrane Database Syst Rev* 2012;**10**:CD000323.

26. **Beavan J, Conroy SP, Harwood R, Gladman JR, Leonardi-Bee J, & Sach Tea.** Does looped nasogastric tube feedng improve nutritional delivery for patients with dysphagia after acute stroke? A randomised controlled trial. *Age Ageing* 2010;**39**(5):624–30.

27. **Oh H & Seo W.** Age differences in fluid balance and serum Na + and K + levels after nasogastric tube feeding in stroke patients: elderly vs. non-elderly. *JPEN J Parenter Enteral Nutr* 2006;**30**(4):321–30.

28. **NCEPOD (National Confidential Enquiry into Patient Outcome and Death).** *Scoping Our Practice: The 2004 Report of NCEPOD.* Available from: https://www.ncepod.org.uk/2004sop.html [Accessed: 26 July 2019].

29. **Williams J.** Exploring ethically sensitive decision-making in acute hospital care: using hand control mittens in adult patients. In: Shaw T & Sanders K (eds.) Foundation of Nursing Studies. 2008. Available from: http://www.fons.org/resources/documents/DissSeriesVol4No8.pdf [Accessed 26 July 2019].

30. **Smithard DG, O'Neill PA, England RE,** et al. The natural history of dysphagia following a stroke. *Dysphagia* 1997;**12**(4):188–93.

31. **Laasch HU, Wilbraham L, Bullen K,** et al. Gastrostomy insertion: comparing the options-PEG, RIG or PIG. *Clin Radiol* 2003;**58**(5):398–405.

32. **Lowe AS, Laasch HU, Stephenson S,** et al. Multicentre survey of radiologically inserted gastrostomy feeding tube (RIG) in the UK. *Clin Radiol* 2012;**67**(9); 843–54.

33. **National Patient Safety Agency.** *Rapid Response Report NPSA/2010/RRR010: Early Detection of Complications After Gastrostomy (Supporting Information)* March 2010. Available from: https://www.gosh.nhs.uk/file/2393/download [Accessed: 26 July 2019].

34. **Alshekhlee A, Ranawai, N, Syed TU, Conway D, Ahmad SA, & Zaidai OO.** National Institutes of Health Stroke scale assists in predicting the need for percutaneous endoscopic gastrostomy tube placement in acute ischaemic stroke. *J Stroke Cerebrovasc Dis* 2010;**19**(5):347–52.

35. **Kumar S, Langmore S, Goddeau RP Jr,** et al. Predictors of percutaneous endoscopic gastrostomy tube placement in patients with severe dysphagia from an acute-subacute hemispheric infarction. J Stroke Cerebrovasc Dis 2012;**21**(2):114–20.

36. **Sellars, C Bowie L, Bagg J,** et al. Risk factors for chest infection in acute stroke: a prospective cohort study. Stroke 2007;**38**:2284–91.

37. **Brady M, Furlanetto D, Hunter RV, Lewis S, & Milne V.** Staff-led interventions for improving oral hygiene in patients following stroke. *Cochrane Database Syst Rev* 2006;**4**:CD003864.

38. **Satou Y, Oguro H, Murakami Y, et al.** Gastroesophageal reflux during enteral feeding in stroke patients: a 24-hour esophageal pH-monitoring study. *J Stroke Cerebrovasc Dis* 2013;**22**(3):185–9.

39. **British Society of Gerodontology.** *Guidelines for the Oral Healthcare of Stroke Survivors.* **June** 2010. Available from: https://www.gerodontology.com/content/uploads/2014/10/stroke_guidelines.pdf [Accessed: 26 July 2019].

40. **Brady MC, Stott D, Weir CJ, Chalmers C, Sweeny P, & Donaldson C.** Clinical and cost effectiveness of enhanced oral healthcare in stroke care settings (SOCLE II): a pilot, stepped wedge, cluster randomised, controlled trial protocol. *Int J Stroke* 2015;**10**(6):979–84.

41. **Gosney M, Martin MV, & Wright AE.** The role of selective decontamination of the digestive tract in acute stroke. *Age Ageing* 2006;**35**(1):42–7.

42. **Shi, Z, Xie, H, Wang, P, et al.** Oral hygiene care for critically ill patients to prevent ventilator-associated pneumonia. *Cochrane Database Syst Rev* 2013;**(8)**:CD008367.

43. **Chen S, Xian W, Cheng S, & Zhou C.** Risk of regurgitation and aspiration in patients infused with different volumes of enteral nutrition. *Asia Pacific J Clin Nutr* 2015;**24**(2):212–18.

44. **Warusevitane A, Karunatilake D, Sim J, Lally F, & Roffe C.** Safety and effect of metoclopramide to prevent pneumonia in patients with stroke fed via nasogastric tubes trial. *Stroke* 2014;**46**:454–60.

45. **Herzig SJ, Doughty C, Lahoti S, Marchina S, Sanan N, Feng W, & Kumar S.** Acid-suppressive medication use in acute stroke and hospital-acquired pneumonia. *Ann Neurol* 2014;**6**(5):712–18.

46. **Caldeira D, Alarcao J, Vaz-Carneiro A, & Costa J.** Risk of pneumonia associated with use of angiotensin converting enzyme inhibitors and angiotensin receptor blockers: systematic review and analysis. *BMJ* 2012;**345**;e4260.

47. **Shinohara Y & Origasa H.** Post-stroke pneumonia prevention by angiotensin-converting enzyme inhibitors: results of a meta-analysis of five studies in Asians. *Adv Ther* 2012;**29**(10):900–12.

48. **Westendorp WF, Vermeij JD, & Zock E, et al.** The preventable antibiotics in stroke study (PASS): a pragmatic randomised open label masked end point trial. *Lancet* 2015;**385**(9977):1519–26.

49. **Kalra L, Irshad S, Hodsoll J, et al.; STROKE-INF Investigators.** Prophylactic antibiotics after acute stroke for reducing pneumonia in patients with dysphagia (STROKE-INF): a prospective, cluster-randomised, open-label, masked endpoint, controlled clinical trial. *Lancet* 2015;**386** (10006): 1835–44.

50. **Bradley L & Rees C.** *Reducing Nutritional Risk in Hospital: The Red Tray. Nursing Standard.* Available from: https://journals.rcni.com/doi/abs/10.7748/ns2003.03.17.26.33.c3357 [Accessed: 18 July 2019].

51. **Joint British Diabetes Societies (JBDS) for inpatient care.** *Glycaemic Management During the Inpatient Enteral Feeding of Stroke Patients With Diabetes.* June 2012. Available from: http://www.diabetologists-abcd.org.uk/JBDS/JBDS_IP_Enteral_Feeding_Stroke.pdf [Accessed: 26 July 2019].

52. **Brooke J & Omorogieva O.** Enteral nutrition in dementia: a systematic review. *Nutrients* 2015;**7**:2456–68.

53. **Mann G, Hankey GJ, & Cameron D.** Swallowing function after stroke: prognosis and prognostic factors at 6 months. *Stroke* 1999;**30**(4):744–8.

54. **Hamdy S, Aziz Q, Rothwell JC, et al.** Recovery of swallowing after dysphagic stroke relates to functional reorganization in the intact motor cortex. *Gastroenterology* 1998;**115**(5):1104–12.

55. **Kidd L, Lawson J, Nesbitt R, & MacMahon J.** Aspiration in acute stroke: a clinical study with videofluoroscopy. *Q J Med* 1993;**86**(12):825–9.

56. **Smithard DG, O' Neill PA, England RE, et al.** The natural history of dysphagia following a stroke. *Dysphagia* 1997;**12**(4):188–93.

57. **Hamdy S, Aziz Q, Rothwell J, et al.** The cortical topography of human swallowing musculature in health and disease. *Nat Med* 1996;**2**(11):1217–24.

58. **Suntrup S, Kemmling A, Warnecke T, et al.** The impact of lesion location on dysphagia incidence, pattern and complications in acute stroke. Part 1: dysphagia incidence, severity and aspiration. *Eur J Neurol* 2015;**22**(5):832–8.

59. **Soros P, Inamoto Y, & Martin RE.** Functional brain imaging of swallowing: an activation likelihood estimation meta-analysis. *Hum Brain Mapp* 2009;**30**:2426–39.

60. **Huckabee M, Lamvik K, & Jones R.** Pharyngeal mis-sequencing in dysphagia: characteristics, rehabilitative. *J Neurol Sci* 2014;**343**(1–2):153–8.

61. **Schepp SK, Tirschwell DL, Miller RM, & Longstreth WT.** Swallowing screens after acute stroke: a systematic review. *Stroke* 2012;**43**(3):869–71.

62. **Intercollegiate Stroke Working Party.** *National Clinical Guidelines For Stroke*, 5th edition. London, UK: Royal College of Physicians, 2016.

63. **Hinchey JA, Shephard T, Furie K, Smith D, Wang D, & Tonn S.** Formal dysphagia screening protocols prevent dysphagia. *Stroke* 2005;**36**(9):1972–6.

64. **Lakshiminarayan K, Tsai AW, Tong X, et al.** Utility of dysphagia screening results in predicting pneumonia. *Stroke* 2010;**41**(12):2849–54.

65. **Bray B, Smith CJ, Cloud GC, et al.** The association between delays in screening for and assessing dysphagia after acute stroke, and the risk of stroke-associated pneumonia. *J Neurol Neurosurg Psychiatry*, 2017;**88**:25–30.

66. **Miles A, Zeng I, McLauchlan H, & Huckabee ML.** Cough reaction test in dysphagia: a randomised controlled trial. *J Clin Res Med* 2013;**5**(3):222–3.

67. **Rosenbek JC, Robbins JA, Roecker EB, Coyle JL, & Wood JL.** A penetration-aspiration scale. *Dysphagia* 1996;**11**(2):93–8.

68. **O' Neil KH, Purdy M, Falk J, & Gallo L.** The dysphagia outcome and severity scale. *Dysphagia* 1999;**14**(3):139–45.

69. **Enderby P & John A.** *Therapy Outcome Measures for Rehabilitation Professionals,* 3rd edition. Guildford, UK: J & R Press, 2015.

70. **National Outcomes Measurement System (NOMS).** Available from: https://www.asha.org/noms/national-outcomes-measurement-system [Accessed: 24 April 2019].

71. **Skeat J & Perry A.** Outcome measurement in dysphagia: not so hard to swallow. *Dysphagia* 2005;**20**(2):113–22.

72. **Jayasekeran, V, Singh S, Tyrrell P, et al.** Adjunctive functional pharyngeal electrical stimulation reverses swallowing disability after brain lesions. *Gastroenterology* 2010;**138**:1737–46.

73. **Crary MA, Carnaby Mann GD, & Groher ME.** Initial psychometric assessment of a functional oral intake scale for dysphagia in stroke patients. *Arch Phys Med Rehabil* 2005;**86**(8):1516–20.

74. **Steele CM, Namasivayam-MacDonald AM, Guida BT, et al.** Creation and initial validation of the international dysphagia diet standardisation initiative functional diet scale. *Arch Phys Med Rehabil* 2018;**99**:934–44.

75. **Silbergleit AK, Schultz L, Jacobson BH, Beardsley T, & Johnson AF.** The Dysphagia handicap index: development and validation. *Dysphagia* 2012;**27**(1):46–52.

76. **Rinkel RN, Verdonck-de Leeuw IM, Langendijk JA, van Reij EJ, Aaronson NK, & Leemans CR.** The psychometric and clinical validity of the SWAL-QOL questionnaire in evaluating swallowing problems experienced by patients with oral and oropharyngeal cancer. *Ann Otol Rhinol Laryngol* 2008;**117**(2):919–24.

77. **Belafsky PC, Mouadeb DA, Rees CJ, et al.** Validity and reliability of the Eating Assessment Tool (EAT-10). *Ann Otol Rhinol Laryngol* 2008;**117**(12):919–24.

78. **Langmore SE, Schatz K, Olsen N. Langmore SE, & Schatz K.** Endoscopic and videofluoroscopic evaluations of swallowing and aspiration. *Ann Otol Rhinol Laryngol* 1991;**100** (8):678–81.

79. **Kelly AM, Leslie P, Beale T, Payten C, & Drinnan MJ.** Fibreoptic endoscopic evaluation of swallowing and videofluoroscopy: does examination type influence perception of pharyngeal residue severity? *Clin Otolaryngol* 2006;**31**(5):425–32.

80. **Kelly AM, Drinnan MJ, & Leslie P.** Assessing penetration and aspiration: how do videofluoroscopy and fibreoptic endoscopic evaluation of swallowing compare? *Laryngoscope* 2007;**117**(10):1723–7.

81. **Warnecke T, Teismann I, Oelenberg S**, et al. The safety of fiberoptic endoscopic evaluation of swallowing in acute stroke patients. *Stroke* 2009;**40**(2):482–6.

82. **Langmore SE.** *Endoscopic Evaluation and Treatment of Swallowing Disorders.* New York, NY: Thieme Publishers, 2001.

83. **Aviv JE.** Prospective, randomized outcome study of endoscopy versus modified barium swallow in patients with dysphagia. *Laryngoscope* 2000;**110**(4):563–74.

84. **Steele CM & Miller AJ.** Sensory input pathways and mechanisms in swallowing: a review. *Dysphagia* 2010;**25**(4):323–33.

85. **Robbins J, Butler SG, Daniels SK, Diez Gross R, Langmore S, & Lazarus CL.** Swallowing and dysphagia rehabilitation: translating principles of neural plasticity into clinically oriented evidence. *J Speech Lang Hear Res* 2008;**51**(1):S276–300.

86. **Park JS, Oh DH, Chang MY, & Kim KM.** Effects of expiratory muscle strength training on oropharyngeal dysphagia in subacute stroke patients: a randomised controlled trial. *J Oral Rehabil* 2016;**43**: 364–72.

87. **Hegland KW, Davenport PW, Brandimore AE, Singletary FF, & Troche MS.** Rehabilitation of swallowing and cough functions following stroke: an expiratory muscle strength training trial. *Arch Phys Med Rehabil* 2016;**97**:1345–51.

88. **Carnaby G, LaGorio L, Crary M, & Miller D.** A randomized double blind trial of neuromuscular electrical stimulation + McNeill dysphagia therapy (MDTP) after stroke (ANSRS). *Dysphagia* 2012;**27**:569–620.

89. **Benfield JK, Everton LF, Bath PB, & England TJ.** Does therapy with biofeedback improve swallowing in adults with dysphagia? A systematic review and meta-analysis. *Arch Phys Med Rehabil* 2019;**100**:551–61.

90. **Hamdy S, Jilani S, Price V, Parker C, Hall N, & Power M.** Modulation of human swallowing behaviour by thermal and chemical stimulation in health and after brain injury. *Neurogastroenterol Motil* 2003;**15**(1):69–77.

91. **Logemann JA, Pauloski BR, Colangelo L, Lazarus C, Fujiu M, & Kahrilas PJ.** Effects of a sour bolus on oropharyngeal swallowing measures in patients with neurogenic dysphagia. *J Speech Hear Res* 1995;**38**(3):556–63.

92. **Ebihara T, Ebihara S, Maruyama M**, et al. A randomized trial of olfactory stimulation using black pepper oil in older people with swallowing dysfunction. *J Am Geriatr Soc* 2006;**54**(9):1401–6.

93. **Gatto AR, Cola PC, da Silva RG, Spadotto AA, Ribeiro PW, & Schelp AO.** Sour taste and cold temperature in the oral phase of swallowing in patients after stroke. *CoDAS* 2013;**25**(2):163–7.

94. **Theurer JA, Johnston JL, Fisher J**, et al. Proof-of-principle pilot study of oropharyngeal air-pulse application in individuals with dysphagia after hemispheric stroke. *Arch Phys Med Rehabil* 2013;**94**(6):1088–94.

95. **Sdravou K, Walshe M, & Dagdilelis L.** Effects of carbonated liquids on oropharyngeal swallowing measures in people with neurogenic dysphagia. *Dysphagia* 2012;**27**:240–50.

96. **Sdravou K, Walshe M, & Dagdilelis L.** Effects of carbonated liquids on oropharyngeal swallowing measures in people with neurogenic dysphagia. *Dysphagia* 2012;**27**(2):240–50.

97. **Rosenbek JC, Robbins J, Fishback B, & Levine RL.** Effects of thermal application on dysphagia after stroke. *J Speech Hear Res* 1991;**34**(6):1257–68.

98. **Rosenbek JC, Roecker EB, Wood JL, & Robbins J.** Thermal application reduces the duration of stage transition in dysphagia after stroke. *Dysphagia* 1996;**11**(4):225–33.

99. **Rosenbek, JC, Robbins, J, Willford, WO**, et al. Comparing treatment intensities of tactile-thermal application. *Dysphagia* 1998;**13**:1–9.

100. **Xie Y, Wang L, He J, & Wu T.** Acupuncture for dysphagia in acute stroke. *Cochrane Database Syst Rev* 2008(**3**):CD006076.

101. Wong ISY & Tsang HWH. Acupuncture following stroke: a systematic review. *Eur J Int Med* 2012;4:e141–50.

102. Bath PM, Lee HS, & Everton LF. Swallowing therapy for dysphagia in acute and subacute stroke. *Cochrane Database Syst Rev* 2018;(**10**):CD000323.

103. Fraser C, Power M, Hamdy S, et al. Driving plasticity in human adult motor cortex is associated with improved motor function after brain injury. *Neuron* 2002;**34**(5):831–40.

104. Gow D, Hobson AR, Furlong P, & Hamdy S. Characterising the central mechanisms of sensory modulation in human swallowing motor cortex. *Clin Neurophysiol* 2004;**115**(10):2382–90.

105. Jayasekeran V, Singh S, Tyrell PME, et al. Adjunctive functional pharyngeal electrical stimulation reverses swallowing disability after brain lesions. *Gastroenterology* 2010;**138**(5):1737–46.

106. Bath P, Scutt, P, Love J, Clavé, P, et al., **on behalf of the Swallowing Treatment Using Pharyngeal Electrical Stimulation (STEPS) Trial Investigators**. Pharyngeal electrical stimulation for treatment of dysphagia in subacute stroke: a randomized controlled trial. *Stroke* 2016;**47**:1562–70.

107. Dziewas R, Stellato R, van der Tweel I, Walther E, Werner CJ, & Braun T. Pharyngeal electrical stimulation for early decannulation in tracheostomised patients with neurogenic dysphagia after stroke (PHAST-TRAC): a prospective, single = blinded, randomised trial. *Lancet Neurol* 2018;**17**(10):849–59.

108. Chen Y, Kwang-Hwa C, Hung-Chou C, Wen-Miin L, Ya-Hui W, & Yen-Nung L. The effects of surface neuromuscular electrical stimulation on post-stroke dysphagia: systematic review and meta-analysis. *Clin Rehabil* 2016;**30**(1):24–35.

109. Jefferson S, Mistry S, Singh S, Rothwell J, & Hamdy S. Characterising the application of transcranial direct current stimulation in human pharyngeal motor cortex. *Am J Physiol Gastrointest Liver Physiol* 2009;**297**(6):1035–40.

110. Vasant DH, Mistry S, Michou E, Jefferson S, Rothwell JC, & Hamdy S. Transcranial direct current stimulation reverses neurophysiological and behavioural effects of focal inhibition of human pharyngeal motor cortex on swallowing. *J Physiol* 2014;**592**(4):695–709.

111. Beavan J. Update on management options for dysphagia after acute stroke. *Br J Neurosci Nurs* 2015;**11**:10–19.

112. Jefferson S, Mistry S, Michou E, Singh S, Rothwell JC, & Hamdy S. Reversal of a virtual lesion in human pharyngeal motor cortex by high frequency contralesional brain stimulation. *Gastroenterology* 2009;**137**(3):841–9.

113. Mistry S, Verin E, Singh S, et al. Unilateral suppression of pharyngeal motor cortex to repetitive transcranial magnetic stimulation reveals functional asymmetry in the hemispheric projections to human swallowing. *J Physiol* 2007;**585**:525–38.

114. Du J, Yang F, Lui L, et al. Repetitive transcranial magnetic stimulation for rehabilitation of poststroke dysphagia: a randomised, double-blind clinical trial. *Clin Neurophysiol* 2016;**127**(3):1907–13.

115. Michou E, Williams S, Vidyasagar R, et al. fMRI and MRS measures of neuroplasticity in the pharygngeal motor cortex. *Neuroimage* 2015;**117**:1–10.

116. Doeltgen SH & Huckabee ML. Swallowing neurorehabilitation: from the research laboratory to routine clinical application. *Arch Phys Med Rehabil* 2012;**93**:207–13.

Chapter 13

Communication disorders post-stroke

Dee Webster and Sally Knapp

Introduction

Communication disorders post-stroke are varied in presentation and severity. Impairments such as aphasia, dysarthria, and apraxia of speech have a significant and often long-lasting impact on an individual's daily communication; the ability to express wants, needs, opinions, and decisions. As communication is so central to how we live our lives, it is not surprising that these changes can profoundly affect the individual, their social relationships, their role within society, and their confidence, self-esteem, and overall quality of life.

This chapter describes common communication disorders that can arise following a stroke. It discusses theoretical models, assessment considerations, goal setting, approaches to delivering rehabilitation, and considers factors of particular relevance to older adults.

Aphasia

Aphasia is an acquired language disorder affecting around a third of individuals post-stroke.[1,2] It results from a cerebral infarction or haemorrhage affecting cortical or subcortical structures associated with language production in the dominant hemisphere. In over 95% of right-handed individuals and over 75% of left-handed individuals with aphasia, the lesion will be situated in the left hemisphere.[3]

Aphasia can affect all four language modalities: auditory comprehension (understanding spoken language), reading, producing words and sentences, and spelling. Distinct to cognitive changes affecting memory or attention, aphasia does not affect intelligence. Although historically aphasia has been used to define a total loss of language, with dysphasia referring to a partial loss, the terms can be used interchangeably, with aphasia now the preferred term.

The following examples demonstrate how individual severity of aphasia can vary widely:

Margaret

Margaret is 75 years old. She had a stroke 2 months ago affecting both her understanding and expression. She is able to understand conversations providing her conversation partner uses less complex language and speaks at a steady rate. She continues to read the newspaper and can fill in forms and complete the crossword.

She has occasional word-finding difficulties which are exacerbated when under pressure or when fatigued. She finds that she can accommodate for this by choosing an alternative word or focusing on the first letter of the word. She has begun to return to some of her regular activities and also enjoys spending time with her family.

David

David is 78 years old. He had a stroke 4 months ago resulting in aphasia. Prior to his stroke he lived alone and has no family nearby. He has recently been discharged to a care home as he now has long-term nursing and care needs.

He finds understanding words very difficult and relies heavily on the context of conversation, and the non-verbal communication (such as facial expression and gestures) of his conversation partner to understand. He is able to read his own name but is unable to read single words reliably.

He has a few 'automatic' phrases such as ' thank you; that's right' but has difficulty expressing himself verbally. He is unable to write.

He depends greatly on the skills of those caring for him to support communication and provide opportunities to engage in activities.

As you can see from the previous examples, both the type and severity of aphasia can vary significantly; varying from mild difficulties in one modality, such as occasional difficulties in finding words only, to severe difficulties in all four modalities; with a significant impact on both understanding and expression.

We will now consider how language processing can be affected by aphasia and how the various processes involved in understanding and producing language can break down.

Disorders of auditory comprehension

Models of single word (lexical) processing describe the way that we understand words as a multistaged process.[4] In order to understand a word we hear, we first perceive speech sounds from the acoustic signal, and we then access our mental dictionary or lexicon, enabling word recognition for familiar words, which then leads to word understanding via access to the semantic representation (or meaning) associated with the word (Fig. 13.1).

If one or more of these stages are affected as a result of aphasia, this can lead to individuals, with otherwise intact hearing abilities, experiencing a deficit in understanding single words.

Difficulty in the initial stage of acoustic analysis (i.e. perceiving speech sounds from the acoustic signal) can result in word *sound* deafness.[5] Because this initial process is impaired, subsequent processing stages are then affected; the ability to recognize words and subsequent access to the semantic (meaning) system in order to understand the word.

Similarly, a deficit in accessing the phonological input lexicon (or word store) will affect an individual's ability to recognize the words they are hearing. This is termed as word *form* deafness.[6]

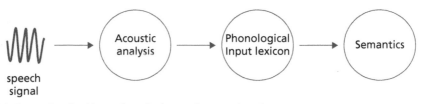

speech
signal

Fig. 13.1 Stages involved in spoken single word comprehension.

Adapted from Whitworth, A., Webster, Janet, & Howard, David. (2014). *A cognitive neuropsychological approach to assessment and intervention in aphasia : A clinician's guide* (Second ed.). By permission of Taylor and Francis Group Ltd, a division of Informa plc.

So, on hearing a list of familiar words (e.g. 'car') and non-words (e.g. 'flaget'), an individual would have difficulty in choosing the familiar words from those that have been invented.

Finally, a deficit in mapping this recognized word from the lexicon to its corresponding representation within the semantic system will result in an individual recognizing a word but being unable to understand its meaning; word *meaning* deafness.[7]

Cases of individuals presenting with a discrete impairment at any one of the stages is rare; commonly in clinical practice individuals will present with multiple deficits at more than one stage of processing. Depending on the site and location of the underlying lesion, the ability to understand words can vary significantly between individuals. This ability can also be influenced by psycholinguistic variables such as word frequency (how commonly a word occurs compared to other words in that language), age of acquisition (the age at which the word is learned), and imageability (or concreteness; how easily the concept represented by a particular word can be mentally imagined).

Is auditory comprehension affected in older age?

In older adults, there are a number of physical, sensory, metabolic, and neurological changes that occur as part of the ageing process that might also impact on communication.[8]

These include changes to non-language or hearing-specific cognitive functions such as working memory and information processing speed.[8,9] A study by Peelle et al.[10] also found that older individuals with 'age-normal' hearing loss demonstrate reduced neural activity for cortical structures that are activated when processing complex language. They concluded that the reduction in sensory information directly increases listening effort, resulting in fewer resources available for higher-level language processing.

Hearing loss of higher frequency sounds is also common in older adults, particularly affecting consonants, and leading to difficulty in speech discrimination of these sounds, meaning that speech perception can become distorted. This can also become more challenging when language is presented with background noise present.[8]

Given the established high incidence of hearing loss in the older population, we might then assume that older individuals with aphasia will also have some degree of age-related cognitive and sensory change, in addition to aphasia, affecting language comprehension. Rankin et al.[11] investigated the relationship between hearing loss and auditory processing in individuals with aphasia. In this study, measures of hearing acuity such as pure tone audiometry did not predict auditory processing ability, suggesting instead that affected processes such as working memory, information processing speed, and higher-order attention, which can also be affected in aphasia, are more influential in contributing to auditory processing ability.

It is clear that age-related changes associated with auditory comprehension are multifaceted, and that the complex interaction between lower level peripheral processes and higher-level cognitive processes affects understanding of spoken language. It is particularly pertinent therefore that we consider these factors in addition to traditional methods of language comprehension assessment when diagnosing type and degree of aphasia.

Disorders of spoken word production

As with comprehension, production of a spoken word involves a series of stages (see Fig. 13.2). It can be helpful to consider each stage as a discrete level of processing, however, we know that there is some interaction and overlap between these different stages.[12,13]

So, how do we produce a word? After generating an idea or message, an activation of a lexical (or word) concept within the semantic system occurs, leading to activation within the output lexicon to retrieve the word, and then production of the relevant speech sounds. Some theories

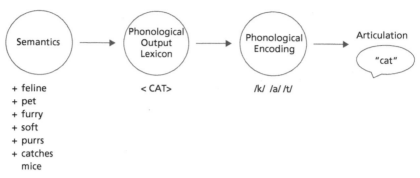

Fig. 13.2 Stages of processing in word production.

Adapted from Whitworth, A., Webster, Janet, & Howard, David. (2014). *A cognitive neuropsychological approach to assessment and intervention in aphasia : A clinician's guide* (Second ed.). By permission of Taylor and Francis Group Ltd, a division of Informa plc.

also support further intermediate stages of processing such as retrieval of the grammatical features prior to the word form.[12,13]

Disorders of word-finding can occur due to an impairment at one or more of these levels of processing. Impairment at any level will result in word-finding errors, and by analysing error type, we can gain an insight into where the level of breakdown is occurring. Disruption to the semantic system, which is involved in both comprehension and expression, will typically result in semantic errors, while disruption to the output lexicon will give rise to word form errors, and impairment to the phonological encoding will result in sound errors. See Table 13.1 for examples of error types.

Sentences and conversation

Individuals with aphasia can present with fluent aphasia or non-fluent aphasia. Fluent aphasia typically consists of long strings of content-light language, with stereotypical and overused phrases, often containing 'jargon' or non-words. Often intonation is appropriate and individuals will typically demonstrate reduced self-monitoring and insight into their difficulties.[14] An example of expressive language in fluent aphasia might be 'it was that way round of course but inkle on the day it kenter for'.

In contrast, individuals with non-fluent aphasia demonstrate comparably greater self-awareness. Expressive language typically contains greater pauses with verbs omitted to a greater extent than nouns. Attempts to self-correct word errors are more likely to be evident. An example

Table 13.1 Examples of word error types in aphasia (in this example, the target word is 'pear')

Semantic	apple
Phonological	bear
Visual	balloon
Semantic + phonological (mixed)	peach
Unrelated	flamingo
Non-word	visobil

Table 13.2 Verbs differ in how many arguments they require

Verb	Example	No. of arguments
Laugh	<u>the boy</u> is laughing	1
Kiss	<u>the princess</u> kissed <u>the frog</u>	2
	(vs. *the princess kissed—this is ungrammatical)	
Give	<u>the woman</u> gave <u>the girl</u> <u>a hug</u>'	3
	(vs. * <u>the woman</u> gave <u>the girl</u>— this is ungrammatical)	

of expressive language in someone with non-fluent aphasia is 'Monday . . . car . . . shops . . . lots . . . time . . . shops . . . busy'.

For some individuals with aphasia, specific difficulties arise as a result of agrammatism; a term which describes a cluster of symptoms including verb production, reduced morphology (i.e. the suffixes in words are omitted), and overall simplified grammatical constructions such as in the example here.

Differing models have been proffered to explain how we produce sentences. Consensus has been reached, however, on the idea that verbs are pivotal to sentence production as they contain information which dictates the structure of the sentence. Verbs differ in their type and complexity (see Table 13.2).

In order to produce a sentence, we first need to generate an idea or message that we want to convey. This leads to verb selection (including specifying how many arguments are required), then construction of the sentence form before the sentence can be produced.

Individuals with aphasia can have difficulties in sentence processing due to impairments affecting: verb retrieval,[15,16] generating the message to be communicated (known as event processing[17]), generating the correct sentence structure (assigning the correct roles, e.g. whether in the aforementioned example it is the woman or the girl giving or receiving the hug),[18] or in assigning suffixes describing tense (e.g. the man walk the dog vs. the man walk<u>ed</u> the dog).[19] Often individuals with sentence production deficits also demonstrate impairments to sentence comprehension.

Clearly, difficulties at a single word and sentence level will inevitably have an impact on an individual's ability to express themselves when retelling a narrative or in conversation. However, there are mechanisms specific to conversation that can also be affected in aphasia. These include the ability to choose the topic to be talked about, keep the conversation going, or change the topic of conversation. If the conversation breaks down, some individuals with aphasia can also find it challenging to 'repair' the conversation. Given the nature of conversation as a dynamic, shared activity between an individual and their conversation partner, research has focused on the conversational features of both individuals and the strategies that might facilitate or prevent successful conversation.[20]

Is expressive language affected in older age?

Studies investigating naming abilities in older adults have investigated 'tip of the tongue' states (ToT); this occurs when an individual is able to access the semantic information about a word but is unable to retrieve the corresponding word form. Overall, research supports the view that older adults tend to exhibit more ToT in comparison with younger adults,[21] particularly for proper nouns (i.e. people's names) comparative to common nouns.[22] Salthouse and Mandell[21] concluded that this phenomenon cannot be explained by age-related episodic memory decline.

Older adults have also been reported to speak more slowly and less fluently than younger adults, pause more frequently, and produce semantically underspecified words or 'filler' words.[23] Belke and Meyer[24], in their comparison of single and multiword tasks in older adults, report that this might be attributed to the overall cognitive demand; the need to divide resources between single word retrieval, connected speech production, and self-monitoring, rather than due to slowed lexical or phonological processing for single words.

Sentence production has also been reported to be vulnerable to ageing, with Sung[25] reporting that in tasks with a higher cognitive load and subsequent demand on working memory, an age-related decline was observed across study participants.

We therefore need to be mindful of these subtle features when assessing older adults, considering for example whether assessment tools have been standardized with older adults, and recognizing that different assessment methods may place a greater cognitive demand on the individual, affecting performance.

Literacy

Individuals with aphasia can also experience reading difficulties (acquired dyslexia or alexia) mirroring those difficulties observed within the auditory modality. For example, individuals can have difficulties in recognizing and perceiving single letters or words, or in accessing the meaning of written words.

Individuals with an acquired alexia might experience a central alexia, such as surface alexia (impaired reading of words with an irregular spelling compared to regular words, e.g. 'pint' read aloud to rhyme with 'mint'), deep alexia (characterized by semantic errors, e.g. 'tea' read aloud as 'coffee', and an inability to read plausible non-words or pseudowords such as 'sprode'), or phonological alexia (resulting in the inability to read pseudowords comparable to real words).

In contrast individuals may experience a peripheral alexia, such as neglect alexia (difficulty in identifying words either at the beginning or ends of sentences distinct to a more general visual neglect or hemianopia, e.g. *butter* → 'otter'), attentional alexia (an inability to identify the spatial characteristics of letters in comparison to neighbouring letters, e.g. *seed* → 'deed'), or visual alexia (difficulty in identifying individual letters leading to visually related errors, e.g. *fan* → 'tan').

Similarly, individuals can experience acquired spelling difficulties, known as dysgraphia.[26] Impairments can mirror those seen in spoken production: difficulties in accessing the meaning and corresponding word form resulting in semantic spelling errors; affected access to the written (or orthographic) output lexicon, or difficulties in spelling novel words or non-words.

Is literacy affected in older age?

There is limited evidence on the literacy abilities of older adults. In general, it appears that older adults do maintain their overall reading and spelling abilities when compared to younger adults.[27] However, they may demonstrate slower processing compared to younger age groups.[28] In keeping with accounts of sentence comprehension and production in older age, Borella et al.[29] also found that age was correlated with decreased performance on reading comprehension tasks requiring a higher cognitive load and subsequent demand on working memory.

Dysarthria

Dysarthria is a motor speech disorder caused by upper or lower motor neuron lesions. It is more common post-stroke in comparison to aphasia, with estimated incidence at around 42%.[30] Various subsystems of speech production can be affected including: respiration, phonation (voice production), prosody or intonation, resonance (hyper or hyponasality), and articulation.

Table 13.3 Dysarthria subtypes associated with stroke

Dysarthria type	Localization	Motor symptoms
Flaccid	Lower motor neurone	Weakness
Spastic	Upper motor neurone	Spasticity
Ataxic	Cerebellum	Incoordination
Hypokinetic	Basal ganglia	Rigidity or reduced range of movement
Hyperkinetic	Basal ganglia	Dystonic or choreaic movements
Mixed	Multiple	Multiple

Source data from Duffy, J. (2005). *Motor speech disorders: Substrates, differential diagnosis, and management*, 2nd edition, Elsevier.

Traditionally, dysarthria has been characterized according to the Mayo clinic classification.[31,32] Dysarthria post-stroke will commonly be classified as spastic, flaccid, ataxic, or mixed depending on the location of the underlying neurological lesion (Table 13.3).

Dysarthria presentation can vary both in type and severity, with some individuals presenting with occasional unintelligible speech to individuals being unable to execute any oral movements necessary for successful speech production (termed anarthria).

Apraxia of speech

Debate exists over the underlying mechanisms involved in apraxia of speech (AoS) (sometimes also referred to as verbal dyspraxia).[33]

In AoS, articulation difficulties exist, but are thought to be due to an impairment of the execution of motor planning required for articulation, rather than as a result of neuromuscular weakness. Apraxia results in observable speech characteristics such as altered prosody, vowel distortions, and prolongations, effortful, 'groping' speech behaviours, and inconsistent articulation patterns. As with aphasia and dysarthria, AoS severity can vary significantly from minor speech errors to a total loss of speech.

How is motor speech production affected in older age?

It is recognized that overall neuromotor function is affected by age,[34] with motor speech changes in elderly adults an emerging area of research. In their exploratory study, Sadagopan and Smith[35] found that the ability to repeat complex non-words accurately and rapidly was affected significantly by age in a group of healthy older adults. Bilodeau-Mercure et al.[36] also found that motor planning for speech production and orofacial movements also declined with age. However, whether ageing is a significant factor does vary according to the type of speech task.[37] Therefore we cannot conclude that older adults necessarily demonstrate compromised motor speech function during functional conversation.

The ICF Framework as a model to guide assessment and intervention

The World Health Organization's International Classification of Functioning Disability and Health (ICF)[38] is a standard framework which describes how any specified health condition might affect

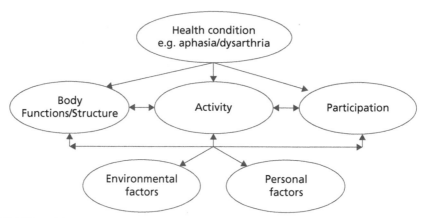

Fig. 13.3 ICF model.

Reproduced with permission from The World Health Organization. *The World health report : 2001 : Mental health : new understanding, new hope*. World Health Organisation International Classification of functioning, disability and health: ICF. Geneva, Switzerland.

the individual in a range of domains. It describes both body functions and structures (anatomy, physiological and or/psychological factors) or impairment and activity and participation, that is, the impact of a particular health condition or disorder (such as aphasia or dysarthria) on the individual's ability to function, such as the ability to communicate within both the immediate and wider social context. It also includes environmental factors external to the client that might in-clude attitudes of others, opportunities, occupational, societal, and cultural factors, and personal factors which include age, gender, educational level, or personal resources, such as coping style or attitude (Fig. 13.3).

Application of the ICF framework is well established within speech and language therapy, including stroke rehabilitation. It forms the basis of standardized outcome measures used in indi-viduals with aphasia, dysarthria, and AoS[39] and can be used to conceptualize client goals, assess-ment emphasis, and the focus of rehabilitation.[40] For example, assessment of aphasia at a body function/structure level might focus on word-finding ability or sentence production; at an activity level would focus on the ability to have conversations with a family member or friend, and at a participation level would consider the impact of aphasia on the individual's occupation, leisure activities, or social networks. The ICF model does not specifically consider an individual's quality of life or well-being, and we will return to this later.

Assessment considerations

So far, we have considered how aphasia, dysarthria, and AoS might present in the individual. Now we turn to considerations in assessing individuals post-stroke.

It is established that communication assessment is good practice within stroke care.[41] Assessment can be used to detect the presence or absence of a communication disorder, estab-lish the level of language breakdown and plan appropriate therapy, identify facilitation strategies to support communication within everyday communication, contribute to differential diagnosis, educate the client and his or her family about the presenting communication disorder, and inform the goal setting or mental capacity assessment process. Choice of assessment will be determined by a range of factors, including clinical setting, model of service delivery, stage of recovery, and the client's own goals and future plans.

Assessment should be carried out by a suitably qualified individual, typically a speech and language therapist. This is in contrast to a communication screen such as the Frenchay Aphasia Screening Test[42] or the Sheffield Screening Test for Acquired Language Disorders.[43] Typically screening tools can be used by a range of health professionals to determine the likely presence of an acquired language disorder and prompt onward referral to speech and language therapy for a more detailed comprehensive assessment.

Where a more detailed assessment is appropriate, language assessment should be undertaken based on a cognitive neuropsychological approach; considering models of single word and sentence processing such as those outlined here. Assessment batteries such as the Psycholinguistic Assessment of Language Processing in Aphasia[44] or the Comprehensive Aphasia Test[45] enable the clinician to assess comprehension and expression, testing out hypotheses regarding the level of underlying language breakdown and establishing which aspects of linguistic processing are a relative strength. If AoS is suspected, assessment using a tool such as the Apraxia Battery for Adults—2[46] can inform differential diagnosis.

When establishing the presence or absence of dysarthria, assessment of motor function should include assessment of respiratory control, voice production, intonation, resonance, and articulation, including a detailed examination of cranial nerve function and orofacial structures such as lips, tongue, face, and soft palate. Examples of assessment tools include the Frenchay Dysarthria Assessment[47] and the Robertson Dysarthria Profile.[48] In addition, measures of intelligibility should be considered such as the Assessment of Intelligibility in Dysarthric Speech.[49]

When considering assessment of older adults, we need to consider any age-related sensory and physical changes such as reduced visual acuity, fatigue, and the psychometric properties of the assessment, including whether normative data is available for the age of the individual being assessed.

Clearly, communication assessment should only be undertaken at a time when it will inform and benefit the individual. For example, in an acute setting where an individual is in the early days and weeks post-stroke, assessment commonly focuses on establishing a communication profile. Knowing how much an individual is able to understand is paramount in ensuring individuals are empowered in decisions surrounding their care and rehabilitation. At this point, the focus of the speech and language therapist will be to inform the multidisciplinary team, support the individual to set goals, educate them regarding the sudden change in their communication, explore suitable techniques to support conversation, monitor changes in communication that might occur due to spontaneous recovery, and establish readiness for therapy.

Speech and language therapists working in the acute sector have reported intervention for communication needs as being deprioritized in preference for dysphagia (swallowing difficulties).[50] This is despite evidence that some individuals would greatly benefit from early impairment-focused, intensive intervention.[51] In considering the factors influencing this situation, Foster et al.[50] suggest that in the acute environment with a prevalent medical model, the perception exists that comparable to dysphagia, the consequences and impact of communication impairment are minimal. However, the authors suggest that given the recognized impact of communication on a range of factors such as increased length of stay, impact on decision-making, and negative health outcomes, this view should be challenged (see Foster et al.[50] for a full discussion).

Within the community and domiciliary settings, communication assessment should, in addition to the reasons just described, include an assessment of the individual's communication environment including the skills of regular conversation partners, and identification of barriers to activity and participation that might be addressed in therapy. Assessment should also consider both the short and anticipated long-term needs of the individual, given that aphasia is a chronic condition.

Spontaneous recovery of communication post-stroke

Recovery of language ability post-stroke is related to a range of factors such as lesion location and size, neuroplasticity, and language reorganization. Evidence suggests that both the left and right hemisphere neural systems are involved in the reorganization of language post-stroke.[52] Aphasia presentation can also change significantly over time, with the most rapid rate of recovery observed in the first 3 months post-stroke.[2]

In their review investigating factors affecting spontaneous aphasia recovery, Watila and Balarabe[53] report that aphasia recovery is correlated with lesion size and location. In Ali et al.'s [54] study investigating spontaneous recovery of dysarthria and aphasia in the first 3 months post-stroke, stroke severity and age were associated with a poor recovery. In their longitudinal study, Laska et al.[2] found that younger individuals demonstrated more spontaneous improvement in aphasia compared to older adults. However, in their review of the literature investigating factors affecting recovery in aphasia, Watila and Balarabe[53] report that due to conflicting evidence in the literature, the influence of age on aphasia recovery is not clear. What may in fact be more crucial for individuals is assessment of their suitability for therapy, and establishing which facilitators and barriers might exist to support communication recovery, rather than their chronological age.

Assessing suitability for therapy

How do we know whether speech and language therapy will be of benefit for the individual post-stroke? There are several factors to consider including neurobiological principles underpinning therapy in addition to factors internal and external to the individual.

Therapy principles

In common with any other form of rehabilitation aimed at improving behaviour by modifying neuronal function, therapy at an impairment level, including linguistic processes, should be based on principles of neuroplasticity in order to maximize effectiveness. Intervention should therefore be of sufficient intensity, include massed practice (a large amount of therapy within a short time period), and of relevance to the individual. In studies where intervention has been based on these principles, changes in behaviour as a result of neurophysiological changes have been observed,[52,55,56] however debate does exist over the degree of intensity required for specific intervention approaches.[57] Clinical guidelines reflect evidence for intensive therapy, with the Royal College of Physicians (RCP) recommending a minimum of 45 minutes therapy for a minimum of 5 days per week.[41]

Similarly, where motor speech recovery is the target of intervention for those individuals with dysarthria, we need to consider principles of motor learning to maximize the impact of therapy, such as intensive, targeted, relevant practice with clear, specific feedback,[58,59] including treating dysarthria using speech rather than non-speech oromotor tasks.[60] Ludlow et al.[58] also concluded that although there is evidence to suggest that neuroplasticity in response to behavioural approaches diminishes with age, the effect of age on dysarthria treatment outcome has not been reported.

Within the aphasia literature there is considerable variability regarding how effective treatments are, not least because differences exist regarding how efficacy is measured, how long effects of intervention are sustained in order to be deemed effective, and whether or not the impact on an individual's overall communication is measured (see Webster et al.[61]). Given this variation, speech and language therapists are best placed to investigate an individual's stimulability, or response to a particular intervention.

Internal factors

It is recognized that while aphasia is distinct from non-linguistic cognitive processes, aphasia can commonly occur alongside cognitive changes as a result of stroke.[62,63] Cognitive processes such as memory, executive function, visuospatial skills, and attention are all involved in the ability to learn and engage in rehabilitation; individual differences in these abilities may explain differences in therapeutic success in individuals with seemingly similar levels of aphasia.[62]

Similarly, where motivation or low mood is a factor, this can also impact adversely on therapy outcome. Older age and aphasia have both been found to be associated with low mood post-stroke.[64]

External factors

Factors external to the client can also influence suitability for therapy. A significant percentage of older adults with communication disorders post-stroke may live alone and lack regular support to provide regular, intensive therapy practice. Similarly, where a conversational approach is recommended, the individual may not have sufficient opportunities with suitably skilled conversation partners, or access to community activities. Older adults may have limited access to technology that might allow for massed practice.

We know that older adults also experience psychosocial changes as they age. It is recognized that social relationships and networks may diminish, and access to leisure and social activities can reduce. Increased social isolation has been associated with higher mortality.[65] Where individuals with aphasia perceive loneliness and a reduction in social network, these have been found to be predictors of low mood post-stroke.[66]

Setting collaborative goals

When delivering patient-centred care, collaborative goal setting is paramount in ensuring that the aspirations and priorities of the individual provide a foundation for rehabilitation planning.

In Worral et al.'s 2011[40] study, individuals with aphasia, including older adults, reported priorities post-stroke encompassing a range of factors including communication and the impact of social life, work, and leisure activities. They also identified goals related to maintaining or developing friendships, and educating others about aphasia. It is clearly important that assessment and intervention should fully encompass the goals and aspirations of people with aphasia.

What does speech and language therapy look like?

In the same way that assessment might include all dimensions of the ICF, intervention in speech and language therapy for the older adult should also address aspects of impairment, activity, participation, and environmental and personal factors. Intervention includes direct therapy (working directly with the individual) or indirect therapy (working with the individual's primary caregivers or family). Individuals may be seen by a stroke-specific service such as an early supported discharge or community stroke team. Where older individuals present with a stroke alongside other comorbidities, they may not receive stroke-specific treatment, as this is often dependent on the locally commissioned speech and language therapy or stroke service.

Impairment-focused intervention

Interventions at an impairment level, typically involve 'retraining' lost skills. Examples include: word-finding therapies,[67,68,69] therapies focusing on sentence processing,[70,71] articulation, and motor planning,[72] or spelling[73]; with the specific type of intervention determined by the results of impairment-focused assessment.

Despite several studies that do include older adults,[68,70] this has tended to be the exception rather than the norm, with older adults being under-represented in the literature. Research participants with any coexisting hearing loss, cognitive change, who have had more than one stroke, or who are unable to access clinics away from the home environment tend to be excluded; leading to a gap in the evidence-base particularly for frail older adults.

Where an impairment-based therapy is the focus of intervention, technology might be used to support the necessary intensity and repetitive practice needed to maximize therapeutic success. There are a number of therapy applications and software packages available targeting a range of areas in aphasia and apraxia. In a recent review of computer-based therapy in aphasia, Zheng et al.[74] reported that again the majority of participants in studies have been under 65 years of age, commenting that generalization to the older population should be limited, given the recognized reduction in neuroplasticity for learning in older age.

We might extrapolate then, that with older adults, impairment-based approaches should be trialled, considering all of the factors discussed just now when deciding on therapy suitability.

Activity and participation-focused intervention

Intervention at addressing social and life participation should include identifying internal barriers to communication success such as motivation, mood, or confidence and external barriers, such as the skills, attitudes and resources of others.

Speech and language therapy can address barriers to successful communication, support access to premorbid interests and activities,[40] or find new roles (e.g. as a conversation partner).[75] Individuals with aphasia have reported 'helping others' as a priority post-stroke[40] and report the importance of 'moving forward'.[76] Individuals have also reported the importance of engagement post-stroke,[77] thus intervention for healthy older adults might focus on return to paid employment or voluntary work, or involvement in groups for people with aphasia.

Conversation approaches to aphasia have been found to be effective in supporting individuals to have more successful communication interactions. In the Supported Conversation™,[78] individuals and their conversation partners are taught strategies such as writing, drawing, and gesture to supplement their verbal communication and increase the methods available to support both understanding and expression. These strategies allow the individual with aphasia's underlying competence to be revealed, which can often be masked as a result of aphasia. This approach can improve psychosocial outcomes by increasing confidence, promoting positive self-identity, and leading to enhanced social relationships.[79]

Digital literacy and participation

It is widely recognized that the way that we interact with the world increasingly involves a digital interaction. Use of the internet as a means to carry out daily activities and maintain social relationships has increased exponentially in recent years. While for some people, technology can increase independence and access to social networks, research is also beginning to recognize the 'digital divide'; that for some people with communication difficulties, or indeed older adults (see [80]), information available in a digital-only format (such as healthcare or financial information) can be inaccessible and disempowering. Speech and language therapy intervention might therefore also include addressing barriers to accessing digital information, in order to enhance social participation and autonomy.[81]

Health-related quality of life and older people with communication impairments

Health-related quality of life is a multifaceted concept and includes a range of factors including physical well-being, psychological and mental health, social activities, social networks, communication, and overall life satisfaction (see [82,83]). Older people with aphasia have reported several core factors that contribute to life quality[84]: the ability to engage in activities or employment, or the opportunity to try new activities; verbal communication and the impact of compromised speaking on activities; support from family; and physical and cognitive changes.

Low mood has also been found to be associated with reduced social networks post-stroke.[66] For some older adults, low mood can result in reduced motivation and reduced engagement in rehabilitation. Where low mood is identified, referral for specialist counselling or psychological support is warranted.

Intervention should therefore aim to increase social participation, including facilitating access to social networks and activities in addition to supporting individuals to find ways to compensate for their communication difficulties (see [85]). One such option is to provide group therapy which directly addresses life participation.[86]

Care homes

Many older people, particularly frail older adults, will reside in care homes in order to have their nursing and physical needs associated with stroke met. This can pose specific challenges for individuals with communication needs. Although the literature describing intervention specifically targeting individuals in care homes is lacking, provided the individual has appropriate support and resources, the care home setting should not preclude individuals from receiving impairment-focused speech and language therapy in addition to functional communication support.

There is evidence to suggest that training care staff in supported conversation techniques[78] can result in increased awareness and skills of care staff.[87] Training volunteer conversation partners to visit individual care homes has also been found to decrease social isolation with potential positive effects on mood.[88]

Conclusion

Aphasia, dysarthria, and AoS are common communication disorders post-stroke, varying significantly in presentation across individuals. Although there is some evidence to support specific age-related changes in language and motor speech function, assessment and differential diagnosis of the presenting communication disorder should be undertaken on an individual basis. Rather than chronological age, more pertinent factors to consider are the individual's own health status and cognitive resource and motivation, in addition to external factors such as the clinical setting, resources, and model of service delivery.

Intervention should be based on focused assessment, and consider all aspects of the ICF model, working with the individual, their family, and health professionals to enable effective communication. This will achieve involvement in decision-making in everyday life and in the context of rehabilitation, and overall have a positive impact on mood and health-related quality of life. Intervention should address the long-term and evolving needs of the individual for enhanced social participation and engagement and recognize the individuality of 'living successfully' with a long-term communication disability.[89]

References

1. **Flowers HL, Silver FL, Fang J, Rochon E, & Martino R.** The incidence, co-occurrence, and predictors of dysphagia, dysarthria, and aphasia after first-ever acute ischaemic stroke. *J Commun Disord* 2013;**46**:238–48.

2. **Laska AC, Hellblom A, Murray V, Kahan T, & von Arbin M.** Aphasia in acute stroke and relation to outcome. *J Int Med* 2001;**249**:413–22.

3. **Pujol J, Deus J, Losilla JM, & Capdevila A.** Cerebral lateralization of language in normal left-handed people studied by functional MRI. *Neurology* 1999;**52**(5):1038–43.

4. **Whitworth A, Webster J, & Howard D.** *A Cognitive Neuropsychological Approach to Assessment and Intervention in Aphasia: A Clinician's Guide*, 2nd edition. Hove, UK: Psychology Press, 2014.

5. **Woolf C, Panton A, Rosen S, Best W, & Marshall J.** Therapy for auditory processing impairment in aphasia: an evaluation of two approaches. *Aphasiology* 2014;**28**(12):1481–505.

6. **Howard D & Franklin S.** *Missing the Meaning?*. Cambridge, UK: MIT Press, 1988.

7. **Bormann T & Weiller C.** 'Are there lexicons?' A study of lexical and semantic processing in word-meaning deafness suggests 'yes'. *Cortex* 2011;**48**(3):294–307.

8. **Aydelott J, Leech R, & Crinion J.** Normal adult aging and the contextual influences affecting speech and meaningful sound perception. *Trends Amplif* 2010;**14**(4):218–32.

9. **Rast P & Eccles J.** Verbal knowledge, working memory, and processing speed as predictors of verbal learning in older adults. *Dev Psychol* 2011;**47**(5):1490–8.

10. **Peelle J, Troiani V, Grossman M, & Wingfield A.** Hearing loss in older adults affects neural systems supporting speech comprehension. *J Neurosci* 2011;**31**(35):12638–43.

11. **Rankin E, Newton C, Parker A, & Bruce C.** Hearing loss and auditory processing ability in people with aphasia. *Aphasiology* 2014;**28**:576–95.

12. **Dell GS, Schwartz MF, Martin N, Saffran EM, & Gagnon DA.** Lexical access in aphasic and nonaphasic speakers. *Psychol Rev* 1997;**104**:801–38.

13. **Levelt W, Roelofs A, & Meyer A.** A theory of lexical access in speech production. *Behav Brain Sci* 1999;**22**(1):1–38.

14. **Sampson M & Faroqi-Shah Y.** Investigation of self- monitoring in fluent aphasia with jargon. *Aphasiology* 2011;**25**(4):505–28.

15. **Cnroy P, Sage K, & Lambon Ralph M.** Towards theory-driven therapies for aphasic verb impairments: a review of current theory and practice. *Aphasiology* 2006;**20**(12):1159–85.

16. **Routhier S, Bier N, & Macoir J.** Smart tablet for smart self-administered treatment of verb anomia: two single-case studies in aphasia. *Aphasiology* 2015;**30**(2–3):1–21.

17. **Dean M & Black M.** Exploring event processing and description in people with aphasia. *Aphasiology* 2005;**19**(6):521–44.

18. **Marshall J, Chiat S, & Pring T.** An impairment in processing verbs' thematic roles: a therapy study. *Aphasiology* 1997;**11**(9):855–76.

19. **Thompson C, Lee J, & Mack J.** Verbal morphology in aphasia: comparison of structured vs. narrative elicitation tasks. *Procedia—Social and Behavioral Sciences* 2012;**61**:228–9.

20. **Beeke S, Beckley F, Johnson F, et al.** Conversation focused aphasia therapy: investigating the adoption of strategies by people with agrammatism. *Aphasiology* 2015;**29**(3):355–77.

21. **Salthouse T & Mandell A.** Do age-related increases in tip-of-the-tongue experiences signify episodic memory impairments? *Psychol Sci* 2013;**24**(12):2489–97.

22. **Juncos-Rabadán O, Facal D, Soledad Rodríguez M, & Pereiro AX.** Lexical knowledge and lexical retrieval in ageing: insights from a tip-of-the-tongue (TOT) study. *Language and Cognitive Processes* 2010;**25**:10:1301–34.

23. **Mortensen L, Meyer AS, & Humphreys GW.** Age-related effects on speech production: a review. *Language and Cognitive Processes* 2006;**21**:238–90.

24. **Belke E & Meyer A.** Single and multiple object naming in healthy ageing. *Language and Cognitive Processes* 2007;**22**(8):1178–211.

25. **Sung JE.** Age-related changes in sentence production abilities and their relation to working-memory capacity: evidence from a verb- final language. *PLoS One* 2015:**10**(4):e0119424.

26. **Thiel L, Sage K, & Conroy P.** Comparing uni-modal and multi-modal therapies for improving writing in acquired dysgraphia after stroke. *Neuropsychol Rehabil* 2016;**26**:3:345–73.

27. **Crowley K, Mayer P, & Stuart-Hamilton I.** Changes in reliance on reading and spelling subskills across the lifespan. *Educ Gerontol* 2009:**35**(6):503–22.

28. **Stuart-Hamilton I & Rabbitt P.** Age-related decline in spelling ability: a link with fluid intelligence? *Educ Gerontol* 1997;**23**(5):437–41.

29. **Borella E, Ghisletta P, & De Ribaupierre A.** Age differences in text processing: the role of working memory, inhibition, and processing speed. *J Gerontol B Psychol Sci Social Sci* 2011;**66**(3):311–20.

30. **Flowers HL, Silver FL, Fang J, Rochon E, & Martino R.** The incidence, co-occurrence, and predictors of dysphagia, dysarthria and aphasia after first ever acute stroke. *J Commun Disord* 2012;**46**:238–48.

31. **Darley FL, Aronson AE, & Brown JR.** Differential diagnostic pat- terns of dysarthria. *J Speech Hearing Res* 1969;**12**:246–69.

32. **Simmons KC & Mayo R.** The use of the mayo clinic system for differential diagnosis of dysarthria. *J Commun Disord* 1997;**30**(2):117–32.

33. **Ziegler W, Aichert I, & Staiger A.** Apraxia of speech: concepts and controversies. *J Speech Lang Hear Res* 2012;**55**:S1485–501.

34. **de Miranda Marzullo AC, Neto OP, Ballard KJ, et al.** Neural control of the lips differs for young and older adults following a perturbation. *Exp Brain Res* 2010;**206**:319–27.

35. **Sadagopan N & Smith A.** Age differences in speech motor performance on a novel speech task. *J Speech Lang Hear Res* 2013;**56**(5):1552–66.

36. **Bilodeau-Mercure M, Kirouac V, Langlois N, Ouellet C, Gasse I, & Tremblay P.** Movement sequencing in normal aging: speech, oro-facial, and finger movements. *Age* 2015;**37**(4):9813.

37. **Pierce JE, Cotton S, & Perry A.** Alternating and sequential motion rates in older adults. *Int J Lang Commun Disord* 2013;**48**(3):257–64.

38. **World Health Organization.** *International Classification of Functioning, Disability and Health: ICF.* Geneva, Switzerland: WHO, 2001.

39. **Enderby P & John A.** *Therapy Outcome Measures for Rehabilitation Professionals.* Guildford, UK: J & R Press, 2015.

40. **Worrall L, Sherratt S, Rogers P, et al.** What people with aphasia want: their goals according to the ICF. *Aphasiology* 2011;**25**(3):309–22.

41. **Intercollegiate Stroke Working Party.** *National Clinical Guideline for Stroke*, 4th edition. London, UK: Royal College of Physicians, 2012.

42. **Enderby P, Wood V, & Wade D.** 2013 *Frenchay Aphasia Screening Test.* Bodmin, UK: Stass Publications.

43. **Syder D, Body R, Parker M, & Boddy M.** *Sheffield Screening Test for Acquired Language Disorders.* Windsor, UK: NFER-Nelson, 1989.

44. **Kay J, Coltheart M, & Lesser R.** *Psycholinguistic Assessments of Language Processing in Aphasia.* Hove, UK: Psychology Press, 2001.

45. **Swinburne K, Porter G, & Howard D.** *Comprehensive Aphasia Test.* London, UK: Routledge, 2004.

46. **Dabul B.** *Apraxia Battery for Adults*, 2nd edition. Austin, TX: Pro.ed, 2000.

47. **Enderby P & Palmer R.** *Frenchay Dysarthria Assessment: Examiner's Manual*, 2nd edition. Austin, TX: Pro.ed, 2008.

48. **Robertson SJ & Thomson F.** *Working with Dysarthric Clients: A Practical Guide to Therapy for Dysarthria.* Tucson, AX: Communication Skill Builders, 1987.

49. **Yorkston K, Beukelman D, & Traynor C.** *Assessment of Intelligibility in Dysarthric Speech.* Austin, TX: Pro.ed, 1984.

50. **Foster A, O'Halloran R, Rose M, & Worrall L.** 'Communication is taking a back seat': speech pathologists' perceptions of aphasia management in acute hospital settings. *Aphasiology* 2016;**30**(5):585–608.

51. **CicconeN, West D, Cream A, et al.** Constraint-induced aphasia therapy (CIAT): a randomised controlled trial in very early stroke rehabilitation. *Aphasiology* 2016;**30**(5):566–84.

52. **Pulvermuller F, Hauk O, Zohsel K, Neininger B, & Mohr B.** Therapy-related reorganization of language in both hemispheres of patients with chronic aphasia. *NeuroImage* 2005;**28**:481–9.

53. **Watila MM & Balarabe SA.** Factors predicting post-stroke aphasia recovery. *J Neurol Sci* 2015;**352**:12–18.

54. **Ali M, Lyden P, & Brady M.** Aphasia and dysarthria in acute stroke: recovery and functional outcome. *Int J Stroke* 2015;**10**:400–6.

55. **Mozeiko J, Coelho CA, & Myers EB.** The role of intensity in constraint-induced language therapy for people with chronic aphasia. *Aphasiology* 2016;**30**(4):339–63.

56. **Bhogal S, Teasell R, & Speechley M.** Intensity of aphasia therapy, impact on recovery. *Stroke* 2003;**34**(4):987–93.

57. **Cherney L, Patterson R, & Raymer J.** Intensity of aphasia therapy: evidence and efficacy. *Curr Neurol Neurosci Rep* 2011;**11**(6):560–9.

58. **Bisklick LP, Weir PC, Spencer K, Kendall D, & Yorkston KM.** Do principles of motor learning enhance retention and transfer of speech skills? A systematic review. *Aphasiology* 2012;**26** (5):709–28.

59. **Ludlow CL, Hoit J, Kent R, et al.** Translating principles of neural plasticity into research on speech motor control recovery and rehabilitation. *J Speech Lang Hear Res* 2008;**51**:S240–58.

60. **Bunton K.** Speech versus non-speech: different tasks, different neural organization. *Semin Speech Lang* 2008;**29**:267–75.

61. **Webster J, Whitworth A, & Morris J.** Is it time to stop 'fishing'? A review of generalisation following aphasia intervention. Aphasiology 2015;**29**(11):1240–64.

62. **Helm-Estabrooks N.** Cognition and aphasia: a discussion and a study. *J Commun Disord* 2002;**35**;171–86.

63. **Seniów J, Litwin M, & Leśniak M.** The relationship between non-linguistic cognitive deficits and language recovery in patients with aphasia. *J Neurol Sci* 2009;**283**:91–4.

64. **Kauhanen ML, Korpelainen JT, Hiltunen P, et al.** Aphasia, depression, and non-verbal cognitive impairment ischaemic stroke. *Cerebrovasc Dis* 2000;**10**:455–61.

65. **Holt-Lunstad J, Smith T, Baker M, Harris T, & Stephenson D.** Loneliness and Social Isolation as Risk Factors for Mortality. *Perspectives on Psychological Science* 2015;**10**(2):227–37.

66. **Hilari K, Northcott S, Roy P, et al.** Psychological distress after stroke and aphasia: the first six months. *Clin Rehabil* 2010;**24**(2):181–90.

67. **Maddy KM, Capilouto GJ, & McComas KL.** The effectiveness of semantic feature analysis: an evidence-based systematic review. *Ann Phys Rehabil Med* 2014;**57**(4) 254–267.

68. **Boyle M.** Semantic feature analysis treatment for anomia in two fluent aphasia syndromes. *Am J Speech Lang Pathol* 2004;**13**(3):236–49.

69. **Wisenburn B & Mahoney K.** A meta-analysis of word-finding treatments for aphasia. *Aphasiology* 2009;**23**(11):1338–52.

70. **Edmonds LA, Obermeyer J, & Kernan B.** Investigation of pretreatment sentence production impairments in individuals with aphasia: towards understanding the linguistic variables that impact generalisation in verb network strengthening treatment. *Aphasiology* 2015;**29**(11):1312–44.

71. **Edmonds L A, Nadeau S, & Kiran S.** Effect of verb network strengthening treatment (VNeST) on lexical retrieval of content words in sentences in persons with aphasia. *Aphasiology* 2009;**23**:402–24.

72. **Ballard K, Wambaugh J, Duffy J, et al.** Treatment for acquired apraxia of speech: a systematic review of intervention research between 2004 and 2012. *Am J Speech Lang Pathol* 2015;24(2):316–37.

73. **Thiel L & Conroy P.** A comparison of errorless and errorful therapies for dysgraphia after stroke. *Neuropsychol Rehabil* 2014;24(2):172–201.

74. **Zheng C, Lynch L, & Taylor N.** Effect of computer therapy in aphasia: a systematic review. *Aphasiology* 2016;30(2–3):211–44.

75. **Swart J & Horton S.** From patients to teachers: the perspectives of trainers with aphasia in a UK Conversation Partner Scheme. *Aphasiology* 2015;29(2):195–213.

76. **Grohn B, Worrall L, Simmons-Mackie N, & Hudson K.** Living successfully with aphasia during the first year post-stroke: a longitudinal qualitative study. *Aphasiology* 2014;28(12):1405–25.

77. **Dalemans R, De Witte L, Wade D, & Van den Heuvel W.** Social participation through the eyes of people with aphasia. *Int J Lang Commun Disord* 2010;45(5):537–50.

78. **Kagan A, Black S, Simmons-Mackie N, & Square P.** Training volunteers as conversation partners using 'supported conversation for adults with aphasia' (SCA): a controlled trial. *J Speech Lang Hear Res* 2001;44(3):624–38.

79. **McMenamin R, Tierney E, & MacFarlane A.** Addressing the long-term impacts of aphasia: how far does the conversation partner programme go? *Aphasiology* 2015;29:889–913.

80. **Hill R, Betts L, & Gardner SE.** Older adults' experiences and perceptions of digital technology: (Dis) empowerment, wellbeing, and inclusion. *Computers in Human Behavior* 2015;48:415–23.

81. **Kelly H, Kennedy F, Britton H, Mcguire G, & Law J.** Narrowing the 'digital divide'—facilitating access to computer technology to enhance the lives of those with aphasia: a feasibility study. *Aphasiology* 2016;30(2–3):133–63.

82. **Hilari K, Needle JJ, & Harrison KL.** What are the important factors in health-related quality of life for people with aphasia? A systematic review. *Arch Phys Med Rehab* 2012;93:S86–95.

83. **Hilari K, Cruice M, Sorin-Peters R, & Worrall L.** Quality of life in aphasia: state of the art. *Folia Phoniatrica Et Logopaedica* 2015;67(3):114–18.

84. **Cruice M, Hill R, Worrall L, & Hickson L.** Conceptualising quality of life for older people with aphasia. *Aphasiology* 2010;24(3):327–47.

85. **Northcott S, Burns K, Simpson A, & Hilari K.** 'Living with aphasia the best way i can': a feasibility study exploring solution-focused brief therapy for people with aphasia. *Folia Phoniatr Logop* 2015;67(3):156–67.

86. **Mackenzie C, Paton G, Kelly S, Brady M, & Muir M.** The living with dysarthria group: implementation and feasibility of a group intervention for people with dysarthria following stroke and family members. *Int J Lang Commun Disord* 2012;47(6):709–24.

87. **Coles R, Lester R, Bryan K, et al.** Coping with communication disability in residential care. *Int J Lang Commun Disord* 1995;30(S1):384–8.

88. **Hickey E, Bourgeois M, & Olswang L.** Effects of training volunteers to converse with nursing home residents with aphasia. *Aphasiology* 2004;18(5–7):625–37.

89. **Brown K, Worrall L, Davidson B, & Howe T.** Snapshots of success: an insider perspective on living successfully with aphasia. *Aphasiology* 2010;24(10):1267–95.

Chapter 14

Early and late complications of stroke

Ganesh Subramanian

Introduction

Medical complications are common after acute stroke and present potential barrier to optimal recovery. In one prospective study,[1] 24% of patients suffered at least one serious medical complication (defined as prolonged, immediately life-threatening, or resulting in hospitalization or death). Another prospective multicentre study[2] found that 85% of patients suffered from a medical complication during their hospital stay, most common being infections (63%—of which 24% were urinary infection, 22% chest infection, and 19% others), confusion (56%), pain (45%—shoulder pain 9% and other pain 34%), psychological (42%—depression 16%, anxiety 14%, and emotionalism 12%), and falls (25%). The same study also found that long-term complications were related to patient dependency and duration after stroke.

Medical complications account for approximately half of stroke mortality. Prospective studies[1,3] of ischaemic strokes suggest that in the first week, direct neurological damage accounted for majority of deaths, but subsequent mortality was predominantly accounted for by medical complications.

Complications after acute stroke can be divided into three groups:

1. Neurological deterioration (early neurological deterioration, seizures, raised intracranial pressure, including malignant middle cerebral artery syndrome and hydrocephalus)

2. True complications (new conditions arising due to the stroke)—cardiac, pulmonary, gastrointestinal, infections, thromboembolism, pressure sores, spasticity, shoulder and other pains, psychological, falls and associated problems, continence issues, sexual dysfunction, and fatigue

3. Long-term complications—infections, pain, psychological problems, and those relating to persisting stroke symptoms like spatial neglect, dysphagia, and cognitive problems

In this chapter, some of the important complications will be discussed in more detail. Issues with pain (including shoulder pain), continence, fatigue, cognitive problems, dysphagia, and nutrition, although important complications, are not dealt with in this chapter as they are discussed elsewhere in this book.

Neurological deterioration

Early neurological deterioration

Early neurological deterioration has been variously termed 'stroke progression', 'stroke-in-progression', 'stroke-in-evolution' and 'early stroke progression'. It is common, occurring in 26–43% of patients; about half of all cases occur within 24 hours of stroke onset.[4,5] The pathophysiology of this is unclear and a number of factors have been proposed—haemodynamic factors, extension of original infarction or haemorrhage, excitotoxicity (e.g. high concentration of cerebrospinal fluid (CSF) glutamate), severe inflammatory response (e.g. severe sepsis), new but remote brain damage, cerebral oedema, hydrocephalus, and others.[6] There is some evidence to suggest that there might be an interaction between CSF glutamate level and pyrexia in patients with early neurological deterioration, raising a possibility that excitotoxicity and pyrexia could synergistically aggravate ischaemic damage and neuronal death.[7]

Organized stroke unit care seems to improve outcome by preventing early deterioration.[8] It is unclear which aspect of stroke unit care improves outcome and it appears it a combination of factors including multidisciplinary specialist input. In terms of medical management, care must be given to maintain oxygen saturations of 94% or above (unless they are at risk of carbon dioxide retention), euthermia, blood glucose between 4 and 11 mmol/litre, hydration, and nutrition.[9] It appears that managing hypertension aggressively in intracerebral haemorrhage may improve outcome[10] but there is a lack of evidence in infarcts (the ongoing ENCHANTED trial[11] is trying to answer this question). It is unclear if active cooling will prevent early neurological deterioration (EURO-HYP[12] trial is currently ongoing to answer this question).

Seizures

Stroke is the commonest cause of seizures in population studies of adults over the age of 35 years of age.[13] 8.9% of patients with stroke suffer from post-stroke seizures, including 8.6% after ischaemic stroke and 10.6% of those with cerebral haemorrhage.[14] Most seizures are focal at the time of onset but secondary generalization is common; however status epilepticus is uncommon.

The pathogenesis of early and late onset seizures appears to be very different. Local ion shifts and neurotransmitter release at the site of damage is the reason in the former, and underlying permanent scarring causing neuronal excitability accounts for the latter. Those who suffer from late onset post-stroke seizure tend to suffer from recurrent seizures—supporting this hypothesis.

While stroke severity and cortical location of lesion were found to be the predisposing factors for early and late onset seizures, young age was found to be a risk factor for late onset post-stroke seizures.[15–18] One study suggested that pre-existing dementia increases the risk of late onset seizures (and not early seizure), it is worth noting that patients with dementia are at risk of epilepsy even if they haven't had a stroke.

There is no clear evidence when (and how) to treat post-stroke seizures in older people. Recurrence is uncommon[19] but many physicians treat if the patient has had more than one seizure of early onset and are also more likely to treat late onset seizures with antiepileptic agents. While choosing an antiepileptic agent in an older patient, care must be taken to take account of polypharmacy, impaired renal or hepatic function, and other comorbidities like dementia and general frailty. Lamotrigine or levetiracetam appear to be a reasonable choice if treatment is indicated.

Raised intracranial pressure

After an acute stroke, almost invariably there is a degree of cerebral oedema (whether it is an infarct or a haemorrhage) but in most instances, this is not clinically relevant. Two clinically important conditions are discussed.

a) *Space occupying middle cerebral artery territory infarction*: This is also referred to as 'malignant middle cerebral artery (MCA) syndrome'. This happens in roughly 10% of patients with ischaemic stroke and is characterized by significant cytotoxic cerebral oedema associated with increased intracranial pressure and brain herniation.[3,20] This is typically seen in those patients who have occlusion of terminal internal carotid artery, carotid-T, or proximal portion of the MCA (M1 segment).

Patients who progress to develop malignant MCA syndrome usually deteriorate rapidly as the oedema increases and clinically characterized by increasing neurological deficit (as identified by National Institute of Health Stroke Scale—NIHSS) and drowsiness. In a retrospective study, patients with fatal brain oedema[21] were predicted by the presence of increased baseline white cell count, early signs of infarction involving more than 50% of MCA territory or involvement of additional vascular territories, history of hypertension, and heart failure.

Malignant MCA syndrome carries a high mortality (as high as 80% if untreated).[22] Mortality is related to increased intracranial pressure causing uncal herniation. The principle of management is to reduce the intracranial pressure before brain herniation occurs. Although tracheal intubation and hyperventilation can transiently (and modestly) reduce the intracranial pressure due to hypocapnia-related cerebral vasoconstriction, the definitive treatment is decompressive hemicraniectomy. Pooled analysis of three small randomized controlled trials[23] suggest that the mortality is significantly reduced if they undergo decompressive hemicraniectomy within 48 hours of the onset of ischaemic stroke. It appears that the more severe the stroke, the more is benefit in terms of survival (number needed to treat (NNT) was 2 if the modified Rankin Scale (mRS) was 4 or more and NNT was 4 if the mRS was 3 or less.

More recently, the DESTINY II trial[24] has confirmed that there is a similar mortality benefit in an older population (age range 61–82) if operated within 48 hours of stroke onset. However, it is worth bearing in mind that the outcome was modified Rankin Scale (mRS) score 4 or 5 in a large number of patients who survived, indicating 'very dependent, needing 24-hour care' or 'moribund', and not a single patient achieved a mRS of 0–2 (independent). This raises quite an important debate about whether this increased morbidity is acceptable to the patient and hence the decision of hemicraniectomy should be made on an individual patient basis.

b) *Hydrocephalus*: There are two mechanisms whereby patients with acute stroke develop hydrocephalus—those who suffer from posterior circulation strokes (either haemorrhage or infarct; see Fig. 14.1) have a risk of developing 'obstructive' or 'non-communicating' hydrocephalus, and those who suffer from deep parenchymal bleed with extension into the lateral or third ventricles (e.g. thalamic bleed) have a risk of developing 'communicating' hydrocephalus. As the name suggests, in the former, the hydrocephalus develops due to blockage

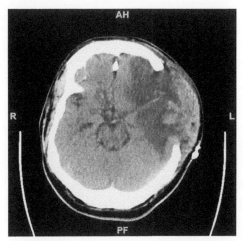

Fig. 14.1 Image showing large (space occupying) left middle cerebral artery territory infarct with evidence of recent hemicraniectomy and brain herniating externally.

of cerebrospinal fluid (CSF) flow around the fourth ventricle (in the posterior cranial fossa) and in the latter it is due to lack of CSF absorption as the arachnoid villi gets coated with blood and blood products. The incidence of hydrocephalus following an acute stroke is not known. Although obstructive hydrocephalus usually develops in the first few days after the stroke (when the peri-infarct oedema or the volume of haematoma is at its worst), communicating hydrocephalus can develop either in the acute phase or even a few weeks later. However, it does appear that the mortality is increased in patients with acute stroke who develop hydrocephalus.[25,26]

Patients who develop acute hydrocephalus usually show a significant deterioration in conscious level; development of papilloedema is a late sign and should not be relied upon to diagnose increased intracranial pressure. There may be deterioration in the neurological deficit as measured by NIHSS score, but one should not rely just on this.

Computed tomography (CT) brain scan is very sensitive and specific in diagnosing acute hydrocephalus (particularly if there is an earlier, recent scan to compare). Lumbar puncture should not be attempted as it significantly increases the chance of cerebellar 'coning'.

There are case reports[27] of patients managed with repeated lumbar puncture for communicating hydrocephalus following subarachnoid haemorrhage but this is not routine practice. The definite treatment would be to relieve the pressure by external ventricular drain[28] (EVD), which is a relatively safe procedure although carries a risk of infection. In most cases of obstructive hydrocephalus, EVD is only needed for a few days after which it can be removed. However, in case of communicating hydrocephalus, one may need to resort to ventriculoperitoneal shunt if the hydrocephalus persists.

True complications

Cardiac complications

Stroke and ischaemic heart disease have a number of risk factors in common; in addition, presence of underlying heart disease (e.g. valvular heart disease, atrial fibrillation, and congestive cardiac failure) increases the risk of stroke substantially. However, in those who have sustained a severe stroke there is also an increase in the risk of myocardial infarction, heart failure, ventricular arrhythmias, and cardiac arrest/sudden cardiac death.[29] Serious cardiac events and death is common[30–33] and also occurs in the early phase after stroke.[33] It is particularly common in those with heart failure, diabetes, chronic kidney disease, and prolonged QTc on electrocardiogram.[34]

Electrocardiographic changes

Electrocardiographic changes are extremely common after an acute stroke. The typical 'cerebral T waves' (large and upright T) are not specific to ischaemic strokes and have been noted in those with transient ischaemic attack (TIA), subarachnoid haemorrhages, and non-vascular cerebral lesions. Of more significance are the repolarization abnormalities which are common and increase the risk of malignant ventricular arrhythmias and may account for the increased risk of sudden death following an acute stroke.

Myocardial infarction and cardiac enzyme increase

Systematic review of cohort studies suggests that there is 2% annual risk of myocardial infarction and non-vascular death in those with stroke and TIAs.[33] The risk is greater soon after stroke.[33] Serum troponin concentrations are often raised after an acute stroke; however, no definitive criterion has been established to differentiate if the increase is due to true myocardial damage or neurally induced[35] (autonomic dysregulation and a physiological stress response may be the aetiology of the neural mechanism of troponin elevation and this is particularly common in those who have infarction affecting the right insular cortex[36]).

Arrhythmias

Cardiac arrhythmias (both supraventricular and ventricular) have been noted in those with acute stroke, but there is little literature on the aetiology or the possible neural mechanisms or their incidence rates. It may, in fact, represent underlying heart disease which had been undiagnosed before the stroke. Right insular cortex damage may lead to increased risk of arrhythmias, but more research is needed in this area. Having prolonged QTc is independently associated with increased risk of cardiac death (irrespective of area or volume of brain damage).[37]

Stroke-related mortality increases if the individual also has congestive heart failure.[33] As with arrhythmias, there is little literature on the incidence of congestive heart failure associated with ischaemic stroke. However, Takotsubo syndrome is a characteristic cardiomyopathy associated with strokes (both ischaemic and haemorrhagic) and subarachnoid haemorrhages[38,39] and it is associated with increased risk of sudden death and congestive heart failure. In those with Takotsubo syndrome, the brain's natriuretic peptide is significantly elevated in the presence of normal troponins. There is a preponderance of females affected particularly if they have strokes affecting the insular cortex or brain stem.

Pulmonary complications

Pneumonia

Pneumonia is one of the most frequent medical complications after an acute stroke[1,2,40,41] and affects between 5% and 9% of patients; it is the commonest cause of fever within the first 48 hours after an acute stroke.[1,42] Patients with stroke-related pneumonia have a higher mortality and a poorer long-term outcome when compared to those without pneumonia[40,41]; pneumonia increased the risk of death by three fold (after adjusting for important confounders).[43] Age (>65), dysarthria or dysphasia, severe stroke-related disability, cognitive impairment, and an abnormal water swallow test are independent predictors for developing pneumonia after an acute stroke.[44] Aspiration is by far the commonest cause of pneumonia, accounting for up to 60%[1], and is related to inhalation of bacteria colonizing the oral cavity. It is very important to differentiate this from aspiration pneumonitis, which causes chemical lung damage due to aspiration of stomach contents, particularly acid, as the aspiration pneumonitis is usually self-limiting and does not need antimicrobial therapy (whereas aspiration pneumonia needs treatment with antimicrobial agents that cover Gram-positive cocci and Gram-negative bacilli). Aspiration pneumonia is more common in those who are on gastric acid suppressants (e.g. H_2-receptor antagonists or proton pump inhibitors)[45] which should be avoided if possible.

Although it can be very difficult to differentiate aspiration pneumonia from pneumonitis, the following criteria (Box 14.1) may be helpful.[46]

These are consensus opinion and are not validated (or robustly evaluated); however, they are based on Centre for Disease Control criteria with the main pragmatic application relating to certainly based on chest X-ray infiltrates.

Appropriate management of dysphagia remains the cornerstone in preventing aspiration pneumonia. Positioning and regular suctioning (in those who cannot manage their own salivary secretions) may help but is not proven in randomized controlled trials. Similarly, a number of other interventions (e.g. prophylactic antibiotics, pneumococcal and influenza vaccinations,

Box 14.1 Recommended diagnostic criteria for Definite and Probable stroke-associated pneumonia (SAP) in patients not receiving mechanical ventilation based on Centre for Disease Control and Prevention (CDC) criteria

At least one of the following:

1. Fever >38°C with no other recognized cause
2. Leukopenia <4000 WBC/mm^3 or leukocytosis >12 000 WBC/mm^3
3. For adults ≥ 70 years, altered mental status with no other recognized cause

And at least two of the following:

1. New onset of purulent sputum or change in character of sputum over a 24-hour period, or increasing respiratory secretions, or increased suctioning requirements
2. New onset or worsening cough or dyspnoea or tachypnoea (respiratory rate >25/min)
3. Rales, crackles, or bronchial breath sounds
4. Worsening gas exchange, for example, oxygen desaturation (e.g. PaO$_2$/FiO$_2$ ≤240), increased oxygen requirements*

And ≥ 2 serial chest radiographs** with at least one of the following:

New or progressive or persistent infiltrate, consolidation, or cavitation

(Note: in patients without underlying pulmonary or cardiac disease, one definitive chest radiograph is acceptable.)

Probable SAP: all CDC criteria met, BUT initial chest X-ray (CXR) and serial/repeat CXR nonconfirmatory (or not undertaken) and no alternative explanation or diagnosis

Definite SAP: ALL CDC criteria met, including diagnostic CXR changes (on at least one).

*Category of increased ventilator demand removed.

**CDC recommendation is for repeat CXR at days 2 ± 7 if initial CXR negative.

Source: data from U.S. Department of Health & Human Services, Centre for Disease Control and Prevention (CDC) criteria.

---

angiotensin converting enzyme inhibitors, and so on) have been tried but there is no evidence to support their routine use.

Oxygen desaturation

Oxygen desaturation is very common although it is generally transient. About 20% of patients with stroke are affected in the first few hours (irrespective of whether it is ischaemic or haemorrhagic stroke) and as many as two-thirds of patients are in the first 48 hours.[47] Oxygen desaturation is more common in those with advanced age, more severe strokes (higher NIHSS score), dysphagia, or pre-existing cardiopulmonary disease.[48] Other factors like aspiration pneumonia, pulmonary embolism, respiratory muscle dysfunction, sleep disordered breathing, and neurogenic pulmonary oedema can increase the likelihood of desaturation. Although it is logical to think that oxygen desaturation would increase the risk of penumbral damage and thus increasing the risk of disability and mortality, in reality it does not appear to be so straightforward. Rowat et al.[49] have shown that major oxygen desaturation occurred mostly in those with cardiopulmonary disease and was associated with higher mortality but not disability.

Neurogenic pulmonary oedema is more common in those with head injury, subarachnoid haemorrhage, or seizures but can be associated with severe strokes. It is usually transient but it can be fatal in severe cases. Typically this condition manifests soon after onset and develops abruptly (in contrast aspiration pneumonia usually takes longer to manifest) but symptoms and signs (as well as imaging) can mimic aspiration pneumonia. This is a diagnosis of exclusion and treatment is largely supportive in nature.

Abnormal respiratory patterns

Abnormal respiratory patterns are common after a stroke and it may be related to the site of brain damage or to underlying cardiopulmonary disease (or a combination of both). The real incidence of abnormal respiratory pattern is not known but advanced age, more severe strokes, and reduced left ventricular systolic function seem to be significantly associated with incidence of this condition (particularly periodic breathing).[50]

1. *Cheyne–Stokes breathing*—this is characterized by recurrent central apnoea alternating with crescendo-decrescendo pattern of tidal volume and is the most commonly recognized abnormal respiratory pattern after a stroke but in majority of patients it relates to underlying cardiorespiratory disease. This pattern of breathing does not have prognostic significance nor has any correlation to the site of brain damage. There is a theoretical possibility that the patient may develop hypocapnia and related cerebral vasoconstriction, causing penumbral damage, but this has never been proven.

2. *Periodic breathing*—this is a variant of Cheyne–Stokes breathing; it is characterized by regular, recurrent cycles of changing tidal volumes and is more common in subarachnoid haemorrhage. This is the most common abnormal breathing pattern directly associated with brain damage.

3. *Ataxic (or Biot's) breathing*—this is rare and is characterized by erratic rate and depth of breathing associated with apnoeic spells (once again not with any regularity). This type of breathing is usually associated with medullary damage but can also be found in patients with neurodegenerative diseases. Surprisingly there is very little correlation between this type of breathing and prognosis. This pathogenesis is thought to be related to dysfunction of dorsal respiratory neurons the medulla that control the rhythmicity of breathing.

4. *Apneustic breathing*—this is typically seen in pontine damage which leads to dysfunction of the inspiratory cut-off mechanism leading to sustained deep breathing followed by a rapid exhalation and a brief pause before the next cycle. If these patients require invasive ventilation, weaning is often difficult.

5. *Sleep apnoea*—both obstructive and central sleep apnoea have been observed in the acute post-stroke setting. Obesity and large neck circumference increase the risk of development of obstructive sleep apnoea (as in the general population) and is not related to stroke severity. Central sleep apnoea, as already discussed here (in different types of breathing patterns), usually improves over time. In the event of significant airway obstruction (particularly soon after the acute stroke), functional outcome tends to be poor.[49] Although continuous positive airway pressure ventilation is a well-proven treatment in those with obstructive sleep apnoea, the evidence is lacking in terms of improving functional outcomes in those who develop this as a consequence of acute stroke.

Gastrointestinal complications

Gastrointestinal (GI) bleeding is a relatively common complication that affects about 3% of stroke patients and it is a serious complication in 2%.[1] It can be a complication of both ischaemic and haemorrhagic stroke. Retrospective data suggest that older age, severe stroke, a history of peptic ulcer disease, cancer, sepsis, and renal or liver dysfunction increase the risk of GI bleeding substantially but there is no correlation with the use of antithrombotic therapy, H_2-receptor antagonist, or proton pump inhibitor, and the risk of GI bleeding.[51,52] 1.5% of patients suffer from GI bleeding during their index hospital admission with a stroke.[52] Although the reasons are not entirely clear, NG feeding seems to be associated with higher risk of GI bleeding but not percutaneous endoscopic gastrostomy (PEG) feeding.[53] Although H_2-receptor antagonists and proton pump inhibitor can reduce the risk of stress ulceration, there is a concern that they may increase the risk of pneumonia and hence are not routinely recommended in those with acute stroke. It may be appropriate to use prophylactic gastric acid suppressants in selected patients who need management in intensive care setting or in exceptional circumstances (e.g. recent GI bleeding, presence of coagulopathy, severe sepsis, and others). In those who have already suffered GI bleeding, there is no good evidence on whether to stop antithrombotic drugs or anticoagulants and it should be decided on an individual basis. The principles of management of GI bleed are the same as in any other individual.

Genitourinary complications

Urinary tract infection is another common complication after a stroke, occurring in as many as 15% of patients in the first 3 months following the index event.[2,41] Although it has a good prognosis when appropriately treated, it can be a serious problem in a small minority of patients[1] and some studies have shown a poor outcome[54,55] but it is possible that the latter is related to other comorbidities (e.g. advanced age and severe stroke). In addition to advanced age, severe stroke, and female sex,[54,55] urinary catheter insertion is an important risk factor for developing urinary infection. The longer the catheter is left *in situ*, the more is the chance of developing an infection.[56] *Escherichia coli* is the commonest organism that is implicated in urinary tract infections; although they are usually sensitive to commonly used antimicrobials, we are starting to see an increase in Enterococcus that are resistant to Vancomycin (VRE) or carbapenem (CRE). Urinary tract infection should be considered in patients who develop bladder symptoms and in those who develop delirium or systemic features of sepsis. Diagnosis of urinary tract infection can be difficult particularly in those with indwelling urinary catheters as they may not have significant systemic inflammatory response and the diagnosis depends on urine cultures (but care should be taken not to treat 'asymptomatic bacteriuria' as it potentially increases the risk of developing antimicrobial resistance).

Unfortunately, indwelling urinary catheters may be unavoidable in frail, immobile patients who are at risk of skin breakdown, particularly in females as the alternate option of 'urinary pouches' are cumbersome, difficult to manage, and not particularly effective when it comes to preventing skin breakdown. In men, if urinary catheterization is necessary, one should consider use of a sheath catheter in the first instance. Should catheterization become essential, meticulous catheter care is paramount to reduce the risk of infection. There is some evidence that antimicrobial-coated catheters may reduce the risk of infection[57] but more research is needed in this area. Early mobilization may help to reduce the risk of developing urinary tract infection. Appropriate antibiotic therapy should be commenced as soon as possible but ideally should be guided by urinary culture and antimicrobial sensitivities.

Deep venous thrombosis (DVT)

DVT is a major and serious problem particularly in patients with hemiparetic stroke as it may lead to potentially life-threatening pulmonary embolism. Studies using radiolabelled fibrinogen suggest DVT in up to 50% of patients, but clinically evident DVT occurs in about 10% of patients.[58,59] DVT may occur as early as the second day after an acute stroke but peak incidence is between 2 and 7 days.[60] Studies using magnetic resonance imaging of the lower limb and pelvis for direct thrombus visualization detected venous thrombosis in 40% of patients and pulmonary emboli in 12% 3 weeks after the onset of acute stroke (in patients given graduated compression stockings and aspirin[61]). Old age, severe paralysis, and dehydration are major risk factors that contribute to the development of venous thromboembolism.[62,63] The risk of death in those with DVT is approximately 15% due to fatal pulmonary embolism. Venograms are rarely needed to establish the diagnosis of DVT as venous duplex studies are very sensitive particularly in those with proximal DVTs.

The CLOTS 3 trial[64] has shown that intermittent pneumatic compression (IPC) stockings are very effective in preventing DVT in immobilized patients with few clinically important side effects. However, IPC is contraindicated in those with significant peripheral vascular disease and leg ulcers (absolute contraindication), severe leg oedema, or dermatitis (relative contraindication). In those in whom IPC is contraindicated, low dose enoxaparin[65] appears to be a safe and effective alternative for DVT prevention in those with acute ischaemic stroke without any significant increase in intracranial or systemic bleeding and mortality (but this is not applicable in those with haemorrhagic stroke). Directly acting oral anticoagulants (dabigatran, rivaroxaban, apixaban, and edoxaban) have not been shown to be effective in DVT prevention in acute stroke although evidence is accumulating in postsurgical settings.

Pulmonary embolism (PE)

Most fatal PE occurs between second and fourth week after acute stroke. Diagnosis can be challenging in those who have significant cognitive problems, dysphasia, or dysphagia. It can be further complicated by coexistent pulmonary disease (e.g. COPD), while aspiration or chemical pneumonitis PE should be considered in those who develop sudden onset of breathlessness or hypoxia in the absence of another explanation. CT pulmonary angiogram is the investigation of choice and is easily available with excellent diagnostic value. In the past, ventilation/perfusion scan was commonly used but has poor specificity.

In those with acute ischaemic stroke and a confirmed PE, anticoagulation must be commenced as soon as possible. Traditionally, a patient was commenced on low molecular weight heparin (e.g. enoxaparin at a dose of 1.5 mg/kg once a day) subcutaneously and subsequently on warfarin orally (aiming for an international normalized ratio—INR—of between 2 and 3) and the low molecular weight heparin discontinued when the INR was in therapeutic range. However, more recently various directly acting oral anticoagulants (DOACs) have been shown to be effective in the management of DVT and PE,[66–68] and these are active almost immediately.

Venous thromboembolism and haemorrhagic stroke

Management is much more complicated in those with intracranial haemorrhage and there is little literature on what to do. While IPC can be used to prevent DVT, an inferior vena cava filter needs to be considered in those with an established diagnosis of DVT to prevent PE. In those with established PE, there are no good data on how best to treat them—one needs to consider the risk:benefit and decision should be made on an individual basis. Some studies suggest that inferior vena cava (IVC) filters reduces the risk of short-term mortality but evidence is incomplete.[69–71] Although it is well accepted that the IVC filters should be removed as soon as the risk of venous thromboembolism reduces, retrospective studies show that it is not the case and unfortunately result in suboptimal outcome and increased risk of venous thromboembolism.[72]

Spasticity

Spasticity is difficult to define; it is not seen in isolation but occurs as part of a spectrum of symptoms of upper motor neuron syndrome (due to damage to pyramidal (corticospinal) and parapyramidal (corticoreticulospinal) tracts) including muscle weakness, spasms, clonus, and reduced postural responses. Lance[73] described spasticity as 'velocity dependent intrinsic resistance to passive movement of a limb in people with upper motor neuron syndrome'. This has been refined by Pandyan et al.[74] as 'disordered sensorimotor control resulting from an upper motor neuron lesion, presenting as intermittent or sustained involuntary activation of muscles' which takes into account the contribution of elasticity of soft tissue, proprioception, and cutaneous neural pathways. One study suggests that spasticity affects 39% of patients at 12 months after first ever stroke[74] (see also [75]); however, a more recent study[76] suggests that 50% of patients have at least one contracture 6 months after their stroke.

There are no high-quality studies which have looked at the natural history of spasticity and contracture development. It can occur as early as 3–6 months. The neural mechanism(s) underlying normal muscle tone are complex and ill-understood. Spasticity may result from a breakdown in control of the spinal stretch reflex mechanisms causing inappropriate muscle overactivity and limitation of joint movements. Spasticity typically affects the flexor muscles of the upper limb (e.g. biceps, brachioradialis, long finger flexors), pectoralis major, and pronator teres; in the lower limb, the hamstrings, knee adductors, and calf muscles are commonly affected. Other muscles (including the small muscles of the hands and feet) are less commonly affected.

The modified Ashworth scale[77] is an assessment method employed to quantify muscle spasticity (Table 14.1). Examination should also include a full neurological examination including power (as this may determine whether spasticity treatment would improve function), presence of soft tissue shortening (passive range of movement) and thorough skin examination (both for identifying trigger factors and hygiene). Gait (while patient is walking barefoot) should be documented if possible. Factors that may aggravate spasticity should be sought (e.g. pressure sores, infections, pain, constipation, urinary retention).

The mainstay of management of spasticity is multidisciplinary therapy including physiotherapist and occupational therapist. One cannot overstate the importance of the '24-hour approach' in positioning; nursing staff play a vital role here as appropriate positioning of patient is crucial

Table 14.1 Modified Ashworth spasticity scale

Grade	Description
0	No increase in muscle tone
1	Slight increase in muscle tone, manifested by a catch or by minimal resistance at the end of the range of motion (ROM) when the affected part(s) is moved in flexion or extension
1+	Slight increase in muscle tone, manifested by a catch followed by minimal resistance throughout the remainder (less than half) of the ROM
2	More marked increase in muscle tone throughout most of the ROM, but affected part(s) easily moved
3	Considerable increase in muscle tone, passive movement difficult
4	Affected part(s) rigid in flexion or extension
9	Unable to test

Reproduced with permission from Bohannon RW, Smith MW. Inter-rater reliability of modified Ashworth scale of muscle spasticity. *Physical Therapy*, 67(2), 206–7. Copyright © 1987, Oxford University Press. https://doi.org/10.1093/ptj/67.2.206

in maintaining 'normal' movement pattern. While the physiotherapists are involved in restoring 'normal' movement patterns and active and passive movement programmes, the occupational therapists are involved with satisfactory seating and splinting to stretch the affected muscles.

Focal therapy has been used very successfully in reducing muscle spasm without the systemic side effects—botulinum toxin type A and B are used for this purpose while at the same time, different muscles can be targeted to provide maximum benefit. Botulinum toxin has to be supplemented by stretching exercises of the muscles involved, and should only be used as part of a multidisciplinary spasticity management plan.

Oral drug treatment of spasticity is mostly unsatisfactory, and often does more harm than good. Pharmacological measures include medications like baclofen (the mechanism of action of this drug is not entirely clear but it works at spinal level) or tizanidine (which is a potent alpha 2 adrenergic receptor agonist and thus reduces stretch reflexes). Other oral medications include those that modulate GABAergic transmission (e.g. gabapentin, or benzodiazepines). Cannabis is reputed to reduce pain and spasticity (but the mode of action is unclear) and is used in those who are refractory to other treatments. However, the side effects of oral therapy include 'relaxation' (or weakness) of normal muscles potentially reducing functional ability, and causing drowsiness and confusion. Intrathecal therapy (e.g. baclofen or phenol) is occasionally used in those who do not respond to oral or focal therapies.

Pressure ulcer

Patients who have suffered a stroke are at high risk of developing pressure ulcers; the usual areas that are affected include sacral and gluteal regions and the heels. Prolonged immobilization (e.g. bed-ridden or wheelchair bound) is the key factor. In addition, those who have nutritional deficiencies, frailty, urinary or faecal incontinence, and comorbidities (e.g. peripheral vascular disease, diabetic neuropathy) are at increased risk.

It is easier to prevent pressure ulcers than to treat once it has developed. Early mobilization, pressure redistribution (e.g. regular turning), and appropriate pressure relieving equipment (e.g. air mattresses and padded heel boot) are effective in preventing pressure ulcers. Care should be taken to prevent friction or shearing while turning. Urinary catheters are not generally recommended to manage urinary incontinence but if the patient is at high risk of developing pressure ulcers, one can make an argument for urinary catheterization to minimize the risk of skin irritation and subsequent maceration which can predispose to further skin breakdown as well as preventing pressure ulcer dressings getting wet. One has to consider the risks associated with the catheter against the benefits on an individual basis. If possible, absorbent pads still remain the preferred choice compared to indwelling catheters.

Musculoskeletal complications

Having suffered a stroke in the past is one of the five major risk factors for a fall in an older person. A number of features contribute to the risk of falls, including limb weakness, cognitive impairment, and visuospatial perceptive problems (including neglect and agnosia). Falls is one of the most common complications of a stroke[2,78]; about a third of patients have had a fall within 3 months of stroke.[79]

Falls are associated with serious complications (e.g. hip fracture) in about 5% of patients.[2] Of all fractures that are suffered by patients after a stroke, 45% are of the hip, being two to four times more common compared to an age-matched population without stroke.[80]

Older adults are at risk of osteopenia, especially women, and this is further exacerbated by increased bone resorption due to weakness and disuse. Disuse osteopenia is disproportionately seen on the paretic side but is noted bilaterally in those who are immobile. Fractures are seen particularly on the paretic side and the most important contributory factors include 'accidental' fall[80,81] and lack of protective response (e.g. outstretched arm to prevent major impact on the hip joint) due to upper limb weakness.

All patients who have had a stroke should have an assessment to prevent falls; vitamin D deficiency should be treated although there is little evidence that vitamin D supplementation reduces the risk of fractures after a stroke.[82] Medications should be reviewed carefully to avoid unnecessary psychotropic agents or other medication that may increase the risk of drowsiness or exacerbate cognitive problems. Judicious use of antihypertensive medication is advocated in frail older people to avoid the development of postural hypotension. Hip protectors may be appropriate in those who are at high risk of sustaining hip fractures but are cumbersome for patients to position appropriately particularly in those who have paretic limbs. Bisphosphonates drugs should be considered in those with high risk and reduces the risk of fractures particularly in females. In those with significant dysphagia, or for whom tablet-burden or administration is a problem, intravenous bisphosphonate can provide an attractive alternative.

Persistent spatial neglect (perceptual deficits)

Spatial neglect represents a cluster of symptoms involving an inability to report, respond, or orient to stimuli generally in the contralesional space. It could be defined as spatial bias leading to functional disability. Disability cannot be attributable purely to primary sensory deficit (e.g. hemianaesthesia, hemianopia) or motor deficit (e.g. hemiparesis). There is a relationship between perceptual deficits and impairment in ability to perform activities of daily living.[82–85] One study[86] suggested that perceptual problems are second only to motor problems in impacting on functional autonomy. Patients with spatial neglect are often significantly disabled.

The biggest impact of spatial neglect is the risk the patient might put themselves under, especially falls. In most instances, those with significant spatial neglect will live in care homes where they are supervised 24 hours a day. Driving ability is a problem and most patients with spatial neglect will not be allowed to drive as they pose a risk to themselves and others (and hence they must be specifically re-evaluated before allowed to drive). Dangerous tools and other environmental risks should be removed from patient's reach if they are unsupervised. Risk of falls (and fractures including hip fractures) is a major concern in this group of people and appropriate precautions must be taken to prevent falls. With left-sided visual neglect, the patient can get 'lost' in unfamiliar surroundings, injure themselves due to not seeing obstacles and occasionally may lead to significant errors in dealing with their finance, reading/writing, or other detail-orientated tasks if they have difficulty reading materials on the left side (so-called neglect dyslexia).

Vocational disability may have significant impact on the psychological well-being of the individual. It is not uncommon to note changes in social behaviour, likely due to complex cognitive, emotional, and behavioural issues.

Sexual dysfunction

This common problem has been subject to little research. Most studies were undertaken in 1970s and 1980s, were small, and predominantly looked at younger ages (<60 years).

The most common sexual problems that have been identified after stroke include decline in libido and coital frequency, decline in vaginal lubrication and orgasm in women, and poor or failed erection and ejaculation in men.[87,88] It is likely that there are a number of factors in play which leads to sexual dysfunction/dissatisfaction including paresis, social activity/family stress,[89] sociodemographic factors, psychological issues (e.g. mood disorder), cognitive deficits, other comorbidities and medications. Hypersexuality can be a rare feature after stroke (e.g. Klüver–Bucy syndrome).

Erectile dysfunction can be treated by a variety of measures (e.g. phosphodiesterase inhibitors like sildenafil and tadalafil, local papaverine injection, or even penile prosthesis). In those whose sexual dysfunction has more of a psychological basis (e.g. decline of libido), psychological therapies like cognitive behavioural therapy may be helpful.

References

1. **Johnston KC, Li JY, Lyden PD, et al.** Medical and neurological complications of ischemic stroke: experience from the RANTTAS trial. RANTTAS investigators. *Stroke* 1998;**29**:447–53.

2. **Langhorne P, Stott DJ, Robertson L, et al.** Medical complications after stroke: a multicentre study. *Stroke* 2000;**31**:1223–9.

3. **Silver FL, Norris JW, Lewis AJ, & Hachinski VC.** Early mortality following stroke: a prospective review. *Stroke* 1984;**15**:492–6.

4. **Britton M & Roden A.** Progression of stroke after arrival at hospital. *Stroke* 1985; **16**:629–32.

5. **Dávalos A, Cendra E, Teruel J, Martinez M, & Genís D.** Deteriorating ischemic stroke: risk factors and prognosis. *Neurology* 1990;**40**:1865–9.

6. **Castillo J.** Deteriorating stroke: diagnostic criteria, predictors, mechanisms and treatment. *Cerebrovasc Dis* 1999;**9**:1–8.

7. **Castillo J, Davalos A, & Noya M.** Aggravation of acute ischemic stroke by hyperthermia is related to an excitotoxic mechanism. *Cerebrovasc Dis* 1999;**2**:22–7.

8. **Langhorne P, on behalf of the Stroke Unit Trialists' Collaboration.** Organized inpatient (stroke unit) care for stroke. *Cochrane Database Syst Rev* 2013(**2**). Available from: http://stroke.ahajournals.org/content/45/2/e14.full.pdf [Accessed: 1 July 2017].

9. **Intercollegiate Stroke Working Party.** *National Clinical Guideline for Stroke*, 5th edition. London, UK: Royal College of Physicians, 2016.

10. **Anderson CS, Heeley E, Huang Y, et al., for the INTERACT2 investigators.** Rapid blood-pressure lowering in acute intracerebral haemorrhage. *N Engl J Med* 2013;**368**(25):2355–65.

11. **Anderson CS, Robinson T, Lindley RI, et al.** Low-dose versus standard-dose intravenous alteplase in acute ischemic stroke. *N Engl J Med* 2016;**374**(24):2313–23.

12. **van der Worp HB, Macleod MR, Bath PM, et al.** EuroHYP-1: European multicenter, randomized, phase III clinical trial of therapeutic hypothermia plus best medical treatment vs. best medical treatment alone for acute ischemic stroke. *Int J Stroke* 2014;**9**(5):642–5.

13. **Hauser WA, Annegers JF, & Kurland LT.** Incidence of epilepsy and unprovoked seizures in Rochester, Minnesota: 1935–84. *Epilepsia* 1993;**34**:453–68.

14. **Bladin CF, Alexandrov AV, Bellavance A, et al.** Seizures after stroke: a prospective multicentre study. *Arch Neurol* 2000:**57**:1617–22.

15. **Graham NS, Crichton S, Koutroumanidis M, Wolfe CD, & Rudd AG.** Incidence and associations of poststroke epilepsy: the prospective South London Stroke Register. *Stroke* 2013;**44**:605–11.

16. **Lossius MI, Ronning OM, Slapø GD, Mowinckel P, & Gjerstad L.** Poststroke epilepsy: occurrence and predictors—a long term prospective controlled study (Akershus Stroke Study). *Epilepsia* 2005;**46**:1246–51.

17. **Camilo O & Goldstein LB.** Seizures and epilepsy after ischemic stroke. *Stroke* 2004;**35**:1769–75.

18. **Heuts-van Raak L, Lodder J, & Kessels F.** Late seizure following a first symptomatic brain infarct are related to large infarcts involving the posterior area around the lateral sulcus. *Seizure* 1996;**5**:185–94.

19. **Bladin CF, Alexandrov AV, Bellavance A, et al.** Seizures after stroke: a prospective multicentre study. *Arch Neurol* 2000;**57**:1617–22.

20. **Moulin DE, Lo R, & Barnett HJ.** Prognosis in middle cerebral artery occlusion. *Stroke* 1985;**16**:282–4.

21. **Kasner SE, Demchuk AM, Berrouschot J**, et al. Predictors of fatal brain oedema in massive hemispheric ischemic stroke. *Stroke* 2001;**32**:2117–23.

22. **Hacke W, Schwab S, Horn M**, et al. 'Malignant' middle cerebral artery territory infarction: clinical course and prognostic signs. *Arch Neurol* 1996;**53**:309–15.

23. **Vahedi K, Hofmeijer J, Juettler E**, et al. **for the DECIMAL, DESTINY and HAMLET investigators.** Early decompressive surgery in malignant infarction of the middle cerebral artery: a pooled analysis of three randomised controlled trials. *Lancet Neurol* 2007;**6**:215–22.

24. **Juttler E, Unterberg A, Woitzik J**, et al. Hemicraniectomy in older patients with extensive middle-cerebral-artery stroke. *N Engl J Med* 2014;**370**:1091–100.

25. **Ruscalleda J & Periro A.** Prognostic factors in intraparenchymatous haematoma with ventricular haemorrhage. *Neuroradiology* 1986;**28**:34–7.

26. **Young WB, Lee KP, Pessin MS**, et al. Prognostic significance of ventricular blood in supratentorial haemorrhage. *Neurol* 1990;**40**:616–19.

27. **Hasan D, Lindsay KW, & Vermeulen M.** Treatment of acute hydrocephalus after subarachnoid haemorrhage with serial lumbar puncture. *Stroke* 1991;**22**:190–4.

28. **Adams RE & Diringer MN.** Response to external ventricular drainage in spontaneous intracerebral haemorrhage with hydrocephalus. *Neurol* 1998;**50**:519–23.

29. **Kumar S, Selim MH, & Caplan LR.** Medical complications after stroke. *Lancet Neurol* 2010; **9**:105–18.

30. **Oppenheim SM & Hachinski VC.** The cardiac consequences of stroke. *Neurol Clin* 1993; **10**:167–76.

31. **Daniele O, Caravaglios G, Fierro B, & Natalè E.** Stroke and cardiac arrhythmias. *J Stroke Cerebrovasc Dis* 2002;**11**:28–33.

32. **Touze E, Varenne O, Chatellier G, Peyrard S, Rothwell PM, & Mas JL.** Risk of myocardial infarction and vascular death after transient ischaemic attack and ischaemic stroke: a systematic review and meta-analysis. *Stroke* 2005;**36**:2748–55.

33. **Liao J, O'Donnell MR, Silver FL**, et al. In-hospital myocardial infarction following acute ischaemic stroke: an observational study. *Eur J Neurol* 2009;**16**:1035–40.

34. **Prosser J, MacGregor L, Lees KR**, et al., **on behalf of VISTA investigators.** Predictors of early cardiac morbidity and mortality after ischaemic stroke. *Stroke* 2007;**38**:2295–302.

35. **Jensen J, Atar D, Mickley H**, et al. Mechanism of troponin elevation in patients with acute ischaemic stroke. *Am J Cardiol* 2007;**99**:867–70.

36. **Ay H, Koroshetz WJ, Benner T**, et al. Neuroanatomic correlates of stroke-related myocardial injury. *Neurol* 2006;**66**:1325–9.

37. **Wong KY, MacWalter RS, Douglas D**, et al. Long QTc predicts future cardiac death in stroke survivors. *Heart* 2003;**89**:377–81.

38. **Bybee KA, Kara T, Prasad A**, et al. Systematic review: transient left ventricular apical ballooning: a syndrome that mimics ST segment elevation myocardial infarction. *Ann Int Med* 2004;**141**:858–65.

39. **Lee VH, Connolly HM, Fulgham JR, Manno EM, Brown RD Jr, & Wijdicks EF.** Tako-tsubo cardiomyopathy in aneurysmal subarachnoid haemorrhage: an unappreciated ventricular dysfunction. *J Neurosurg* 2006;**105**:264–70.

40. **Finlayson O, Kapral M, Hall R**, et al. Risk factors, inpatient care and outcomes of pneumonia after ischaemic stroke. *Neurology* 2011;**77**:1338–45.

41. **Ingeman A, Andersen G, Hundborg HH, Svendsen ML, & Johnsen SP.** In-hospital medical complications, length of stay and mortality among stroke unit inpatients. *Stroke* 2011;**42**:3214–18.

42. **Grau AJ, Buggle F, Schnitzler P, Spiel M, Lichy C, & Hacke W.** Fever and infection early after ischaemic stroke. *J Neurol Sci* 1999;**171**:115–20.

43. **Katzan IL, Cebul RD, Husak SH, Dawson NV, & Baker DW.** The effect of pneumonia on mortality among patients hospitalised for acute stroke. *Neurology* 2003;**60**:620–5.

44. Sellars C, Bowie L, Bagg J, et al. Risk factors for chest infection in acute stroke: a prospective cohort study. *Stroke* 2007;**38**:2284–91.

45. Herzig SJ, Doughty C, Lahoti S, et al. Acid-suppressive medication use in acute stroke and hospital-acquired pneumonia. *Ann Neurol* 2014;**76**:712–18.

46. Smith CJ, Kishore AK, Vail A, et al. Diagnosis of stroke associated pneumonia: recommendations from the Pneumonia in Stroke Consensus group. *Stroke* 2015;**45**:1202–9.

47. Rowat AM, Dennis MS, & Wardlaw JM. Hypoxaemia in acute stroke is frequent and worsens outcome. *Cardiovasc Dis* 2006;**21**:166–72.

48. Sulter G, Elting JW, Stewart R, den Arend A, & De Keyser J. Continuous pulse oximetry in acute hemiparetic stroke. *J Neurol Sci* 2000;**179**:65–9.

49. Basetti CL, Milanova M, & Gugger M. Sleep disordered breathing and acute ischaemic stroke: diagnosis, risk factors, treatment, evolution and long-term clinical outcome. *Stroke* 2006;**37**:967–72.

50. Turkington PM, Allgar V, Bamford J, Wanklyn P, & Elliott MW. Effect of upper airway obstruction in acute stroke on functional outcome at 6 months. *Thorax* 2004;**59**:367–71.

51. Davenport RJ, Dennis MS, & Warlow CP. Gastrointestinal haemorrhage after acute stroke. *Stroke* 1996;**27**:421–4.

52. O'Donnell MJ, Kapral MK, Fang J, et al. (investigators of the Registry of the Canadian Stroke Network). Gastrointestinal bleeding after acute ischaemic stroke. *Neurol* 2008;**71**:650–5.

53. Dennis MS, Lewis SC, Warlow C, & FOOD Trial Collaboration. Effect of timing and method of enteral tube feeding for dysphagic stroke patients (FOOD): a multicentre randomised controlled trial. *Lancet* 2005;**365**:764–72.

54. Stott DJ, Falconer A, Miller H, Tilston JC, & Langhorne P. Urinary tract infection after stroke. *QJM* 2009;**102**:243–9.

55. Aslanyan S, Weir CJ, Diener HC, et al. for GAIN International Steering Committee and Investigators. Pneumonia and urinary tract infection after acute ischaemic stroke: a tertiary analysis of the GAIN International trial. *Eur J Neurol* 2004;**11**:49–53.

56. Sedor J & Mulholland SG. Hospital-acquired urinary tract infections associated with indwelling catheter. *Urol Clin North Am* 1999;**26**:821–8.

57. Drekonja DM, Kuskowski MA, Wilt TJ, & Johnson JR. Antimicrobial urinary catheters: a systematic review. *Expert Rev Med Devices* 2008;**5**:495–506.

58. Dennis M, Mordi N, Graham C, Sandercock P, & CLOTS trials collaboration. The timing, extent, progression and regression of deep vein thrombosis in immobile stroke patients: observational data from the CLOTS multicentre randomised trials. *J Thromb Haemost* 2011;**9**:2193–200.

59. Amin AN, Lin J, Thompson S, & Wiederkeht D. Rate of deep-vein thrombosis and pulmonary embolism during the care continuum in patients with acute ischemic stroke in the United States. *BMC Neurol* 2013;**13**;17.

60. Kelly J, Rudd A, Lewis R, & Hunt BJ. Venous thromboembolism after acute stroke. *Stroke* 2001;**32**:262–7.

61. Kelly J, Rudd A, Lewis RR, Coshall C, Moody A, & Hunt BJ. Venous thrombembolism after acute ischaemic stroke: a prospective study using magnetic resonance direct thrombus imaging. *Stroke* 2004;**35**:2320–5.

62. Landi G, D'Angelo A, Boccardi E, et al. Venous thromboembolism in acute stroke. *Arch Neurol* 1992;**49**:279–83.

63. Kelly J, Hunt BJ, Lewis RR, et al. Dehydration and venous thromboembolism after acute stroke. *QJM* 2004;**97**:293–6.

64. Clots in Legs Or sTockings after Stroke (CLOTS) trials collaboration, Dennis M, Sandercock, P, et al. Effectiveness of intermittent pneumatic compression in reduction of risk of deep vein thrombosis

in patients who have had a stroke (CLOTS 3): a multicentre randomised controlled trial. *Lancet* 2013;**382**:516–24.

65. **Sherman DG, Albers VW, Bladin C, et al.** The efficacy and safety of enoxaparin versus unfractionated heparin for venous thromboembolism in patients with acute ischaemic stroke (PREVAIL study): an open-labelled randomised comparison. *Lancet* 2007;**369**:1347–55.

66. **Schulman S, Kearon C, Kakkar AK, et al., for the RE-COVER study group.** Dabigatran versus warfarin in the treatment of acute venous thromboembolism. *N Engl J Med* 2009;**361**:2342–52.

67. **The EINSTEIN investigators.** Oral rivaroxaban for symptomatic venous thromboembolism. *N Engl J Med* 2010;**363**:2499–510.

68. **Agnelli G, Buller HR, Cohen A, et al., for the AMPLIFY investigators.** Oral apixaban for the treatment of acute venous thromboembolism. *N Engl J Med* 2013;**369**:799–808.

69. **White RH, Brunson A, Romano PS, Li Z, & Wun T.** Outcomes after vena cava filter use in non-cancer patients with acute venous thromboembolism: a population-based study. *Circulation* 2016;**133**: 2018–29.

70. **Muriel A, Jimenez D, Aujesky D, et al., for RIETE investigators.** Survival effects of inferior vena cava filter in patients with acute symptomatic venous thromboembolism and a significant bleeding risk. *J Am Col Cardio* 2014;**63**:1675–83.

71. **Stein PD & Matta F.** Vena caval filters in unstable elderly patients with acute pulmonary embolism. *Am J Med* 2014;**127**: 222–5.

72. **Sarosiek S, Crowther M, & Sloan MJ.** Indications, complications and management of inferior vena caval filters. The experience in 952 patients at an academic hospital with a level 1 Trauma centre. *JAMA Intern Med* 2013;**173**(7): 513–17.

73. **Lance JW.** The control of muscle tone, reflexes and movement: Robert Wartenberg Lecture. *Neurology* 1980;**30**:1303–13.

74. **Pandyan AD, Gregoric M, Barnes MP, et al.** Spasticity: clinical perception, neurological realities and meaningful measurement. *Disabil Rehab* 2005;**27**:2–6.

75. **Watkins CL, Leathley MJ, Gregson JM, Moore AP, Smith TL, & Sharma AK.** Prevalence of spasticity post-stroke. *Clin Rehab* 2002;**16**:515–22.

76. **Kwah L, Harvey L, Diong JHL, et al.** Half of adults who present to hospital with stroke develop at least one contracture within 6 months: an observational study. *J Physiotherapy* 2012;**58**:41–7.

77. **Bohannon RW & Smith MW.** Inter-rater reliability of modified Ashworth scale of muscle spasticity. *Phys Ther* 1987;**67**:206–7.

78. **Minet LR, Peterson E, von Koch L, & Ytterberg C.** Occurrence and predictors of falls in people with stroke: six-year prospective study. *Stroke* 2015;**46**:2688–90.

79. **Ramnemark A, Nyber L, Borssén B, Olsson T, & Gustafson Y.** Fractures after stroke. *Osteopor Int* 1998;**8**:92–5.

80. **Myint PK, Poole KE, & Warburton EA.** Hip fractures after stroke and their prevention. *QJM* 2007;**100**:539–45.

81. **Nevitt MC & Cummings SR.** Type of fall and risk of hip and wrist fractures: the study of osteoporotic fractures. The study of Osteoporotic Fractures Research Group. *J Am Geriatric Soc* 1993;**41**:1226–34.

82. **Brockman RK & Van Deusen J.** Relation of perceptual and body image dysfunction to activities of daily living in persons after stroke. *Am J Occup Ther* 1995;**49**:551–9.

83. **Bernspang B, Vutamen M, & Eriksson S.** Impairments of perceptual and motor functions: their influence on self-care ability 4 to 6 years after stroke. *Occup Ther J Res* 1989;**9**:27–37.

84. **Lincoln NB, Drummond AE, & Berman P.** Perceptual impairment and its impact on rehabilitation outcome. *Disabil Rehab* 1997;**19**:231–4.

85. **Titus MND, Gall NG, Yerxa EJ, Roberson TA, & Mack W.** Correlation of perceptual performance and activities of daily living in stroke patients. *Am J Occup Ther* 1991;**45**:410–18.

86. **Mercier L, Audet T, Hébert R, Rochette A, & Dubois MF.** Impact of motor, cognitive and perceptual disorders on ability to perform activities of daily living after stroke. *Stroke* 2001;**32**:2602–8.

87. **Monga TN, Lawson JS, & Inglis J.** Sexual dysfunction in stroke patients. *Arch Phys Med Rehab* 1986;**67**:19–22.

88. **Boldrini P, Basaglia N, & Calanca MC.** Sexual changes in hemiparetic patients. *Arch Phys Med Rehab* 1991;**72**:202–7.

89. **Angeleri F, Angeleri VA, Foschi N, Giaquinto S, & Nolfe G.** The influence of depression, social activity and family stress on functional outcome after stroke. *Stroke* 1993;**24**:1478–83.

Chapter 15

Occupational therapy in older people with stroke

Rowena Padamsey and Avril Drummond

Introduction

This chapter will detail the role of the occupational therapist (OT) in stroke rehabilitation for the older person. Following the process that OTs use in their daily practice, it will outline how OTs assess patients with stroke, including the various methods available such as functional and formal assessments. A checklist for an informal bedside assessment will be discussed in detail, providing a foundation for all other OT interventions. A case study will guide the reader through the process (see Box 15.1), giving an example of an initial interview and also the assessment of daily activities to identify any impairment. Following on from the initial assessment process, goal setting will be examined and the two main approaches for OT treatment explored with case examples.

The role of the OT in the rehabilitation of the upper limb and vision will be covered briefly. Moreover, the OT's key role in the rehabilitation of cognition and perception is detailed, including some of the main areas of impairment impacting on a person's ability to function. Finally, the discharge process is discussed, with reference to some of the common challenges experienced in discharging an older person with stroke from hospital.

OT assessment

OTs use assessment to gain an understanding of a person's level of function and performance during the completion of an activity. It often includes a variety of standardized and non-standardized measures which can inform the therapist about the extent of the impairment and limitations on function, within the social and environmental contexts.[1]

Standardized assessments are a formal method of assessment. They are used in practice to identify and quantify problem areas, and can also be used as outcome measures.[2] Standardized assessments form part of the OT's toolkit, and as time constraints in the acute setting may limit the extent to which these are used, brief assessments are becoming more commonplace. There are many assessments available for the assessment of cognition and perception. For example, the Montreal Cognitive Assessment (MoCA)[3] is a brief screening tool designed to identify mild cognitive impairment and early Alzheimer's disease. It assesses several cognitive domains, including immediate and delayed recall, attention, executive function, and language. It gives a score out of 30 (adjusted for previous levels of education), with a score of 26 indicating 'normal' cognition. This screen can be a useful tool to identify potential areas of impairment for further assessment, and can be repeated after 3 months to be used as an outcome measure.

The Oxford Cognitive Screen (OCS)[4] has been specifically designed for use with stroke survivors. The test is aphasia and neglect friendly and assesses all the major domains of cognition. Scoring of the OCS results in a Cognitive Profile, which gives a visual indication of the areas of impairment. The use of standardized assessments with older patients requires careful consideration.

Box 15.1 Case study: Introduction

Mr Bob Garner, 71, has been admitted to the hospital with a 1-day history of sensory changes in his left arm and leg, onset of confusion, and headaches. He has previously had a transient ischaemic attack (TIA) and has a history of diabetes and hypertension. A CT scan has revealed a right middle cerebral artery infarct. He has a dense weakness of his left arm and leg and is unable to sit unaided.

Following his admission, he is being nursed in the bed, and is awaiting assessments from the multidisciplinary team (MDT). The nursing team have assessed his swallow and placed him on a soft diet and normal fluids, due to his difficulty swallowing food and potential risk of aspiration.

For some, they are reminded of completing exams at school and find the assessment process upsetting and patronizing; this may affect performance.[5]

A more global view of a person's functioning is taken using non-standardized assessments such as observing someone getting washed or dressed. This approach to assessment examines functioning in context, and allows the therapist to understand what is important and meaningful to the individual. Completion of a functional assessment (e.g. making a cup of tea), with an older person can sometimes be more meaningful and less threatening than a formal assessment. The therapist's skills in activity analysis enable them to identify areas of impairment within the task and to treat those impairments in context.

Most OTs use a combination of standardized and functional assessments in planning the rehabilitation programme of the older person following a stroke. Both have their merit, and combined, they can strengthen the therapist's decision-making for their interventions with an individual.

The OT's initial interview (see Box 15.2) aims to gain an understanding of how the person functioned prior to their stroke and consequent admission to hospital. This information provides a baseline for interventions, and gives a level of function for the person and multidisciplinary team (MDT) to aim for, in rehabilitation. It is essential at this stage to discuss what is important to the patient. This will help to direct the approach taken within therapy, and assists in tailoring interventions to the individual needs and wants of the patient. If the patient has communication problems, writing phrases down on paper with yes/no options can help to facilitate the conversation. Alternatively, background information can be gained through discussion with family members. Ensuring interactions with patients are meaningful is at the core of rehabilitation.

The therapist will use their clinical experience to decide what further level of assessment the person can tolerate. Those who have had a severe stroke are likely to receive a bedside assessment, to build a picture of their current level of function, and identify any impairment sustained as a result of the stroke. The bedside assessment is an example of a non-standardized assessment of a person's level of function. The OT will use familiar objects and the environment to assess the patient's level of arousal, awareness, vision, cognition, and perception. Using personal items belonging to the patient during assessments aims to increase levels of interest and motivation, and may elicit a response where something unfamiliar may not.

Checklist of points for the OT to consider during a bedside assessment

Arousal and alertness: Does the patient respond to their name or a physical stimulus? Do they acknowledge your presence? Are they making spontaneous or voluntary movements of their

Box 15.2 Initial interview with Bob

Awareness: Where are you now? What happened to bring you into hospital?

'I don't know where I am' 'I think I had a fall'

Social situation: *lives with wife and dog in owner-occupied house. His wife has reduced mobility but is otherwise fit and well, daughter visits weekly. Two steps to get into the house, manages independently. Independent on stairs (straight, one rail to right side ascending).*

Care package? No key-safe? No

Pendant alarm? No warden aided? No

ACTIVITY	Pre-admission level of function	Current level of function
Personal ADL (location, type of shower/ bath, assistance required)	*Independent with daily showering. Has shower cubicle upstairs with step, no seat* *Independent dressing*	*Requires assistance of two for full washing and dressing* *Able to sit out in wheelchair to complete top half in bathroom*
Transfers **Bed** (type of bed, equipment), pressure care	*Double divan bed, standard firm mattress. Independent on/off*	*Requires assistance of two to get from lying to sitting*
Chair (type of chair, equipment, pressure care)	*Three-piece suite armchair, quite low but manages independently. No pressure cushion*	*Sit to stand with standing hoist to normal wheelchair*
Toilet (location of toilet, equipment, continence)	*Toilets up and downstairs. Use the sink to help get on/off. Passes urine ×2 a night*	*Doubly incontinent*
Domestic ADL Making hot drinks/meals/ transport of food/ drinks Eating and drinking, shopping, cleaning, and laundry	*Wife does most of the cooking, independent with hot drinks and snacks if needed. Eats at table and chairs in kitchen* *Good appetite* *Shares with wife, drives to shops once a week*	*Not assessed yet*

Box 15.2 Initial interview with Bob *(continued)*

ACTIVITY	Pre-admission level of function	Current level of function
Driving (including car transfers)	*Independent driving, wife doesn't drive*	*Unable to drive for 4 weeks following his stroke. However, will need longer before considering a return to driving due to the level of his impairments*
Leisure activities	*Enjoys reading, watching sport on TV, and walking dog (Yorkshire terrier) gardening*	*Attends gardening group on the ward. Plan to refer to community rehab team to engage in leisure activities once home*
Occupation (including reading and writing ability)	*Retired shop manager*	*Reading impaired by hemianopia-review with anchor line. Bob is right hand dominant*
Self-medication	*Manages own medications independently*	*Nursing staff to discuss with Bob and wife closer to discharge*

ACTIVITY	Pre-admission level of function	Current level of function
Vision (including do they wear glasses, fields, tracking)	*Reading and distance glasses, no other eye history*	*Left homonymous hemianopia* *Oculomotor movements intact* *Will require orthoptics referral*
Cognition (including the MoCA, attention, memory)	*Some difficulties with short-term memory but uses a diary to help remember appointments, and so on*	*Disorientation to location and reason for admission. Poor delayed recall, MoCA 19/30, reduced attention to task, becomes easily distracted* *Neglect to left: personal and peripersonal* *Apraxia noted—difficulty initiating and sequencing tasks*
Perception (and hearing)	*Good hearing, no concerns*	*No concerns noted*
Mood (including anxiety/distress, depression)	*Normally quite bright, no previous history of low mood or anxiety*	*Feeling frustrated at lack of movement in arm and leg, but otherwise feeling okay*

limbs? Can they focus on a dominant stimulus and maintain their focus? How long can they maintain eye contact for?

Awareness: Does the patient know where they are? Do they know they are in hospital and do they have an awareness of what happened to bring them into hospital? Are they aware they have had a stroke? Do they know how the stroke has affected them (i.e. can they identify their deficits?).

Orientation: Are they orientated to the time of day? Date?

Attention: Consider to what extent they are able to focus on you—are they easily distracted? Can they maintain attention only briefly before losing focus? Can they focus on the person talking to them? Can they be reorientated to your conversation? Are they able to switch attention between two stimuli (i.e. two therapists?).

Memory: Can they recall parts of your conversation when asked? Can they recall their address? If you told them the date earlier can they recall this after a delay?

Vision: Do they open their eyes to stimulus? Are they able to focus on you as you are talking to them? Are both eyes in alignment? Can they track you moving around their bed space or do they have a limitation in their oculomotor movements? Can they track your moving finger/pen across their field of vision? Do they orientate to you or objects presented in both hemifields? Do they report any changes to their vision (i.e. double vision, reduced acuity, or field reduction?).

Cognition and perception

◆ Are they able to follow 1/2/3 stage commands (e.g. *Can you touch your nose? Can you touch your right ear with your left hand? Touch your nose then your head? Copy my movements with your right hand).*

◆ Can they tell you what's on their table/select 10 objects in the bay? *Look at the location of the items they select, are they mainly in one area? Are they attending to both sides of space?*

◆ Can they pour a glass of water from the jug? (do not complete if on modified fluids). *Review their depth and distance perception.*

◆ Select some objects on their table, can they identify whether one is in front or behind of the other? Whether one is on top of or underneath another object? Can they name the objects?

◆ Object recognition: present them with two objects in their central visual field. Ask them to select the correct object with a verbal prompt (*i.e. which one is the comb?*).

◆ Present them with an object from their locker/table, ask them to show you how to use it (e.g. comb, toothbrush). *Cue 1: demonstrate if they cannot initiate, Cue 2: guide their hand to their head/face, Cue 3: facilitate their movements then see if they can follow (praxis).*

Mood: Do they appear to be engaging with their environment? Are they making eye contact with people around them? Are they anxious during interventions? Are they tearful or crying out? Are they able to indicate their mood on a visual scale of 0–10 (0 = happy, 10 = distressed/feeling depressed)?

Fatigue: How long can they tolerate before they become tired and close their eyes? Are they drowsy or alert during the session?

Motor/sensory: Can they identify touch to their affected arm and leg? Do they know where their limbs are in space? Can they move their arm/leg? Can they move their limbs against gravity or resistance? Have they got any tone (increased/decreased)? How are they positioned in bed (symmetrical/asymmetrical)?

Some of these aspects can be observed simultaneously in the patient during the assessment, which can save time in the fast-paced setting of the hospital.

In addition to the bedside assessment, the therapist may choose to complete some pen- and paper-based tasks with the patient. These can help to inform the treatment plan by providing further information about the person's visual and perceptual skills. Examples of this may include the assessment of 2D construction by asking the patient to copy shapes and images and to draw familiar items on a piece of paper (Chessington Occupational Therapy Neurological Assessment Battery) (see Fig. 15.1). Drawing a clock provides a useful way of assessing a person's attention

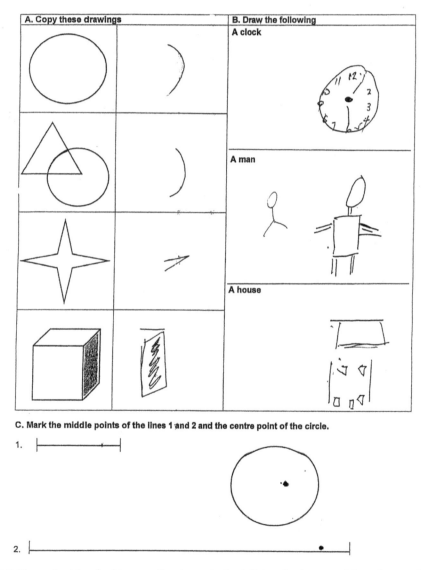

Fig. 15.1 The patient is asked to copy the shapes in the left-hand column and then draw a clock, man, and house. They are then asked to mark the midline points of the lines and circle at the bottom. This example demonstrates a left hemianopia and potentially a left neglect.

to both sides of space, the interaction between their visual, perceptual, and motor functions, memory, and executive functions. The Broken Hearts test[4] offers an assessment of hemianopia and neglect, and with the use of the timing criteria, can be used as a stand-alone standardized assessment or as part of the full OCS.

Assessment of function

Alongside the bedside assessments and pen and paper tasks, functional tasks provide an ideal opportunity to collect additional information.

Mealtime assessment: Provided the person is not 'nil by mouth', the mealtime observation can inform the therapist of the person's ability to initiate and sequence a task, bilateral use of the upper limbs, visual and perceptual function, ability to follow instructions, safety, attention, and many other functions. The OT can also recommend the use of adapted cutlery or other small adaptations to promote independence.

Grooming: A grooming task can be used when a full personal care assessment is not appropriate. This may be because the patient remains very dependent, fatigues easily, or has limited attention to the task. Dependent on the patient's level of function, their ability to plan, set-up, and complete a grooming task can be explored. This may include washing/drying face, shaving, brushing teeth, or applying make-up. Personal grooming is an important activity. This is something that people engage in on a daily basis, and being able to tend to their own appearance can improve their self-esteem and dignity, and can be motivating for the individual.

Washing and dressing: An assessment of ability to perform a personal care task is a key area of practice in OT (see Box 15.3). Not only does this provide information regarding their ability to get themselves washed and dressed, which can inform the discharge process, but also offers an opportunity to identify cognitive, perceptual, or visual impairments impacting on function. The task of washing and dressing can be broken down into its component parts: grooming (see earlier), top half, bottom half, or full washing and dressing.

Hot drink/meal preparation: Assessing the person's ability to make a hot drink serves a number of purposes. This is an activity familiar to many, and therefore provides an ideal opportunity to identify task performance errors which can then be generalized to other activities of daily living (ADL). To assess a person's function in a more complex task, preparation of a hot snack or meal can also be used. These tasks offer information about whether someone will be safe to make a hot drink and/or meal on discharge from hospital, or whether they will require support from family members or social care.

Social skills/money management/road safety: The acute setting of a hospital does not offer many opportunities to assess higher level cognition in function (however, this can be assessed using standardized assessments). Use of the wider hospital environment can offer a solution to this. Taking a patient to the shop to purchase some items enables the therapist to explore the patient's ability to manage money, search and locate items on shelves, negotiate social situations, and locate their way back to the ward. Concerns regarding road safety can be explored by taking the patient off the ward to negotiate the roads within the hospital grounds. A person's ability to use pedestrian crossings safely and their insight into road safety can inform decisions around discharge, particularly if they live alone.

Calling for help: For patients who have aphasia, or reduced insight into their level of function, ascertaining whether they are able to call for help is essential when planning their discharge. For many people on discharge from hospital, a package of care to support with personal and domestic ADLs will mean there will be gaps during the day where the person is on their own, unless they

Box 15.3 Case study: Washing and dressing assessment

Bob required assistance to initiate and sequence the whole task of washing and dressing. His bottom half was completed in bed with assistance of two to roll him from left to right and wash his lower legs. With encouragement and facilitation, he was able to wash and dry his groin area and the tops of his legs. Bob required the assistance of two to dress his lower half on the bed, but with facilitation was able to lift his hips and assist in pulling his lower clothing over his bottom.

Bob transferred from lying to sitting on the edge of the bed with the assistance of two. He had poor awareness of midline in sitting and was leaning to the left. Using the standing hoist and two staff he transferred into a normal wheelchair to complete his top half washing and dressing in the bathroom. The use of the correct environment for this task will provide cues to the task to be performed.

Bob required ongoing prompts to initiate and sequence the top half washing and dressing task. He was provided with a washcloth with soap on it and his hand brought to his face to initiate washing. Once initiated, he was able to continue this task, but needed another prompt to rinse and dry his face. He used his right hand throughout the task; his left hand was placed on the arm of the wheelchair. Bob did not wash his left arm or the left side of his face. His right arm and back were washed with assistance, due to his dense arm weakness. Bob had great difficulty putting his top on as he was trying to put his head in through the arm hole. He was given assistance to put it on.

Grooming: Bob needed assistance to set up his grooming tasks, for example, help to put toothpaste on his toothbrush and take it to his mouth, and needed 'hand over hand' facilitation to comb his hair.

Analysis: Bob has a dense left-sided weakness and personal neglect of his left side. He requires prompts to initiate and sequence the task, indicating a potential apraxia. He has a poor awareness of where his body is in space and had reduced insight into the difficulty he had getting washed and dressed.

have family support. Exploring what they would do if they had a fall, required the toilet, or if there was a fire will inform the hospital and community teams of their needs and safety on discharge.

Rehabilitation of the older person

Goal setting

Following the completion of the initial assessments, the therapist, patient, and their family will be able to have a discussion regarding goals for rehabilitation (see Box 15.4). Goal setting is a collaborative process which involves education and negotiation.[1] Both short- and long-term goals can be discussed and set; these offer the patient an opportunity to put forwards their aspirational goals for the future, but also for the therapist to assist in setting realistic and achievable short-term goals for their initial phase of rehabilitation. Setting goals can provide a patient with the motivation to engage in therapy, and offer a method of measurement for both the patient and the therapist by which to chart their progress.

Box 15.4 Case study: Goal setting

Bob was fully independent prior to having his stroke. His wife would be able to support with some activities on discharge but cannot offer too much physical assistance. During the goal setting discussion, Bob stated that he wants to be able to walk his dog again and go home.

The therapist and Bob discussed what he needs to be able to do in order to leave hospital. Through discussion, it was agreed that he would prefer to manage his own personal care, rather than relying on his wife or social carers. He would also like to read a newspaper again, something which he really enjoys. Bob would like to be able to transfer himself from bed to chair/toilet, without assistance. The goals that follow next demonstrate the short-term goals necessary for Bob to achieve his overall goals of independence with personal care and transfers. As these are achieved, new goals can be set in order to progress his rehabilitation.

Goal 1: Bob to wash his bottom half in the bed, with minimal assistance to roll to the left, in 2 weeks

Goal 2: Bob to independently dress his top half, in 1 week

Goal 3: Using an anchor line to the left border of a newspaper, Bob to independently read a paragraph, in 2 weeks

Goal 4: Bob to sit unaided for 5 minutes on the edge of the bed, in 4 days

---

Rehabilitation treatment approaches

The OT uses a number of approaches in treating the person with stroke. This enables interventions to be tailored to the individual, and promotes a flexible and patient-centred approach to rehabilitation. While the overall aim of therapy is for the patient to regain independence or function in ADLs, there will be cases when the patient is not able to achieve a particular level of function during their inpatient stay, or their sub-optimal pre-morbid function necessitates the provision of equipment to assist in their daily functioning. The OT will provide equipment essential for a hospital discharge, for example, moving and handling equipment, toileting equipment, or hospital bed packages. Bathing equipment, ramps, and major adaptations will be assessed by community teams to ensure the patient's long-term care needs are met.

Upper limb management and rehabilitation

Approximately 70% of people experience altered arm function after a stroke, and this persists in about 40%.[5] The treatment of the upper limb (UL) is addressed by both physiotherapy and OT. The focus of the OT is on function, using meaningful activities to treat motor and sensory impairments. A thorough neurological assessment of the upper limb will identify any areas of weakness, sensory loss, increased tone or subluxation, and the therapist will then work with the patient to promote self-management of the UL. The use of intensive, repetitive, and task-orientated training is fundamental in the management of the UL following stroke. People with stroke should be given every opportunity to practice functional activities using their UL,[6] and where able, the use of mental practice is showing some promise as an adjunct to traditional therapies (see Box 15.5).

> ## Box 15.5 Case study: Management of the upper limb
>
> Bob has a dense left hemiplegia. He has reduced sensation in his left arm and reduced attention to his arm and the left of his body. As a result of this, his arm often becomes trapped and is at risk of injury. Therapy will focus upon increasing his attention to his arm and his sensation, and maintaining range of movement through the joints to prevent stiffening and oedema. Other adjuncts to therapy would be suitable for Bob, including use of a mirror box, which can 'trick' the brain into perceiving movement in his left arm. This, alongside mental practice, would be an activity that Bob could complete independent of a therapy session as self-practice.

Decreased muscle tone: It is important to ensure that the arm is well supported and deweighted using a pillow or arm rest. This will prevent further damage to the shoulder joint and reduce the risk of shoulder pain because of dislocation or subluxation. The patient, family, and carers should be shown how to correctly handle the UL to prevent injury.

Increased muscle tone: The management of increased tone requires an MDT approach. The medical team will ensure that the patient is receiving the correct medication to manage spasticity and pain and the physiotherapist and OT will work together to maintain range of movement and prevent contractures. The correct positioning and handling of the arm will also support the management of increased tone.

Splinting

Any joint that does not move frequently is at risk of developing shortening of surrounding tissues leading to restricted movement.[6]

Splinting for low tone: The evidence for splinting indicates that splints should not be used routinely to prevent loss in range of movement at the wrist and hand, but may be beneficial in selected cases, especially where there is a risk of injury.[7] Splinting and positioning can be used to protect the joints in the wrist and hand from damage caused by poor positioning or neglect. As recovery of activity occurs, there can be a resulting increase in tone in specific muscle groups which may lead to muscle shortening and malalignment. Ensuring the hand and wrist are well supported, aligned, and positioned in mid-range, with accompanying passive movements, can help to maintain the structures and architecture of the hand.

Splinting in increased tone: It is suggested that splints, used in conjunction with botulinum toxin, may reduce spasticity in selected cases. Splints should not be used routinely to correct contractures, but again, may be beneficial in selected cases (i.e. in the presence of pain).[7] The decision to splint should be made by a senior therapist who has a good understanding of the person's posture, medical condition, pain, cognition, skin integrity, musculoskeletal, and neurological function. The subsequent daily management of a splint is the responsibility of the MDT, patient, and family, to ensure it is worn according to the regime set by the therapist and with the appropriate rest periods.

Oedema management: Oedema can occur as a result of reduced movement in a limb following stroke. Oedema results in enlargement and swelling of the hemiplegic UL and can limit rehabilitation progress through restriction of mobility and function.[8] The long-term effect of oedema may be reduced range of movement and pain in the limb. Evidence has shown significant improvements in oedema following the use of compression gloves and active/passive range of movements,[9] however, there is still a need for further research on the efficacy of retrograde massage in reducing oedema. Education and advice are important in managing oedema; patients and family members can be encouraged to position the limb and complete passive movements throughout the day to reduce the effects of the swelling.

Visual impairment following stroke

The assessment and rehabilitation of visual impairments is covered in great detail in Chapter 21. Alongside the key specialists in the management of vision, the OT also has a role in screening for visual impairments and consideration of the impact of this impairment on the persons function (see Box 15.6 for an example of this).

Cognition

Cognition refers to those mental functions which allow us to acquire, organize, manipulate, and use information, and can be described as our thinking processes.[10] Cognition therefore guides much of human performance, and the impact of cognitive impairment on functioning can be considerable. Age-related changes can occur in memory, attention, processing, and executive function; furthermore, cognitive impairment is found in a substantial number of stroke survivors, affecting more than one-third of stroke survivors at 3 and 12 months after stroke. These impairments persist in many individuals for years and are associated with poor long-term survival, higher disability, and greater institutionalization rates.[11]

Attention

Attention forms the foundation for many of the cognitive functions, including memory. It is one of the most common cognitive impairments to occur following a stroke, and can affect the person's ability to function in all tasks of daily living. Often the therapist sets goals around improving attention as a priority within the initial stages post-stroke. Higher cognitive functions such as information processing, memory, and executive function are often more evident and pose more of an impact on functioning in the community setting.

In order to engage in a meaningful activity, a person must be able to focus and maintain their attention, blocking out other competing stimuli, but also shift their focus onto other stimuli as needed. This manipulation of attention enables us to concentrate on a task and commit information to both short-term and long-term memory for use later. Reduced attention means that information cannot enter the brain correctly for processing, which is likely to result in reduced

---

Box 15.6 Case study: Management of visual impairment

Following assessment, it was identified that Bob has a left homonymous hemianopia: damage to the visual pathway of his brain means that he cannot see the left half of his visual field in both eyes. This combined with his neglect means that his attention to the left half of space is severely impaired, and this will affect his mobility, social interactions, and function. Education will be an important intervention with Bob, as the explanation that the damage has happened to his brain rather than his eyes often helps people take on board strategies to manage their deficit.

Bob will be referred to the orthoptist for formal field testing and therapeutic intervention and the OT will continue to work with him to develop compensatory strategies, such as head turning and scanning to reduce the impact of his visual impairment on his function.

understanding and poor recall of information. Reducing distractions in the environment, allowing time for the processing of information and having shorter therapy sessions can assist the person with reduced attention to focus on their daily activities. Working to improve their attention can include the use of graded tasks, and providing cues encouraging the patient to describe the task and the steps required to complete it before initiating it.

Insight/awareness

A person's level of awareness varies from situation to situation. Insight or awareness can be affected by a stroke, whereby the person lacks or has partial understanding of their situation (see Box 15.7). They may have an understanding of how the stroke has affected them physically, but lack insight into their cognitive or language impairments. As a result of this lack of insight, they may not be able to consider how the impairment affects their function, and therefore put into place strategies to manage these difficulties. A lack of awareness is a potential barrier to successful rehabilitation following a stroke. People with reduced awareness may find it challenging to set realistic goals or engage in rehabilitation, if they do not believe they have any problems. They may display poor judgement in risky situations and fail to see the need to employ compensatory strategies. Often increasing insight into a person's condition and impairments can result in decreasing mood: as the person becomes more aware of how the stroke has affected them, they may find it more difficult to adjust to these changes. The involvement of Clinical Psychology is essential in supporting patients with these changes, and the whole MDT should have an understanding of strategies which can be used with patients struggling to adjust following a stroke.

There are a variety of ways to assess insight, including behavioural observations, questionnaires, and self-rating scales. Education is a key strategy to use in facilitating awareness; educating the patient and their family regarding the brain, how a stroke happens, which parts of their brain have been affected, and how the brain repairs itself enables them to put their stroke and recovery into context. Appreciating how improvement can be made has been shown to maintain a person's effort and performance in rehabilitation.[12] Other strategies to improve awareness include giving consistent feedback following task completion and facilitating a safe failure at a task, so that they can appreciate the effects of their impairment on their functioning.

Neglect

Bob's lack of attention to his left side suggests the presence of neglect (see Box 15.8 for a description of this). The existence of neglect can predict a longer inpatient stay and a lower functional outcome on discharge.[13] Neglect is an attentional deficit, whereby an awareness of one side of space or the person is affected, in the absence of a primary sensory or motor deficit. This usually occurs in the space opposite the site of the stroke and is more commonly found in right sided strokes (with left-sided weakness). Neglect can occur in some or all of the following domains: personal

---

Box 15.7 Case study: Managing a lack of insight

Bob has demonstrated a lack of insight into his impairments following the stroke, as he believed his admission was due to a fall, rather than the stroke. At an intellectual level, he can appreciate that a level of impairment exists, but not that these difficulties are linked together and caused by the stroke. Regular brain injury education can be used with Bob and his family, including feedback following therapy sessions to give real-time examples of his functioning.

Box 15.8 Case study: Management of neglect

Bob has a neglect of his personal and peripersonal space. This was confirmed during the washing and dressing assessment as he did not wash or dry his left arm or leg. He is also unable to pay attention to stimuli positioned within arm's reach in his left space.

Rehabilitation will focus on increasing Bob's awareness of his left side (body and space) through sensory stimulation to his arm, providing cues to his left side and encouraging him to use his arm in functional tasks. A brightly coloured 'anchor' line can be used to draw his attention to the left side of his peripersonal space and will help him with his visual field loss. The mirror box can also be used as an adjunct to the functional activities. Bob would not be appropriate for constraint-induced movement therapy (CIMT) due to the lack of activity in his left hand.

space (the person's body itself), peripersonal space (the space within arm's reach of them), and extrapersonal space (the wider environment). Neglect can be extremely disabling, as the person is unable to attend to one-half of their space, and objects within it. A patient experiencing neglect has reported the following:

'My arm doesn't feel as if it belongs to me. It feels like I am lying in bed next to a corpse.'

Neglect can be assessed using a variety of techniques. An observation of the patient in function can offer a clear indication of a neglect, as the patient may be neglecting one-half of their body, or the space around them. Use of pen and paper tasks is also a common way of highlighting this impairment, as the person may begin their drawing to the right side of the paper, or omit one-half of the drawing (see Figs. 15.1 and 15.2).

In addition to this, standardized assessments offer a formal way of assessing neglect. The Catherine Bergego Scale (1995) is an observational measure, where the patient is observed doing 10 different daily activities, including grooming and eating, and they are scored depending on the amount of neglect they show. Other assessments include the Behavioural Inattention Test (1987), which is a battery of tests comprising both pen and paper tasks and behavioural tasks, and the Baking Tray Test, which asks patients to spread wooden cubes across a board as evenly as possible.

In OT, the treatment of neglect can include the following strategies:

- Cueing the person to their inattentive side using auditory, visual, and sensory cues
- Videoing the patient completing a functional task to provide feedback on their performance
- Limb activation, or encouraging voluntary movements of the affected hand and arm
- Visual scanning training. The person is encouraged to visually explore the neglected side of space, by setting up activities in this area and using a visual target to anchor their attention

There is interest in but less evidence for:

- Constraint-induced movement therapy can be used if the person meets the criteria (i.e. has an appropriate amount of activity in the affected limb and understands the concept of the approach)
- Mirror box therapy to 'trick' the brain into thinking that limb is moving and increase attention to that limb

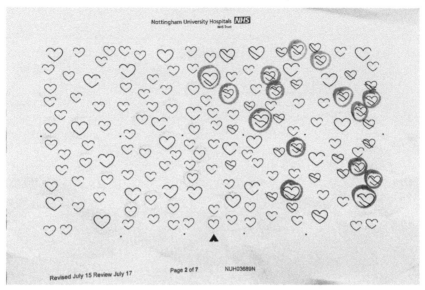

Fig. 15.2 Broken hearts test demonstrating severe left-sided visual neglect.

Apraxia

Apraxia is a neuropsychological disorder, which affects the ability to perform learned and purposeful skilled movements. Apraxia can be very disabling for people following a stroke (see Box 15.9 as an example of this). They may have the idea or concept behind a movement but have difficulty performing the physical aspect of it. Alternatively, they may have the physical means to complete a movement but struggle to use objects correctly, plan, and complete the task. It is likely that some level of apraxia will persist following rehabilitation, but patients can adopt compensatory strategies to learn how to complete tasks, including following cues, performing the task in the correct environment (i.e. washing and dressing in the bathroom, rather than by the bedside) and imitating the movements of others.

Box 15.9 Case study: Management of apraxia

Bob has demonstrated elements of apraxia during his functioning in washing and dressing. His difficulty in initiating and sequencing the task (putting the parts of the task together to make a whole) and producing the correct movements to comb his hair both indicate an apraxia. These errors in performing the washing task are likely to present themselves in other activities—these will be identified through further assessment in function.

To promote independence in this task, a prompt card can be developed with Bob, giving him written prompts to begin washing and dressing and cue him to move onto the next part of the task. Due to his visual impairment, an anchor line can be used down the left-hand column of the sheet to draw his attention to that side. All further washing and dressing practice would be completed in the bathroom, to ensure that Bob can take cues from the environment. Giving him hand-on-hand support to comb his hair will also help him to relearn the movement required for this task.

Perception

Perception is the ability to make sense of or interpret knowledge gained from the senses, and in particular, the visual system provides the majority of the information to the brain. Due to the close relationship between vision and perception, age-related visual changes can impair the older person's perceptual abilities.[14] The older person may experience reduced acuity, changes to their visual fields, visual memory, and depth perception problems. Perception can be categorized into the following three areas: body scheme, visual discrimination, and agnosia.[14]

Body scheme is the representation of the spatial relations of body parts within the brain. Through the integration of the senses, it provides a foundation from which movement, balance, and posture occur, and is crucial for interaction with the environment. Someone with impaired body schema may present with difficulty identifying body parts, their relations with each other, or discriminating right from left. Encouraging the person to name their body parts in function and providing sensory stimulation to the affected areas can assist the person in rebuilding the representation of their body within the cortex.

Visual discrimination is the ability to discriminate between different forms. Understanding the various properties of objects enables you to recognize objects so that you can use them functionally and move around within the environment. If someone has difficulty perceiving depth, foreground from background, or relations between objects, they may be at risk of falls, have reduced mobility, and require assistance with everyday tasks. The use of contrast in colours and textures can help people to discern between the different forms, and verbally describing the objects location assists in difficulties perceiving the differences in depth and distance.

Agnosia is the disorder of the recognition of an object, affecting the analysis of the object or recognition of its meaning.[15] Objects are identified through their visual properties, colour, weight, shape, orientation, and movement, and the incorrect identification of an object may result in its improper use. A person with agnosia may not be able to recognize an object and therefore use it correctly. Utilizing the intact senses to recognize an object and providing labels to help identify the object can support someone to use them independently.

Group work in OT

Treating patients in a group setting facilitates a number of benefits for patients, including enhancing their communication and socialization skills, and enables them to mirror others' physical and functional abilities. Examples of groups that can be run within the acute setting are UL groups, gardening, baking, exercise, and relaxation groups. These offer an opportunity for patients to leave their immediate ward environment which is important for mood and motivation. It provides an opportunity for people to share experiences with others and engage in leisure activities, which can be especially important for older people (see Box 15.10).

The 24-hour approach to rehabilitation is key within stroke services. Patients should be given every opportunity to practice functional activities and complete exercises central to their rehabilitation. The support of the wider MDT is essential, as they can support patients and their families to engage in rehabilitation activities throughout the day, and promote recovery and independence in the evenings and overnight. Involving the family is an important part of promoting 24-hour rehabilitation. Family members are often eager to support their relative in their progress and their encouragement can be motivating for the person with stroke. Demonstrating activities or exercises that they can do with the patient can help this, and may help to reduce feelings of helplessness that relatives can often experience.

Self-management and self-efficacy in stroke patients have been seen to have a positive effect on a person's physical functioning, engagement in daily activities, psychosocial functioning, and

Box 15.10 Case study: Group work

Bob agreed to attend a weekly upper limb rehabilitation group on the ward. This time enables him to focus purely on his upper limb, and practice exercises with the supervision of a therapist. He enjoys getting to socialize with people from different wards and finds it useful to see how others function varies from his.

Bob also attends a weekly gardening group. He enjoyed spending time in his garden at home and finds that the group means that he can relax away from the ward and spend time working on his sitting balance, orientation to midline, and placement of his arm in a different context.

reduced levels of depression. Encouraging patients to problem-solve, reflect upon their functioning, engage in activities, set their own goals, and improve their knowledge and understanding are all aspects of promoting self-efficacy and should be seen as central to stroke rehabilitation. Providing a patient with a pack of appropriate exercises or activities for them to use in their time on the ward can help to give them control over their rehabilitation and progress.

Discharge planning

Supportive discharge planning

Developing an understanding of a person's functioning over a 24-hour period is key to planning a safe discharge. Therapists will largely be present during working hours whereas nursing staff have an overview of a patient's needs day and night. Completion of a 48-hour care chart provides detailed information to the MDT about the patient's care and behavioural needs. This information will often be used in family meetings to give an insight into how their relative functions and to develop insight into care needs for the patient themselves. One of the added complexities of an older person with stroke is the age of their relatives/spouses, or the fact that they lived alone prestroke. For those patients who wish to aim for discharge to their own home, an overnight stay by relatives may be recommended. The spouse or carer of the patient is invited to spend the night at the hospital observing and providing care for the patient as required. Nursing staff are there to support both parties, and in this supportive environment the family and patient are able to see whether they will be able to manage on discharge from hospital. This goes some way to reduce the number of discharges which result in readmissions or emergency respite due to the breakdown of the care plan.

If the patient has agreed to receive social care on discharge in the form of a care package, then a simulation of care calls on the ward will prepare them for how this will be delivered once at home. Following thorough discussion and agreement with the patient and family as required, the MDT will deliver care to the patient in line with the agreed package of care, for example, toileting, repositioning and meals/drinks, and so on would only be completed four times a day to replicate a four-call care package. Any care required outside of these 'calls' would be discussed with the patient.

Insight and capacity to make a decision regarding discharge plans

Impaired insight can be a common impairment following a stroke. While a lack of insight does not automatically mean a lack of capacity, the person's understanding of their needs must be taken into account. A lack of understanding may suggest the need for a formal assessment of capacity. Capacity is covered in more detail in Chapters 17 and 18.

Family meetings

It is good practice to ensure regular communication with patients' relatives during their hospital stay. This ensures everyone is informed of the progress of the patient and the plans for discharge. This is especially important if the older person's needs place demands on the family on discharge.

Social support on discharge

People over 65 may be caregivers themselves, with nearly 1.4 million people aged over 65 providing unpaid care for family or others in 2011.[16] The support of carers following a stroke is immeasurable. Having support on discharge from hospital can sometimes mean the difference between living at home and being discharged to a residential/nursing home. Having regular contact with the patient's relatives or support network predischarge will give the OT an idea of their capabilities and considerations for discharge. The ability of the patient's family or relatives to support them on discharge must be considered and discussed as part of discharge planning. Social care packages can be used to support people on discharge, especially when their needs cannot be met by their spouse or family.

Challenges

Patients who live alone will often need to be functioning at a higher level in order to manage at home safely. Alternatively, those who wish to return home may require an increased package of support from social services in order to make this happen.

For patients who cared for their spouses pre-admission, the OT and the MDT will need to make sure the relative is safe and cared for by the family following the patient's admission. If there is no additional family support available, social services will need to place the relative into emergency respite care until home care can be formally organized.

Access and home visits

An access visit is a predischarge visit made to the patient's property without the patient present. This is usually completed to assist with discharge planning, as the therapist can assess the environment; what space is available, access into the property, and any hazards or safety concerns. The access visit can inform what kind of equipment the patient will need on discharge and also gives an insight into the person's life before stroke. Additionally, this provides an opportunity to discuss with the relatives the potential set-up on discharge, and prepare them for how life will be.

Home visits : A change in environment is likely to impact further on the person's ability to function, and therefore when considering their needs, the optimal environment in which to work with them is a key decision to be made. Enabling the person to complete a task in their own environment will reduce the variables created by the unfamiliar environment of the hospital rehabilitation areas. Home visits can be completed for a number of reasons. A home visit enables the therapist to view the person functioning in their own environment and also problem-solve any issues that may arise during this assessment. For those patients who may have dementia or confusion, performing everyday tasks in their own environment may be more appropriate and enabling to their abilities. Evidence suggests that performance in ADLs is impaired in an unfamiliar environment.[17]

Box 15.11 gives an example of planning Bob's discharge from hospital.

Conclusion

Stroke is a potentially chronic condition which affects all aspects of a person's life and function. Rehabilitation does not end in hospital, but extends into the community, with many people making functional gains for many years afterwards. While this book is aimed towards the older

Box 15.11 Case study: Planning discharge from hospital

Bob has spent 3 weeks in hospital and is now able to step around transfer from bed to chair with supervision of one. He has made good progress but will still require minimal support of one person for washing and dressing on discharge.

An access visit to his home showed adequate space for a bed downstairs, and with two reception rooms, he will be able to sleep in one room and have family time in the second room. Bob will be provided with a commode for bedside toileting but is otherwise able to use his existing furniture. For times when his wife needs to go out and do the shopping, Bob has agreed to have a pendant alarm, so that he can alert her/family members in case he has a fall or needs medical assistance.

Bob doesn't feel he requires a social services care package, and his wife has spent some time in therapy with him and feels able to support him with his personal care needs on discharge. A community team will continue his rehabilitation and progress his mobility as able.

Although Bob has not achieved his long-term goals, he is happy to be discharged from hospital and continue his rehabilitation in his own home. His awareness of the stroke and how it has affected him has improved and he is developing strategies to manage some of his cognitive impairments.

person with stroke, the emphasis of OT is on treating each person as an individual; therapy approaches should not merely be dictated by a person's age.

The role of the OT is essential in stroke rehabilitation. The OT will work with the patient and their family to identify areas of function which are particularly important to them, and will aim to enable people to complete these activities as independently as possible. This chapter has only skimmed the surface of the diverse and varied role of the OT working with this complex condition; however, it gives an insight into key fundamental therapeutic interventions with the older person following a stroke.

References

1. Mew M & Ivey J. The occupational therapy process. In: Edmans J (ed.) *Occupational Therapy and Stroke*, p. 49. London, UK: Wiley-Blackwell, 2010.
2. **Wolff S, Jackson T, & Reid L.** Management of motor impairments. In: Edmans J (ed.) *Occupational Therapy and Stroke*, p. 90. London, UK: Wiley-Blackwell, 2010.
3. **Nasreddine ZS, Phillips NA, Bédirian V,** et al. The Montreal Cognitive Assessment, MoCA: a brief screening tool for mild cognitive impairment. *J Am Geriatr Soc* 2005;**53**(4):695–9.
4. **Demeyere N, Riddoch M, Slavkova E, Bickerton W, & Humphreys G.** The Oxford Cognitive Screen (OCS): validation of a stroke-specific short cognitive screening tool. *Psychol Assess* 2015;**27**(3):883–94.
5. **Ivey J & Mew M.** Theoretical basis. In: Edmans J (ed.) *Occupational Therapy and Stroke*, p. 36. London, UK: Wiley-Blackwell, 2010.
6. **Royal College of Physicians.** *National Clinical Guidelines for Stroke.* Available from: http://guideline. ssnap.org/2016StrokeGuideline/index.html p83 [Accessed: 29 June 2017].
7. **Royal College of Occupational Therapists and the Association of Charted Physiotherapists in Neurology.** *Splinting for the Prevention and Correction of Contractures in Adults with Neurological Dysfunction. Practice Guideline for Occupational Therapists and Physiotherapists,* 2015 Available from: https://www.rcot.co.uk/file/926/download?token=ZyFUmQMR [Accessed: 28 July 2019].

8. **Jackson T, van Teijlingen E, & Bruce J.** Light retrograde massage for the treatment of post-stroke upper limb oedema: clinical consensus using the Delphi technique. *Br J Occup Ther* 2012;**75**(12):549–54.

9. **Giang T, Ong A, Krishnamurthy K, & Fong K.** Rehabilitation interventions for poststroke hand oedema: a systematic review. *Hong Kong J Occup Ther* 2016;**27**:7–17.

10. **Jackson T & Wolff S.** Management of cognitive impairments. In: Edmans J (ed.) *Occupational Therapy and Stroke*, p. 144. London, UK: Wiley-Blackwell, 2010.

11. **Winstein CJ, Stein J, Arena R**, et al. Guidelines for adult stroke rehabilitation and recovery: a guideline for healthcare professionals from the American Heart Association/American Stroke Association. Stroke 2016;**47**(6):e98–e169.

12. **Blackwell L, Trzesniewski K, & Dweck C.** Implicit theories of intelligence predict achievement across an adolescent transition: a longitudinal study and an intervention. *Child Dev* 2007;**78**(1):246–63.

13. **Gillen R, Tennen H, & McKee T.** Unilateral spatial neglect: relation to rehabilitation outcomes in patients with right hemisphere stroke. *Arch Phys Med Rehabil* 2005;**86**(4):763–7.

14. **Zoltan B.** *Vision, Perception, and Cognition: A Manual for the Evaluation and Treatment of the Adult with Acquired Brain Injury*, 4th edition. Thorofare, NJ: SLACK Inc., 2007.

15. **De Renzi, E.** Disorders of visual recognition. In: Zoltan B (ed.) *Vision, Perception, and Cognition. A Manual for the Evaluation and Treatment of the Adult with Acquired Brain Injury*, 4th edition, p. 171. Thorofare, NJ: SLACK Inc., 2007.

16. **Age UK.** *Later Life in the United Kingdom.* Factsheet. 2017 [Updated May 2019]: 14. In: UK Census, 2011, as reported by the Office for National Statistics. Available from: https://www.ageuk.org.uk/globalassets/age-uk/documents/reports-and-publications/later_life_uk_factsheet.pdf Accessed: 28 July 2019].

17. **Geusgens C, van Heugten C, Hagedoren E, Jolles J, & van den Heuvel W.** Environmental effects in the performance of daily tasks in healthy adults. *Am J Occup Ther* 2010;**64**(6):935–940.

Chapter 16

Physiotherapy of the older stroke patient

Dawn Hicklin and Clair Finnemore

Introduction

Regardless of any disease or age process, the aim of physiotherapy is to restore movement and function in order either to enhance or maintain physical performance. Good practice must be holistic in its breadth of knowledge and attitude to the individual but meticulous in attention to detail in examination of the older person.

This chapter will introduce concepts in physiotherapy and provide an insight into the complexities of rehabilitation within this population.

The invisible burden of stroke

In the United Kingdom 7% of NHS budget is spent annually on stroke care provision and there are 1.2 million people living post stroke in the United Kingdom. The burden of stroke now disproportionately affects individuals living in resource-poor countries with evidence suggesting that the overall incidence of stroke in low to middle income countries, are far greater than those of high-income countries, by at least 20%.[1]

Traditionally we consider the physical impact of stroke (such as limb weakness) that limits function which in turn, affects the ability to contribute to the economy, live independently, and self-provide. What it often fails to consider are the unseen physical factors such as loss of visual fields, continence, and development of physiological fatigue among others (Fig. 16.1).

The impact of age

Working with older people affected by stroke can present the physiotherapist with a set of challenges unseen in other areas of practice. We must consider the ageing process and unique individual patterns of ageing and how their particular stroke has affected their abilities to not only move but how they process this movement into functional gain—no two strokes ever present the same.

Many physiological changes occur as individuals increase in age. When rehabilitating an individual, consideration of the degree of physiological decline is reflected at different physiological levels as seen in Table 16.1.

The degree to which these alterations in function are present in any given individual is influenced by how physically fit they were at the time of the stroke. The perceptions or presumptions of clinicians may unjustifiably dictate the management of the older person. A clinical example can be seen in Box 16.1.

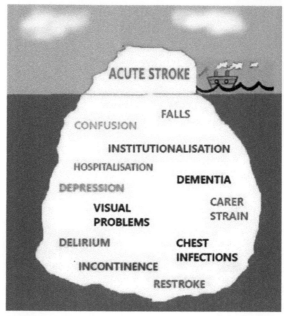

Fig. 16.1 The invisible burden of stroke; cerebrovascular disease as an iceberg.

This demonstrates not only a need to educate broadly about stroke but also to quash the assumption that older age and stroke equates to an inability to regain function, movement, and return to their previous lifestyle.

Recent literature has identified that while some of these physiological changes are present as early as 50 years of age, they are considerably less pronounced in individuals who have an active lifestyle, especially if this includes regular exercise. An old adage states that 'age is merely a number'. In clinical practice we are faced with 80-year-old people who work, holiday abroad, and remain physically active and there are others that have many comorbidities, require support to walk, and suffer cognitive decline. Ageing means we must consider an individual's capacity to learn and physical capacity to function within the constraints of physiological decline. To illustrate this, Box 16.2 provides comparative presentation.

This illustrates that the older person cannot be assumed to be retired and dependent. Age alone is not an indicator of abilities, health, or lifestyle.

Table 16.1 Neurological changes with ageing that affect motor function

Decline in muscle power	Reduced interhemispheric communication
Reduced fine motor control	Reduced sensorimotor feedback
Earlier onset of muscle fatigue in sustained function	Reduced cognition
Dysfunction of the neuromuscular junction	Reduced stability during complex tasks
Progressive cerebral atrophy	Increased reliance on our prefrontal cortex during simple tasks

Box 16.1 Case study: When you perhaps care too much?

An 82-year-old female attended hospital with suspected delirium of unknown cause. She was diagnosed as having stroke but due to other medical conditions taking priority was unable to access a stroke unit immediately. As a result, the stroke multidisciplinary team saw her on an elderly care ward. On arrival, the therapy team discovered that the staff were doing everything for the patient. She was being physically supported for all personal care needs, including transfers. When questioned, the staff explained that the combination of her age and diagnosis made them feel she was far too frail to help herself, had a high risk of fall and therefore required maximal assistance with all care. The patient's perception was that she was in hospital to be 'looked after' and as such did not question why she was being offered so much support. On reviewing the patient's history this lady was self-caring and independent, regularly used public transport, attended social events, and entertained others in her own home. Her stroke had left her with minimal physical weakness and some affects to balance. The treatment was to educate the staff around her, provide an opportunity to move and as such explore her physical abilities. This lady left hospital 2 weeks later having regained all of her mobility, ability to self-care, and continues to proceed with her previous stroke event lifestyle.

Frailty

One-quarter to a half of people older than 85 years are 'frail'.[2]

Frailty and the older person are often considered interchangeable terminology for health professionals. Growing old is inevitable, but at what point are we considered frail?

Xue (2011)[3] defined frailty as a 'clinically recognizable state of increased vulnerability resulting from ageing-associated decline in reserve and function across multiple physiologic systems such that the ability to cope with every day or acute stressors is comprised'.

Frailty does not have a single definition or criteria to guide diagnosis. As such, identifying frailty within the older person is often dependent on the perception of the health professional.

Identifying true frailty is important for providing appropriate medical attention required and to recognize early on in their care the risk of increased dependency.[4] There is an assumption that if you have had a stroke you should be considered frail; however, it is important to differentiate

Box 16.2 Case study: Do only older people have multiple diseases?

A 64-year-old female presented with right middle cerebral artery infarct. Known diabetes, hypertension, and vascular dementia. Has resided in a residential home for 18 months. Normally has assistance of one carer with mobility and personal hygiene and requires close observation at mealtimes.

An 85-year-old male presented with right middle cerebral artery stroke. Lives alone. Completes all household chores and shops independently. Works each morning for 1 hour as a school crossing warden. Has an allotment he tends to daily. Three times a week collects his 8-year-old grandson from school.

between the effects of the stroke and frailty. Interventions such as strengthening programmes and nutritional supplementation may slow or reverse the frailty process. As clinicians we must take account of the ageing body and frailty and the effects of stroke if we are to maximize recovery.

Falls

Falls risk and frequency is a huge focus in preventative medicine in the field of geriatrics. Given the likely comorbidities following stroke in the older person, coupled with the physical, cognitive, or psychosocial affect that the stroke has left them with, this group of patients are even more susceptible to falls than their non-stroke counterparts. Particularly in the older population, falls can have serious adverse consequences both in terms of cost to the patient and cost to the health service when considering, for example, the financial and physical implications for post-fall fractures.

While this is true for stroke patients in longitudinal studies—10 years post stroke—recent studies[5] indicate that in the short term (1–3 years) there is little difference between those who have had a stroke and those who have not.[6] Despite this, the frequency of falls in older people after a stroke is as high as 37% in the first 6 months[7] which, given the number of stroke patients, represents a significant public health problem. This can be attributed to the fact that this is the time when gait patterns are continuing to evolve and where balance is the least reactive in those patients who are mobilizing.

In order to prevent falls, we must first consider the potential causes of falls in this group of patients.

Typical considerations include motor deficits, increased dependency levels, and sensory deficits. These go hand in hand with perceptual, cognitive, and visual impairments that have developed as a result of stroke. There is a variety of other considerations that are not so obvious. Poor upper limb function has been identified as a factor in post-stroke falls, due to the lack of automatic righting reactions on the affected side, and the inability to use the arm during a fall as a protective mechanism.[8]

What is physiotherapy?

Physiotherapy has been defined in many different ways:

'treatment of disease, injury or deformity by physical methods such as massage, heat treatment and exercise rather than drugs or surgery.' (Oxford Dictionaries, 2017)[9]

'physiotherapists help people affected by injury, illness or disability through movement, exercises, manual therapy, education and advice. The profession helps to encourage development and facilitate recovery enabling people to stay in work while helping to maintain independence for as long as possible.' (Chartered Society of Physiotherapy, 2017)[10]

'restore movement and function when affected by injury, illness or disability. Help reduce risk of injury, illness in the future.' (NHS Choices, 2017)[11]

'physiotherapists assess, diagnose, treat and prevent a wide variety of conditions and movement disorders.' (Australian Physiotherapy Association, 2017)[12]

'physical medicine and rehabilitation using mechanical force and movements to remediate impairments and promote mobility, function and QOL through examination, diagnosis and physical intervention.' (American Physical Therapy Association, 2017)[13]

Definitions vary; but how does this translate into recovery from stroke for an older population. Do we restore function? Do we reduce risk of a recurrence? Do we help people to stay in work?

Research into the effectiveness of physiotherapy intervention identifies that it improves health, well-being, function, and independence. A systematic approach to care including medical, nursing, and allied health professional input undoubtedly improves outcomes. However, very little of this research has been able to identify the best approach for the rehabilitation of an individual post stroke. Current evidence of effectiveness of individual interventions is inconclusive or absent. As physiotherapists we should consider the best available evidence, in conjunction with contextual information. It is essential to assess, measure, and formulate treatment plans taking these factors into account while being careful not to limit treatment options due to the lack of evidence base when you know that in practice these options can be effective for a given individual in the right context.

There is still much we do not know about the brain and how it compensates for damage caused by stroke. We know from evidence[14] that early intervention post stroke can be effective. However, we must consider the type of event—catastrophic/minor stroke—coupled with the patient's physiological state, comorbidities, and disease state.

It is not always possible, despite early and intensive input, that full or part recovery is realized.

Research supports the hypothesis that augmented exercise has a favourable effect on activities of daily living (ADL), particularly if therapy input is augmented at least 16 hours in the first 6 months after stroke. However, it does not indicate 'type of therapy' or the skills and experience pertaining to the individual therapist in these trials.

There is no one detailed algorithm we can utilize to treat an individual stroke survivor. There is no recipe for recovery.

Therapy by nature will consider the patient as a whole and will naturally absorb information regarding how the individual presents and will individualize therapy around bespoke clinical findings.

Much literature describes the different methodological approaches.[15,16] Nowadays, most therapists are not dogmatic purists in one particular 'school' of physiotherapy; sometimes therapists utilize one approach or combine many to achieve the desired outcome in a realistic timeframe. These approaches are there to guide the process of rehabilitation through the interpretation of how learning and relearning of every day movement occurs.

We must consider activity as a performance and as such a 'skill'. 'The learned ability to bring about predetermined results with the maximum certainty, often with minimum outlay of time or energy or both'.[17] As such we must consider practice, but this has to be the correct practice at the correct time, with the therapist facilitating this practice and not simply doing it unto the patient receiving treatment. Enabling learning in an enriched environment is the key to recovery. Physical rehabilitation is dynamic, not just preparatory, delivering regained activity into a functional context and altering the environment to increase understanding and learning. It is not just a series of exercises but the ability to adapt afferent input to gain positive alterations in outcome.

As clinicians we have the capacity to alter physiological pathways and assist the brain to respond to afferent stimuli. Every movement, every moment in the 24-hour care of a patient can have an impact on outcome, good or bad. However, there are times when the environment itself limits progression and recognition of this is important. Without the psychological drive to self-motivate and actively participate, rehabilitation is futile.

Consideration must be given to all avenues of therapy as demonstrated in Box 16.3. Traditionally we provide exercises and treatment for patients, but it can be argued that we err on the side of caution when it comes to the older patient, fearing the ageing process and its physiological consequences may create increased risk of harm such as falls, and cardiac and respiratory events.

Our approach should be individual to the patient and should provide sufficient challenge and intensity as any other patient regardless of age. Without challenging the individual, we fail to

---

Box 16.3 Case study: Self-directed rehabilitation

A 67-year-old gentleman was admitted after a middle cerebral artery infarct affecting his left side. He had significant spasticity in his left arm and no functional use. He spent 3 months in hospital. The multidisciplinary team felt that further inpatient rehabilitation was required to maximize outcome, however, the psychological impact of being away from his wife and family for more time was too great for him and affecting his psychological health. He had never previously spent time apart from his wife in their 42 years of marriage.

The gentleman went home with community therapy follow-up, downstairs living, and wheelchair dependent when he was manoeuvred out of his property. He loved gardening but was unable to access it. An opportunity arose following cessation of his community therapy to trial an unconventional patient-led intensive exercise programme (guided self-rehabilitation, GSR). This encompassed graded stretching exercises to facilitate muscle length and range in his right arm and was very different to hands-on therapy that he had been receiving. Performance could be tracked by the therapists and the patient in terms of repetition and outcomes.

Two months after using the GSR, this gentleman had returned to independent mobility with a stick (indoors), he stopped his antidepressants as he felt he no longer required them and he had started sleeping upstairs again and accessing his garden. He reported that his improvement had been a result of him taking control of his own recovery. He felt that he was simply a part in the rehabilitation process, whereas the GSR had allowed him to be leading it. If he worked, he saw results, through the tracking of his exercise and the results it yielded for him. He felt that he could challenge himself beyond the level therapists had challenged him because he was aware of his own limits and wasn't scared to push the boundaries.

---

encourage neuroplastic changes which further hamper recovery. Without enabling the individual to control their recovery and take responsibility for the outcome we limit their potential to achieve. Age should not play a part in the decision-making; the individual and our ability to enhance recovery as therapists are central to the rehabilitation process.

How much physiotherapy is enough?

There is much debate surrounding the amount and frequency of therapy required after stroke. Rehabilitation is an adaptive process where repetition and practice are likely key components needed to optimize outcomes. It is plausible that increased intensity may accelerate recovery but timing and what is actively delivered should be carefully considered. Immobility and/or bed rest are well-documented to have detrimental effects on hospital patients in general. Early mobilization (e.g. activities such as sitting out of bed, transfers, standing, and walking) aims to minimize the risk of the complications of immobility and improve functional recovery. However, the AVERT trial (2015) showed that very early, more frequent, higher dose mobilization focused on out-of-bed activities in addition to usual care was worse than usual care alone. Very early mobilization led to greater disability at 3 months with no effect on immobility-related complications or walking recovery.

There is little evidence to guide precisely how much or what type of therapy should be regarded as a minimum.[18] The development of the Royal College of Physicians of London Stroke guidelines have provided recommended levels of intensity and a guide on evidence based treatment that may be appropriate, enabling service users to gain access to a significant amount of therapy. However not everyone will require the same intensity.

Ultimately physiotherapy utilizes a variety of approaches to enhance physical function which can only be achieved through appropriate guidance of physiological change at a cellular level. Therefore, despite the lack of evidence perhaps it is fair to conclude that the greater potential there is for neuronal change—affected in part by how 'physiologically fit' the elderly individual is—the more effective intense and frequent treatment would be in gaining functional improvements.

Neuroplasticity

How each individual learns best is specific to that individual. The older person's ability to relearn may be compounded by multiple factors that are associated with the ageing process and individual lifestyle choices.[19–21]

It was a common conception that connections in our brains only developed and formed in our early years of life and are then fixed as we age.

Today we recognize that the brain continues to reorganize itself by forming new neuronal connections throughout life—a phenomenon called neuroplasticity—where the brain continues to adjust and reorganize. This can therefore facilitate recovery.

Existing pathways that are inactive or used for other purposes can take over 'lost' activities and there is evidence that reorganization in the adult brain can even involve the formation of new connections.[22]

Understanding the brain's ability to dynamically reorganize helps us to understand how people recover function after damage (such as a stroke) and why appropriate stimulation and activity promote brain reorganization to improve motor function.[23,24]

The ability to adapt may be doubted among older people, even with the most appropriate environment and therapy. Synaptic connections are continuously modified in response to demand, but an ageing brain may have less capacity to respond or may respond in a different way. As age increases, there is a reduction in brain white matter and neuronal volume within the brain.[25] If this is the case, how can we rehabilitate the older person post stroke? Experience in clinical practice demonstrates daily that we can alter performance with therapy regardless of age.

More recent research has highlighted that while the volume of specific structures within the brain may decrease, the functionality does not necessarily alter. As we age there is evidence of a greater breadth of function and recruitment of additional sites to facilitate performance that is not seen in the younger population but enhances performance significantly, arguably highlighting a more efficient functionality at a cellular level.[26]

Neuroplasticity remains relevant in the rehabilitation of the older person and can produce functional gains in all aspects of physical and cognitive performance—it is not age dependent.

We can conclude that lifestyle, the presence of comorbidities, and frailty will have far more influence on outcome post stroke in the older person than physiological change.

Types of therapeutic treatments

In order to cause neuroplastic change (either to restore or compensate for loss of function) various types of therapy are available to enhance motor recovery or provide a compensatory adjunct. Table 16.2 highlights the most common interventions.

The extent to which some of the treatments are available depends upon the health system of any given country and the financial capacity of the individual to source their treatments.

Table 16.2 Common physiotherapy approaches

Treatment	Indication
Constraint-induced movement therapy (CIMT)	A form of rehabilitation therapy that improves upper extremity function by increasing the use of their affected upper limb. In the United States, the prolonged duration of the therapy has resulted in restricted reimbursement.
'Modified' CIMT	As above but with a less restrictive more clinically relevant protocol for use. Can be delivered as an outpatient and has enjoyed high success rates internationally when compared to conventional CIMT.
Specific therapeutic handling	The therapist combines and applies their understanding of alignment, lever length, physiological understanding of what muscles, and cortical relearning to actively facilitate movement through the use of learnt techniques encouraging implicit and explicit learning.
Specific exercise and strengthening	The therapists identify focal weakness within a specific muscle or specific muscle group. Aerobic training is encouraged to enhance motor relearning.
Gait re-education	Specific analysis and physical handling are utilized to facilitate normal patterns of movement.
Robotics	Upper limb robotics to mimic normal movement, lower limb to facilitate gait (Re-walk). Limited currently and dependent on financial capability of the health system used.
Treadmill deweighting systems	Allows the patient to stand and practice gait while partly deweighted; facilitating normal function prior to being able to fully weight bear.
Virtual gaming	Wii/X-box utilized to encourage normal movement. If unfamiliar with this type of technology, it can be used with the older person as a novel task to enhance attention and therefore learning.
Splinting/Casting	To maintain tissue length, dampen spasticity, facilitate alignment during function.
Therapeutic taping	Applying dynamic tape directly to the skin in order to facilitate normal alignment and movement through range of muscles during activity. This is also used as a source of sensory input.
Functional electrical stimulation (FES)	Use of small electrical signals to directly stimulate muscles to contract. Facilitate sensation, movement, and help maintain muscle bulk/health.
Ankle foot orthosis (AFO)	Prevents foot drop during transfers/gait which in turn may prevent falls. Adjunct to gait re-education.

Treatment cessation

'Most stroke survivors do not get anything like the amount of therapy they need on the NHS to enable them to recover their independence and return to work, and they can't afford to pay privately for the often lengthy treatment required' (Andrew Marr; TV presenter and stroke survivor).

How many times do we hear 'my physio has stopped', 'can I have more physio?', and 'if I had more physio, I would get much better'?

The goal of any treatment programme is to help relearn skills that were lost to the best of the individual's capability. But how much intervention is enough?

The Stroke Association have stated that 'It is recommended if you have ongoing difficulties resulting from your stroke; you should continue to have rehabilitation (including physiotherapy) for as long as you need'.[27]

While we always hope for a full recovery and share the same desire as a stroke survivor to regain all function, sometimes the damage to the brain is so severe that the brain is irreparable and the neuroplasticity required is too great a demand; or the patient at this point in time has remained unchanged for a protracted period despite therapy input—rehabilitation has reached a limit where significant gains can no longer be expected. This is where there is a mismatch between desired recovery and actual recovery.

Balancing the prognostic indicators, patient perceptions, socioeconomic constraints, individual finances, and health insurance models, commissioned models of care, and autonomy of treating clinicians all impact on the cessation of therapy to varying degrees depending on where and how you live.

The identified goal to attain as an outcome of therapy is important and it must be remembered that not all goals will revolve around physical functionality, but rather quality of life (see Box 16.4).

We might assume that this is a terrible outcome for anyone. However, this individual continues to access some of his favourite pastimes and continues to have a quality of life. Everyone involved will have hoped for a full recovery, but this could not be achieved due to the severity of brain damage. Despite this, he continues to enjoy a good quality of life; often the ability to still be part of life through socialization and human interaction can be more important than regaining physical function. Formal 'therapy' involves a personal cost in terms of time, effort, and possibly repeated experience of failure. Other avenues of care may become more appropriate. Cessation of therapy is not always a bad thing.

Therapy shopping

Even when individuals may be informed of the minimal likely gains that further therapy will provide, as therapists serving both inpatient and community-based caseloads it has been our experience that there are many people who want more and 'therapy shop'. This occurs where there is a lack of understanding of what physiotherapy is and can achieve, an outlook of 'I want to return to my normal self before my stroke', and a perception that receiving more (or different) therapy will lead to a full recovery. For the older person, it is sometimes argued that as a lifelong taxpayer

---

Box 16.4 Case study: Quality of life

A 77-year-old male was a stroke survivor of three stroke events all within 6 months of each other. From the first two strokes he recovered independent mobility and returned to home and general life. Unfortunately, his third stroke affected him profoundly. It made him physically totally dependent for all care. His third stroke also affected his communication, cognition, visual fields and, as such, despite intensive therapy input he made very little recovery. The main objective for this gentleman was to ensure he could achieve supported sitting so that he could socialize with family and friends. Despite achieving this goal, he was unable to return home and was admitted to a nursing home. Despite being physically dependent for all his physical needs, he went on to marry his fiancé of 3 years. He continues to access his barber's for regular hair trims and wet shave, family events, and goes on regular outings with his new wife.

they are entitled to as much therapy as they perceive they need because they have paid for it. There is also a degree of self-entitlement to an abundance of physical therapy, despite the therapist knowing that this would yield minimal additional recovery.

While those who are financially able to invest in private therapy and can therefore pursue optimistic goals for as long as a therapist is willing to treat them, despite there being little progression or benefit that can be seen by the treating therapist, less affluent patients rely on the care systems to provide whatever is available in the face of competing demands on the resource.

It is at this stage that we urge any health professional to consider, during their consultation with their patient, investing time to explore interventions the patient has already received and provide and manage their patients' unrealistic expectations. Communication between health professionals is paramount prior to promising 'I will refer you for a bit more therapy'.

Extended roles

There are many different therapists in the world of stroke with extended roles, one of whom is that of the independent prescriber.

Within the United Kingdom, Allied Health Professionals (AHPs, including physiotherapists) can be licensed to prescribe independently within their competencies, following rigorous training. In the context of older people who have had a stroke, this can enhance the multidisciplinary management of patients and provide responsive care.

It shares the burden of medicines management across acute and community services, ensuring that we are minimizing adverse drug reactions and maximizing cost effectiveness through careful monitoring at every point of contact. However, it raises the issue of who is in overall strategic control of prescribing; in hospital this will usually be the medical consultant, and in the community the general practitioner, making clear lines of responsibility and communication very important.

Understanding the physiological process of ageing and disease processes that may be associated with the older person is paramount to rehabilitation. At every contact, there is an opportunity to understand not only the patient's physical abilities, but also concordance with medication which then provides an opportunity there and then to adjust, add, or omit medication to enhance optimal recovery (Box 16.5).

As AHPs continue to advance in prescribing, this skill can only serve to improve multidisciplinary therapy (MDT) as a whole, and thus the patient's experience of rehabilitation and ultimately provide a more responsive service.

Box 16.5 Case study: A successful use of the extended role

An 81-year-old lady suffered a stroke 10 years previously. A physiotherapist was asked to see her as she required recurrent antibiotics treatment to tackle infections in her right palm due to spasticity and contracture. Surgical opinion was sought regarding severing her tendons, but this was declined due to anaesthetic risk and conservative management was requested.

The physiotherapist prescribed and delivered botulinum toxin A to her finger flexors as part of a spasticity management programme. The outcome was life-changing for the patient. Although there was no gain in hand function, the patient reported less pain, fewer infections, increased access to the palm for hygiene and the reduced use of antibiotics.

This example demonstrates that the role of understanding the physiological effects of spasticity in this case was best place with the prescribing physiotherapist, skilled in this extended role.

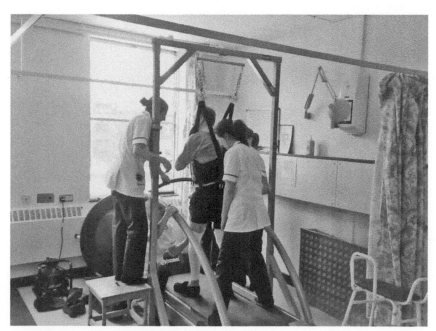

Fig. 16.2 Coordinating technology and therapy.

Box 16.6 Case study: Against all odds

A 71-year-old gentleman (previously independent, self-caring, a musician and writer; ex-army; physically very fit and lived a relatively healthy lifestyle; car driver; very driven to recover), suffered a right middle cerebral artery infarct resulting in significant left-sided weakness. He developed spasticity 2 weeks post stroke affecting the left side; the arm more than the leg.

Protracted length of stay to maximize rehabilitation potential (6 months). Discharged from hospital to home being able to transfer independently, mobilize with a tripod, and wearing an ankle foot support (AFO) indoors only. Required a wheelchair for outdoor mobility and needed carers for personal activities of daily living.

Therapy on discharge consisted of brief spell with a community team and then he paid privately for ongoing one-to-one therapy. He attended spasticity management clinic for upper and lower limb alongside surgical intervention for his left forearm (tendon transfers) coupled with further physiotherapy.

Eight years later he was mobile independently in- and outdoors using a stick as required outdoors. He returned to driving in an adapted car, writing books/plays, playing the guitar, and writing music. He has discovered that he is far more capable than he ever realized, leading to the current aspiration of representing GB in the 2020 Tokyo para-Olympic games. This would make him one of the oldest para-Olympians.

Regardless of the ongoing considered disability this shows that you can still strive for aspirations that initially seem beyond our expectations on every level.

This demonstrates that a winning formula for rehabilitation in older people requires a wide consideration of the individual and removal of stereotypical thinking that can restrict the potential for recovery before our patients have even begun their rehabilitation journey.

This gentleman remains evidently disabled to the untrained eye; however, internal drive, MDT support, and optimism not only from the patient but the clinicians involved in their care will inarguably produce a positive, age-defiant successful outcome.

Conclusion

This chapter has introduced the role of physiotherapy in stroke and the older person. The authors have attempted to provide an insight of the influencing factors for stroke management from a therapy perspective, identify the challenges surrounding the perception of the older person, and facilitate understanding of the treatments available.

Physiotherapy (alongside the rest of the MDT) is essential to enhancing recovery after a stroke. Age should not be a factor in delivery of care, merely a consideration of the presenting patient if it is relevant. Ongoing technological advancement and the ever-increasing developments in treatment options continue to inspire clinicians worldwide (Fig. 16.2). Physiotherapists provide the skills required to reduce or manage complications (such as spasticity and falls), maximize function, and enhance quality of life, and form a core component of the stroke multidisciplinary team. Box 16.6 provides a shining example of age being exactly what it is—just a number.

References

1. Truelsen T, Heuschmann PU, Bonita R, et al. Standard method for developing stroke registers in low-income and middle-income countries: experiences from a feasibility study of a stepwise approach to stroke surveillance (STEPS Stroke). *Lancet Neurol* 2007;6:134–9.

2. Buckinx F, Rolland Y, Reginster J-Y, Ricour C, Petermans J, & Bruyère O. Burden of frailty in the elderly population: perspectives for a public health challenge. *Arch Public Health* 2015;73(1):19.

3. Xue, Q.-L. The frailty syndrome: definition and natural history. *Clin Geriatr Med* 2011;27(1):1–15.

4. Clegg A, Young J, Iliffe S, Rikkert MO, & Rockwood K. Frailty in elderly people. *Lancet* 2013;381:752–62.

5. Mackintosh SF, Goldie P, & Hill K. Falls incidence and factors associated with falling in older, community-dwelling, chronic stroke survivors (>1 year after stroke) and matched controls. *Aging Clin Exp Res* 2005;17:74–81.

6. Goh HT, Nadarajah M, Hamzah NB, Varadan P, & Tan MP. Falls and fear of falling after stroke: a case-control study. *PM & R* 2016;8(12):1173–80.

7. Kerse N, Parag V, Feigin VL, et al. Auckland Regional Community Stroke (ARCOS) Study Group. Falls after stroke: results from the Auckland Regional Community Stroke (ARCOS) Study, 2002 to 2003. *Stroke* 2008;39:1890–3.

8. Ashburne A, Hyndman D, Pickering R, Yardley L, & Harris S. Predicting people with stroke at risk of falls. *Age Ageing* 2008;37:270–6.

9. Oxford Dictionaries. Available from: https://languages.oup.com/ [Accessed: 28 July 2019].

10. Chartered Society of Physiotherapy. *What is Physiotherapy?* 2017. Available from: https://www.csp.org.uk/careers-jobs/what-physiotherapy [Accessed: 28 July 2019].

11. NHS Choices 2017. *Overview: Physiotherapy*. Available from: https://www.nhs.uk/conditions/physiotherapy/ [Accessed: 28 July 2019].

12. Australian Physiotherapy Association. What is physio? 2017. Available from: https://choose.physio/what-is-physio [Accessed: 28 July 2019].

13. American Physical Therapy Association. Available from: http://www.apta.org/ [Accessed: 28 July 2019].

14. Intercollegiate Stroke Working Party. *National Clinical Guideline for Stroke,* 5th edition. London, UK: Royal College of Physicians, 2016.

15. Carr JH & Shepherd RB. *A Motor Relearning Programme for Stroke.* Oxford, UK: Butterworth-Heinemann, 1982.

16. British Bobath Association. Available from: https://www.bbta.org.uk [Accessed: 28 July 2019].

17. Knapp BH. *Skill in Sport: The Attainment of Proficiency.* London, UK: Routledge and Kegan Paul, 1963.

18. **Kwakkel G, van Peppen R, Wagenaar RC,** et al. Effects of augmented exercise therapy time after stroke: a meta-analysis. *Stroke* 2004;**35**:2529–39.

19. **Lang CE, Lohse KR, & Birkenmeier RL.** Dose and timing in neurorehabilitation: prescribing motor therapy after stroke. *Curr Opin Neurol* 2015;*28*(6):549–55.

20. **Park DC & Reuter-Lorenz P.** The adaptive brain: aging and neurocognitive scaffolding. *Ann Rev Psychol* 2009;**60**(1):173–96.

21. **Hedden T & Gabrieli JDE.** Insights into the ageing mind: a view from cognitive neuroscience. *Nat Rev Neurosci* 2004;**5**(2):87–96.

22. **Brown CE, Aminoltejari K, Erb H, Winship IR, & Murphy TH.** In vivo voltage-sensitive dye imaging in adult mice reveals that somatosensory maps lost to stroke are replaced over weeks by new structural and functional circuits with prolonged modes of activation within both the peri-infarct zone and distant sites. *J Neurosci* 2009;**29**:1719–34.

23. **Carmichael ST.** Cellular and molecular mechanisms of neural repair after stroke: making waves. *Ann Neurol* 2006;**59**:735–42.

24. **Dimyan MA & Cohen LG.** Neuroplasticity in the context of motor rehabilitation after stroke. *Nat Rev Neurol* 2011;**7**(2):76–85.

25. **Braver TS & West R.** Working memory, executive control, and aging. In: Craik FIM, & Salthouse TA (eds.) *The Handbook of Aging and Cognition*, 3rd edition, pp. 311–72. New York, USA: Psychology Press, 2008.

26. **Goh JO & Park DC.** Neuroplasticity and cognitive aging: the scaffolding theory of aging and cognition. *Rest Neurol Neurosci* 2009;**27**(5):391–403.

27. **Stroke Association.** *Physiotherapy After Stroke.* April 2012. Available from: https://www.stroke.org.uk/sites/default/files/physiotherapy_after_stroke.pdf [Accessed: 28 July 2019].

Chapter 17

Ethical and moral dilemmas including do not attempt resuscitation orders, advanced care planning, and end-of-life care

Rowan H. Harwood

What is ethics?

Ethics is the study and practice of correct decision-making, distinguishing right from wrong, and the moral principles that govern behaviour. No single set of rules adequately covers all human activity, including medical practice, but ethical frameworks can help us analyse and understand difficult situations, and resolve or address them through better understanding.

Ethics is close to, and overlaps, with other influences on behaviour, including the law, professional accountability, and culture. These vary over time and place, but are often based on ethical ideas. This account draws on the current position in England, but in the field of medical practice, the principles are broadly similar across developed societies and jurisdictions.

Laws are rules created by countries or communities that aim to regulate the actions of their members and which are enforced by means of penalties or sanctions. Laws define who may practice as a doctor, prescription of medicines, consent, and compulsory treatment, mental capacity to take decisions, financial remuneration, redress for errors, and handling of human tissues. Particularly important laws confer rights (so-called human rights), such as the right to life, private and family life, and freedom from degrading or inhumane treatment, and control the handling and confidentiality of personal data.

A profession is an occupation with a particular training and implying a position of responsibility and trust. Professions are regulated, primarily to ensure that public confidence is maintained, and vulnerable people protected. Regulators determine who can practice, stipulate ongoing education, and often publish 'ethical guidance'. For example, in the United Kingdom, the General Medical Council has a library of advice (https://www.gmc-uk.org/guidance).[1]

'Culture' describes the attitudes and behavioural characteristic of a social group. Quite apart from law and regulation, and sometimes in contravention to it, people have expectations about healthcare, who should be consulted over decisions, and how we should approach death and dying. Problems in delivering medical care may have as much to do with culture as it does with ethics and law.

Difficult decisions in stroke medicine

All aspects of stroke medicine (prevention, acute care, and rehabilitation) include the need to make decisions, and these can be among the most challenging in all of medicine. Some examples are given in Table 17.1.

Table 17.1 Difficult decisions in stroke medicine

Decision	Issues
Anticoagulants for atrial fibrillation	Effective prevention vs. burden of taking medication and monitoring, risk of bleeding
Carotid endarterectomy for stenosis	Perioperative stroke risk vs. longer-term stroke prevention; variation in surgical performance, rapid loss of efficacy with time after index TIA
Thrombolysis for acute infarction	Better functional outcomes vs. risk of bleeding; sensitivity to time- and protocol-compliance; need for system redesign
Hemicraniectomy for malignant infarction	Risk of survival with severe disability
Surgery for intracranial haemorrhage	Uncertainty. Efficacy data are lacking, but trials may have excluded those most likely to benefit. Risk of survival with severe disability
Admission to intensive care units. Intubation and ventilation	Enabling physiological normalization or support. Unlikely effectiveness. High cost. Risk of survival with severe disability
Feeding tube insertion	Unlikely effectiveness. Cost. Risk of survival with severe disability
Cardiopulmonary resuscitation	Unlikely effectiveness. Cost. Risk of survival with severe disability
Secondary prevention medication	Prevention of recurrence vs. tablet and side effect burden. High numbers needed to treat (population vs. individual ethics)
Lifestyle choices (smoking, activity, body weight)	Risk of recurrence, individual responsibility, medical paternalism
Continuation or cessation of rehabilitation	Uncertain effectiveness; possibility of late functional gains; cost, effort, access
Discharge home	Respect of identity with return to symbolically important and familiar environment; risk of falls, isolation, need for adaptations and human help

Ethical systems

There are many systems of ethical analysis (known as 'normative ethics') which fall into four main groups. These have been developed over many centuries dating back to the Chinese masters, classical Greece, the theology of many faiths, the philosophy of the enlightenment, and twentieth-century insights into social psychology and feminism. The four groups are:

1. *Consequentialism.* Whether an action is right or wrong depends on its outcomes, or consequences. The intended or likely benefits of an action must justify the burdens and risks involved. An example is utilitarianism, which holds that the right action is the one which results in the greatest good for the greatest number. The limit to consequentialism comes when the good end is achieved by means of actions that are fundamentally bad for some other reason (such as deliberately taking life, or compromising someone else's well-being or liberty).

2. *Rights and duties (deontology).* This approach holds that all people have fundamental rights, such as the right to life, to have personal information kept confidential, or to be consulted about

medical treatment. Many of these rights are enshrined in declarations, such as the European Convention on Human Rights, and statute laws.

3. *Virtues*. Ethical action results from the display of personal characteristics or predispositions, such as honesty, courage, compassion, forgiveness, and generosity. These form the basis of many religious teachings, and cultural expectations.

4. *Communication and relationships*. The right action is the one that results from exchange of information and views from the perspectives of all stakeholders, and seeks to maintain and develop relationships between them.

'Practical ethics' describes how practitioners decide on actions in practice.

These ethical approaches can all lead to contradictions or conflicts, and none is wholly adequate for all situations. Analysing difficulties using different systems can bring clarity about why problems arise, a first step towards resolution.

Principlism

The most important contemporary framework for medical decision-making, known as 'principlism', was set out by Beauchamp and Childress (1979),[2] and combines two approaches, consequentialism and deontology. Together the principles allow decisions to be made in most medical situations, and are consistent with most cultures.

The four principles are:

1. Benefits (beneficence)

2. Avoiding burdens and harms (non-maleficence)

3. Autonomy

4. Justice

Each should be respected as far as possible. Benefits are actual or potential physical, psychological, or social gains, in terms of prevention or cure of disease, lengthening life, relieving symptoms, improving function, giving information, or supporting families and other carers. Burdens are adverse effects, complications, risks, debility, and time expended. Benefits and burdens may be uncertain or unpredictable.

Autonomy is the right to self-determination, or for an individual to make informed choices for themselves. Justice is about non-discrimination (on the basis of characteristics not pertinent to the decision), and the duty to make the best use of limited resources. In fee-for-service healthcare systems, the 'right' to a share of resources is far from guaranteed. Assessing 'opportunity cost' asks what else might have been done with resources if they are not used as they were? Age and personal characteristics, such as smoking, may or may not be grounds for limiting access to healthcare, including where the characteristic is strongly associated with adverse outcomes; for example, some neurosurgery among the very old. UK equality law defines 'protected characteristics' on the basis of which access to public services must be fair (age, sex, disability, race, religion, marital status, pregnancy or maternity, and sexual orientation).

Some sort of balancing between principles must take place in the course of practical decision-making. It is rarely possible to avoid all burdens and risk, but the anticipated benefits should justify them. Different individuals may make different decision in drawing this balance, based on personality, experiences, beliefs, values, hopes, and fears (e.g. 'risk-takers' vs. 'risk averse'). The exercise of autonomy may, therefore, contribute to drawing the balance about what is acceptable in terms of burden and potential gain.

Principlism is a useful and practical framework, but does not always provide conclusive guidance on how to act. There are two fundamental limits to the application of principlism:

◆ There is no definitive way of balancing conflicting principles. We often presume that autonomy takes precedence. However, decisions can be complex, abstract, or intangible, and some people struggle with ideas such as probability or futility. In cases where healthcare professionals think that intervention is highly unlikely to deliver benefits, or recklessly risky, or requires resources that are not available, relying on autonomy alone is insufficient.

◆ Autonomy cannot be expressed where mental capacity to understand the issues involved in making a decision is lacking. In an attempt to respect self-determination, we invoke proxy or substitute decisions, which introduces further uncertainty and potential conflict.

Communication and relationship-based ethics

Communication between stakeholders is central to all ethical decision-making, but some ethical thinking makes a virtue of building and maintaining relationships in its own right, including respect for emotions, and caring as a disposition (a virtue).

This approach can be useful in difficult situations involving people who lack mental capacity. It can involve a lot of explanation and information-giving, negotiation, and consensus-building, including explicitly recognizing, and trying to accommodate or mitigate, divergent or opposing points of view. An example is the recently popular approach of 'shared decision-making'.

Communication and relationship-based approaches also have limitations. It is not sufficient simply to do as the patient, family, or concerned others, want, in order to keep them happy. They may lack sufficient knowledge, and need guidance in interpreting and applying it to a particular case. Prejudice or strong emotions can be a barrier to rational thought. It may be reasonable to try something, even when the chances of success are small, but equally, vulnerable patients (or families) need protection from misinformation, deception, exploitation, or false hope.

Consent

Consent is agreement to have an examination, investigation, treatment, care, or surgery (or outside of medicine, to do anything else, such as enter into a contract, marry, or engage in sexual relations). Consent is an expression of autonomy, the right to choose. To be valid, consent must be:

◆ Capacitous (the person must understand what they are doing)

◆ Informed (the person must have enough information on which to base a decision)

◆ Un-coerced (freely given)

◆ Ongoing (consent can be withdrawn at any time)

Consent can be explicit (asked for and granted) or implicit (implied through behaviours, such as coming to the doctor for advice, or cooperating with a test). Explicit consent may be verbal or written. Both are equally valid, but verbal consent is harder to prove after the event.

Treatment without consent may be considered an assault, a criminal offence.

Mental capacity (also known as mental competence)

Mental capacity describes the ability of an individual to make decisions. Assessing mental capacity is a prerequisite for legal and ethical decision-making, as the approach varies according to whether it is present or not.

Having mental capacity requires the ability to retain, understand, and use information related to the decision, and communicate that decision. The person must be able to understand the nature, purpose, and consequences of the proposed intervention, any alternatives, and the consequences of refusal.

There are various tests for specific decisions such as making a will, or giving a power of attorney (authority for someone else to make decisions on your behalf).

Mental capacity is decision- and time-specific. Patients may be able to consent to some things, but not others, and capacity may fluctuate, for example, due to delirium or severe anxiety. Strictly mental capacity should be assessed for every decision about every examination, test, care procedure, or treatment, but usually this will be informal and implicit, reserving formal assessment for important or potentially contentious decisions.

Assessing mental capacity in practice can be difficult. While some cases are clear, others are borderline or uncertain. Questions that arise include:

◆ How much understanding must be shown?

◆ How long information must be retained?

◆ How is reasoning or use of information to be demonstrated?

◆ Which possible consequences or alternatives should be revealed?

The threshold for each of these is arbitrary. Aphasia and severe illness can make assessment difficult. Speech and language therapists may help with decision-making for patients with aphasia by assessing level of comprehension, or explaining procedures (such as percutaneous endoscopic gastrostomy (PEG) insertion) in the optimal way, including use of picture cards ('supported conversation'). A translator (professional or family) is required if patient and healthcare professional do not share a common language.

An approach might include the following:

◆ assess communication (comprehension and expression)

◆ assess cognition

◆ describing the problem and proposed treatment

◆ ask the patient for their opinion, to recap the information given, the reasons for the decision, and appreciation of risks and consequences

In English Law, understanding need only be in 'broad terms', and 'sufficient to be able to make a decision'.

The main problems after a stroke are:

◆ coma

◆ aphasia

◆ cognitive impairment or delirium due to stroke

◆ comorbid dementia or learning disabilities

◆ other communication problems such as deafness

Medical interventions without consent in conditions which may only be temporary should be limited to those required to preserve life and immediate health. In practice, this rarely applies in stroke:

◆ We may not know how reversible the condition will be (e.g. cognitive impairment or aphasia)—or how quickly it might reverse.

◆ Sometimes, if you are going to treat something at all, you need to treat quickly—such as antibiotics or rehydration.

As a general rule, if someone has presented to hospital, it is reasonable to give nursing and medical care (i.e. anything short of operative procedures), as you think is best practice and in their best interests, unless or until someone objects. At that point you can reassess more formally:

◆ Formally consider someone's capacity to consent

◆ The nature of the objection

◆ The likely alternatives

◆ The closeness of the relationship with the person

◆ Whether someone else has relevant information or views which must be sought prior to making a decision

◆ What best interest comprises

Any proposed operative procedure (such as placing a feeding tube) should trigger the same process.

Best interests

Assessment of best interests attempts to respect the autonomy of the person lacking capacity, by trying to identify what they would have wanted if they had capacity. The process is open to uncertainty. In the United Kingdom, if a person lacks mental capacity, a treatment may be legally given if it is in the patient's best interest.

In assessing best interests, we should:

◆ try to involve the person in the discussion

◆ take account of their current and previously expressed wishes, beliefs, preferences, and values

◆ seek the opinions of family members and others close to or concerned for the well-being of the patient (in the United Kingdom 'next of kin' has no legal status in this context)

◆ use the least restrictive alternative

The technical issue of effectiveness still holds—the benefits of treatment must justify the burdens. As with people having mental capacity, this balance may vary from one person to another.

Some people might have made advance care plans, such as a written statement of wishes and preferences. These can be useful in giving a general indication of what might or might not be wanted. Otherwise the role of family members or informants is crucial. They are asked both for their report of what the person may have said in the past, and what they think they would have said if they were able to.

In emergency situations, treatment may be given without consent to a person lacking mental capacity if it is necessary to preserve life or health, if there is no clear reason to believe that they would not have wanted it. In some jurisdictions, doctors may be under an obligation to act in these circumstances.

Proxy and substitute decision-makers

A *proxy* is someone who speaks on behalf of the person, and can to tell you what the patient would have said, because they had discussed the issues previously. The degree of uncertainty is greater when the exact circumstances have not been discussed, but opinions may still be known in general terms. This is equivalent to asking 'knowing the person as you do, what do you think they would have wanted?'

A *substitute judgement* asks what the informant (relative, friend, or staff member) would want in this situation. This may be useful when someone is of a particular religious faith, where general principals are well known. Staff making this judgement are essentially saying 'as a fellow human being, what would I have wanted?' This has some validity, but opinions vary widely. People with a condition generally view it as less bad than do healthcare staff, relatives, or members of the general population (who are the most averse to descriptions of severe disability). Most the population, when asked, rate living with a severe stroke as bad as death, or worse than death. A minority disagrees, however, some strongly.

Lasting (or durable) power of attorney is a legal device to give a person authority to act as a proxy to make decisions (medical, welfare, financial, or property) on behalf of another. At the time of making a power of attorney, the person giving it must have mental capacity to do so, but the arrangement can persist even after the loss of capacity. If one of these is not in place, a Court may appoint a person (deputy) to act in the same way.

Advance care planning

This is a means for someone who has mental capacity to promote and extend patient autonomy, in advance of a time when it may be lost. It may take the form of a statement of wishes or preferences, an advance decision to refuse treatment, or the appointment of a Lasting Power of Attorney.

The context should generally be a long-standing, trusting professional relationship. The time after a stroke will not usually be a good one for advance care planning:

◆ Health and function may be changing rapidly.

◆ Psychological consequences of stroke, including depression and cognitive impairment, may compromise judgement.

◆ The process of psychological adjustment may lead to dramatic changes in attitudes and values.

◆ The professional relationship will often be too short, and potentially open to conflicts of interest.

Some people may, however, choose the time after a stroke to consider how they would like to plan for future healthcare. The patient's GP or care home manager should be invited to contribute. Plans are usually most useful for someone who is very disabled, and would prefer to avoid re-admission to hospital in the case of deterioration. Unfortunately, many people in this situation lack mental capacity to engage in the process. The Royal College of Physicians has published sensible guidelines.[3]

Shared decision-making

Shared decision-making attempts to improve the match between what clinicians offer and what patients want in healthcare, and may be considered an application of communication-based ethics. The ideas support the desire for greater patient and family engagement in decision-making and avoidance of dissatisfaction with medical care. It can be applied to screening, investigation strategies, and other care arrangements (such as moving to a care home or not).

A condition is 'preference-sensitive' when there are several treatment options that might produce different results. The 'right' decision depends on patient-specific factors such as different priorities and values.

The process requires:

◆ at least two participants, including the clinician and patient, and possibly family or advocates

◆ parties share information, reflecting their different areas of expertise (Table 17.2)[4]

Table 17.2 Clinician and patient expertise in shared decision-making

Clinician's expertise	Patient's expertise
Diagnosis	Experience of illness
Disease aetiology	Social circumstances
Prognosis	Values
Treatment options	Preferences
Outcome probabilities	Attitude to risk
Uncertainties	

Source data from Coulter A, Collins A. *Making shared decision-making a reality*. London, Kings Fund. Copyright © 2011, The King's Fund. http://www.kingsfund. org.uk/publications/making-shared-decision-making-reality.

◆ patients or families are supported to deliberate about choices and their consequences

◆ reaching consensus on the treatment or care

◆ a system for recording, communicating, and implementing the decision

  A shared decision-making conversation should:

◆ support patients to understand and articulate what they want to achieve from the treatment (their preferred outcome or goal)

◆ help them articulate their current understanding of their condition

◆ inform them about their condition, the treatment options available, and the benefits, burdens, and risks of each

◆ where information is uncertain or lacking

◆ a means of helping people clarify their preferences

◆ support them in making trade-offs between goals

◆ ensure that patients and clinicians arrive at a decision based on mutual understanding.

  Many people struggle to make a decision in the face of:

◆ a mass of unfamiliar, complex, and technical information

◆ uncertainties and risks

◆ priorities and fears, which may be conflicting

◆ anxiety

◆ time pressure

A counselling approach with a clinician or health coach is required. The main obstacles are that clinicians do not always have counselling skills (tending instead to adopt an informing approach), nor the time. In which case, others can help (often trained nurses or allied health professionals). Decision support tools may be available, including information sheets, more detailed written material or computer programmes, DVDs, or interactive websites that include filmed interviews with patients and professionals. These are different from more traditional patient information materials because they do not tell people what to do, but aim to set out the facts and help people to deliberate about options.

Empirical evidence suggests that shared decision-making is effective, in:

- improved knowledge and understanding
- developing more accurate risk perceptions
- increasing comfort with decisions
- greater participation
- better treatment adherence
- improved confidence and coping skills
- improved health behaviours
- fewer patients choosing major surgery
- more appropriate service use

Quantified decision-making

'Prevention is better than cure'. But there may be a cost. Anticoagulation for atrial fibrillation (AF) and endarterectomy for carotid artery stenosis are examples where intervention, on average over a population of patients, does more good than harm, yet some individuals will be harmed (by bleeding or perioperative stroke).

These conditions have been well-researched, and the size of risks and benefits quantified. This enables numbers (or decision-aid diagrams indicating probabilities) to be used when deciding on treatments with patients. Three factors must be considered:

- Individual baseline risk: most treatments reduce risk by a set proportion (the relative risk). How much benefit is expected depends on both this and the baseline risk (the absolute risk reduction). In the case of AF, this can be determined from a risk score such as CHA2DS2VASc. In carotid stenosis, degree of narrowing, other risk factors including age and time since the index transient ischaemic attack (TIA), determine risk of subsequent stroke. This can be used to calculate number needed to treat NNT = 1/absolute risk reduction = 1/(RR × baseline risk).
- Expected risks. Risk scores such as HASBLED, or a corresponding number needed to harm (NNH), can be calculated.
- How well the treatment is delivered. For carotid surgery, this includes timing of surgery and surgeon-specific complication rates. For AF it is drug choice or anticoagulation control.

Cardiopulmonary resuscitation (CPR)

Making anticipatory decisions about CPR as an important part of good clinical care. This allows practitioners to avoid delivering care that may not be wanted or may have no chance of success. The usual principals apply—except that CPR and do not attempt resuscitation (DNAR) orders have become subject to ill-informed press and political opinion, and, in the United Kingdom, prescriptive legal decisions, that may jeopardize ethical practice.

People with cerebral vascular disease often have coronary artery disease as well. If primary neurological death is not expected, and in the absence of severe comorbidities or complications, there is no reason to expect that people with mild or moderate stroke might not benefit from CPR if they collapse unexpectedly with cardiac arrest. In these cases, a 'presumption of active treatment' is reasonable, unless we have information to the contrary.

For patients who have had a severe stroke or who are frail, the main issue is futility—where a treatment cannot, or is highly unlikely, to achieve its end. Resuscitation is successful when cardiac arrest is due to ventricular tachyarrhythmias or ventricular fibrillation, which most often occurs shortly after myocardial infarction. Success rate to discharge after CPR attempts on coronary care units are about 50%. On general medical wards, they are perhaps 5%. A third or more of survivors develop new hypoxic brain damage.

A long list of conditions is associated with poor (or negligible) chances of success. These include:

- severe stroke
- systemic sepsis
- severe metabolic derangements
- renal failure
- disseminated malignancy
- severe anaemia
- severe lung disease
- pulmonary embolism
- 'severe general frailty'

In these cases, death is not due to an acute arrhythmia, and CPR is futile. For example, in severe stroke death is due to brain damage, or oedema, raised intracranial pressure, and tentorial herniation, pulmonary embolism, or sepsis.

A patient may tell you that they would not want a CPR attempt, which should be respected under the general rules of consent. Otherwise, you will have to ask. If a patient with capacity is at foreseeable risk of cardiac or respiratory arrest, and the healthcare team has doubts about whether the benefits of CPR would outweigh the burdens, or whether the level of recovery expected would be acceptable to the patient, this should be discussed with the patient.

Some clinicians argue that it is unduly worrying to approach all patients about their wishes routinely. Unfortunately, the issues are often not well understood. The success of CPR is generally overestimated, patients discussing CPR may feel they are being told they are going to die, or fear they are not valued, or might be denied other treatments. Written information sheets can help introduce the subject in a non-threatening way. Current UK guidance and legal rulings require, however, that if the patient has mental capacity, they should be told if a DNAR order is made.

For patients who are not able to give their own opinions, we can ask family or close friends what the patient would have wanted were they able to say. This information can best be appended to discussions about other things. If CPR is likely to be futile it may be more a matter of 'telling' than 'asking'. Avoid concentrating on asking the family what they want (although you may still ask their view). It is the patient's best interest that concerns you. This is informed by what the family say, but not determined by it. Be aware that some people value life almost at all costs (e.g. some orthodox Jews and Muslims).

Dementia, in particular, is a distressing condition, and you should think very carefully about resuscitation attempts on anyone with moderate dementia or worse.

Current UK guidelines from the British Medical Association, Resuscitation Council (UK) and Royal College of Nursing, are sensible and measured.[5]

Drips and feeding tubes

A balance sheet of potential goods and potential harm is given in Table 17.3

Table 17.3 Benefits and burdens balance sheet for feeding decisions

Potential good	Potential harm
Relieve thirst and hunger	Risk of death or complications during insertion of PEG
Prolong life	Prolong the process of dying
Ensure best chance of making a recovery	Survival in a distressing, highly dependent state
Minimize muscle catabolism, preserving muscle mass	
Ease of nursing, delivery of medication	

If the patient is in a position to give an opinion about the desirability of inserting a gastros-tomy tube, it should be discussed with them. Often they are not: the main problem in deciding is *uncertainty*, about:

◆ Recovery. Patients admitted with swallowing problems, which do not resolve within a couple of weeks usually have had severe strokes. We know that for patients with total anterior circula-tion strokes, 60% will be dead within a year, and only 4% will recover to independence (fewer, if we exclude patients with initially severe deficits which recover quickly).

◆ How people feel about the value or worth of the likely outcomes. Most people (but not all) con-sider life with a severe stroke to be at least as bad as death. We are relatively poor at predicting who will do well.

◆ The quality of the evidence on the individual's views. We are usually dependent on what family or friends say the person's opinion would have been, based on what they said before, or what they think they would have said before.

An alternative way of looking at the problem from the standpoint of 'best interest' and autonomy is to consider what the individual would give up to achieve what they want as a final outcome:

◆ If we want to give people their best chance of a survival and recovery, we should feed as many as possible, in order not to miss those who do well despite initially poor signs.

◆ If the person had strong feelings about not surviving in a dependent state, they might be willing to trade the small chance of a good recovery for the avoidance of the much larger probability of surviving but being dependent.

Strictly, the arguments for and against gastrostomy apply to nasogastric feeding, and intravenous or subcutaneous fluids (except that these options have necessarily time-limited reviews, since cannulae must be resited and tubes replaced).

Experience shows that if there has been difficulty deciding whether or not to insert a feeding tubes, most patients die within a few weeks. This suggests we err on the side of intervention. The FOOD trials demonstrated that decisions about type and timing of tube feeding have relatively little effects on outcome.[6]

Tube feeding is legally a 'medical treatment'. Ordinary feeding by mouth is not. If we are not feeding someone, or intending to do so, it is illegal to deny them free access to food and drink, even if their swallow is 'unsafe'. Clearly if any attempt at swallowing leads to distressing aspiration, it cannot be considered in their interests. Most likely the patient would not want to try after one bad experience. However, if able to communicate, that should be up to the patient. Sips of water are unlikely to cause undue problems. In any case, mouth care is especially important for any pa-tient who is not swallowing.

End-of-life care

Around 15–20% of people suffering a stroke will die within a month. Several clinical features of strokes are associated with a poor outcome, including unconsciousness, haemorrhages, total anterior circulation stroke, dysphagia, gaze palsy, breathing abnormalities, heart disease, severe comorbidity, or pre-existing disability, hyperglycaemia, pyrexia, AF, and delirium. However, no single feature, or prognostic score, determined soon after stroke onset, is sufficiently accurate to allow us to predict death (or survival) with certainty in an individual patient.

Knowing that a patient is going to die can be useful, even if little can be done to prevent it.

◆ Sometimes the patient can make choices about care, settle affairs, and say goodbye.

◆ Families can gather and are prepared for the worst.

◆ Staff can prioritize symptom relief and can avoid futile and burdensome treatments.

◆ It may be possible to arrange discharge home for end-of-life care if that is what everyone wants.

'Palliating' is 'alleviation without cure'. By this definition, much medical care is palliation. It is not non-treatment, or withdrawal of treatments, rather a prioritization of treatments with the aim of relieving distress, minimizing treatment-related burden, and maintaining as much independence, autonomy, and control as possible. 'Terminal care' is the management of patients in whom death is thought to be certain, and not far off, and for whom medical effort is wholly directed at relief of symptoms, and psychological support of patient and family rather than cure or prolongation of life.

All other things being equal, prolonging life is a good thing. However:

◆ We may be over-optimistic and intervene too vigorously when death is likely.

◆ We can initiate a self-fulfilling prophesy—not treating someone because we think they are dying, and they die for lack of a treatment which would otherwise have saved them.

◆ Sometimes palliative and potentially curative approaches must proceed together, as so-called twin track care. We may still want to attempt life-prolonging treatment when the chances of success are small, but not completely hopeless. However, we may have to treat many people unsuccessfully to save one life, which may not be justified if the treatment is unpleasant, uncomfortable, or compromises dignity.

◆ A balance must be drawn between falsely raising expectations and not extinguishing hope. 'Hope for the best, but plan for the worst'.

Some other patients 'fail to thrive' or 'turn their head to the wall' after initial survival. Beware the possibility of severe depression, undiagnosed physical comorbidity, or complications, but consider if these patients too are dying.

The timeframe over which palliative stroke care occurs is from a few hours to several months, and these determine how the problem is approached:

◆ Severe stroke, leading to rapid neurological death

◆ Complications of stroke (e.g. pneumonia, in the early or recovery phase)

◆ 'Stroke presentation' of tumour, inoperable abscess, or subdural haematoma

◆ 'Incidental' stroke occurring in someone dying from another condition, such as cancer or severe heart or respiratory failure

The key principals of palliative medicine are:

◆ Meticulous management of symptoms

◆ Open communication

- Psychological, emotional, and spiritual support of the patient and of those close to them
- Advance care planning

Symptoms may be stroke related, including aspiration pneumonia or seizures, or more general, such as pain, delirium, breathlessness, or nausea. Guidance on drug management of symptoms at the end of life is widely available, for example, in the United Kingdom's Palliative Care Formulary. Fortunately, severe pain is rarely an issue for a dying stroke patient.

Managing uncertainty can be difficult. Supportive care, such as intravenous hydration, may be necessary to temporize, while nature takes its course towards death or improvement. Uncertainty should be acknowledged, and a decision may change in the light of events. This may look like indecision and prevarication, but it is inevitable.

Proactive family engagement is important to gather information about previous health, attitudes, beliefs, and preferences; to inform them about diagnosis, treatment, and prognosis, and to help meet their psychological, emotional, and spiritual needs. If the patient is aware, the family will be important in providing company and comfort, and they may engage in practical tasks such as mouth care.

A framework for such discussions includes:

- Ascertaining from patient or family what their understanding of the illness and its prognosis is, and informing or correcting if needed
- Identifying priorities for expected time remaining
- Identifying fears
- Negotiating what can be traded-off to achieve the priorities and avoid the fears (e.g. use of feeding tubes or antibiotics)

Clear plans should be agreed on action to be taken if deterioration occurs (escalation or palliation), including a DNACPR order, and on criteria for readmission to hospital if a discharge home or to a care home is contemplated.

Managing decision-making

Information and explanations should be primarily directed to the patient if they are able to comprehend. Decisions should be made by the person to whom they apply. Who else they want told, or to help or support them in making decisions (even a spouse or children), is up to them. Avoid telling relatives something that you have not told a patient who is in a position to be told.

An extreme view of confidentiality, however, does not represent good practice either. Confidentiality has to be traded-off against pragmatism and courtesy. If a patient is severely ill, unable to communicate, or otherwise speak for themselves, close relatives will naturally be concerned and want to know what is going on. Moreover, family members are likely to be the best source of information about someone's medical past, and their likely wishes.

Taking the lead on decision-making has traditionally fallen to doctors, but there is no particular reason why this should be so. Senior medical staff should be available and willing to support others in this role. Sometimes a problem can be introduced by one professional and followed up by another, if a difficult decision needs to be broken gently, if time is needed to think the problem through, or consult others.

Summary

Healthcare professionals should be, and almost always are, motivated by a desire to do good and avoid harm. Stroke care raises situations where the best course of action is not clear. Ethical theory helps to understand these dilemmas but applying them in practice needs knowledge (about stroke and about people), time, skills in communication, teamwork, and managing situations, compassion and sensitivity, and broad-mindedness. This only comes from experience, professionalism, and the support of teams and colleagues.

Practitioners must be adept at thinking about benefits, burdens, autonomy, mental capacity, developing communication skills, and building trusting relationships, should respect fundamental rights, and show virtues of honesty, compassion, and courage.

References

1. **General Medical Council.** 'Good Medical Practice' and 'A-Z of ethical guidance'. Available from: https://www.gmc-uk.org/guidance [Accessed: 29 July 2019].
2. **Beauchamp TL & Childress JF.** *Principles of Medical Ethics.* New York, NY: Oxford University Press, 1979.
3. **Intercollegiate Stroke Working Party.** *National Clinical Guideline for Stroke,* 5th edition. London, UK: Royal College of Physicians, 2016.
4. **Kings Fund, Coulter A,** & **Collins A.** Making shared decision-making a reality. London, Kings Fund 2011. Available from: http://www.kingsfund.org.uk/publications/making-shared-decision-making-reality [Accessed: 29 July 2019].
5. **British Medical Association, the Resuscitation Council (UK) and the Royal College of Nursing.** *Decisions Relating to Cardiopulmonary Resuscitation, A Joint Statement,* 3rd edition, 2014. Available from: http://www.resus.org.uk/pages/dnar.pdf [Accessed: 29 July 2019].
6. **FOOD triallists** (2005). Effect of timing and method of enteral tube feeding for dysphagic stroke patients (FOOD): a multicentre randomised controlled trial. *Lancet* 2005;**365**:764–72.

Chapter 18

Assessing capacity and decision-making

Thomas McGowan and Adrian Blundell

What is capacity?

We all make multiple decisions in the course of a day, from minor choices such as what to wear through to potentially more significant ones such as whether to accept or decline specific medical treatments. Mental capacity is this ability to make autonomous decisions, and this chapter will deal with the practical, legal, and ethical components of dealing with this common situation based on the legal situation in England and Wales (the legal position in Scotland and Northern Ireland will be dealt with at the end of the chapter).

The Mental Capacity Act 2005[1] (MCA) provides a framework for decision-making on behalf of adults over the age of 16 who are found to lack capacity to make their own decisions. The MCA sets out five statutory principles (Box 18.1). In addition, capacity assessments are both decision specific (e.g. a person may have capacity to decide what to eat for lunch, without necessarily having capacity to decide whether or not to accept complex medical treatments or understand the risks of an unsupported discharge) and time specific (e.g. a person may not have capacity when distracted by severe pain). Assessment of capacity should be delayed, where possible, if it is thought that the person may regain capacity.

Suffering a stroke may lead to impairment of higher cortical function which can lead to a diminution of a person's ability to make independent decisions. This can subsequently mean difficulty for health and social care professionals in assessing a patient's ability to make their own decisions, both with regards to their medical care and their discharge.

Box 18.1 Statutory principles of the Mental Capacity Act 2005

1. A person must be assumed to have capacity unless it is established that they lack capacity.

2. A person is not to be treated as unable to make a decision unless all practicable steps to help him to do so have been taken without success.

3. A person is not to be treated as unable to make a decision merely because he makes an unwise decision.

4. An act done, or decision made, under this Act for or on behalf of a person who lacks capacity must be done, or made, in his best interests.

5. Before the act is done, or the decision is made, regard must be had to whether the purpose for which it is needed can be as effectively achieved in a way that is less restrictive of the person's rights and freedom of action.

Reproduced from the Mental Capacity Act 2005 c.9 (Eng). Contains public sector information licensed under the Open Government Licence v3.0.

Capacity does not depend on the wisdom of that decision, as the Act also states that 'A person is not to be treated as unable to make a decision merely because he makes an unwise decision'. This means that the MCA cannot be used to modify patient decisions that the medical team disagrees with unless that team are satisfied the patient cannot make the decision themselves. The legal case exemplifying this was a patient known as C, who was detained under the Mental Health Act at Broadmoor due to paranoid schizophrenia. He developed gangrene in his leg, which in the opinion of the medical team was likely to be fatal if he did not undergo an amputation of his leg, which he refused. The court upheld the right of C to refuse this treatment and refuse the amputation.[2]

Assessing capacity

Assessing capacity follows a two-stage process as shown in Fig. 18.1.

This second stage of capacity assessment is broken down into four further stages, as shown in Fig. 18.2.

Assessing capacity in an older person who has suffered a stroke follows the same principles as any other patient, although most patients will, by definition, have had a disturbance of brain function. This requires health and social care professionals to be mindful of this, as capacity assessments are likely to be more commonplace in such patients.

It is essential to remember that poor performance on cognitive assessments does not automatically mean that a person lacks capacity and while cognitive assessments can provide useful background information, they do not allow a decision to be made on the score alone.[3] Capacity to make decisions may well fluctuate with time, and determining this may need repeated assessments with decisions being made when the patient is most likely to be able to make these decisions independently. Capacity assessment is not specifically a medical domain, but rather should be performed by each member of the multidisciplinary team (MDT) for the decisions relevant to them (e.g. the social worker may decide capacity for place of discharge decisions while the doctor should decide capacity for proposed medical treatments).

Emergency decisions, such as the decision whether or not to thrombolyse a patient presenting to hospital with a stroke, fall into an area of medicine in which decisions on capacity must be made very quickly. Medical professionals would still be expected to perform assessments of capacity in these situations, but if the patient was felt to need further support in order to be able to make a decision, the code of practice makes it clear that 'in some situations treatment cannot be delayed while a person gets support to make a decision'.[4] It suggests that in these cases the only practical step might be to make a decision in the best interests of the patient and 'keep [the] person informed of what is happening and why'.[4]

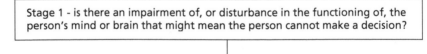

Stage 1 - is there an impairment of, or disturbance in the functioning of, the person's mind or brain that might mean the person cannot make a decision?

Stage 2 - Is the impairment or disturbance sufficient that the person is unable to make that particular decision?

Fig. 18.1 Two-stage capacity assessment.

Can the patient understand the information (***Receive***)?

- For example, does a receptive dysphasia lead to a difficulty understanding verbal information? If so, can this information be understood by any other route, such as pictorially?
- Is the patient's cognition so impaired that they do not understand the information in any meaningful way?
- The patient needs to understand the decision they are being asked to make, the reason a decision is needed and the likely consequence of deciding one way or the other, or of not making a decision.

Can the patient ***Retain*** the information?

- This only needs to be long enough to come to a decision, so a short term memory that only lasts 5 minutes may be adequate.

Can the patient weigh up and use the information (***Rationalise***)?

- The patient must be able to use the information provided to influence their conclusion. This will require a grasp of benefit versus risk and the potential consequence of their decision

Can the patient communicate their decision (***Relate***)?

- It is rare that a patient is felt to lack capacity based solely on this aspect, as most communication difficulties can be overcome with aids, patience with or without specialist help, and normally lack of communication leading to a lack of capacity is only relevant to patients with "locked in" syndrome or in a coma, such as many of those on intensive care units.

Fig. 18.2 Details of how to assess second stage of the capacity assessment.

Capacity assessment in older patients suffering a stroke can present specific challenges in view of the potential for sudden changes in cognition as a direct result of the stroke and also due to specific communication issues such as dysphasia. In addition, strokes are increasingly prevalent in older adults and so are more common in people with multimorbidity and up to 15% of patients presenting with a stroke have a pre-existing dementia.[5] These factors present challenges for health and social care professionals meaning capacity assessments are often more time consuming but the MCA is clear that all practicable steps must be taken to aid the patient to make a decision.[1] Some patients may initially appear cognitively intact and only after more detailed assessment can deficits such as dysexecutive function be revealed.[6] In these cases, involvement of occupational therapists and/or neuropsychologists should be considered. For older patients with communication deficits, speech and language therapists have a vital role to play in facilitating capacity assessments by supporting conversations, tailored to the specific patient and their communication difficulties. This can be through aiding verbal or written communication (ensuring questions are concrete and active, not abstract or passive), using appropriate yes/no questions (ensuring questions are repeated with the same meaning varying between yes and no answers), and using pictorial aids (photos or line drawings, with or without text).

Fig. 18.3 provides a summary of capacity assessment.

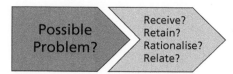

Fig. 18.3 Summary of capacity assessment.

Making decisions for patients lacking capacity

The conclusion that an older patient lacks capacity to make a specific decision can only be made once all practicable steps have been taken to help the patient make the decision themselves, and the healthcare professional has developed a 'reasonable belief' that the patient lacks capacity.[1] This means that there does not need to be certainty of a lack of capacity, only a belief that this is the case and the ability to evidence this if challenged.

If, after all practicable steps have been taken, it is still concluded that a patient lacks the capacity to make a necessary decision, the next question must be whether or not that decision can be delayed until a patient regains capacity. If it can be delayed, then this course of action should be taken. If the decision cannot be delayed until capacity is regained, then a decision must be made in the patient's 'best interests', in the least restrictive manner possible (see Box 18.2 for an example). The MCA[1] suggests four guiding principles to help with making this best interests decision:

- Make the care of your patient your first concern
- Treat patients as individuals and respect their dignity
- Support and encourage patients to be involved, as far as they want to and are able, in decisions about their treatment and care
- Treat patients with respect and do not discriminate against them.

Determining a patient's best interests is often a complex area, and one in which family and friends can be uniquely placed to help you make this judgement. However, the relatives' views have no

---

Box 18.2 Case study 1

Mr Humbers is an 81-year-old gentleman with a background of vascular dementia, who has been admitted with a right-sided partial anterior circulation ischaemic stroke yesterday. He has been consistently refusing all medications since admission, despite both the nurses and his son trying to explain the importance of taking them. The nurse looking after him has asked if she can covertly administer the medications in his food. Dr Andrews, the consultant looking after Mr Humbers, assesses his capacity to refuse medications, and explains in simple language what the medications are for. However, Mr Humbers only replies by saying that he 'doesn't want them', and is unable to explain what any of the medications are for or what problems he might develop if he does not take them. Dr Andrews therefore decides that he is unable to understand, retain, or weigh up any information regarding his medications, and therefore lacks capacity to refuse them. He agrees with the nurse, the pharmacist and Mr Humbers' son that it would be in the best interests of Mr Humber to administer any essential medications covertly. Dr Andrews clearly documents the capacity assessment and best interests process and a clear care plan for medication administration is drawn up.

legal standing in English law, and the decision must be made by the responsible professionals. If the decision made by the health and social care professionals in the best interests of the patient is challenged by the relatives, it is good practice for the team to review the original decision. If this does not resolve the issue, the next step would be to obtain a second opinion from a fellow healthcare professional or, failing that, mediation or even a decision from the Court of Protection.[7]

Trying to enact this decision in the least restrictive manner possible should be straightforward, but at times can have resource implications. For example, two options of how to ensure that a patient does not pull out a nasogastric tube could be sedation and one-to-one nursing with use of safety mittens. One-to-one nursing with safety mittens would be the less restrictive of these two options, but obviously has significantly higher immediate costs. However, the MCA is clear that this is the path that should be followed.

Advance care planning

There are a variety of methods people use to express their wishes for medical treatment in the future should they lose the capacity to decide upon them. These can vary from somebody having an informal conversation with family members about the types of treatments they might not want in certain circumstances, through to the legal transfer of their decision-making should they lose capacity to make decisions for themselves.

Statements of preferences (often referred to as advance statements) of the types of treatments that a patient would and would not want to receive in specific circumstances (written or verbal) can be very useful to the healthcare team in making decisions in the patient's best interests. They provide an insight into the values that the patient has, and allow the healthcare team to make a far more individualized decision than would otherwise be the case. However, these statements are not legally binding, and act only as advice to the healthcare team when a best interests decision is being considered.

Advance decisions are legal documents that set out what treatment the patient would or would not want to receive in specific examples (e.g. 'if I suffer with dysphagia due to a stroke I have decided that I do not wish to accept percutaneous endoscopic gastrostomy (PEG) feeding as an alternative or to supplement oral feeding, and accept the risks involved including loss of life'). They must be written while the patient has capacity, and refusing life-sustaining treatment it must be:

◆ In writing
◆ Signed and witnessed
◆ State clearly that the decision applies even if life is at risk[1]

Often healthcare professionals are provided with these by relatives, and have to make decisions on whether or not they believe them to be valid and relevant. Pertinent points to consider are if the patient:

◆ Has done anything that clearly goes against their advance decision
◆ Has withdrawn their decision
◆ Would have changed their decision had they known more about the current situation

If the advance decision is valid and relevant, then healthcare professionals must follow it or be liable to criminal prosecution. However, if the advance decision is not valid, it may well still be a relevant statement of the patient's wishes, which will need to be considered in a best interests decision.

A lasting power of attorney (LPA) is a legal document that allows one or more people(the attorneys) authority to make decisions on behalf of another (the donor) when the donor lacks

---

Box 18.3 Case study 2

Mr Smith is a 75-year-old gentleman admitted with a left-sided total anterior circulation ischaemic stroke 2 weeks ago. Since that time, he has started to slowly recover and has been fed through a nasogastric tube, but the speech and language therapists report he still has an unsafe swallow with little evidence of this improving and suggests percutaneous endoscopic gastrostomy (PEG) insertion. His consultant, Dr Jones, assesses Mr Smith's capacity to decide on PEG insertion with the help of the speech and language therapist, but Mr Smith is not following any instructions and is not communicating, even with the help of the therapists. Dr Jones explains the decision and the options, but Mr Smith does not appear to follow any of the information, so Dr Jones decides that Mr Smith is unable to understand, retain, or weigh up the information given on the possible feeding options. Dr Jones and the multidisciplinary team feel that it would be in the best interests of Mr Smith to proceed with a PEG insertion for feeding, but are aware that Mr Smith had previously arranged a lasting power of attorney with his daughter. After frank discussions with Mr Smith's daughter, she does not wish for her father to receive a PEG but would like him to be allowed to eat and drink as he is able and accept the risks of aspiration. The medical team agree to proceed with this plan after confirming the detail of the lasting power of attorney.

---

capacity to make these decisions themselves.[1] There are two types of LPA—property and financial affairs, and health and welfare, and only an LPA covering health and welfare is relevant to consent for medical treatments. For it to be valid, it must be written when the donor has capacity to make decisions, must be in the statutory form, and registered with the Office of the Public Guardian. An LPA covering health and welfare allows the attorney(s) to make decisions as if they were the donor themselves (providing the donor lacks capacity to make that decision), but are only allowed to consent to or refuse life-sustaining treatment if specified in the LPA. The attorney(s) must also act in the 'best interests' of the donor at all times and if this does not seem to be the case, the Court of Protection can remove the attorney from the LPA if appropriate. If the healthcare professional has good reason to doubt the validity of an LPA or have not been shown the document, particularly in the emergency setting, they must act in the best interests of the patient until this has been clarified. It is essential that health and social care professionals determine if a person has a LPA and if so that this has been witnessed, a copy provided, and that the LPA has been properly registered with the Office of the Public Guardian. See Box 18.3 for a case study with a LPA.

IMCAs, DOLs, and Court of Protection

Independent mental capacity advocates (IMCAs) are trained, independent individuals who are *required* to be consulted when a patient lacks capacity, has no-one else (such as friends, family, or neighbours—excluding paid professionals) who is willing to advocate for them, and one of the following apply:

- A decision needs to be made on serious medical treatments
- Do not attempt resuscitation (DNAR) decisions are made
- A hospital stay of longer than 28 days is proposed
- A care home placement for longer than 8 weeks is proposed[1]

They have no power to make decisions, but do have the right to view the medical notes, speak up for what they believe the patient would have wished if they had capacity, and have these views taken account of. See Box 18.4 for an example of a situation in which an IMCA is required.

Deprivation of liberty safeguards (DOLs) aim to provide a level of independent scrutiny to ensure that patients who lack capacity are managed in the least restrictive manner possible while in a care home or hospital.[1,8] Authorization should be applied for from the local authority in situations when:

◆ The patient lacks capacity

◆ There is continuous supervision and control

◆ The patient is not free to leave (irrespective of whether they physically can leave or wish to leave)

It is clear that this is not meant to delay emergency treatment, and is not designed for situations when the patient is only likely to be subject to deprivation of liberty safeguards (DOLs) for a negligible length of time (meaning that this is primarily applicable for rehabilitation wards rather than hyperacute stroke wards). In scenarios when recurrent restraint (including sedation) are used, visits from relatives and carers are restricted, or the relatives and carers are refused permission to remove the patient from the hospital, it is extremely likely that DOLs authorization will need to be applied for (providing the patient lacks capacity for these decisions). The hospital will normally provide an urgent authorization for the first 7 days of deprivation of liberties, and then the local authority will place a standard authorization for the DOLs for up to 12 months thereafter, which can be renewed if needed. In view of the vulnerable state of these patients, any deaths while under a standard authorization for DOLs must be reported to the coroner, who may wish to investigate further.

The law underlying DOLs is currently being updated, with the Mental Capacity (Amendment) Bill currently being scrutinized by MPs in the committee stage. This proposes to abolish DOLS and instead replace them with liberty protection safeguards (LPS), with introduction expected in 2020. The major changes from DOLS are that LPS would allow the hospital to authorize the

Box 18.4 Case study 3

Mrs Abrahams is a 78-year-old lady with a background of learning difficulties, who has been admitted after a left-sided total anterior circulation ischaemic stroke 4 weeks ago. Since then, she has undergone intensive inpatient rehabilitation and is now transferring with the aid of a rotunda with two people. However, the multidisciplinary team do not feel Mrs Abrahams would be able to manage back in her supported living accommodation and have advised discharge to a nursing home as a long-term placement. Dr Rowlands, her consultant, assesses her capacity to decide on her discharge destination but after multiple simple explanations of the benefits and risks of each option with the support of the learning disabilities nurses, Mrs Abrahams is still unable to give any disadvantages to her returning home, or any advantages to a nursing home placement. Dr Rowlands therefore decides that Mrs Abrahams is unable to understand, retain, or weigh up the different options and therefore lacks capacity to decide on her discharge destination. Mrs Abrahams has no living relatives and does not have any friends or neighbours who are willing to be consulted on this decision, therefore Dr Rowlands applies for an independent mental capacity advocate to aid in the decision-making process.

deprivation of liberty (rather than the local authority), and makes more explicit the ability to treat people and deprive them of their liberty in a medical emergency without prior authorization. It is expected to maintain the same definition of DOL, but to clarify the requirement for the person to lack capacity, be of unsound mind and be subject to necessary and proportionate arrangements to restrict liberty (rather than the 'best interests' required for DOLS). However, these proposals are still subject to debate and change.

Capacity and research

Participating in research is a difficult area with patients who lack capacity. The MCA[1] suggests most research on those who lack capacity should have some chance of benefiting the person who lacks capacity, and that the benefit must be in proportion to any burden caused by taking part. Alternatively, the research may be to provide knowledge about the cause of, or treatment or care of people with the same impairing condition—or a similar condition with the following requirements:

◆ The risk to the person who lacks capacity must be negligible;

◆ There must be no significant interference with the freedom of action or privacy of the person who lacks capacity; and

◆ Nothing must be done to or in relation to the person who lacks capacity which is unduly invasive or restrictive.

Clearly, any research will need approval from an ethics committee, who will consider if these conditions have been met. If research is approved, there should then be a discussion with a personal consultee (such as a family member) for each person without capacity that is approached to join the trial, to advise the research team if they feel the person would have wished to take part in the research. If they do not feel the potential participant would have wished to take part, then no further attempt should be made to enrol the person in the research.[9,10]

Scotland and Northern Ireland

The law differs in Scotland and Northern Ireland with regards to capacity. In Scotland, the Adults with Incapacity (Scotland) Act 2000[11] states that when a patient is found to lack capacity, a certificate of incapacity must be issued (except for emergency situations), stating the decision to be made, the likely duration of incapacity, and the duration of the certificate (up to 1 year). In Northern Ireland, new legislation covering mental capacity is planned to be implemented in 2020. Meanwhile, medical practice is based upon common law with no specific legal power of LPA or advance directives, but it is felt that the courts would most likely uphold the views in an advance direction as representing the wishes of the patient and therefore being in their best interests.[12]

References

1. *Mental Capacity Act 2005*. Available from: https://www.legislation.gov.uk/ukpga/2005/9/section/27 [Accessed: 29 July 2019].

2. **Great Britain. England. High Court of Justice, Family Division**. *Re C (Adult: refusal of treatment) [1994] 1 All ER 819*. Available from: https://www.4pb.com/case-detail/re-c-refusal-of-medical-treatment/ [Accessed: 29 July 2019].

3. **Kim SY & Caine ED**. Utility and limits of the mini mental state examination in evaluating consent capacity in Alzheimer's disease. *Psychiatr Serv* 2002;**53**(10):1322–4.

4. **Mental Capacity Act** 2005. *Code of Practice.* Available from: https://www.gov.uk/government/uploads/system/uploads/attachment_data/file/224660/Mental_Capacity_Act_code_of_practice.pdf [Accessed: 26 November 2015].

5. **Pendlebury ST & Rothwell PM.** Prevalence, incidence, and factors associated with pre-stroke and post-stroke dementia: a systematic review and meta-analysis. *Lancet Neurol* 2009;**8**(11):1006–18.

6. **Leskela M, Hietanen M, Kalska H**, et al. Executive functions and speed of mental processing in elderly patients with frontal or nonfrontal ischaemic stroke. *Eur J Neurol* 1999;**6**:653–61.

7. **General Medical Council.** *Consent: Patients and Doctors Making Decisions Together*, 2008. Available from: http://www.gmc-uk.org/guidance/ethical_guidance/consent_guidance_index.asp [Accessed: 16 December 2015].

8. **The Law Society.** *Deprivation of Liberty—A Practical Guide.* Available from: http://www.lawsociety.org.uk/support-services/advice/articles/deprivation-of-liberty/ [Accessed: 26 November 2015].

9. **The Law Society.** *Mental Capacity and Deprivation of Liberty. A Consultation Paper.* Consultation No. 222. Available from: http://www.lawcom.gov.uk/wp-content/uploads/2015/07/cp222_mental_capacity.pdf [Accessed: 30 December 2015].

10. **The Law Society.** *Outline of the Proposed Protective Care Scheme.* Available from: http://www.lawcom.gov.uk/wp-content/uploads/2015/07/cp222_mental_capacity_short_outline.pdf [Accessed: 30 December 2015].

11. **Scottish Parliament.** *Adults with Incapacity (Scotland) Act 2000.* Available from: https://www.legislation.gov.uk/asp/2000/4/section/74 [Accessed: 29 July 2019].

12. **General Medical Council.** *Treatment and Care Towards the End of Life: Good Practice in Decision Making.* Available from: http://www.gmc-uk.org/guidance/ethical_guidance/end_of_life_binding_advance_refusals.asp [Accessed: 26 November 2015].

Chapter 19

Urinary incontinence after stroke

Amy Hillarious, Sunil K. Munshi,
and Rowan H. Harwood

Introduction

Incontinence is a scourge of frail older people, caused by many illnesses associated with older age, and causing humiliation, dependency, and cost. Between three and six million people in the United Kingdom are affected by urinary incontinence.[1] Prevalence varies between 5% and 69% in women[2] and 11–34% in men,[3] and 30–60% among UK care home residents. Variation is due to age, differing definitions, the population studied, and measurement method used.[4–7] Incontinence is under-reported due to embarrassment and social stigma, with many people waiting a significant time before seeking help.[6,8] Urinary incontinence is common after stroke and is an independent predictor of mortality, dependency, and need for institutional care. It can affect 40–60% of people admitted to hospital after a stroke, with 25% still having problems on hospital discharge and 15% remaining incontinent after 1 year.[9]

In this chapter, we describe different types of urinary incontinence, the types prevalent after a stroke, and consider comorbid incontinence.

General considerations and some definitions

Maintaining continence is a complex chain of events: being aware of the need to void, getting to and recognizing the toilet, manipulating clothing, inhibiting bladder contractions until ready to void, using the toilet (or an alternative such as a urinal or commode), cleaning, and dressing. This requires neurological bladder control, mobility, dexterity, communication, and cognition, including planning and anticipation, the taking of medication, using devices or pads, or accessing help to do so.

The main functions of the urinary bladder are to store and expel urine. Appropriate voiding of urine requires coordination between detrusor muscle activity (inhibition or contraction) and the urethral sphincter closure or relaxation, controlled by the nervous system. The innervation of the bladder is from the S2–S4 segments of the spinal cord. The parasympathetic system is dominant, but the sympathetic and somatic systems are also involved. In normal function, the bladder tends to contract as it fills, via a 'long reflex' (up the spinal cord to the brain stem, and back again). Voluntary control over voiding is exerted by inhibiting the reflex until voiding is intended, at which point the reflex is 'dis-inhibited', allowing the bladder to contract and the sphincter to relax. Central nervous control includes the cerebral cortex (second medial frontal convolution), and subcortical structures in the anterior cingulate cortex, thalamus, caudal hypothalamus, insula, midbrain, and the medulla).[10–12] Impairment of any of these can lead to incontinence. The neurotransmitter in the parasympathetic and somatic nerves is acetylcholine; in sympathetic neurones noradrenaline is released.[13–15] The internal and external sphincters provide (short-term) support in the control of voiding, and are controlled by involuntary (sympathetic) and voluntary (somatic) nerves, respectively.

Clinical assessment (symptoms, examination, and simple tests) is usually sufficient to guide management, especially in frail older people. Definitive assessment, to distinguish types of incontinence, or evaluate comorbidity (especially prostate disease) requires cystometry (also called urodynamics, bladder pressure studies), which estimates detrusor muscle pressure by taking the difference between bladder pressure and abdominal pressure while the bladder is artificially filled, and then during voiding. Video contrast X-rays can be used to assess anatomy. These tests are time-consuming and moderately unpleasant (requiring two catheters in the bladder and one in the rectum or vagina).

Urinary urge incontinence is leakage of urine that is caused by a sudden and often uncontrollable urge to void urine, due to an inability to inhibit bladder contractions during filling. It results in the frequent passage of small quantities of urine, including at night. Urge incontinence is part of a larger symptom complex known as the 'overactive bladder syndrome', defined as urinary urgency with or without incontinence. Urinary frequency is defined by the International Continence Society as voiding more than seven times in 24 hours, while nocturia is passing urine more than once during the sleeping hours. Together, these symptoms suggest of detrusor overactivity, but they can also result from urinary retention, and other forms of urethrovesical dysfunction (such as atrophic urethritis).[14] Around 10% of the general population, and 20% over the age of 70 years, has an overactive bladder, of varying degrees of severity. The cause is often idiopathic, but many neurological diseases including stroke and dementia, and procholinergic drugs (such as donepezil) can be responsible.

Stress incontinence presents with leakage of (usually small amounts of) urine caused by activity that increases intra-abdominal pressure, such as standing up, running, coughing, or sneezing, and represents a failure of the bladder neck sphincter mechanism. This commonly occurs due to a pudendal neuropathy following childbirth, uterine prolapse, alpha-adrenergic antagonist drugs, or after radical prostatectomy in men. Small volume urinary leakage without a feeling of urgency is usually due to stress incontinence.

Mixed urinary incontinence is where involuntary leakage is associated with urgency and stress incontinence. Interpretation can be difficult: stress manoeuvres can induce an unstable bladder contraction, and stress leaks may be interpreted as urgency by the person. Definitive assessment requires cystometry.

Incomplete emptying of the bladder occurs if the bladder muscle fails to contract (or contracts inefficiently), or the outflow is obstructed. Obstruction occurs usually at the level of the prostate gland, but can also result from urethral stricture, or incoordination between detrusor contraction and sphincter relaxation (dyssynergia). The detrusor muscle loses some of its contractility and efficiency with age and at least 5–10% of older adults have poor bladder contractility regardless of stroke. Anticholinergic drugs can cause incomplete emptying; faecal impaction may also contribute.

Overflow incontinence occurs when there is difficulty emptying the bladder, with leakage of urine due to distortion of the bladder neck (sphincter), or unstable contractions of the full and stretched bladder. Patients in this group present with continuous urinary leakage or dribbling of urine. The bladder may or may not feel full.

Functional incontinence is voiding in an inappropriate place due to inability to recognize the need to void, find, get to and use the toilet, undress, or adequately clean, with or without concurrent bladder dysfunction. Those with overactive bladders need greater access to toilets, mobility, and dexterity to remain dry.

Nocturnal enuresis is the involuntary leakage of urine at night, which can be associated with overactive bladder, chronic retention, any cause of polyuria, insomnia, or sleep apnoea.

Lower urinary tract symptoms (LUTS) is a non-specific term used to describe voiding and storage problems including urinary frequency, urgency, nocturia, dysuria, poor or intermittent stream, or incomplete emptying,[16,17] with or without urinary incontinence.

Bladder problems in the general older adult population

Most stroke patients are from the older age group, and bladder problems in the general older population often become manifest when a stroke occurs. Both LUTS and incontinence are more prevalent with increasing age, due to declining bladder capacity, an increase in involuntary contractions, and various pathologies. In women, laxity of the pelvic floor causes reduced resistance at the bladder neck and urethra, resulting in stress incontinence. Atrophic vaginitis and urethritis caused by oestrogen deficiency after the menopause cause dysuria, urinary urgency, and proneness to urinary infection. Prostatic enlargement in men decreases urine flow rates and may cause incomplete emptying or 'irritability' (overactivity, involuntary contractions of the bladder) leading to urge or overflow incontinence. Age- or disease-related increase of secretion of atrial natriuretic peptide, and loss or reversal of diurnal variation in arginine vasopressin peptide (anti-diuretic hormone, ADH), diabetes, heart failure, and other causes of oedema can lead to nocturnal polyuria and night-time incontinence.[18]

Specific bladder problems occurring after stroke

Bladder dysfunction after a stroke varies greatly, and includes bladder overactivity, hyporeflexia, and dyssynergia, suggesting that there is no one mechanism that precipitates incontinence.[19] Some people become incontinent despite normal bladder function.

The prevalence of new-onset urinary incontinence after a stroke ranges from 21% to 56%, and is higher among older adults. In the Copenhagen Stroke Study of 935 acute stroke patients admitted consecutively over 19 months, about half were incontinent of urine. The proportion declined to one-fifth of the surviving patients after 6 months. Increasing age, stroke severity, diabetes, and other disabling diseases increased the risk of incontinence.[20]

'Impaired awareness' urinary incontinence is particularly common. Diminished consciousness, delirium, or a specific denial or awareness of illness (anosognosia) can be a consequence of stroke and may contribute to incontinence. This type of incontinence is associated with damage to parietal lobe or subcortical damage, and impaired cognition. 'Impaired awareness' urinary incontinence can be due to inability to recognize or respond to bladder fullness or contractions. It is associated with higher functional dependence and poor outcome after 3 and 12 months after a stroke.[21–23] Petterson and colleagues showed that extensive supratentorial white matter lesions, particularly in the right parietal region, new basal ganglia involvement, and new lesions involving two or more lobes or regions were all strong independent risk factors for 'impaired awareness' urinary incontinence; older age was a weaker factor (Box 19.1). Other studies showed that older people with white matter lesions on computed tomography (CT) were more likely to have incontinence than age-matched controls without white matter lesions.[24–26] The influence of other frontal regions, particularly the orbitofrontal cortex, on conscious attention to bladder sensations and voluntary suppression of the voiding reflex has been repeatedly demonstrated in clinical and experimental studies.[27–29]

On admission to post-acute stroke rehabilitation, double (urinary and faecal) incontinence was more prevalent (33%) than isolated urinary (12%) and isolated faecal incontinence (8%). By the time of discharge, prevalence was somewhat reduced, due to recovery, and selective mortality of those most severely affected (double incontinence, 15%; isolated urinary, 8%; isolated faecal, 5%).

Box 19.1 Clinical and neuroradiological factors related to 'impaired awareness' urinary incontinence with odds ratios

1 Age > 80 (OR 2.8)

2 Right-sided lesions (OR 2.3)

3 Parietal lobe stroke (OR 2.8)

4 Frontal lobe lesions (OR 2.1)

5 Acute basal ganglia involvement (OR 3.1)

6 Total stroke lesion volume >1.5 cm^3 (OR 3.5)

7 White matter lesions (OR 3.7)

8 Cognitive impairment

Adapted with permission from Pettersen R, et al. Post-stroke urinary incontinence: One-year outcome and relationships with measures of attentiveness. *Journal of the American Geriatrics Society*, 55(10), 1571–7. Copyright © 2007, The American Geriatrics Society. https://doi.org/10.1111/j.1532-5415.2007.01396.x

---

Impaired awareness-associated incontinence was more prevalent (12% in 'young old' to 58% in 'oldest old' age groups) than urgency (9–42%).[30]

Urinary urge incontinence is caused by damage to the neuronal pathways inhibiting bladder contraction (sometimes called 'hyperreflexia'); estimates suggest 37–90% of cases due to this mechanism, depending on setting and case mix. However, other pathologies are also seen, with prevalence of overflow incontinence between 21% and 35%.[21] Functional incontinence is common after a stroke due to mobility or communication problems; maybe accounting for 25% of inpatient incontinence after a stroke.

In the Copenhagen Stroke Study, the multiple logistic regression analysis found age, severity of stroke (Scandinavian Stroke Scale score and lesion volume), diabetes mellitus, hypertension, and comorbidity of other disabling diseases were significant risk factors for urinary incontinence.[20] Other variables associated with greater risk of incontinence include: age over 75 years, motor weakness, dysphasia, cognitive difficulties, neglect, and visual field defects. Poor cognition has the greatest negative impact.[30] Overall, there is no clear association between the site of infarct and incontinence.[31] However, people with frontal lobe lesions and larger infarcts affecting frontal and parietal lobes have been suggested to be at especially high risk.[31-33]

Assessment of urinary incontinence

Incontinence after a stroke may or may not recover. A reversible cause may be found and treated. If not, symptoms may still be reduced and impact minimized if it is managed well. Identification and treatment of transient factors that contribute to incontinence is required as part of this assessment (Table 19.1). If symptoms of incontinence persist beyond 2 weeks after a stroke, a detailed further assessment should be undertaken (Table 19.2).

A thorough history of urinary symptoms prior to the stroke should be obtained in order to identify comorbid diseases and contributory factors such as prostate disease, cognitive impairment, diabetes, and medications.

The type of incontinence can often be suspected from the symptoms (Table 19.2), although this is imprecise ('the bladder is an unreliable witness'). Further studies including simple tests

Table 19.1 Transient causes of urinary incontinence: identification and treatment

Transient cause	Diagnostic method	Treatment strategy
Urinary tract infections	Symptoms, urinalysis, culture, inflammatory markers	Antibiotics as per culture and sensitivities
Atrophic vaginitis/ urethritis in women	Physical examination	Topical vaginal oestrogens
Constipation	Physical examination/ stool charts	Disimpaction, stool softeners, bulking agents, laxatives
Drugs	Drug review	Discontinuation/dose reduction
Excessive fluid or caffeine intake	Fluid chart monitoring	Moderating fluid intake, caffeine-free drinks
Delirium	Clinical, investigations for cause	Treat underlying cause

(postvoid bladder ultrasound scanning, frequency-volume chart, urine flow rate) or more complex urodynamic testing may be needed in cases where there is significant clinical doubt as to underlying aetiology, and a likely impact on management (especially surgery).

Management of urinary incontinence

Management will vary according to diagnosis, time after stroke, alertness and awareness, and level of disability or dependency. It requires a multidisciplinary approach, with nursing, medical, speech and language therapy (communication), physiotherapy (mobility, dexterity), and occupational therapy (aids, appliances, adapted clothing) elements.

Sometimes nurses resort to containment of incontinence without proper assessment or treatment.[34–35] This can occur after stroke, the main reasons being shortage of staff time and knowledge, competing priorities (including pressure area care), the difficulty in doing anything other than containment in severely ill, semi-conscious, or dependent stroke patients, and perceived disappointing results from intervention. But this represents a missed opportunity for health gain.

In general, indwelling urethral catheters are best avoided, unless there is a specific indication, as they are always associated with complications. Containment with absorptive pads (diapers) is often possible, even in very dependent patients, but they should not be used without prior

Table 19.2 History taking to determine type of urinary incontinence

Questions to ask the patient/or carers	Type of incontinence
Is the patient alert enough to be aware of the need to void, or ask for help?	Impaired awareness incontinence
Is there a frequent need to void small volumes with inability to reach toilet on time	Urge incontinence
Are there any impairments of cognition, mobility, or dexterity that may impede toileting?	Functional incontinence
Is there leakage of urine painless related to change in position which may be continuous	Overflow incontinence

assessment. However, it is sometimes difficult to argue against short-term containment using a sheath or catheter in the early days after stroke for a very immobile, 'heavy' patient.

Best practice will be to treat what is treatable without undue patient burden, while awaiting recovery of awareness, function, and bladder, and optimizing containment to minimize distress, hygienic problems, and protect skin.

Research suggests that structured assessment, in conjunction with specialist continence nursing, reduces rates of post-stroke incontinence. However, studies looking at physical or behavioural complementary therapies, and anticholinergic drug use in isolation, have been inadequate in guiding treatment.[9,19,36]

Treat 'transient' and comorbid causes of incontinence

'Transient' causes should be addressed first (Table 19.3). Moderation of fluid intake (to about 2 litres per day) and caffeine restriction should be considered.[37–38] Urinary tract infections should be treated with antibiotics (but should not be overemphasized as a potential causative mechanism). Constipation, stool impaction, atrophic urethritis, and causes of delirium should be treated. Poorly controlled diabetes causes polyuria, which is improved by blood sugar control using oral agents or insulin. Advice about weight loss if body mass index is over 30 kg/m^2.[39]

Indwelling or clean intermittent catheterization is required for urinary retention (postvoid residual volume >400 ml). Incomplete emptying may resolve, with the withdrawal of a culprit drug, relief of constipation, or improving mobility. Residual volumes should be monitored, and several attempts made to remove the catheter ('trial without catheter', 'TWOC').

Polypharmacy is frequent in older persons, and adverse effects are common.[40] This includes effects on bladder function and continence. Drugs associated with incontinence include sedative-hypnotics, diuretics, anticholinergics, antispasmodics, analgesics, antihistamines, antipsychotics, alpha-adrenergic agonists, alpha-antagonists, calcium channel blockers, ACE inhibitors (cough),

Table 19.3 Management strategies for post-stroke incontinence

Types of post-stroke incontinence	Cause	Symptoms	Possible treatment strategies
Urge incontinence	Disruption of micturition neural pathways	Urge accompanies or precedes involuntary incontinence. Frequency, nocturia	Lifestyle modification; bladder training; medications for BPH (alpha blockers, finasteride); vaginal oestrogens, antimuscarinics
Impaired awareness incontinence	Reduced consciousness, or awareness of desire to void	Sudden or unexpected urge to void	Containment until clinical improvement; prompted voiding
Overflow incontinence	Decreased bladder contractility or outflow obstruction	Continuous leakage, urinary retention	Intermittent catheterization; indwelling catheterization; urology referral
Functional incontinence	Deficits in cognition, communication, and mobility	Inability to find or reach toilet in time	Rehabilitation, timed, or prompted voiding

Adapted with permission from Mehdi Z, et al. Post-stroke urinary incontinence. *International Journal of Clinical Practice*, 67(11), 1128–1137. Copyright © 2013, John Wiley & Sons Ltd. https://doi.org/10.1111/ijcp.12183

and antiparkinsonian medications.[41-43] In particular, anticholinergic drugs can cause chronic urinary retention.[44]

Urospecific alpha-blocker drugs (e.g. tamsulosin) and 5-alpha reductase inhibitors (e.g. finasteride) constitute medical management of benign prostatic hypertrophy. This may improve flow, reduce incomplete emptying, and may relieve secondary overactivity. The side effects of alpha-blocker drugs include orthostatic hypotension. Men with benign prostatic hyperplasia (BPH) often have secondary detrusor overactivity, so there may be need for concomitant antimuscarinic therapy as well, provided the bladder empties well (postvoid residual volume <100 ml).[45] Prostate cancer may be identified incidentally, and will require specific referral and management by a urologist.

If haematuria is present, urine culture, renal imaging, and cystoscopy are indicated, but full investigation can wait until after the immediate post-stroke period if the person is very unwell or debilitated.

Non-pharmacological management

Scheduled toileting or prompted voiding aims to achieve 'dependent-continence' by anticipating or pre-empting voiding, or 'independent continence' by re-establishing awareness and an independent habit of going to the toilet. Caregivers use verbal prompts and positive re-enforcement to encourage regular toileting. Systematic reviews of trials of prompted voiding suggested some benefits in the short term, but are inconclusive in the longer term.[46] This is a main management strategy for people with cognitive impairment, especially if there is relatively preserved mobility.

Bladder training aims to progressively increase the amount of urine held in the bladder and increase the duration of time before emptying the bladder. Many people with overactive bladders remain continent by going to the toilet frequently or 'just in case'. This is believed to reduce the functional bladder capacity, exacerbating the problem. A programme of bladder training involves voiding 'by the clock', progressively increasing the time between voids, starting with a period that can be comfortably achieved (such as 1 or 2 hours, determined from a voiding diary). This allows bladder inhibition to be practised or trained. The programme can be completed rapidly (over a few days), or more usually nowadays, over several weeks. It is often used in conjunction with anticholinergic drug treatment to try to reduce urgency. Time between voids can certainly be increased in some by bladder retraining, however, symptoms often relapse or return. A Cochrane review of randomized controlled trials showed that bladder training may be beneficial for treatment of urge incontinence; however, supporting data are limited. In the review, pharmacological therapy was not demonstrated to be superior to bladder training or helpful in conjunction with it.[47] Bladder retraining is often difficult or impossible for people who have had a stroke, especially in the acute phase, but may be appropriate for some.

Treatment of persisting urge incontinence

Pelvic floor exercises can be tried, especially in women; the sphincter cannot withstand a strongly contracting bladder for more than 10–20 seconds, but pelvic floor contraction reflexively inhibits detrusor contractions. Avoiding caffeinated drinks, weight loss, and smoking cessation may improve symptoms.[39] Procholinergic drugs should be avoided. Bladder training may be of benefit.[48]

The mainstay of pharmacological treatment is antimuscarinic anticholinergic drugs. These block the muscarinic receptors on the detrusor muscle, thereby relaxing it. They reduce urgency and increase bladder capacity, but on average only by a small amount—about 25–50 ml, or 10%. The effect is rapid after drug initiation, and maximum within a month (so if ineffective, can be discontinued at that stage). Urinary retention is a possible side effect, so it is advisable to perform a postvoid bladder scan after a few weeks. Compliance is affected by adverse effects with the most common being dry mouth, blurred vision, constipation, oesophageal reflux, and cognitive impairment or delirium. Anticholinergic drugs may precipitate angle closure glaucoma in those who are predisposed.

There are a number of different anticholinergic drugs licensed for overactive bladder treatment in the United Kingdom. NICE (2015a) recommends: immediate release oxybutynin or tolterodine (but these are both very prone to adverse effects and the inconvenience of multiple doses per day), or modified release darifenacin.[6] Older patients are more susceptible to central nervous system effects, which can be avoided by using an agent that does not cross the blood–brain barrier (trospium)[49] or a uroselective agent such as darifenacin. The high rate of adverse effects leads to poor compliance, and reported discontinuation rates of 43–83%.[50]

Anticholinergic drugs undergo hepatic metabolism (with cytochrome P450 in particular CYP3A4 and CYP2D6) and renal excretion, requiring additional care in cases of renal or hepatic impairment. Many other medications have anticholinergic properties, including as tricyclic antidepressants and antihistamines, which can aggravate the risk of side effects.[51]

Where antimuscarinic drugs are not tolerated, prove ineffective, or are contraindicated, beta-adrenergic agonists like mirabegron can be used. This acts by activating the beta 3-adrenergic receptor in the detrusor muscle causing muscle relaxation and increased capacity. Efficacy is similar to antimuscarinic drugs. Dose can be titrated over several weeks if needed. Combination therapy with antimuscarinic and beta-3 agonist makes logical sense, and is sometimes used, but in the United Kingdom the combination is not licensed.[6,14,52]

Treatment of impaired awareness incontinence

A patient who is unaware because they are very ill or not fully conscious will be managed by containment pending clinical improvement. An extreme version impaired awareness, where the subject experiences sudden or imminent need to void ('precipitancy'), is associated with stroke affecting the frontal lobe. A prompted or timed voiding regimen can be tried.

Treatment of overflow incontinence

This is often due to a comorbidity, or an anticholinergic drug, which must be addressed. Detrusor underactivity can be associated with stroke *per se*, and may recover over time. Clean intermittent catheterization may be used if practical; alternatively, an indwelling catheter may be used, preferably temporarily.

Treatment of functional incontinence

Treatment compromises multidisciplinary rehabilitation, to improve mobility, communication, dexterity, and dressing ability, and modification of the environment to enable good access to the toilet, or modification to clothing, or use of aids such as urinals, commodes, or sheath catheters. Timed or prompted voiding may be used.

Treatment of nocturnal symptoms (nocturia, polyuria, and enuresis)

Medical causes of polyuria should be addressed, including diabetes, heart failure, peripheral oedema, hypercalcaemia, diuretic, or lithium therapy.

Some drug approaches aim to reduce nocturnal urine production, but none is wholly effective, and some are little known about.

Desmopressin is a synthetic analogue of vasopressin or ADH, which acts on the renal tubules to reabsorb water.[6] When given at night it reduces nocturnal urine production. It is relatively less effective in older people, and can cause severe hyponatraemia, due to free water retention. For this reason it is given six nights out of seven, or three weeks out of four, to allow excretion of any accumulating free water load. It should be avoided in people with cardiovascular disease or hypertension. In the United Kingdom desmopressin is not licensed for people over 65 years. Serum sodium should be measured 3 days after the first dose, and periodically thereafter, especially if the person becomes acutely unwell.

An alternative is to use loop diuretic, often given at noon or late afternoon, which can reduce night-time urine output by about 200 ml.[6] High-dose chlorthalidone (50 mg bd) can also be tried, also at risk of electrolyte disturbances (by sensitizing renal tubules to ADH). Drugs that stimulate ADH secretion may also be tried, including tricyclic antidepressants, but these are rarely used in older people nowadays due to risk of adverse effects.

Specialized interventions can be used in selected or intractable cases

Injection of botulinum toxin into the detrusor muscle can give better relief than conventional pharmacological treatment, while avoiding systemic anticholinergic adverse effects. Botulinum toxin type A has been shown to reduce urinary symptoms of overactive bladder by 35–50% compared with placebo.[6] The effect lasts weeks to months, and can be repeated. Unfortunately, in some cases the toxin paralyses the bladder, leading to urinary retention; around 20% of patients will need to perform self-catheterization afterwards.

Sacral nerve stimulation is a minimally invasive surgical option, involving placement of a sacral electrode and a subcutaneous generator (a bit like a pacemaker), used for the treatment of severe overactive bladder, with good results over 6 months compared with medical treatment alone.[53] However, it is expensive, and undertaken in specialist centres only.

Containment

Often urinary incontinence after a stroke cannot be cured. In this case, adequate containment can allow better hygiene, less embarrassment, reduced laundry, and improved social function.

Incontinence pads comprise a waterproof shell, a water absorbing gel to increase capacity, and a hydrophilic surface material to keep the skin dry. Fitted and used properly they are highly effective. They are available in a variety of shapes and sizes, including some held in place by pants, and 'pull up' versions. Different designs are preferred by men and women, and a high capacity pad can be used at night (maximum capacity is 1.2 litres). Small pads similar to a sanitary towel may be used by women with mild stress incontinence. Men may use a 'dribble pouch' if struggling with postmicturition dribbling.

Absorbent sheets may also be used in bed, usually as a failsafe in conjunction with pads; a waterproof mattress protector is also useful.

Indwelling urethral catheters and external (sheath) urinary catheters are most commonly used during the acute phase after a stroke. Indwelling catheters may be indicated in those with incomplete bladder emptying, hemodynamically unstable patients where urine output needs monitoring, or as an initial management strategy for immobile patients who are at high risk of developing pressure sores. However, indwelling catheters can be associated with urethral trauma, infections, bladder spasm, and stones. If indwelling catheters are used as part of initial treatment, their continued use needs to be reviewed regularly with attempts of trial without catheter. However, dogmatism must be avoided; if a duly informed patient wishes to use a catheter for containment, there is no absolute reason not to, especially if the stakes are high; for example, allowing a return home. Penile sheaths (external urinary catheters) have a lower associated morbidity rate; however, these are not feasible in those with a retracted penis, and need frequent fitting. Spouses, partners, and carers can be taught how to apply and remove penile sheaths if the patient is unable to do this themselves.

Outcomes

Urinary incontinence is a marker of stroke severity, but also has a severe negative impact on quality of life, mood, functional dependence, and discharge destination. It also causes increased carer strain.

Urinary incontinence occurring in the first few days after a stroke is associated with a 6-month mortality rate of 52% versus the 7% mortality rate for those who remain continent. The presence of incontinence is a predictor of poor functional recovery; newly diagnosed incontinence in those younger than 75 years is associated with risk of disability 3 months later.[31] Patients with incontinence are more likely to require institutional care.

Impact on quality of life is rarely formally assessed.[54] The International Continence Society advises assessing symptom severity and quality of life using standardized questionnaires, including the ICIQ, I-QOL, and KHQ. I-QOL and KHQ have been used in clinical trials and have good psychometric properties. The ICIQ has fewer validation reports and is used less in clinical trials, but is a more practical tool for the busy practitioner. The Bristol Female Urinary Tract Symptoms questionnaire (BFLUTS) and the Stress and Urge Incontinence and Quality-of-Life Questionnaire (SUIQQ) may also be useful.[55–59]

Following publication of the Francis Report[60] and a national audit of continence care,[61] it was recommended that healthcare professionals should proactively ask individuals about symptoms of bladder incontinence to identify those who have a problem. This is especially true of stroke patients as they are often very dependent and frail.[60,61]

Summary

Half of patients suffering a stroke will be initially incontinent of urine; 20% of survivors will remain so. It is caused by neurological damage, or comorbidity. A variety of pathologies are responsible, most often bladder overactivity, but also incomplete emptying, and functional problems such as mobility or communication impairment alongside a bladder that may or may not function normally. Continence will tend to improve with time and functional recovery after a stroke, but proper assessment and optimal management increases the chances of recovery. However, specific treatments are not always effective, and aids, appliances and means of containment are also important in achieving the best outcomes and quality of life for patients.

References

1. Irwin DE, Milsom I, Kopp Z, Abrams P, & Cardozo. L. Impact of overactive bladder symptoms on employment, social interactions and emotional wellbeing in six European countries. *BJU Int* 2005;**97**:96–100.
2. Hunskaar S, Lose G, Sykes D, & Voss S. The prevalence of urinary incontinence in women in four European countries. *BJU Int* 2004;**93**(3):324–30.
3. Markland AD, Goode PS, Redden DT, Borrud LG, & Burgio KL. Prevalence of urinary incontinence in men: results from the National Health and Examination survey. *J Urol* 2010;**184**(3):1022–7.
4. Buckley BS & Lapitan MCM. Prevalence of urinary incontinence in men, women and children-current evidence: findings of the fourth international consultation on incontinence. *J Urol* 2009;**76**(2):265–70.

5. **Thom D.** Variation in estimates of urinary incontinence prevalence in the community: effects of differences in definition, population characteristics, and study type. *J Am Geriatr Soc* 1998;**46**:473–80

6. **National Institute for Health and Care Excellence (NICE).** *Urinary Incontinence in Women: Management. NICE guideline CG171.* London, UK: NICE, 2015.

7. **National Institute for Health and Care Excellence (NICE).** *Lower Urinary Tract Symptoms: Management. NICE clinical guideline CG97,* London, UK: NICE, 2015.

8. **Strickland R.** Reasons for not seeking care for urinary incontinence in older community-dwelling women: a contemporary review. *Urol Nurs* 2014;**34**(2):63–94.

9. **Thomas L, Barrett J, Cross S,** et al. Prevention and treatment of urinary incontinence after stroke in adults. *Cochrane Database Syst Rev* 2005;**3**:CD004462.

10. **Sampselle CM & DeLancey JO.** Anatomy of female continence. *J Wound Ostomy Continence Nurs* 1998;**25**:63–74.

11. **Ouslander J.** Management of overactive bladder. *N Engl J Med* 2004;**350**(8):786–99.

12. **Getliffe C & Dolman M.** *Promoting Continence: A Clinical and Research Resource.* 3rd edition. London, UK: Elsevier (Churchill Livingstone), 2007.

13. **de Groat WC, Griffiths D, & Yoshimura N.** Neural control of the lower urinary tract. *Compr Physiol* 2015;**5**(1):327–96.

14. **Abrams P, Andersson KE, Birder L,** et al. 4th International Consultation on Incontinence 2010: Recommendations of the International Scientific Committee: Evaluation and Treatment of Urinary Incontinence, Pelvic Organ Prolapse and Faecal Incontinence. Paris, France: International Continence Society.

15. **Fowler CJ, Griffiths D, & de Groat WC.** The neural control of micturition. *Nat Rev Neurosci* 2008;**6**:453–66.

16. **McVary K.** Lower urinary tract symptoms and sexual dysfunction: epidemiology and pathophysiology. *BJU Int* 2006;**97**(2):23–8.

17. **Tibaek S, Gard G, Klarskov P,** et al. Prevalence of lower urinary tract symptoms (LUTS) in stroke patients: a cross-sectional, clinical survey. *Neurourol Urodyn* 2008;**27**:763–71.

18. **Kane R, Ouslander J, & Abrass I.** *Essentials of Clinical Geriatrics,* 7th edition. New York, NY: McGraw Hill: 2013, pp. 191–2.

19. **Linsenmeyer TA.** Post-CVA voiding dysfunctions: clinical insights and literature review. *NeuroRehabilitation* 2012;**30**(1):1–7.

20. **Nakayama H, Jorgensen HS, Pederson PM,** et al. Prevalence and risk factors of incontinence after stroke—the Copenhagen Stroke Study. *Stroke* 1997;**28**:58–62.

21. **Mehdi Z, Birns J, & Bhalla A.** Post-stroke urinary incontinence. *Int J Clin Pract* 2013;**67**(11):1128–37.

22. **Pettersen R & Wyller TB.** Prognostic significance of micturition disturbances after acute stroke. *J Am Geriatr Soc* 2006;**54**:1878–84.

23. **Pettersen R, Saxby BK, & Wyller TB.** Post-stroke urinary incontinence: one-year outcome and relationships with measures of attentiveness. *J Am Geriatr Soc* 2007;**55**:1571–7.

24. **Tarvonen-Schroder S, Roytta M, Raiha I,** et al. Clinical features of leuko-araiosis. *J Neurol Neurosurg Psychiatry* 1996;**60**:431–6.

25. **Sakakibara R, Hattori T, Yasuda K, & Yamanishi T.** Micturitional disturbance after acute hemispheric stroke: analysis of the lesion site by CT and MRI. *J Neurol Sci* 1996;**137**(1) 47–56.

26. **Hirono N, Kitagaki H, Kazui H,** et al. Impact of white matter changes on clinical manifestation of Alzheimer's disease—a quantitative study. *Stroke* 2000;**31**(9):2182–8.

27. **Griffiths D, Derbyshire S, Stenger A,** et al. Brain control of normal bladder. Brain control of normal and overactive bladder. *J Urol* 2005;**174**:1862–7.

28. **Blok BF, Willemsen AT, & Holstege G.** A PET study on brain control of micturition in humans. *Brain* 1997;**120**:111–21.

29. **Griffiths D.** Clinical studies of cerebral and urinary tract function in elderly people with urinary incontinence. *Behav Brain Res* 1998;**92**:151–5.

30. **Kovindha A, Wyndaele JJ, & Madersbacher H.** Prevalence of incontinence during rehabilitation in patients following stroke. *Curr Bladder Dysfunct Rep* 2010;**5**:32.

31. **Brittain KR, Peet SM, & Castleden CM.** Stroke and incontinence. *Stroke* 1998;**29**(2):524–8.

32. **Khan Z, Hertanu J, Yang WC, Melman A, & Leiter E.** Predictive correlation of urodynamic dysfunction and brain injury after cerebrovascular accident. *J Urol* 1981;**126**(1):86–8.

33. **Srikanth VK, Quinn SJ, Donnan GA,** et al. Long-term cognitive transitions, rates of cognitive change, and predictors of incident dementia in a population-based first-ever stroke cohort. *Stroke* 2006;**37**:2479–83.

34. **Booth J, Kumlien S, Zang Y, Gustafsson B, & Tolson D.** Rehabilitation nurses practices in relation to urinary incontinence following stroke: a cross-cultural comparison. *J Clin Nurs* 2009;**18**(7):1049–58.

35. **Ostaszkiewicz J, O'Connell B, & Millar L.** (2008). Incontinence: managed or mismanaged in hospital settings? *Int J Nurs Pract* 2008;**14**(6):494–502.

36. **Thomas LH, Cross S, Barrett J,** et al. Treatment of urinary incontinence after stroke in adults. *Cochrane Database Syst Rev* 2008;**23**(1):CD004462.

37. **Lohsiriwat S, Hirunsai M, & Chaiyaprasithi B.** Effect of caffeine on bladder function in patients with overactive bladder symptoms. *Urol Ann* 2011;**3**(1):14–18.

38. **Maserejian NN, Wager CG, Giovannucci EL, Curto TM, McVary KT, & McKinlay JB.** Intake of caffeinated, carbonated, or citrus beverage types and development of lower urinary tract symptoms in men and women. *Am J Epidemiol* 2013;**177**(12):1399–410.

39. **Lucas MG, Bedretdinova D, Berghmans LC,** et al. EAU guidelines on surgical treatment of urinary incontinence. *Eur Urol* 2012;**62**(6):1118–29.

40. **Duerden M, Avery T, & Payne R.** *Polypharmacy and Medicines Optimisation.* London, UK: The King's Fund, 2013.

41. **Porter MD & Kaplan KKL.** *The Merck Manual of Diagnosis and Therapy,* 19th edition. Kenilworth, NJ: Merck Sharp and Dohme Corp, 2013.

42. **Tsakiris P, Oelke M, & Michel MC.** Drug-induced urinary incontinence. *Drugs Aging* 2008;**25**:541–9.

43. **British Medical Association and the Royal Pharmaceutical Society.** *Nurse Prescribers Formulary for Community Practitioners.* London, UK: British Medical Association and the Royal Pharmaceutical Society, 2016.

44. **Selius BA & Subedi R.** Urinary retention in adults: diagnosis and initial management. *Am Fam Physician* 2008;**77**(5):643–50.

45. **Oelke M, Baard J, de la Rosette J, Jonas U, & Hofner K.** Age and bladder outlet obstruction are independently associated with detrusor overactivity in patients with benign prostatic hyperplasia. *Eur Urol* 2008;**54**(2):419–26.

46. **Eustice S, Roe B, & Paterson J.** Prompted voiding for the management of urinary incontinence in adults. *Cochrane Database Syst Rev* 2000;(2):CD002113.

47. **Wallace SA, Roe B, Williams K, & Palmer M.** Bladder training for urinary incontinence in adults. *Cochrane Database Syst Rev* 2004;(1):CD001308.

48. **Tibaek S, Gard G, & Jensen R.** Is there a long-lasting effect of pelvic floor muscle training in women with urinary incontinence after ischemic stroke? A 6-month follow-up study. *Int Urogynecol J* 2007;**18**:281–7.

49. **Widemann A, Fusgen I, & Hauri D.** New aspects of therapy with trospium chloride for urge incontinence. *Eur J Geriatrics* 2001;**3**(1):41–5.

50. **Sexton CC, Nottle SM, Maroulis C, Dmochowski RR, Cardozo L, & Subramanian D.** Persistence and adherence in the treatment of overactive bladder syndrome with anticholinergic therapy: a systematic review of the literature. *Int J Clin Pract* 2011;**65**(5):567–85.

51. **Robinson D & Cardozo L.** Antimuscarinic drugs to treat overactive bladder. *BMJ* 2012;**344**:e2130.

52. **Abrams P, Kelleher C, Staskin D,** et al. Combination treatment with mirabegron and solifenacin in patients with overactive bladder: efficacy and safety results from a randomised, double-blind, dose-ranging, phase 2 study (symphony). *Euro Urol* 2015;**63**(3):577–88.

53. **Kohli N & Patterson D.** InterStim therapy: a contemporary approach to overactive bladder. *Rev Obstet Gynecol* 2009;**2**(1):18–27.

54. **Robinson D, Anders K, Cardozo L, & Bidmead J.** Outcome measures in urogynaecology: the clinicians' perspective. *Int Urogynecol J* 2007;**18**:273–9.

55. Abrams P, Cardozo L, Wein A, et al. (eds.) Incontinence. 3rd International Consultation on Incontinence, Monaco, 26–29 June 2004. Paris, France: Health Publication, 2005.

56. **Avery K, Donovan J, Peters TJ, Shaw C, Gotoh M, & Abrams P.** ICIQ: a brief and robust measure for evaluating the symptoms and impact of urinary incontinence. *Neurourol Urodyn* 2004;**23**:322–30.

57. **Wagner T.** Quality of life of persons with urinary incontinence: development of a new measure. *Urology* 1996;**41**:(1):67–71.

58. **Kelleher CJ, Cardozo LD, Khullar V, & Salvatore S.** A new questionnaire to assess the quality of life of urinary incontinent women. *Br J Obstet Gynaecol* 1997;**104**:1374–9.

59. **Staskin D & Kelleher C.** Initial assessment of urinary and faecal incontinence in adult male and female patients. In: Abrams P, Cardozo L, Wein A, et al. (eds.) *Incontinence. 4th International Consultation on Incontinence*, Paris 5–8 July 2008. Paris, France: Health Publication, 2009, pp. 331–412.

60. **Department of Health.** *Independent Inquiry into Care Provided by Mid Staffordshire NHS Foundation Trust January 2005—March 2009*, Volume 1, Chaired by Robert Francis QC. London, UK: Department of Health, 2010.

61. **Healthcare Quality Improvement Partnership (HQIP) & Royal College of Physicians.** *National Audit of Continence Care: Combined Organisational and Clinical Report*. London, UK: Healthcare Quality Improvement Partnership (HQIP) & Royal College of Physicians, 2010.

Chapter 20

Fatigue and the older stroke patient

Ian I. Kneebone and Daniel Kam Yin Chan

Derick

Derick was 82 when he woke in the night, attempted to go to the toilet and found he could not move his left side. He woke his wife, a retired nurse, who immediately applied the FAST—Face, Arm, Speech test—and rang for an ambulance. Derick was seen immediately in an accident and emergency department and a computed tomography (CT) scan was performed. On this basis Derick was diagnosed with a right hemisphere ischaemic stroke. Derick had left hemiplegia, mild dysarthria, and a left-sided attentional neglect. Anaemia was also evident on a blood test. Within 3 hours of his stroke Derick was admitted to an acute stroke unit.

Two days post-stroke, adequate cognition was evident on the basis of a screen using the Montreal Cognitive Assessment (MOCA)[1,2] test. Most notably, good language/communication skills were preserved. Screens using the Geriatric Anxiety Inventory (GAI)[3,4] and the Patient Health Questionnaire—9 item (PHQ-9)[5,6] failed to identify significant anxiety or depression.

Once assessed on the acute stroke unit, an immediate goal was mobilization. Unfortunately, this proved extremely difficult. Derick initially felt unable to participate at all. He fatigued 'within moments' of attempting to move from lying to sitting at the side of his bed: the first steps to standing at a plinth. Therapy sessions became confined to a maximum of 15 minutes on account of this and progress was slow. Staff were frustrated by this as indeed was Derick and his wife. His wife had read up about this on online websites, and appreciated early activity and reduced bed rest were associated with better stroke outcomes.

What is fatigue?

Defining 'clinical fatigue' is a challenge. Where does tiredness end and debilitating fatigue begin? The transition point between these states appears to be related to whether the condition is a consequence of effort and responds substantially to a period of rest.[7,8] Fatigue can be considered to be on a continuum from non-pathological proportionate fatigue to that which is disproportionate, chronic, and disabling. Importantly in stroke, it is fatigue that interferes substantially with rehabilitation progress that is a concern. Notably fatigue after stroke is associated with morbidity, lower quality of life, and poorer mental health.[9-11] A number of groups have suggested criteria to establish clinical fatigue in a stroke population (Box 20.1).

Fatigue in stroke: A model

Fig. 20.1 displays a conceptual model proposed to elucidate fatigue occurring post-stroke. Unsurprisingly perhaps, a predisposing factor to both early and late fatigue is prestroke fatigue.[12] In addition, prestroke depression and general white matter changes on neuroimaging seem to make a difference. With respect to 'stroke as a trigger', brain lesion hypotheses abound, but at this point the evidence is inconclusive with respect to both location and size of lesion.[13] By contrast

---

Box 20.1 Proposed criteria for post-stroke fatigue

The following symptoms should be present every day or nearly every day during a 2-week period in the past month:

Significant fatigue (defined as overwhelming feelings of exhaustion or tiredness), diminished energy or increased need to rest, disproportionate to any recent exertion levels, plus any three of the following:

Experience of sleep or rest as unrefreshing or non-restorative

Disrupted balance between motivation (preserved) and effectiveness (decreased)

Perceived need to struggle to overcome inactivity

Difficulty completing or sustaining daily tasks attributed to feeling fatigued

Postexertional malaise lasting several hours

Marked concern about feeling fatigued

Reproduced with permission from de Groot MH, et al. Fatigue associated with stroke and other neurologic conditions: implications for stroke rehabilitation. *Arch Phys Med Rehab.*, 84(11), 1714–1720. Copyright © 2003, American Congress of Rehabilitation Medicine and the American Academy of Physical Medicine and Rehabilitation. Published by Elsevier Inc. All rights reserved. doi:https://doi.org/10.1053/S0003-9993(03)00346-0

---

the association with mood (anxiety and depression) is much more robust. Evidence is available for associations from both cross-sectional, longitudinal, and systematic review studies.[14,15]

With respect to inflammatory and neuroendocrine factors, an association has been found with cytokines,[16] though little else. A systematic review was unable to conclude one way or another about a connection between fatigue and cognitive factors such as memory, attention, speed of information processing, and reading speed after stroke.[17]

Psychosocial, behavioural, and affective factors have also been assessed with a view to considering their role in the aetiology of fatigue after stroke. Those implicated include social support, depression, anxiety, sense of control, alertness, inappropriate laughing, and coping. In the latter case, fatigue appears associated with emotion-focused distraction and self-blame coping styles.[14] Unsurprisingly, sleep disturbance is related to fatigue after stroke and pain may also impact fatigue.[18] Energy expenditure is naturally included in any model of fatigue.

The main difficulty with such a model is the potential for confounding. To a degree this is accounted for, in that residual neurological deficits are conceptualized as influencing post-stroke fatigue *through* their effects on psychological factors.

Derick

Derick's initial assessment had ruled out reduced social support, depression, and cognitive factors as likely contributors to his fatigue levels. Closer psychological review however detected an attitude that recovery was more up to staff input that his own efforts (an external locus of control). A sleep chart identified insomnia. Derick was consistently awake at night, partly as a result of urinary frequency, a further issue he had encountered post-stroke.

Fatigue in the older stroke patient

It is common to consider fatigue a normal consequence of ageing, but the scientific evidence for this is inconsistent. Some studies support the stereotype,[19,20] others do not.[21,22] A number of

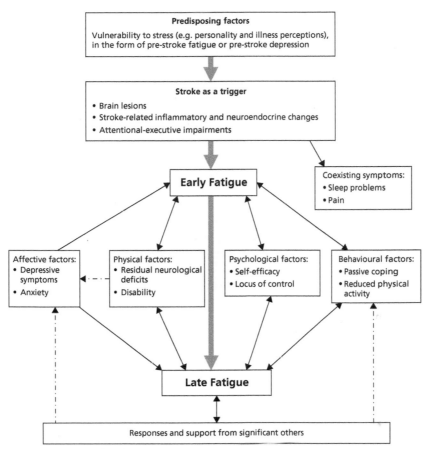

Fig. 20.1 A conceptual model of poststroke fatigue. The unidirectional arrows indicate a causal direction; the bidirectional arrows indicate unknown direction of the association; the dotted arrows indicate potential interactions between factors. Other symptoms may coexist with and maintain symptoms of fatigue.

Reproduced with permission from Wu S, et al. Model of Understanding Fatigue After Stroke. *Stroke*, 46(3), 893–898. Copyright © 2015, American Heart Association, Inc. doi:10.1161/STROKEAHA.114.006647

studies have failed to find a relationship between age and fatigue after stroke,[23–25] while some have found increasing age associated with fatigue.[10] However at least two have identified younger age as associated with higher fatigue.[26–27]

Certainly, a problem with research is the confounding that arises due to comorbidity in the context of older adults with stroke. Older adults are more likely to have multiple medical problems, many of which can cause tiredness and/or fatigue, including cardiac failure and anaemia.[28] Medical illnesses also predispose older people to depressive symptoms, a consistent associate of fatigue. Clinical experience suggests fatigue may be presented as an explanation for low participation in rehabilitation, when the underlying cause is reduced motivation in the context of depression.

Derick

Routine blood work identified Derick's anaemia could be a contributor to fatigue. Investigations established this was likely due to bleeding in his stomach on account of non-steroidal anti-inflammatory drugs (NSAIDs) he was taking for arthritis. His medication was revised and his iron levels stabilized. Bladder overactivity, more common in older adults and after stroke, was considered the cause of his nocturia.

Assessing and treating fatigue in the older stroke patient

Assessing post-stroke fatigue in the older patient needs to consider a range of contributing factors. General to stroke are those indicated in the fatigue model (Fig. 20.1) including activity levels, cognitive impairment, mood disorders, and social support. Additional considerations for older patients can include attention to bereavement—understandably older adults are at higher risk in this respect. Physical screening should include nutritional and systemic factors. Particularly relevant on the older patient would be cardiovascular, respiratory, and musculoskeletal assessment. Excluding heart failure, anaemia, chronic obstructive pulmonary disease, as well as muscle deconditioning and osteoarthritis (especially those of the back, hips, and knees) is important.[28]

Systematic interviewing to proposed criteria (e.g.[29]) is one way of identifying post-stroke fatigue. The Detection List Fatigue (DLF) has recently been developed to support such interviewing. Items include sleep problems, subjective fatigue experience (including mental fatigue), irritability, activity level, motivation, and physical complaints.[30] While it can be argued that no measure is fully psychometrically robust and meets relevant clinical utility criteria in this area,[31] interview assessments can be supported by the use of validated measures. Few measures are validated to assess fatigue in stroke, however, let alone validated for use with older people post-stroke. The failure to establish whether there are true differences in fatigue between older and younger people with stroke also means cut-offs have not been established for older people with stroke as they have been, for instance, for measures of mood.[4, 32] Nor have age-referenced norms been defined. Nonetheless, measures recommended for this purpose include; the Profile of Mood States fatigue subscale, the Short Form-36 item Health Survey (SF36v2) vitality component, Fatigue Severity Scale (FSS), the Multidimensional Fatigue Symptom Inventory general subscale, and the Fatigue Assessment Scale (FAS).[29] The FAS[33] consists of ten statements such as 'I don't do much during the day', that respondents rate from 1 'never' to 5 'always'. Criterion validity for the scale is good, concurrent validity moderate, and test-re-test reliability 'weak to good'.[31] The FSS[34] has the responder consider fatigue in nine situations over the previous week. Items such as 'exercise brings on my fatigue' are rated on a scale from 1 'strong disagreement' to 7 'strong agreement'. The FSS demonstrated excellent internal reliability and discriminant validity in a sample of 852 neurological patients, around 16% of whom had recently experienced an ischaemic stroke.[35]

Possibly one of the best instruments currently available to assess fatigue after stroke is the Neurological Fatigue Index for Stroke (NFI-Stroke; [36]). The NFI-Stroke comprises physical, cognitive, and summary subscales and conforms to the Rasch[37] measurement model. While sound psychometrics and the dimensional aspect of the scale are attractive, of interest in a concern for the older stroke patient is the fact its development was potentially compromised by a selection bias. Of the 999 people mailed questionnaires, those who responded were younger than those who did not[36] and younger than typical for stroke patients.[38] If those who participate in studies of post-stroke fatigue are younger, it is no wonder that differences due to age are not observed.

Cognitive and communication problems post-stroke mean that all those with stroke cannot be routinely assessed with questionnaires. For those significantly affected, simpler instruments can be used. Visual analogue scales (VAS) are commonly used for such assessments (Fig. 20.2). A vertical numerical rating scale is supplemented with faces to evaluate fatigue after stroke. Chuang et al.'s[39] work supports the validity and reliability of this scale; for instance, compared with a traditional numerical rating scale, sensitivity with the NRS-FRS was 94% and specificity 92%.

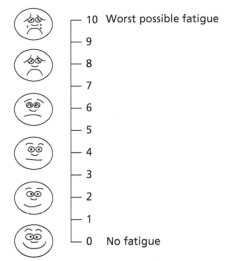

Fig. 20.2 Numerical rating scale supplemented with a faces rating scale for self-reported fatigue intensity.

Derick

Derick was assessed using the FSS two weeks after his stroke. At that time, he endorsed every item of the scale at its highest possible level (i.e. level 7, scoring a total of 63).

Treating fatigue after stroke

Evidence for specific interventions for fatigue is slim. Despite identifying 12 trials of adequate design quality that included 703 participants, via a systematic review, Wu et al.[40] were unable to determine if there was sufficient evidence to support the use of any intervention either to treat or prevent fatigue in people with stroke. Eight of the trials considered had reduction of fatigue as their primary outcome. The interventions included medications: fluoxetine, enerion, (-)-OSU6162 (a monoaminergic stabiliser), as well as a trial of a combination of Chinese herbs. Three non-pharmacological interventions were considered: mindfulness-based stress reduction and fatigue education. The reviewers noted that while fatigue improved overall in the treatment groups relative to controls, benefits were not seen in studies that had used adequate 'allocation concealment'.

The systematic review considered four trials including 248 participants where the primary outcome was not fatigue, but other symptoms after stroke. Continuous positive airway pressure for sleep apnoea, tirilazad mesylate, antidepressants, and a self-management programme for recovery from chronic diseases were not supported for fatigue reduction. None of the trials considered by Wu et al.[40] could validly consider age as a predictor of treatment response as younger people post-stroke dominated the treatment trials (Table 20.1).

Psychological treatment for post-stroke fatigue

The psychological approach to fatigue has its origins in the treatment of chronic fatigue syndrome.[41–48] It is based on the principle that avoidance of activity and excessive rest maintains

Table 20.1 Studies included in a Cochrane review of treatments for fatigue after stroke where fatigue was the primary concern of the intervention

Study	Intervention	Age of participants in years
Choi Kwon (2007)[50]	Fluoxetine	$M = 56$
Clarke (2012)[40]	Group psychoeducation	$M = 72$
Guo (2012)[52]	Chinese medicine	$M = 66$
Gurak (2005)[54]	Enerion (sulbutiamine)	$M = 51$
Johansson (2012)[53]	OSU6162	$M = 50$
Johansson (2012)[47]	MBSR	30 to 65
Zedlitz (2012)[41]	GCT, GCT + treadmill	$M = 55$
Zhou (2010)[51]	Sertraline, electroacupuncture plus cupping	M = 57

Note: OSU6162, oral monoaminergic stabilizer; MBSR, mindfulness-based stress reduction; GCT, group cognitive therapy.

a fatigued state. The cycle is perpetuated when in response to feeling better a person overdoes their activity 'to make up for lost time', with 'collapse' a consequence. A 'boom and bust' cycle can emerge. Cognitive behaviour therapy is one of the most favoured interventions in this context. This considers what people do and how they think about their behaviour and their environment. Typically, intervention includes a graded return to activity, balanced with regular rest breaks. Cognitive elements include education on the nature of the 'boom and bust' cycle to support the graded activity and rest as well as attention to self-defeating thoughts such as 'If I'm having a good day I need to do as much as possible before the fatigue hits' or 'I need to rest all the time so as to prevent another stroke'. This approach is probably used most clinically in stroke rehabilitation but the evidence base is limited to one study in a younger stroke sample (mean 55 years).[47] Pertinent to the needs of the older stroke survivor, cognitive behavioural interventions modified for use with older adults, appears useful.[49,50]

Another psychological approach to fatigue after stroke that has been subject to empirical investigation is mindfulness-based stress reduction (MBSR). Mindfulness exploits attentional processes to benefit the individual through the practice of meditation and mental training. Two key processes are involved: self-direction of attention to immediate experience, allowing awareness of present moment events, and developing openness and acceptance of current experience.[51] Mindfulness has support for its utility in a range of health conditions[52] though evidence for its use with older people is mixed.[53] One randomized controlled trial (RCT) has been conducted using MBSR for fatigue after stroke. While supportive, this was with a mixed sample of stroke and traumatic brain injury patients, and those included in the group were only aged in their mid-fifties.[46] Mindfulness can be blended with cognitive behaviour therapy.[54] This combination shows promise with an older adult population,[55] though at this stage a trial in older people with stroke is awaited.

Derick

Derick was reviewed by an occupational therapist and physiotherapist. They devised a graduated exercise programme for him. This consisted of brief (maximum 15 minutes) but relatively frequent (four times a day) sessions as a starting point to his rehabilitation. Goals were those set in line with normal mobilization procedures employed post-stroke but took into account his arthritis. These included timetabled periods with respect to his sitting up, standing for increasing time periods, and walking. Derick was also seen by the clinical psychologist. The psychologist provided education about fatigue management and addressed Derick's view of his recovery being up to staff rather than himself. Further, the psychologist trained Derick in a meditative strategy to support his sleep. A continence nurse provided support via bladder training.

Medical management of post-stroke fatigue

Treatment of the medical/physical cause(s) of fatigue can include treatment of heart failure, correction of anaemia, and reversal of the cause(s) of anaemia, treatment of chronic respiratory pulmonary disease (via medication, oxygen), treatment of hypothyroidism, hypercalcaemia, vitamin D deficiency, and a drug review (excessive statins, beta-blockers). The association of depression with fatigue has meant antidepressant drugs have been trialled.[41,48] The medications are considered to address underlying serotonin dysfunction responsible for fatigue. Qi 'vital energy' deficiency is the basis for the prescription of Chinese herbal remedies, acupuncture, and cupping for post-stroke fatigue.[43,48] The use of monoaminergic stabilizers is based on the view that mental fatigue is a consequence of reduced function of the prefrontal cortex, that is in turn dependent on a well-balanced catecholaminergic input.[45] It follows monoaminergic stabilizers offer the opportunity to reduce mental fatigue when catecholaminergic input may have been disrupted by stroke. Enerion (sulbutiamine) is man-made thiamine analogue that is thought to stimulate brain activity, though its specific mechanism of action is unknown. It has some limited support for treatment of post-stroke fatigue.[44]

Derick

Derick's NSAID medication was revised to address gastrointestinal bleeding. An anticholinergic, was prescribed to reduce urinary frequency.

Conclusions

While fatigue is common after stroke, research into its management is in its infancy. With respect to the older person there is in particular a deficiency in research not only into fatigue management but also its nature and origins in this age group; many studies have included no or few older people. Older people often have multiple medical comorbidities that can also cause fatigue and these need to be addressed appropriately. Nonetheless clinically both psychological and medical management offer treatments that at the individual level may be worthwhile. Further rigorous empirical research particularly considering older people after stroke might assist in refining understanding and treatment of fatigue in this population.

Derick

Over the course of his treatment Derick gradually improved. His iron levels stabilized and urinary frequency reduced. At discharge he could walk short distances with a quad stick, toilet, dress, and wash himself with standby support. His score was much improved on the FSS (33) and he could tolerate two physiotherapy sessions a day of between 30 and 45 minutes and occupational therapy to address functional goals every second day for up to 45 minutes.

After 42 days as an inpatient Derick was followed up by the Stroke Team for Early Discharge (STED). His improvement with the help of the team was such that by 3 months post-stroke he could tolerate, and enjoy bi-weekly outings to his local club for up to an hour ... on occasions staying on for lunch. Travel time to his club with seniors' transport meant he needed to also manage 30 minutes of sitting prior to and after his club visit. His wife continued to provide him with occasional activities of daily life (ADL) assistance. At STED discharge Derick's five-factor score (FFS) was 19, indicating a dramatic improvement.

References

1. **Nasreddine ZS, Phillips NA, Bedirian V**, et al. The Montreal Cognitive Assessment, MoCA: a brief screening tool for mild cognitive impairment. *J Am Geriatr Soc* 2005;**53**:695–9.

2. **Koski L.** Validity and applications of the Montreal cognitive assessment for the assessment of vascular cognitive impairment. *Cerebrovasc Dis* 2013;**36**:6–18.

3. **Pachana NA, Byrne GJ, Siddle H, Koloski N, Harley E, & Arnold E.** Development and validation of the geriatric anxiety inventory. *Int Psychogeriatrics* 2007;**19**:103–14.

4. **Kneebone II, Fife-Schaw C, Lincoln NB, & Harder H.** Validity and reliability of the Geriatric Anxiety Inventory in screening for post stroke anxiety in older people. *Clin Rehabil* 2016;**30**(12):1220–8.

5. **Kroenke K, Spitzer RL, & Williams JB.** The PHQ-9. *J Gen Intern Med* 2001;**16**(9):606–13.

6. **Williams LS, Brizendine EJ, Plue L**, et al. Performance of the PHQ-9 as a screening tool for depression after stroke. *Stroke* 2005;**36**:635–8.

7. **de Groot MH, Phillips SJ, & Eskes GA.** Fatigue associated with stroke and other neurologic conditions: implications for stroke rehabilitation. *Arch Phys Med Rehab* 2003;**84**(11):1714–20.

8. **Piper BF.** Fatigue: current bases for practice. In: Funk SG, Tornquist EM, Champagne MT, Copp LA, & Wiese RA (eds.) *Key Aspects of Comfort: Management of Pain, Fatigue and Nausea*, pp. 187–9. New York, NY: Springer; 1989.

9. **Glader EL, Stegmayr B, & Asplund K.** Poststroke fatigue: a 2-year followup study of stroke patients in Sweden. *Stroke* 2002;**33**:1327–33.

10. **Mead GE, Graham C, Dorman P**, et al; **UK Collaborators of IST.** Fatigue after stroke: baseline predictors and influence on survival. Analysis of data from UK patients recruited in the International Stroke Trial. *PLoS One* 2011;**6**:e16988.

11. **van de Port IG, Kwakkel G, Schepers VP, Heinemans CT, & Lindeman E.** Is fatigue an independent factor associated with activities of daily living, instrumental activities of daily living and health-related quality of life in chronic stroke? *Cerebrovasc Dis* 2007;**23**:40–5.

12. **Naess H, Lunde L, Brogger J, & Waje-Andreassen U.** Fatigue among stroke patients on long-term follow-up. The Bergen Stroke Study. *J Neurol Sci* 2012;**312**:138–41.

13. **Kutlubaev MA, Duncan FH, & Mead GE.** Biological correlates of poststroke fatigue: a systematic review. *Acta Neurol Scand* 2012;**125**:219–27.

14. **Wu S, Barugh A, Macleod M, & Mead G.** Psychological associations of poststroke fatigue: a systematic review and meta-analysis. *Stroke* 2014;**45**:1778–83.

15. **Wu S, Mead G, Macleod M, & Chalder T.** Model of understanding fatigue after stroke. *Stroke* 2015;**46**:893–8.

16. **Ormstad H, Aass HC, Amthor KF, Lund-Sørensen N, & Sandvik L.** Serum cytokine and glucose levels as predictors of poststroke fatigue in acute ischemic stroke patients. *J Neurol* 2011;**258**:670–6.

17. **Lagogianni C, Thomas S, & Lincoln N.** Examining the relationship between fatigue and cognition after stroke: a systematic review. *Neuropsychol Rehabil* 2016;**28**(1):1–60.

18. **Wu S, Mead G, Macleod M, & Chalder T.** Model of understanding fatigue after stroke. *Stroke* 2015;**46**(3):893–8.

19. **Cupido CM, Hicks AL, & Martin J.** Neuromuscular fatigue during repetitive stimulation in elderly and young adults. *Eur J Appl Physiol Occup Physiol* 1992;**65**(6):567–72.

20. **McNeil CJ & Rice CL.** Fatigability is increased with age during velocity-dependent contractions of the dorsiflexors. *J Gerontol A Biol Sci Med Sci* 2007;**62**(6):624–9.

21. **Allman BL & Rice CL.** Incomplete recovery of voluntary isometric force after fatigue is not affected by old age. *Muscle Nerve* 2001;**24**(9):1156–67.

22. **Lindstrom B, Lexell J, Gerdle B, & Downham D.** Skeletal muscle fatigue and endurance in young and old men and women. *J Gerontol A Biol Sci Med Sci* 1997;**52**(1):B59–B66.

23. **Appelros P.** Prevalence and predictors of pain and fatigue after stroke: a population-based study. *Int J Rehabil Res* 2006;**29**:329–33.

24. **Choi-Kwon S, Han SW, Kwon SU, & Kim JS.** Poststroke fatigue: characteristics and related factors. *Cerebrovasc Dis* 2005;**19**:84–90.

25. **Schepers VP, Visser-Meily AM, Ketelaar M, & Lindeman E.** Poststroke fatigue: course and its relation to personal and stroke-related factors. *Arch Phys Med Rehabil* 2006;**87**:184–8.

26. **Parks NE, Eskes GA, Gubitz GJ**, et al. Fatigue impact scale demonstrates greater fatigue in younger stroke survivors. *Can J Neurol Sci* 2012;**39**:619–25.

27. **Snaphaan L, van der Werf S, & de Leeuw FE.** Time course and risk factors of post-stroke fatigue: a prospective cohort study. *Eur J Neurol* 2011;**18**:611–17.

28. **Evans JG, Williams TF, Beattie BL, Michel JP, & Wilcock GK** (eds.) *Oxford Textbook of Geriatric Medicine*, 2nd edition. Oxford, UK: Oxford University Press, 2002.

29. **Lynch J, Mead G, Greig C, Young A, Lewis S, & Sharpe M.** Fatigue after stroke: the development and evaluation of a case definition. *J Psychosom Res* 2007;**63**:539–44.

30. **Kruithof N, Van Cleef MHM, Rasquin SMC, & Bovend'Eerdt TJH.** Screening poststroke fatigue; feasibility and validation of an instrument for the screening of poststroke fatigue throughout the rehabilitation process. *J Stroke Cerebrovasc* 2016;**25**(1):188–96.

31. **Tyson SF & Brown, P.** How to measure fatigue in neurological conditions? A systematic review of psychometric properties and clinical utility of measures used so far. *Clin Rehabil* 2014;**28**(8):804–16.

32. **Healey A, Kneebone I, Carroll M, & Anderson S.** A preliminary investigation of the reliability and validity of the Brief Assessment Schedule Depression Cards and the Beck Depression Inventory—Fast Screen to screen for depression in older stroke survivors. *Int J Geriatr Psych* 2008:**23**;531–6.

33. **Michielsen HJ, De Vries J, & Van Heck GL.** Psychometric qualities of a brief self-rated fatigue measure: the fatigue assessment scale. *J Psychosom Res* 2003;**54**:345–52.

34. **Krupp LB, Larocca NG, Muirnash J, & Steinberg AD.** The Fatigue Severity Scale—application to patients with multiple sclerosis and systemic lupus-erythematosus. *Arch Neurol* 1989;**46**:1121–3.

35. **Valko PO, Bassetti CL, Bloch KE, Held U, & Baumann CR.** Validation of the Fatigue Severity Scale in a Swiss Cohort. *Sleep* 2008;**31**:1601–7.

36. **Mills RJ, Pallant JF, Koufali M**, et al. Validation of the neurological fatigue index for stroke (nfi-stroke). *Health Qual Life Out* 2012;**10**:51.

37. **Rasch G.** Probabilistic Models for Some Intelligent and Attainment Tests. Chicago, IL: University of Chicago, 1980.

38. **Feigin VL, Lawes CM, Bennett DA, & Anderson CS.** Stroke epidemiology: a review of population-based studies of incidence, prevalence, and case-fatality in the late 20th century. *Lancet Neurol* 2003;**2**(1):43–53.

39. **Chuang L, Lin K, Hsu A**, et al. Reliability and validity of a vertical numerical rating scale supplemented with a faces rating scale in measuring fatigue after stroke. *Health Qual Life Outcomes* 2015;**13**:91.

40. **Wu S, Kutlubaev MA, Chun HYY**, et al. Interventions for post-stroke fatigue. *Cochrane Database Syst Rev* 2015;**7**:CD007030.

41. **Choi-Kwon S, Choi J, Kang D-W, & Kim JS.** Fluoxetine is not effective in the treatment of post-stroke fatigue: a double-blind, placebo-controlled study. *Cerebrovasc Dis* 2007;**23**:102–108.

42. **Clarke A, Barker-Collo S, & Feigin V.** Poststroke fatigue: does group education make a difference? A randomized pilot trial. *Top Stroke Rehabil* 2012;**19**:32–9.

43. **Guo YH, Chen HX, & Xie RM.** Effects of qi-supplementing dominated Chinese materia medica combined with rehabilitation training on the quality of life of ischemic post-stroke fatigue patients of qi deficiency syndrome[Chinese]. *Zhongguo Zhong Xi Yi Jie He Za Zhi* 2012;**32**:160–3.

44. **Gurak SV & Parfenov VA.** Asthenia after stroke and myocardial infarction and its treatment with Enerion. *Klinicheskaya Gerontologia* 2005;**8**:9–12.

45. **Johansson B, Carlsson A, Carlsson ML, Karlsson M, Nilsson MKL, & Nordquist-Brandt E.** Placebo-controlled cross-over study of the monoaminergic stabiliser (-)-OSU6162 in mental fatigue following stroke or traumatic brain injury. *Acta Neuropsychiatrica* 2012;**24**:266–74.

46. **Johansson B, Bjuhr H, & Rönnbäck L.** Mindfulness-based stress reduction (MBSR) improves long-term mental fatigue after stroke or traumatic brain injury. *Brain Injury* 2012;**26**:1621–8.

47. **Zedlitz AMEE, Rietveld TCM, Geurts AC, & Fasotti L.** Cognitive and graded activity training can alleviate persistent fatigue after stroke: a randomized, controlled trial. *Stroke* 2012;**43**:1046–51.

48. **Zhou Y, Zhou GY, Li SK, & Jin JH.** Clinical observation on the therapeutic effect of electroacupuncture combined with cupping on post-stroke fatigue [Chinese]. *Zhen Ci Yan Jiu* 2010;**35**:380–3.

49. **Gould RL, Coulson MC, & Howard RJ.** Efficacy of cognitive behavioral therapy for anxiety disorders in older people: a meta-analysis and meta-regression of randomized controlled trials. *J Am Geriatr Soc* 2012;**60**(2):218–29.

50. **Laidlaw K & Kishita N.** Age-appropriate augmented cognitive behavior therapy to enhance treatment outcome for late-life depression and anxiety disorders. *GeroPsych* 2015;**28**(2):57–66.

51. **Carlson LE & Garland SN.** Impact of mindfulness-based stress reduction (MBSR) on sleep, mood, stress and fatigue symptoms in cancer outpatients. *Int J Behav Med* 2005;**12**(4):278–85.

52. **Gotink RA, Chu P, Busschbach JJ, Benson H, Fricchione GL, & Hunink MM.** Standardised mindfulness-based interventions in healthcare: an overview of systematic reviews and meta-analyses of RCTs. *PLoS One* 2015;**10**(4):e0124344.

53. **Geiger PJ, Boggero IA, Brake CA,** et al. Mindfulness-based interventions for older adults: a review of the effects on physical and emotional well-being. *Mindfulness* 2016;**7**(2):296–307.

54. **Segal ZV, Williams JM, Teasdale JD.** *Mindfulness-Based Cognitive Therapy for Depression.* New York, NY: Guilford Press, 2012.

55. **O'Connor M, Piet J, & Hougaard E.** The effects of mindfulness-based cognitive therapy on depressive symptoms in elderly bereaved people with loss-related distress: a controlled pilot study. *Mindfulness* 2014;**5**(4):400–9.

Chapter 21

Visual disorders in stroke

Deborah Plunkett and Sushma Dhar-Munshi

Introduction

A significant proportion of stroke patients have unrecognized visual problems resulting in little or no advice or treatment. The aim of this chapter is to discuss the mechanisms, clinical features, and management of these disorders to facilitate diagnosis and treatment for the stroke physician, the ophthalmologist who may suspect stroke aetiology, and the general practitioner to identify cases for referral.

Visual disorders following stroke are common. Up to 30% of stroke patients experience visual impairment. In occipital strokes the frequency is up to 70%.[1-4] As the population is ageing, cerebrovascular disease is on the rise and consequently visual impairment after stroke is going to be an increasing problem in the future. The main focus in stroke rehabilitation is often motor impairment; on the National Institutes of Health Stroke Scale (NIHSS) a homonymous hemianopia scores quite low.[5] In a review of 61 studies (n = 25 672), overall prevalence of visual impairment early after stroke was 65%, ranging from 19% to 92%. Visual field loss reports ranged from 5.5% to 57%, ocular motility problems from 22% to 54%, visual inattention from 14% to 82%, and reduced central vision reported in up to 70%. Recovery of visual field loss varied between 0% and 72%, with ocular motility between 7% and 92%, and visual inattention between 29% and 78%.[6]

Fig. 21.1 shows the mechanisms of the central visual processing.[7] The visual field projects onto the retina through the lens and falls on the retinae as an inverted, reversed image. The topography of this image is maintained as the visual information travels through the visual pathway to the cortex.

The functional neurological architecture of vision has been well described. Area V1 (striate cortex) is the primary cortical processing area for macular retinal images. Areas V2 and V3 (extrastriate cortex) are the primary cortical processing areas for peripheral retinal images. Areas V4/V8 (occipito-temporal region corresponding to lingual and fusiform gyri) is the centre for colour processing. A lesion here leads to achromatopsia (defect in colour perception). Area V5 (temporo-parietal-occipital junction) is the motion detection area. Lesions here leads to akinetopsia (disorder of motion perception). The centre for visual object recognition is midway along the medial-lateral plane of the inferior occipital-temporal surface. A lesion here leads to agnosia (loss of object recognition). The lateral inferior occipito-temporal fusiform gyrus is responsible for familiar face recognition. A lesion here leads to prosopagnosia (deficit for recognition of familiar faces, such as those of family, friends, and colleagues). Place recognition is controlled by the medial inferior occipito-temporal parahippocampal gyrus and a lesion here leads to difficulty in recognition of familiar environment. The caudal portion of the intraparietal sulcus is for stereoscopic processing. The rest of the intraparietal sulcus is the 'reach area' which tells the motor cortex where to move to produce a desired effect. A lesion here leads to optic ataxia (impairment of reaching for objects in the environment) and oculomotor apraxia (impairment of voluntary

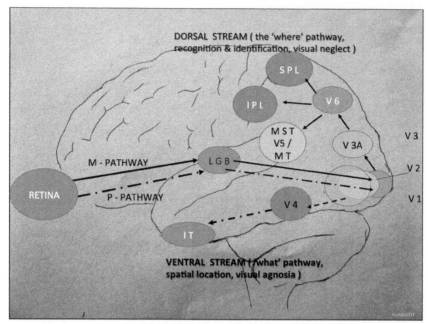

Fig. 21.1 Mechanisms of central visual processing.

Diagram showing principal visual pathways in the cortex. V1, V2, V3, V3A, V4, V5, V6 are the visual cortical areas. MST, medial superior temporal, MT, middle temporal; SPL, superior parietal lobule; IPL, inferior parietal lobule; LGB, lateral geniculate body; IT, inferior temporal lobule; M-pathway, magnocellular; P-pathway, parvocellular.

eye movements to command). The spatial awareness of the body is controlled by the superior and inferior parietal lobules. A lesion here results in hemineglect.

Fig. 21.2 showing the visual fields and pathway.

Post-stroke visual impairment

There are four main types of visual disorders, which may occur individually or in combination.[8-12] These are central loss of vision, peripheral loss of vision, or visual field loss, eye movement disorders, and visual processing disorders (see Table 21.1). The various strategies used for 'neurovisual rehabilitation' can be grouped under three main strategies—restitution, compensation, and substitution.[13] Restitution focuses on areas of residual vision and an attempt is made to identify these areas using high-resolution perimetry. The strategy is based on exploiting the 'plasticity' of the central nervous system.[9]

Disorder of central vision

Central loss of vision may occur in one or both eyes. It is therefore important to test this accurately. In adult ophthalmology practice it is routine to test distance uniocular visual acuity using a LogMAR Chart.[10] The person is asked to read the smallest letters possible and this is recorded in LogMAR units. A person only able to read the largest top line of five letters would have 1.00 compared with normal visual acuity of 0.00 LogMAR. Visual acuity is tested with distance glasses, if these are worn. Pertinent questions about the age of the glasses and when the last optometrist check was performed are important.

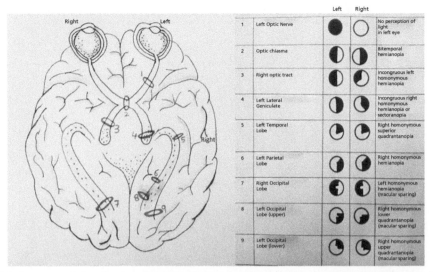

Fig. 21.2 Anatomy of the visual pathways and visual field correlation (view of underside of brain).

Many people affected by stroke are not able to perform the visual acuity LogMAR Chart. This may be due to other disorders following a stroke such as speech problems or due to language barriers or cognitive disabilities. To test visual acuity in a person who is aphasic, a matching lap card with the complimentary letters on the chart is used. The use of interpreters is essential in situations where there is a language barrier for use in the testing and treatment and in discussing findings. Where there is evidence that a person has learning difficulties, whether this is congenital or acquired such as in people with dementia, the visual acuity test appropriate to the ability of the person should be selected. This may range from Keeler Uncrowded LogMAR where there are only two letters presented on one page at once, or the Kay Picture Test where pictures are used instead of letters. In people with more severe learning disabilities where verbal communication is not possible, the use of preferential looking techniques is the best choice for testing visual acuity. This may be by Cardiff Acuity Cards[11] or Keeler Forced Choice Preferential Looking Test.

Near vision is tested with the correct glasses. This may be with bifocals, varifocals, or separate reading glasses. Testing may use individual letters, text, or pictures depending on the ability of the person. If an impairment of visual acuity is detected, it is important to give advice on the correct use of glasses. In adults with presbyopia correction, using reading glasses may only be required. If necessary, a simple labelling of distance and reading glasses may be required where confusion arises and relatives or carers do not know what the glasses are for. If the wrong glasses are used by a person, the visual acuity will be reduced even more causing distress and slowing rehabilitation.

Where visual acuity remains reduced despite the correct glasses, refer to an ophthalmologist for a thorough ocular examination. This includes the adnexal system, the cornea, the crystalline lens, the aqueous and vitreous humours, and the fundus including the optic disc and the macula.

When the visual acuity in a person is so impaired that they are unable to read the largest letters on the LogMAR Chart, other tests are utilized for examination. This may include checking to see if the largest 1.00 LogMAR letter can be seen by reducing the distance between the tester and the examiner. If a letter is not seen at a 1-metre distance, then the person is asked if they can see to

Table 21.1 This table shows common visual disorders after stroke, their important features and management strategies

Visual disorder	Cause	Investigations	Management
Central visual loss	CRA occlusion, BRA occlusion, bilateral cortical infarcts, CRVO, temporal arteritis, and anterior ischaemic optic neuropathy, Terson's syndrome[8]	LogMAR chart, VA testing, fundoscopy, matching lap card in aphasia, Keeler Uncrowded LogMAR, Kay Picture Test, Cardiff acuity cards, or Keeler forced choice preferential looking test	Glasses, magnifiers, minifiers, antiglare, and overlays to decrease contrast and glare; registration as sight impaired with ophthalmologist, referral to low vision clinic
Eye movement disorders	Gaze palsy, third, fourth, and sixth N palsy, nystagmus, oscillopsia, head posture abnormality, internuclear ophthalmoplegia, diplopia, squint, impaired depth perception, Parinaud's midbrain syndrome, Weber's syndrome, ptosis (partial or total), facial palsy with dry eye		Fresnel prisms, scanning, and tracking strategies, typoscopes, patch, exercises, artificial tear drops, lubricants
Visual perceptual disorders	Visual neglect agnosia anosognosia (Anton Babinski syndrome—bilateral V1 lesions) Balint's syndrome (bilateral posterior cerebral artery, PCA strokes), optic ataxia, apraxia, and asimultagnosia; visual hallucinations (Charles Bonnet syndrome)[12]; colour agnosia (central achromatopsia), colour anomia, and metamorphopsia; Prosopagnosia Akinetopsia Vertical and topographical disorientation Riddoch syndrome[9]	Informal line bisection Albert's Test Clock drawing Patient asked to identify five common objects	Explanation to patient and carers Promote affected side Visual scanning Fresnel prisms Adaptive strategies Patches Mirrors
Peripheral visual disorder	Homonymous hemianopia Quadrantanopia scotomas	Confrontation visual fields Perimetry Humphrey's VFA	Optical aids, prism glasses, visual scanning training (card-based exercises and electronic), visual restorative treatment, education leaflets, separate reading glasses, lighting, coloured ruler, Typoscope, Fresnel prisms, referral to low vision clinic

Table 21.1 Continued

Visual disorder	Cause	Investigations	Management
Pre-existing eye disorder or worsening of previous ocular symptoms	Presbyopia, hypermetropia, myopia, astigmatism, cataracts, glaucoma, diabetic retinopathy, age-related macular degeneration, amblyopia, optic nerve disease, anoxia, or other neurological or myogenic disorders		Appropriate management by ophthalmologist

CRA, central retinal artery; BRA, branch retinal artery; CRVO, central retinal vein occlusion; PCA, posterior cerebral artery.

count the number of fingers being held by the examiner in front of them. If this is not seen, then the use of hand movements and finally perception of light is used. Perception of light and dark is the most primitive form of vision. In cases of impaired vision, the person should be offered sight impairment registration by a consultant ophthalmologist and a low vision assessment by a specialist trained in this area.

Registration as sight impaired or severely sight impaired will enable extra statutory support. Referral to a low vision clinic will enable strategies to be given to help the person to make the best use of any remaining vision and overcome difficulties caused as a consequence of low vision.

Eye movement defects

Eye movement defects are common following a stroke. They are distressing to a person and usually affect the speed of recovery from a stroke. This may be due to diplopia, gaze palsy, nystagmus and oscillopsia, and an abnormal head posture. A person may have one or a combination of these symptoms.[6,14,15] It is important to explain why the problem is present so that the person can understand the problem and strategies formulated to treat the symptoms.

Conjugate eye deviations and inattention often occur together and result in reduced fast eye movements (saccades), which are important for daily activities (e.g. reading, walking, and visual exploration). Some of the movement disorders include saccadic dysmetrias, impaired gaze holding, saccadic palsy, gaze palsy, smooth pursuit palsy, sixth and third nerve palsies, Internuclear ophthalmoplegia, Parinaud's dorsal midbrain syndrome,[16] reduced depression, Weber's syndrome,[17] one and a half syndrome and fourth nerve palsy.

Intractable diplopia is usually the presenting symptom and requires examination by a specialist orthoptist. This is caused by strabismus (squint or dysconjugate gaze) resulting from a sixth, fourth, or third cranial nerve palsy or a stroke involving the cerebellum or one of the cerebellar connections. It can give rise to reading problems, difficulty walking, misjudging distance, nausea, and anxiety. The person may have already involuntarily learnt that by closing one eye the diplopia is resolved but this in itself leads to further symptoms. The constant contracture of the orbicularis muscle to close the eye gives rise to a tension headache around the eye and over the ipsilateral temporal and occipital region.

In some cases an abnormal head posture can temporarily relieve the diplopia. Most abnormal head postures when maintained for several hours result in neck muscle spasm and an occipital tension headache. Small change to the head posture is sometimes the preferred choice but commonly the diplopia is treated using Fresnel prisms. The orthoptist measures the strabismus at near and distance and then selects the most appropriate prism strength. Fresnel prisms range from 1 to 40 prism dioptres in strength. The amount required is usually half the horizontal measurement due to the presence of horizontal fusional reserves. The ability of the eyes to converge on a near object and diverge when a target is moved away allows fusional reserves of the eyes to maintain binocular single vision when the eyes are moving. The vertical fusional reserves are smaller resulting in the amount of the vertical measurement to be corrected by two-thirds using a Fresnel prism. It is possible to tilt the Fresnel prism to correct a horizontal and vertical deviation. In the presence of a total unilateral or bilateral fourth cranial nerve palsy torsional diplopia may be present. Occlusion of one eye using a black eye patch or frosting one spectacle lens is the required treatment. The use of Fresnel prisms or occlusion eliminates diplopia relieving the person of their symptoms.

The diplopia is corrected by the Fresnel prism looking in the straight-ahead position but may still be evident looking horizontally or vertically. It is important to teach the use of head movements when tracking and explain that although the Fresnel prism may cause a small reduction in the visual acuity and cause chromatic aberrations, this far outweighs having intractable diplopia. Also, the person must be aware that the Fresnel prism is only temporary. Recovery from cranial nerve palsy can be partial or full, therefore regular assessment is necessary to diagnose any changes and treat accordingly. Where recovery takes place, it may be necessary to decrease the strength of the Fresnel prism. In some instances, the Fresnel can be discarded over time when binocular single vision is regained and in others a prism can be incorporated into the spectacles by a dispensing optician as a permanent treatment.[18]

Third cranial nerve palsy causes impaired vertical eye movement, lateral diplopia, for near vision tasks, dilatation of pupil, and impaired accommodation with total or partial ptosis. This can lead to anxiety due to the changed facial appearance. Total ptosis may be an advantage as it may eliminate diplopia without the need for a Fresnel prism. Where the ciliary muscle has been affected by the paralysis of the third cranial nerve, a dilated pupil may be present and the near vision may be blurred even wearing reading glasses. If this is unilateral then the unaffected eye can usually focus clearly to read but if it is bilateral or the dominant eye is affected, then additional convex lenses may be required in order to read small print.[19]

In trochlear nerve palsy there is impaired downward and lateral eye movement, and vertical diplopia for near vision tasks. In abducens nerve palsy there is impaired lateral eye movement and lateral diplopia for far vision tasks. A face turn right for a right sixth cranial nerve palsy and in the case of a right fourth cranial nerve palsy, which results in a vertical strabismus, a face turn and head tilt to left and chin depression is evident.[20]

In gaze palsies there is an inability to move both eyes either horizontally or vertically. In horizontal or vertical gaze palsies the eyes may be deviated to one side causing the person to turn their head significantly in the opposite direction to enable them to look in the primary position.[21] The use of Fresnel prisms on each lens of the spectacles can be used to move the images to a straight-ahead position thus eliminating the need for a large head turn or chin elevation or depression. The underlying gaze palsy causes an inability of the eyes to move horizontally giving rise to symptoms of unsteadiness and reading problems. Scanning and tracking strategies are necessary to enable progress with rehabilitation. Moving the head to fix on objects may be taught. This requires time and patience as it is a voluntary adaptation to overcome the absent reflex saccadic eye movement. It is important to work as a multidisciplinary team as discussion with the physiotherapist and occupational therapist is essential regarding the visual disorder. Strategies can then be put in place to overcome the difficulties. Difficulties in reading can be managed by the use of a typoscope where a black card is used to cover a block of text, which shows one or two words at a time in a gap in the card. The typoscope is moved along the text and as the print from other lines does not jumble and appear to obscure the individual words being read this allows the person to read again. In vertical gaze palsies where the eyes are not able to move vertically, this can cause problems with walking as the eyes are not able to saccade vertically to allow a person to see when they are walking on uneven surfaces and negotiating steps. Training is necessary to use repeated head scanning strategies, to look down first then undertake the movement then to look straight ahead to see where the body is moving too. This all takes extra time for the person but is essential in the rehabilitation process and in the prevention of falls.

Nystagmus is an involuntary oscillation of the eyes either horizontally, vertically, rotatory, or in combination.[22] It can cause reduced vision, unsteadiness, and nausea. Oscillopsia is a debilitating symptom where the affected person feels that their environment is constantly moving due to the involuntary movement of the eyes. There is usually a null position of gaze where the nystagmus is less or appears absent. The orthoptist can identify this on testing the ocular movements and can explain this to the patient and carers. Training in the use of an abnormal head posture to maximize the null position of gaze can improve the visual acuity and sometimes alleviate the oscillopsia. Reassurance that the oscillopsia usually resolves is important in the rehabilitation of the person as it can relieve anxiety and depression. Where the null position of gaze is only achieved by a large abnormal head posture, the use of Fresnel prisms can aid in the management by deviating the image thus reducing the need to deviate the eyes as much to achieve the desired null position of gaze. The use of Fresnel prisms is temporary and may be required for up to a year until recovery from the visual disorder following stroke. Prisms may be incorporated into glasses as a permanent treatment. It is important to inform the dispensing optician about the strength of the prisms and the direction of the prism in front of each eye. It may be recommended that bifocal and varifocal glasses are no longer suitable and that single vision lenses for distance and reading are required. Reduced convergence may be seen in a sizeable proportion of stroke patients. Separate spectacles for using a computer or reading music may also be required as these activities require the person to have their corrective lenses for a set distance which is further than the near reading position.

Visual field defects

The peripheral vision or visual field is affected by stroke in a significant number of people.[5,6,23] The visual field is the whole area seen by each eye horizontally and vertically when the eye is looking straight ahead. The importance of the peripheral vision is underestimated which is why it can cause disorientation and debilitating symptoms. The person may complain of an inability to see to one side, giving rise to a blind side. This gives rise to symptoms of bumping into objects on one side, tripping or falling over objects, and problems reading and writing. Loss of confidence is common as objects appear to suddenly jump in front of a person causing anxiety. Crowded areas are particularly troublesome, with the sudden appearance of people in front of a person or the frustration of constantly walking into people and objects. Assessment of the visual field is therefore important so that an understanding of the type of visual field defect is recognized and shared with the person and their carers. Management can be challenging.[24-28] Treatment can be given and a management plan formulated and shared with the multidisciplinary team.[29] The visual field can be assessed by confrontation testing. A more formal visual field assessment can be performed using a perimeter. The most common one is the Humphrey visual field analyser. A full field 80 or 120 test is recommended from the menu depending on the ability of the person. Small flashes of white light are presented randomly in the field of vision and the person is instructed to press a trigger when a light is observed. A printout for each eye tested is produced for diagnostic purposes and for monitoring any recovery on repeated testing (Fig. 21.3).

Homonymous hemianopia is the most common visual field defect in a person affected by stroke. This is where half of the vision is affected in each eye on either the right or left side. The right or

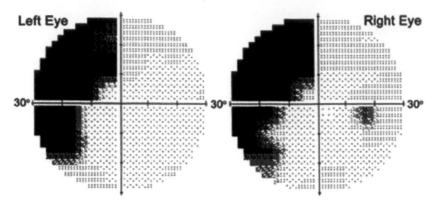

Fig. 21.3 Perimetry showing left homonymous hemianopia after a right occipital stroke.

left half of the vision lost is the same side as the weakness to the leg, arm, or face. Management of the symptoms of homonymous hemianopia are initially educating the patient as to why they are having problems, for example, reading and writing and feeling disorientated.[30] Leaflets with pictures showing what a person can see with a visual field defect or simulated glasses are recommended for carers in the understanding of the condition. Advice may be given on strategies to overcome the reading problems through advising on the correct use of separate reading spectacles and the importance of good lighting when reading. Reading strategies may involve use of a vertical line guide, or finger pointing to mark the beginning and end of lines of text. Advice on rotating the text 90 degrees to read vertically is sometimes very beneficial and a simple solution to a person experiencing reading difficulties. Use of a coloured ruler or typoscope can aid reading and writing by highlighting individual lines or words. The use of high contrast and finger pointing to follow the tip of the pen when writing may be beneficial.

The use of head and eye movements to scan the environment can aid the person feeling disorientated. It is advisable in right homonymous hemianopia to inform carers to sit on the left side of a person and vice versa in a left homonymous hemianopia. This enables the person to make use of their remaining field of vision. This is important when visiting a person who is lying or sitting. When approaching a person, it is important to approach from the front or from the seeing side to reduce the chance of startling the person. If this is not possible then the verbal use of what is happening in a person's environment is recommended. If a person is being approached from their blind side, then the person approaching should say their name and clearly state that they are approaching from that side.

The orthoptist may recommend the use of Fresnel prisms in a person with a visual field defect. Fresnel prisms can be used to expand part of the visual field or displace images from the blind side to the seeing side. This can act as a cue for the person to scan to their blind side to properly view the object. This is especially helpful where mobility was good prior to the stroke and confidence in mobility and esteem has been dramatically affected. Three types of visual field expanders are available to help patients with homonymous hemianopsia. These systems include the EP Horizontal Lens, the Gottlieb Visual Field Awareness System, and the Chadwick Hemianopsia Lens (InWave type monocular lens).

Visual field loss may present as a loss of quarter of the visual field in each eye on the same side or random areas of visual field loss called scotomas. Quadrantanopia and scotomas may be less problematic for reading and writing but this depends on the individual person depending on any comorbidity and their individual needs. In some individuals it may result in milder symptoms for reading and writing and mobility and independence. This should be managed the same as homonymous hemianopia through assessment, documentation, treatment, and subsequent monitoring. In some individuals, it may result in devastating consequences through their inability to drive or perform hobbies as easily as before their stroke, such as reading for pleasure.

Visual processing disorders

The first description of visual anosognosia was made by renaissance French writer Michel de Montaigne (1533–1592). He described a nobleman who denied his own blindness.[31] In 1895, the Austrian psychiatrist and neurologist Gabriel Anton (1858–1933) described the case of Juliane Hochriehser, a 69-year-old dairymaid who had anosognosia with cortical deafness due to a lesion on her both temporal lobes.[32] Anton described other cases of patients with objective blindness and deafness who denied their deficits. In 1914 the French-Polish neurologist Joseph François Babinski (1857–1932) used the term 'anosognosia' to describe the unawareness of the deficit in patients with hemiplegia.[33]

Visual perceptual difficulties may affect a person following a stroke.[5, 34–36] This can be identified formally and informally. Carers when questioned may be able to describe that the affected person has visual inattention. They may have observed that the person ignores everything to one side of them. This includes people sitting or standing to one side and cups placed on one side or food that is left on one side of their plate and also includes neglect of one side of their own body. Visual inattention usually affects a person who has had a right-sided stroke. It can be formally assessed using the line bisection test, the Albert test where several lines are required to be bisected or the clock test where a clock face is presented and the person is asked to write in the numbers on the clock face (Maxton).

It is important that visual inattention is explained to the person and carers. Promotion of the affected side is important. This can be through visual scanning or sitting on the persons affected side to encourage them to be aware of this side. Similar to visual field loss, Fresnel prism treatment may be helpful depending on the individual need.[36] Visual hallucinations may be experienced by individuals in the form of Charles Bonnet syndrome.[12] Advice on this condition should be discussed with the person and their carers and multidisciplinary team. It is very distressing but is usually self-limiting. Reassurance and strategies to overcome are recommended such as looking from side to side ten times each time the visual hallucination occurs. Visual agnosia is also another visual perception disorder experienced by some individuals. This is where an object can be seen but is not recognized by the individual. It is important to recognize this so that it can be explained to the person affected and strategies can be advised to deal with this. Name badges on staff and verbal introduction by carers and family members are important. Advice on what an object is used for may be necessary; for example, explaining that the hot cup has been placed on the right side. The affected person should be encouraged to use eye scanning to look for the cup and told how to pick it up and drink from it. When a meal has been eaten and one-half of the plate of food is left due to visual inattention, the person should be encouraged to always rotate their plate by 180 degrees, so that the other half of the food on the plate is seen.

Dry eye

Dry eye is a common after a stroke due to failure to close the eye or eversion of the eyelid. This should be treated with appropriate artificial tear drops and lubricants (Table 21.2).

Table 21.2 A comparison of neglect and visual field deficits

Neglect	Visual field defect
Damage to the visual/sensory/motor processing areas	Damage to a visual pathway
Most frequently associated with right-sided (parietal) lesions	Damage to the optic tract, geniculostriate pathway, or occipital lobe
Decreased awareness of the body and spatial environment on the affected side	A sensory disturbance within the visual field
Search pattern is asymmetrical; initiated and confined to the right side	Search pattern is abbreviated towards the blind field
Patient makes no attempt to direct their search towards the left side	Patient attempts to direct their search towards the blind side
Search pattern is random and generally inefficient	Search pattern is organized and generally efficient
The patient does not rescan to check the accuracy of their search	The patient rescans to check the accuracy of their performance
The patient completes the task quickly, the level of effort applied is not consistent with the difficulty of the task	Time spent on the task is appropriate to the level of difficulty
Poor prognosis, recovery tends to plateau at 12 weeks	Maximal recovery within 4–12 weeks

Reproduced with permission from Maxton C, et al. Don't neglect 'neglect'– an update on post stroke neglect. *International Journal of Clinical Practice*, 67(4), 369–378. Copyright © 2013, Blackwell Publishing Ltd. https://doi.org/10.1111/ijcp.12058

Drug-induced problems

Many stroke patients receive various drugs (e.g. anticholinergics for urinary incontinence which may lead to worsening of glaucoma or paralysis of accommodation).

Pre-existing eye disorders

Thirty-one per cent (31%) of stroke patients who report visual problems have low vision attributable to associated ocular pathology and not as a result of stroke.[35] A detailed history and ophthalmic examination can determine the extent of the visual disorders. Common visual disorders such as refractive errors (hypermetropia, myopia, astigmatism, and presbyopia), cataracts, glaucoma, diabetic retinopathy, hypertensive retinopathy, and age-related macular degeneration may already exist, and it is important to arrange appropriate management and follow-up.

Prognosis

Peripheral visual field loss can recover in some but not all people following a stroke. In 10% full recovery is seen within the first 2 weeks after stroke. Where full recovery does not take place within 2 weeks, recovery may continue for up to 6 months in 50% of people.[37]

Visual disorders in stroke can range from mild to severe and can be transient of recover fully. The visual disorder should be diagnosed promptly and treatment given so that information can be shared with the individual concerned and the multidisciplinary team involved in the rehabilitation process. This can lead to a speedier discharge from hospital and enable the person to come to terms with their visual disorder, which is often accompanied by multifactorial general health problems prior to the stroke or a consequence of the stroke especially in older people. The aim is to improve the quality of life for the individual and to prevent further health-related problems arising; for example, from physical injuries due to falls, or mental health issues due to anxiety and depression. Often simple solutions, such as new distance glasses for myopia can benefit the distance vision; reassurance that the recovering visual field defect may take up to 6 months; advice that tunnel vision results in good central visual acuity but poor peripheral vision similar to looking through a spy hole in a door; or an explanation as to why a picture can be seen and traced with the finger but not recognized and named as an object, are required. Other patients may require further specialist treatment such as Fresnel prisms by an orthoptist.

Driving and visual problems after stroke

The ability to drive may also be affected after a stroke and is a critical issue. A person should not drive for one month following a stroke. If there is a visual field defect, advice should be given that they should not drive and should contact the Driver and Vehicle Licencing Authority (DVLA).[38] The visual field should be monitored for up to 6 months so that the affected person can be informed of any improvement. It can be very distressing to a person to be informed that they are no longer able to drive as this may lead to loss of independence, depression, and be a barrier to rehabilitation. It is important to diagnose a significant visual field defect as this may allow the person the benefits entitled to then from becoming registered as 'sight impaired'. These benefits range from financial and practical support at home to emotional support and counselling, as most people with visual disorders will experience a grieving process through their loss of previous normal vision.

Stroke patients who drive are more likely to suffer from impaired contrast sensitivity and peripheral vision as well as a reduced 'useful field of view', and are more prone to accidents.[39]

Quality of life, psychological problems, and support strategies after visual loss in stroke

The risk of falls and postural instability increases considerably with visual impairment and impacts profoundly on the quality of life. The visual impairment and the social isolation both cause a reduction in the quality of life. In patients with cortical blindness due to bilateral damage in primary visual cortex or postchiasmal afferents there is often severe deterioration of visual acuity, often complicated by coexistence of cognitive, sensory, physical, and behavioural impairments, which in turn affect rehabilitation.[40–46] Many patients are unaware of visual field loss resulting in increased risk of accidents.

Recognition of loneliness, depression, and inability to cope is essential so that help can be offered whether this is in the form of counselling, referral for specialist counselling, or referral to voluntary local and national support groups and charity groups.[47] Individuals may benefit from talking books and talking newspapers, and audio-description on their televisions.

Visual perceptual deficits like agnosia and neglect can be very distressing by impairing the rehabilitation process of a person due to communication difficulties, loss of social interaction, reduced independence, anxiety, frustration, and depression.

Magnifiers may be used to enlarge reading text and for enabling daily living skills such as reading, dials on the cooker or microwave or central heating, and reading prices of labels when shopping and seeing to count money. These come in a variety of strengths and designs depending on the individual's needs. They can be hand-held, pocket, stand, or free-standing magnifiers. They can be illuminated or non-illuminated or electronic magnifiers. They can clip on to spectacles if a person requires their hands to be free, to enable them to participate in hobbies such as model-making, sewing, and painting. Stand magnifiers are useful for writing and undertaking cross-words. Telescopes or monoculars are beneficial to aid distance vision and to enable continued independence; for example, when looking for an approaching bus number or the platform of a train.

Mobility training may be required through a specialist local mobility officer and referral to Guide Dogs for the Blind may be beneficial to some individuals. The training in safeguarding vulnerable adults is essential so that strategies can be put in place according to the local guidelines.

There is no doubt that targeted treatment or advice with an orthoptist or ophthalmologist and retraining can be invaluable to explore the plasticity of the brain.[48,49] More than a quarter of stroke survivors living with visual impairment do not receive adequate support.

The report *Care Provision and Unmet Need for Post Stroke Visual Impairment (Vision 2020)* reveals that a third of practitioners do not supply vision information to patients or carers, despite an estimated three in five (60%) stroke survivors in the United Kingdom living with visual impairment.[50]

References

1. **Allen CMC, Harrison MJG, & Wade DT.** *The Management of Acute Stroke.* Baltimore, MD: Johns Hopkins University Press, 1989, pp. viii, 215.

2. **Pambakian AL & Kennard C.** Can visual function berestoredin patients wih homonymous hemianopia? *Br J Ophthalmol* 1997;**81**:324–8.

3. **Suchoff IB, Kapoor N, Ciuffreda KJ, Rutner D, Han E, & Craig S.** The frequency of occurrence, types, and characteristics of visual field defects in acquired brain injury: a retrospective analysis. *Optometry* 2008;**79**:259–65.

4. **Papageorgiou E, Hardiess G, Schaeffel F,** et al. Assessment of vision-related quality of life in patients with homonymous visual field defects. *Graefes Arch Clin Exp Ophthalmol* 2007;**245**:1749–58.

5. **Sand KM, Midelfart A, Thomassen L, Melms A, Wilhelm H, & Hoff JM.** Visual impairment in stroke patients—a review. *Acta Neurol Scand Suppl* 2013;(196):52–6.

6. **Hepworth LR, Rowe FJ, Walker MF,** et al. Post-stroke visual impairment: a systematic literature review of types and recovery of visual conditions. *Ophthalmol Res* 2015;**5**(1):1–43.

7. **Kravitz DJ, Saleem KS, Baker CI, & Mishkin M.** A new neural framework for visuospatial processing. *Nat Rev Neurosci* 2011;**12**:217–30.

8. **Terson A.** 'De l'hémorrhagie dans le corps vitre au cours de l'hémorrhagie cerebrale'. *Clin Ophthalmol* 1900;**6**:309–12.

9. **Zeki S & Ffytche DH.** The Riddoch syndrome: insights into the neurobiology of conscious vision. *Brain* 1998;**121**:25–45.

10. **Bailey IL & Lovie JE.** New design principles for visual acuity letter charts. *Am J Optom Physiol Opt* 1976;**53**(11):740–5.

11. **Johansen A, White S, & Waraisch P.** Screening for visual impairment after stroke: validation of the Cardiff Acuity Test. *Arch Gerontol Geriatr* 2003;**36** (pg. 289–293)

12. **de Morsier G.** 'Le syndrome de Charles Bonnet: hallucinations visuelles des vieillards sans deficience mentale' [Charles Bonnet syndrome: visual hallucinations of the elderly without mental impairment]. *Ann Med Psychol* 1967;**125**:677–701.

13. **Lotery AJ, Wiggam MI, Jackson AJ,** et al. Correctable visual impairment in stroke rehabilitation patients. *Age Ageing* 2000;**29**:221–2.

14. **Rowe F.** Prevalence of ocular motor cranial nerve palsy and associations following stroke. *Eye* 2011;**25**(7):881–7.

15. **Fowler MS, Wade DT, Richardson AJ, & Stein JE.** Squints and diplopia seen after brain damage. *J Neurol* 1996;**243**;86–90.

16. **Parinaud H.** Paralysie des mouvements associés des yeux. *Archives de Neurologie, Paris* 1883;**5**:145–72.

17. **Weber HD.** A contribution to the pathology of the crura cerebri. *Med Chir Trans* 1863;**46**:121–39.

18. **Flanders M & Sarkis N.** Fresnel membrane prisms: clinical experience. *Can J Ophthalmol* 1999;**34**:335–40.

19. **Miller NR & Newman NJ** (eds.) *Walsh & Hoyt's Clinical Neuro-Ophthalmology—The Essentials*, 5th edition. Baltimore, MD: Williams & Wilkins, 1998.

20. **Tamhankar MA, Ying G, & Volpe J.** Success of prisms in management of diplopia due to fourth nerve palsy. *J Neuroophthalmol* 2011;**31**:206–9.

21. **Leigh RJ & Kennard C.** Using saccades as a research tool in the clinical neurosciences. *Brain* 2004;**127** (Pt 3):460–77.

22. **Danchaivijitr C & Kennard C.** Diplopia and eye movement disorders. *J Neurol Neurosurg Psychiatry* 2004;**75**:iv24–iv31.

23. **Gilhotra JS, Mitchell P, Healey PR, Cumming RG, & Currie J.** Homonymous visual field defects and stroke in an older population. *Stroke* 2002;**33**:2417–20.

24. **Poggel DA, Kasten E, & Sabel BA.** Attentional cueing improves vision restoration therapy in patients with visual field deficits. *Neurology* 2004;**63**:2069–76.

25. **Peli E.** Field expansion for homonymous hemianopia by optically induced peripheral exotropia. *Optom Vis Sci* 2000;**77**:453–64.

26. **Pollock L.** Managing patients with visual symptoms of cerebro-vascular disease. *Eye News* 2000;**7**:23–6.

27. **Pambakian AL, Mannan SK, Hodgson TL, & Kennard C.** Saccadic visual search training: a treatment for patients with homonymous hemianopia. *J Neurol Neurosurg Psychiatry* 2004; **75**:1443–8.

28. **Zhang X, Kedar S, Lynn MJ, Newman NJ, & Biousse V.** Natural history of homonymous hemianopia. *Neurology* 2006;**66**:901–5.

29. **Freeman CF.** Collaborative working on a stroke-rehabilitation ward. *Parallel Vis (Br Ir Orthopt Soc)* 2003;**56**:3.

30. **Rowe F, Wright D, Brand D,** et al. Reading difficulty after stroke: ocular and non-ocular causes. *Int J Stroke* 2011;**6**(5):404–11.

31. **de Montaigne M.** In: Book 2, Chapter 12. Langelier A (ed.), 1595.

32. **Anton G.** Über die Selbstwahrnehmung der Herderkrankungen des Gehirns durch den Kranken bei Rindenblindheit und Rindentaubheit. *Arch Psychiatrie Nervenkrankh* 1899;**32**:86–127.

33. **Babinski J.** Contribution a l'étude des troubles mentaux dans l'hémiplégie organique (anosognosie). *Revue Neurol* 1914;**27**:845–8.

34. **Maxton C, Dineen RA, Padamsey RC, & Munshi SK.** Don't neglect 'neglect'—an update on post stroke neglect. *Int J Clin Pract* 2013;**67**(4):369–78.

35. **Rowe F, Brand D, Jackson CA,** et al. Visual impairment following stroke: do stroke patients require vision assessment? *Age Ageing* 2009;**38**:188–93.

36. **Frassinetti F, Angeli V, Meneghello F, Avanzi S, & Ladavas E.** Long lasting amelioration of visuospatial neglect by prism adaptation. *Brain* 2002;**125**:608–23.

37. **Warren M.** *Brain Injury Visual Assessment Battery for Adults: Test Manual.* Birmingham, AL: VisAbilities Rehab Services, 1998: pp. 4–43.

38. **Driver and Vehicle Licensing Agency (DVLA).** *Assessing Fitness to Drive: A Guide for Medical Professionals.* 2016. Available from: https://www.gov.uk/government/publications/assessing-fitness-to-drive-a-guide-for-medical-professionals [Accessed: 30 July 2019].

39. **Fisk GD, Owsley C, & Mennemeier M.** Vision, attention, and self-reported driving behaviors in community-dwelling stroke survivors. *Arch Phys Med Rehabil* 2002;**83**:469–77.

40. **National Stroke Association**. *Stroke and Vision Loss*. Available from: https://www.stroke.org/stroke-and-vision-loss/ [Accessed: 2 November 2016].

41. **Corriveau H, Herbert R, Raiche M, & Prince F.** Evaluation of postural stability in the elderly with stroke. *Arch Phys Med Rehabil* 2004;**85**:1095–101.

42. **Marx MS, Werner P, Cohen-Mansfield J, & Feldman R.** The relationship between low vision and performances of activities of daily living in nursing home residents. *J Am Geriatr Soc* 1992;**40**:1018–20.

43. **West CG, Gildengorin G, Haegerstrom-Portney G, Schneck ME, Lott L, & Brabyn JA.** Is vision function related to physical functional ability in older adults?. *J Am Geriatr Soc* 2002;**50**:136–45.

44. **Marmamula S, Ravuri CSLV, Boon MY, & Khanna RC.** A cross-sectional study of visual impairment in elderly population in residential care in the South Indian state of Andhra Pradesh: a cross sectional study. *BMJ Open* 2013;**3**(3):e002576.

45. **Ramrattan RS, Wolfs RC, Panda-Jonas S,** et al. Prevalence and causes of visual field loss in the elderly and associations with impairment in daily functioning: the Rotterdam Study. *Arch Ophthalmol* 2001;**119**:1788–94.

46. **Tsai Tsai SY, Cheng CY, Hsu WM, Su TP, Liu JH, & Chou P.** Association between visual impairment and depression in the elderly. *J Formos Med Assoc* 2003;**102**:86–90.

47. **Wagenbreth C, Franke GH, Sabel BA, & Gall C.** [Impairments of vision- and health-related quality of life in stroke patients with homonymous visual field defects depend on severity of visual function loss]. *Klin Mona- tsbl Augenheilkd* 2010;**227**:138–48.

48. **Pollock A, Hazelton C, Henderson CA,** et al. Interventions for visual field defects in patients with stroke. *Stroke* 2012;**43**(4):e37–8.

49. **Sabel BA.** Residual vision and plasticity after visual system damage. *Restor Neurol Neuros* 1999;**15**:73–9.

50. **Roe F.** *Care Provision and Unmet Need for Post Stroke Visual Impairment (Vision 2020)*. Available from: https://www.stroke.org.uk/sites/default/files/final_report_unmet_need_2013.pdf [Accessed: 30 July 2019].

Chapter 22

Discharge from hospital and early supported discharge

Catherine Gaynor

Introduction

Discharge from hospital following a stroke is an important milestone in a stroke patient's journey. It marks the end of the acute hospital episode, and the start of a new life living with and adjusting to the stroke and its sequelae. It can be a stressful time for patients and their carers, but careful and thorough discharge planning can help to ease the transition from hospital to home.

Discharge planning should start soon after a patient is admitted to hospital. It involves the input of the patient, their family and carers, their doctor, nurse, physiotherapist, occupational therapist, speech and language therapist, and social worker. Many hospitals also employ discharge coordinators who support the nursing, medical, and therapy teams in the efficient and timely discharge of patients. The patient's prestroke abilities and home circumstances should be ascertained, as well as the patient and family's expectations for discharge. A family meeting should be held once the multidisciplinary team have had a chance to assess the patient's rehabilitation potential, and a realistic date for discharge can be set.

When can a patient be discharged?

A stroke patient can be discharged when the multidisciplinary team feel that their care and rehabilitation (if appropriate) can be safely and effectively provided elsewhere. The patient should be medically stable and on appropriate secondary prevention medications. They will have completed any important medical investigations, or any outstanding tests can be performed as an outpatient. Their rehabilitation needs can be met by appropriate community services. Any swallowing or feeding issues will have been addressed, or a permanent non-oral route of feeding will have been established if necessary. An 'access' visit (the occupational therapist visits the patient home to assess the environment and access into and inside the property) or a home visit (both the patient and the therapist visit the patient's home) may have been carried out to assess the discharge environment and any adaptations or equipment needs will have been addressed. Any ongoing personal or domestic care needs will have been identified and addressed with input from a social worker.

Length of hospital stay following a stroke has decreased steadily over the last 10 years with many patients now discharged after less than 1 week. Conventionally stroke patients received most of their rehabilitation in hospital. However, economic pressures, and the growing evidence that many patients do better with rehabilitation in their own homes[1] has led to the development of community services which can offer stroke-specific rehabilitation at home.

Unfortunately, there is no single model of stroke care in the community setting and as a result the provision of community-based rehabilitation has been variable throughout the United Kingdom. Some areas offer a responsive early supported discharge (ESD) service followed by a community stroke rehabilitation team input if necessary. Other areas have little or no access to specialist stroke community rehabilitation.

Early supported discharge

ESD teams provide early, intensive rehabilitation for stroke patients allowing them to leave hospital and return home more quickly. ESD should be stroke specific, delivered by teams with specialist stroke skills, and provide the same intensity of rehabilitation as inpatient care. ESD teams can set rehabilitation goals, identify any stroke complications, and signpost to other services as appropriate. Not all patients will be suitable for ESD, because of either their level of physical disability or significant prior morbidity. In practice, most patients eligible for ESD have a Barthel activities of daily living (ADL) index score of between 10 and 17 and are able to transfer from bed to chair independently, or with the aid of one person. NICE recommends that adults who have had a stroke are offered ESD if the core multidisciplinary stroke team assess that it is suitable for them.[2]

Trials have evaluated the role and efficacy of ESD teams. A Cochrane review published in 2012 identified 14 trials with 1957 participants. Patients tended to be a selected elderly group (average age ranged from 66 to 80 years) with mild to moderate disability. Many of the trials excluded those with cognitive impairment, severe disability, or those who were institutionalized prior to admission. Patients receiving ESD services were more likely to be independent and living at home six months after stroke than those who received conventional (hospital-based) services. The authors concluded that appropriately resourced ESD services provided for a selected group of stroke patients can reduce long-term dependency and admission to institutional care, as well as reducing length of stay by approximately 7 days. Earlier discharge of these patients did not have a negative impact on their mood or subjective health status, and their carers were similarly unaffected.[3]

Many ESD teams have been set up around the United Kingdom in the past few years. The Sentinel Stroke National Audit Programme (SSNAP) run by the Royal College of Physicians is a national clinical audit programme which collects information on stroke services in England, Wales, and Northern Ireland. It reports its findings to healthcare professionals, commissioners, and the public. A total of 142 ESD teams participated in the SSNAP Post-Acute Organisational Audit published in December 2015.[4] Team composition varies from team to team; most have physiotherapists, occupational therapists, and rehabilitation support workers. Some also have nurses, mental health nurses, speech and language therapists, and medical input (a stroke physician). The National Guidelines for Stroke 2012[5] recommend that services such as ESD should be stroke specific and should be delivered by specialist professionals. The SSNAP audit found that 94% of the ESD teams who participated in the audit were stroke specific. Some ESD teams are based in the hospital but most are based in the community, with close working links to the acute hospital. In 2011 a team of CLAHRC (Collaboration for Leadership in Applied Health Research and Care) researchers in the East Midlands developed a consensus document with input from 10 of the original ESD trialists.[6] Using a modified Delphi technique an agreed list of statements regarding team composition, model of team work, intervention, and success was created. The trialists agreed that ESD teams should be multidisciplinary and have specialist knowledge in stroke care. A representative guide for team composition was also agreed for a caseload of 100 patients per year (Box 22.1). The trialists felt that intervention was beneficial for a subset of the population; those with mild to moderate stroke who were able to transfer independently or with one carer, and who were safe at home. They agreed that both hospital and ESD staff should identify patients suitable for ESD and that the length of ESD intervention could be influenced by the presence of other community-based stroke services. The trialists agreed that ESD teams should use

---

Box 22.1 Team composition (whole time equivalent per 100 patients/year caseload) as per reference

1.0   Physiotherapist

1.0   Occupational therapist

0.4   Speech and language therapist

0.1   Stroke physician

0–1.2   Nurse

0–0.5   Social worker

NB: Consensus not reached on role of rehabilitation assistant.

Adapted from *Stroke*, 42(5), Fisher RJ, Gaynor C, Kerr M et al., A consensus on stroke: ESD, pp. 1392–97, Copyright (2011), with permission from Wolters Kluwer Health.

---

standardized assessments (Barthel score, ADLs, patient's subjective health status and quality of life, patient, and carer satisfaction) to monitor outcomes and effectiveness, and that teams should also monitor their impact on length of hospital stay and readmission rates. This consensus provides clear guidelines for commissioners and healthcare professionals on what an evidence-based ESD service comprises.

A further CLAHRC study examined whether the health benefits of ESD seen in the research trials were reproduced when applied to everyday practice.[7] The study compared two groups of patients discharged from two acute hospital trusts. One group in each hospital trust received ESD intervention, the other received standard practices for discharge and onward referral. The combined ESD group had a significantly shorter length of hospital stay and reported higher levels of satisfaction with services. They had significantly higher odds of having a Barthel Index ≥90/100 after 6 weeks, 6 months, and 12 months. Carers of patients in the ESD group showed significant improvement in mental health scores when compared to those in the control group. However, another study found that although patients in the ESD group tended to be more independent than controls at 3 and 6 months, the differences were not statistically significant.[8]

Approximately 36% of stroke patients are suitable for ESD. In practice, between July and October 2015 32% of patients received ESD input in England, Wales, and Northern Ireland.[9] The national standard for waiting times stipulates that ESD teams should triage and treat the next day, or within 24 hours of hospital discharge. The SSNAP post-acute organizational audit published in December 2015 showed that the median waiting time from referral to triage/treatment for the 142 ESD teams who participated in the audit was 1 day. Only 28% of ESD teams provided a 7-day service, with most providing a service 5 day or less per week. Considering the national agenda around providing a 7-day service in the NHS in England, it appears likely that ESD teams will need to increase the number of days they work in the future.

ESD teams also vary in the duration of their intervention, with most teams providing a fixed maximum intervention of between 4 and 6 weeks. The existence of alternative community rehabilitation teams is important as it is obviously easier to end intervention if there is a community stroke team to hand the patient over to for ongoing rehabilitation. Unfortunately, many ESD teams do not have this luxury. This lack of ongoing support can make care difficult after ESD; the patient and their carers may often struggle with the fact that there is no prospect of further rehabilitation once early rehabilitation finishes.

Alternative community rehabilitation teams

Many patients will not fit the criteria for ESD intervention because of stroke severity, home circumstances, or other reasons. However, most patients will still require some rehabilitation after they leave hospital. There is a variety of community rehabilitation teams available around the country (e.g. community stroke teams, intermediate care, or community therapy teams) which are not stroke specific. The type of intervention delivered by these teams is distinct from, and complimentary to, that offered by an ESD service. These teams are less time-responsive and less intensive than ESD; assessment should be provided within 72 hours of referral, with therapy starting within 7 days. Referrals can be accepted from a variety of sources including acute hospital, ESD, out-patients, planned 6-month review, and GPs. Team composition is similar to ESD teams although community teams are less likely to include nurses or doctors. Intensity and duration of the intervention should be agreed between the stroke specialist and the stroke patient and should be based on clinical need tailored to goals and outcomes.

Some patients are seen in outpatient rehabilitation units, which are usually located on the acute hospital site. However, this requires that a patient is able to sit for up to 6 hours and tolerate transport to and from home. Many patients do not meet these criteria and therefore often do not receive any rehabilitation after discharge. A team of therapists in Nottingham ran a 12-month pilot service to meet the rehabilitation needs of the more disabled patients in the community.[10] They provided an in-reach service to the acute hospital, facilitated the transfer of care, and up to ten flexible sessions of rehabilitation after discharge. For those patients who had made minimal recovery from their stroke, the team educated carers (at home or in a care home) and established ongoing therapy regimes (e.g. splinting and positioning). They also supported the family and carers with the transition from hospital to home. Feedback from stakeholders was excellent.

Patient and carer support

The transition from hospital to home can be frightening for both patients and carers. Many patients worry that they will have another stroke and miss the reassurance of being in a 'safe' hospital environment. They can worry about not managing, facing a 'new life' with changed abilities and expectations, as well as the impact that their disability will have on their families and carers. They may feel unsure of what rehabilitation or help they will receive on discharge, or who they can call upon if they develop a problem following discharge. Many of these concerns can be minimized with the right support and input from both hospital and community teams.

Failure to provide 'joined-up' services after discharge is a major concern raised by patients. The NICE guidelines on stroke rehabilitation in adults[11] recommend that before discharge a health and social care plan is discussed and agreed upon by the patient and their family (or carers). This should include planned discharge date, details of planned community rehabilitation, and contact details. It should provide a snapshot of their current level of functioning (mobility, ADLs, continence, swallowing, mood, and cognition) as well as future rehabilitation goals. It also gives details of any equipment or care package to be provided on discharge, as well as planning a review after 6 months.

Approximately 40% of stroke patients who are discharged home need some help with ADLs. Nearly 20% of these patients receive help solely from unpaid carers. The impact of stroke on a carer should not be underestimated—there can be change in roles and relationships and many carers have to come to terms with coping with long-term disability. Family carers often receive very little support or training for their new role, and this can lead to increased stress with negative impacts on both the carer and the patient.

Many hospitals provide some form of training and education for carers to help prepare them for their role post-discharge; however, a multicentre randomized trial of inpatient delivery of a structured training programme to carers found that it was not more cost-effective than usual care in reducing carer burden or in improving the functional outcome of stroke survivors.[12] In clinical practice, however, most carers will be shown how to assist with dressing, transfers, gastrostomy (PEG) feeding, and so on, prior to discharge. Families and carers should also be made aware of their right (in the United Kingdom) to have a carer's needs assessment. This examines the impact that caring for someone has on the carer's health, work, and family commitments. The assessment is usually carried out by the local authority social work team and aims to offer whatever support is available to help the carer.

The Stroke Association in the United Kingdom provides excellent information to patients and carers including guidance after discharge.[13] Likewise, excellent information about local guidance in other countries is available on their respective forums (e.g. Stroke Association Scotland, Stroke Foundation (Australia), Heart and Stroke Foundation (Canada), National Stroke Association (US), and American Stroke Association). In less developed countries such as Africa or on the Indian subcontinent, there is a greater variability with more reliance on input from family members of the patient. Community stroke services in such settings are quite variable and in some places are non-existent. What can be provided after discharge is often dependent on the local services and the financial and socioeconomic situation of the family.

Institutionalization

Some patients will have greater care needs than can be provided in their own homes. These patients will require admission to a residential or nursing home. Institutionalization rates are falling—a retrospective United Kingdom audit of 2778 admissions with stroke in 2005 found the rate of new institutionalization (i.e. if previously living at home) to be 14%,[14] whereas recent SSNAP data suggests a figure of 8%.[9] Older patients are more likely to be discharged to a care home. Other factors which increase the risk of institutionalization include low Barthel score on discharge, PEG feeding, cognitive impairment,[15] previous living circumstances/marital status, and size of cerebral infarct.[16] Some patients who are discharged home following a stroke will eventually be admitted to a residential or nursing home, especially those with cognitive impairment, more severe disability, or more severe stroke. The cumulative risk of institutionalization in the 5-year period following a stroke is about 19%.[17]

Capacity and discharge destination

It is important to assume that a patient has mental capacity unless there are good reasons to suspect otherwise. A diagnosis of stroke does not automatically mean that the patient lacks capacity and is therefore unable to make important decisions regarding their health, finances, or discharge destination. Going against the advice of the multidisciplinary team and making an 'unwise' decision does not necessarily signify lack of capacity. If concerns regarding capacity are raised, a formal assessment of capacity regarding discharge destination should be made. Capacity assessments can be undertaken by any healthcare professionals involved in the patients care; social workers may be the most appropriate for social care decisions including discharge destination. It is vital that the stroke patient is fully supported during these assessments, especially those with aphasia. The use of photographs, pictures, or supported conversation with a speech and language therapist is extremely useful in these circumstances.

If there are safety concerns regarding discharge home but the patient has capacity, then any concerns should be clearly communicated to the patient, and documented, and the patient should be given as much support as possible to minimize any risks on discharge. If the patient lacks capacity, a decision should be made in their best interests. This will involve close discussion with family members and carers to try to ascertain any wishes that the patient may have previously expressed. Sometimes these discussions will result in the patient being transferred to a residential or nursing home, but often it is deemed that a trial of discharge home (although potentially unsafe) may be in the patient's best interest. If this is the case, the patient and their family should receive full support to try to minimize any risks on discharge.

If a patient lacks capacity but does not have any family or friends who are willing to advocate for them, and the multidisciplinary team (MDT) feel they are unsafe to be discharged back to their home, in the United Kingdom an independent mental capacity advocate (IMCA) should be appointed. An IMCA is someone who supports a person so that their views are heard and their rights are expressed. IMCAs are independent and have no connections to the carers or services involved in looking after the patient. The IMCA will meet the patient and ascertain their views, consult with staff, professionals, and anyone else involved in the patient's care, attend meetings as the patient's representative, present information to the decision-maker (usually the hospital consultant) in verbal and written form, remain involved until a decision is made, and challenge that decision if necessary.

Driving

Do not assume that an older person does not drive. It is important to ask about driving, and to make the patient aware of the Driver and Vehicle Licensing Authority (DVLA) guidelines for driving after a stroke.[18] These guidelines state that a person may not drive for 1 month following a stroke. If after this time they have made a full recovery, then they may resume driving without having to inform the DVLA. If there are residual neurological deficits at 1 month (particularly visual field defects, cognitive defects, and impaired limb function) the patient needs to notify the DVLA and continue to desist from driving. All patients who drive should be given the Stroke Association leaflet 'Driving after Stroke' on discharge from hospital. A specialized assessment using a simulator or an off-road test track may be required.

Communication with primary care

Details of the hospital episode are communicated to the patient's GP. The discharge summary should contain the dates of admission and discharge and the name of the consultant who cared for the patient. It should state the current diagnosis as well as any other relevant past diagnoses. It should clearly state if the patient received thrombolysis. There should be a description of events that occurred during the admission, as well as results of all relevant investigations. Any complications (pneumonia, DVT, and others) should be mentioned. Relevant neurological impairments and functional ability should be described. There should be a list of medications, as well as details of drugs which were changed or stopped in hospital with reasons why. It should specify any actions required by the GP (e.g. monitoring and treatment of hypertension), and follow-up arrangements should be described. Any community rehabilitation team involvement should be mentioned. Most discharge summaries are now done electronically. The discharge summary should be emailed or posted to the GP on the day of discharge with a copy given to the patient to take home. If possible, a copy should also be sent to the ESD team or community therapy team involved in the patients care. Remember that in a patient who is newly institutionalized the GP details may change.

The discharge summary not only conveys vital information for the GP, it is also the definitive electronic record of the hospital admission. If it is done correctly it can provide an excellent concise summary which can be useful for future hospital admissions or clinic reviews.

Follow-up

Stroke is a long-term condition and survivors will experience changes in their needs over time. The 2007 National Stroke Strategy stipulates that all stroke patients should have a review of their health and social care status and secondary care needs at 6 weeks and 6 months after discharge from hospital, followed by an annual health and social care check thereafter. The 6-week review is usually carried out by the acute hospital team where the emphasis may be more focussed on outstanding medical investigations and secondary prevention. Six-month reviews for stroke survivors help to identify any unmet needs at this point, and to signpost stroke survivors to any appropriate, targeted support that is available to meet their needs. The 6-month review can be carried out by a number of different providers—acute hospital, rehabilitation teams, voluntary providers (e.g. the Stroke Association), although increasingly there is a move away from the acute hospital trusts. A number of nationally recognized standardized tools have been developed to ensure that the patient receives a suitably in-depth review.[19] The majority of 6-month reviews are conducted in person with a smaller number conducted over the telephone. Annual reviews are usually undertaken by GPs.

All reviews should not only cover medical and secondary prevention issues, but should also address mood, cognition, and behaviour. Any needs should be identified and appropriately supported.

Summary and learning points:

1. Good discharge planning and proper communication can ease transition from hospital to home.

2. ESD teams provide intensive rehabilitation in a stroke patient's home.

3. Other community rehabilitation teams can provide less intensive rehabilitation over a longer period of time.

4. There is a need for community services nationally to amalgamate, creating a smooth pathway whereby the patient receives intensive ESD intervention followed by community stroke team intervention as required.

5. Older patients are more likely to be institutionalized following a stroke.

6. Remember to involve an IMCA where a patient lacks capacity and has no family or friends.

7. Attention should be paid to all 'activities of daily living' and 'instrumental activities of daily living', including driving and return to work where appropriate.

References

1. **Mayo N, Wood-Dauphinee S, Cote R**, et al. There's no place like home. An evaluation of early supported discharge for stroke. *Stroke* 2000;**31**:1016–23.

2. **National Institute for Health and Care Excellence (NICE).** *Stroke in Adults. Quality standard [QS2].* 2010 [updated 2016]. Available from: https://www.nice.org.uk/guidance/qs2 [Accessed: 30 July 2019].

3. **Fearon P, Langhorne P; Early Supported Discharge Trialists.** Services for reducing duration of hospital care for acute stroke patients. *Cochrane Database Syst Rev* 2012;(9):CD000443.

4. **Sentinel Stroke National Audit Programme (SSNAP).** *Results—Post-Acute Audit*, 2015. Available from: https://www.strokeaudit.org/results/PostAcute.aspx [Accessed: 30 July 2019].

5. **Intercollegiate Stroke Working Party.** *National Clinical Guideline for Stroke*, 5th edition. London, UK: Royal College of Physicians, 2016. Available from: https://www.rcplondon.ac.uk/guidelines-policy/stroke-guidelines [Accessed: 30 July 2019].

6. **Fisher RJ, Gaynor C, Kerr M, et al. A consensus on stroke: early supported discharge.** *Stroke* 2011;**42**(5):1392–7.

7. **Fisher RJ, Cobley CS, Potgieter I, et al.** Is stroke early supported discharge still effective in practice? A prospective comparative study. Clin Rehabil 2015; **30**(3):268–76.

8. **Hofstad H, Gjelsvik BE, Næss H, Eide GE, & Skouen JS.** Early supported discharge after stroke in Bergen (ESD Stroke Bergen): three and six months results of a randomised controlled trial comparing two early supported discharge schemes with treatment as usual. *BMC Neurol* 2014;**14**:239.

9. **Royal College of Physicians (RCP).** *Sentinel Stroke National Audit Programme (SSNAP).* Clinical audit July–September 2015. Available from: https://www.strokeaudit.org/Documents/National/Clinical/JulSep2015/JulSep2015-PublicReport.aspx [Accessed: 30 July 2019].

10. **Russell L, Caldwell K, & Sturt R. Complex Stroke Outreach.** Poster presentation at UK Stroke Forum, Liverpool, UK, December 2015.

11. **National Institute for Health and Care Excellence (NICE).** *Stroke Rehabilitation in Adults. Clinical guideline [CG162].* 2013. Available from: https://www.nice.org.uk/CG162 [Accessed: 30 July 2019].

12. **Atteih S, Mellon L, Hall P, et al.; ASPIRE-S study group.** Implications of stroke for caregiver outcomes: findings from the ASPIRE-S study. *Int J Stroke* 2015;**10**(6):918–23.

13. **Stroke Association.** Available from: https://www.stroke.org.uk [Accessed: 30 July 2019].

14. **Portelli R, Lowe D, Irwin P, Pearson M, & Rudd AG; Intercollegiate Stroke Working Party.** Institutionalization after stroke. *Clin Rehabil* 2005;**19**(1):97–108.

15. **Pasquini M, Leys D, Rousseaux M, Pasquier F, & Hénon H.** Influence of cognitive impairment on the institutionalisation rate 3 years after a stroke. *J Neurol Neurosurg Psychiatry* 2007;**78**(1):56–9.

16. **Mees M, Klein J, Yperzeele L, Vanacker P, & Cras P.** Predicting discharge destination after stroke: a systematic review. *Clin Neurol Neurosurg* 2016;**142**:15–21.

17. **Luengo-Fernandez R, Paul N, Gray A, et al., on behalf of the Oxford Vascular Study.** Population-based study of disability and institutionalization after transient ischemic attack and stroke: 10-year results of the Oxford Vascular Study. *Stroke* 2013;**44**:2854–61.

18. **Driver and Vehicle Licensing Agency (DVLA).** *Assessing Fitness to Drive: A Guide for Medical Professionals.* 2016. Available from: https://www.gov.uk/guidance/current-medical-guidelines-dvla-guidance-for-professionals-conditions-s-to-u#stroketia [Accessed: 30 July 2019].

19. **NIHR in partnership with the Stroke Association.** Support programmes and research. Available from: https://www.clahrc-gm.nihr.ac.uk/stroke [Accessed: 30 July 2019].

Chapter 23

Secondary prevention and revascularization in the older person

Jatinder S. Minhas, Amit K. Mistri, and Thompson G. Robinson

Strategies for secondary prevention in ischaemic stroke

Secondary prevention strategies will be considered under three headings: lifestyle modification, pharmacological strategies, and surgical intervention for carotid disease. Relevant guidance, underpinning evidence and pragmatic application of interventions, will be considered.

Lifestyle approaches

Lifestyle modification is an important aspect of a patient-centred approach for both the primary and secondary prevention of cardiovascular disease, including stroke. This was reinforced by the INTERSTROKE study,[1] where most risk factors for stroke were adverse lifestyle behaviours (see Table 23.1). However, much of the underpinning evidence is from primary preventions studies in unselected populations.

Smoking prevalence falls dramatically in the over 65s,[2] but smoking cessation remains of importance with conservative evidence suggesting that tobacco-associated risk is significantly reduced within 5 years of cessation.[3] The risk of stroke is dose-related and smoking any amount at least doubles the risk of ischaemic stroke.[4] This suggests that a reduction in smoking burden is also important if complete cessation is not feasible. The pathogenic mechanism seems to be due to acceleration of atherosclerotic plaques, as demonstrated by a correlation between carotid intima-media thickness and smoking burden (in current and former smokers).[2] Smoking cessation support delivered by nursing staff can significantly increase success rates.[5] Meta-analysis supports a modest but positive effect for smoking cessation intervention by nurses.[5]

Exercise can dramatically reduce stroke risk.[6] The Royal College of Physicians recommends that secondary prevention strategies should encourage adoption of 'tailored exercise programmes' with '150 minutes of moderate-intensity exercise every week', presumably to continue indefinitely.[7] However, the ability to participate in an exercise programme among older people may be limited due to comorbidities and persisting disability. Nonetheless, older patients with stroke do benefit from specialized inpatient neurorehabilitation and intensity to the same degree as younger patients.[8] Importantly comorbidity is acknowledged, and the advice recommends that for those 'at risk of falls, additional activity which incorporates balance and coordination, at least twice per week' should be undertaken. Systematic review data has shown long-term adherence is based on factors including higher socioeconomic status, living alone, better health status, better physical ability, better cognitive ability, and fewer depressive symptoms.[9]

Table 23.1 Risk factors for all stroke in the INTERSTROKE study

	Odds ratio, 99% CI	Population attributable risk (%), 99% CI
History of hypertension	2.64, 2.26–3.08	34.6, 30.4–39.1
Current smoking	2.09, 1.75–2.51	18.9, 15.3–23.1
Waist-to-hip ratio	1.65, 1.36–1.99*	26.5, 18.8–36.0
Diet risk score	1.35, 1.11–1.64*	18.8, 11.2–29.7
Regular physical activity	0.69, 0.53–0.90	28.5, 14.5–48.5
Diabetes mellitus	1.36, 1.10–1.68	5.0, 2.6–9.5
Alcohol intake	1.51, 1.18–1.92 for >30 drinks per month or binge drinking	3.8, 0.9–14.4
Psychosocial stress	1.30, 1.06–1.60	4.6, 2.1–9.6
Depression	1.35, 1.10–1.66	5.2, 2.7–9.8
Cardiac causes	2.38, 1.77–3.20	6.7, 4.8–9.1
Ratio of apolipoprotein B to A1	1.89, 1.49–2.40*	24.9, 15.7–37.1

* highest vs. lowest tertile.

Reproduced with permission from O'Donnell MJ, et al. Risk factors for ischaemic and intracerebral haemorrhagic stroke in 22 countries (the INTERSTROKE study): a case-control study. *The Lancet*, 376(9735), 112–123. Copyright © 2010 Elsevier Ltd. All rights reserved. https://doi.org/10.1016/S0140-6736(10)60834-3

While there is uncertainty as to the magnitude of any effect from dietary modifications, it is reasonable to assume that evidence-based primary preventative interventions are applicable to secondary prevention populations. Recommended dietary modifications include reduced sodium intake,[10] increased consumption of fish/fish oils,[11] and increased consumption of fruit and vegetables.[12]

Pharmacological approaches

Antithrombotic

Several antithrombotic agents are available for the prevention of recurrent stroke and other major cardiovascular events. As monotherapy, aspirin and dipyridamole have similar efficacy,[13] with clopidogrel being slightly superior to aspirin[14] and of equivalent efficacy to aspirin plus dipyridamole.[15] National Institute for Health and Care Excellence (NICE) deemed clopidogrel monotherapy to be the most cost-effective antiplatelet for secondary prevention.[16] However, studies have been focused on younger stroke patients (median age 64 years), and thus efficacy and adverse event profiles may not be representative of an older stroke population.[17,18]

In the setting of transient ischaemic attack (TIA) and minor ischaemic stroke, short-term dual antiplatelet therapy (DAPT) with aspirin and clopidogrel is beneficial. DAPT was associated with reduction of 90-day vascular event (absolute risk reduction: ARR 1.5%)[19] or stroke risk (ARR 3.5%),[20] and a small (0.5% absolute increase)[19] or no[20] increase in major bleeding. A 21-day course is recommended,[20] prior studies reporting increased risk of bleeding complications with longer term use (1.3% absolute increase).[21] The benefit is amplified in those with multiple acute brain infarcts.[22] Triple antiplatelet therapy was associated with increased bleeding risk, and no reduction of recurrent stroke or TIA at 90 days, and is not recommended.[23] An individualized decision will need to be made for older people, keeping in mind individual risk factors for bleeding.

Blood pressure reduction

Hypertension is the most prevalent risk factor for stroke, and BP reduction has been convincingly demonstrated to reduce future stroke risk. However, there remains uncertainty about BP management in the first 2 weeks after acute stroke, where elevated BP is a common reactive phenomenon (~75%), with BP reducing to prestroke values by week two. Overall, there is no convincing evidence to guide management strategy immediately after stroke, with varying recommendations in guidelines (see Table 23.2). A consideration within the acute phase is whether to continue prestroke antihypertensive therapy. An individual patient data meta-analysis incorporating data from the COSSACS[24] and ENOS[25] studies concluded that pre-existing antihypertensive treatment could be restarted after 24 hours, assuming that the patient is medically stable, and oral or nasogastric administration is feasible.[26] Furthermore, the CHHIPS study examined the safety of a treatment strategy in hypertensive patients (systolic >160 mmHg) postacute stroke (both ischaemic and haemorrhagic subtypes). Importantly, a comparable older cohort was included—mean age 74 (SD 11). The treatment strategy using either labetalol or lisinopril was well-tolerated with no adverse events and a borderline reduction in 3-month mortality (HR 0.4, 95% CI 0.2–1.0, $P = 0.05$).[27] Large trials of antihypertensive therapy in the setting of acute stroke have shown no clear benefit, with candesartan,[28] or glyceryl trinitrate (GTN) patches.[29]

The Royal College of Physicians (RCP) guidelines highlighted 'robust evidence' for the importance of long-term BP control in secondary prevention.[7] The PROGRESS study demonstrated that combination therapy substantially reduced the risk of recurrent stroke.[30] With combination therapy, the majority of stroke survivors can achieve and maintain guideline-recommended targets in the longer term.[31]

Strategies targeting individuals with multifactorial interventions have been shown in a meta-analysis to improve systolic blood pressure.[32] The study population was aged between 60 and 70 years; further studies in an older cohort would provide more insight into this group.[32]

Table 23.2 Long-term blood pressure control guidelines for secondary prevention of stroke

Guideline author	Publication year	When to intervene?	Threshold for intervention	How much reduction?	Agent	Ref
ASA	2014	Ischaemic Stroke or TIA	>140/90	<140/90 unless lacunar stroke then <130 systolic	No specific agent	33
ESO	2009	Stroke	No specific value	No specific value	No specific agent	34
RCP	2016	Stroke or TIA	>130/80 (except bilateral carotid stenosis, where target systolic 140–150 is appropriate)	Aim for 130/80	>55, African or Caribbean—CCB or thiazide. <55 ACEi or ARB first choice	7

ASA, American Stroke Association; ESO, European Stroke Organisation; RCP, Royal College of Physicians; ACEi, angiotensin-converting enzyme inhibitors; ARB, angiotensin receptor blocker.

Lipid modification

There is strong randomized controlled trial (RCT) evidence and therefore consensus guidelines supporting lipid-lowering therapy in individuals with cardiovascular risk (see Table 23.3). However, the generalisability to older populations remains an important issue. The Stroke Prevention by Aggressive Reduction in Cholesterol Levels (SPARCL) study investigated high-dose atorvastatin 80 mg for secondary prevention of stroke, and reported a 16% reduction in vascular events at median follow-up of 4.9 years compared to placebo.[35] The mean age of participants was 63 (SD 0.2) years. A small absolute increase in haemorrhagic stroke (0.9%) was noted in the atorvastatin group (HR 1.68, $P = 0.02$), which was associated with older age, male sex, higher BP, and especially if the index event was haemorrhagic (HR 5.81, $P < 0.001$). This suggests that BP treatment should be optimized in the older person alongside consideration for aggressive statin therapy.[36] Similar benefits were reported in a subgroup analysis of the Heart Protection Study (HPS), where simvastatin 40 mg daily was associated with a 28% reduction in risk of ischaemic stroke events.[37] Interestingly, subgroup analysis suggested that the treatment effect was larger in the older age groups. This suggests that the older people should not be denied statin therapy.

The RCP are clear that statin therapy 'should be avoided and only used with caution, if required for other indications, in individuals with a recent primary intracerebral haemorrhage'.[7] However, there is little or no prospective data in the over 70 year olds confirming any association.

In the absence of an RCT, prestroke statin therapy should normally be continued in non-dysphagic patients. Pre-existing statin therapy is associated with better outcomes following stroke, and one study reported worse outcomes (in terms of dependency and early neurological deterioration) with statin withdrawal in acute stroke.[38] Thus, NICE recommend continuation of pre-existing statin therapy.[39] *De novo* statin therapy in acute disabling stroke is not generally advised (in the first 48 hours), due to lack of direct evidence from RCTs.[39] However, early statin therapy as part of a multiple risk factor approach should be considered following TIA or minor stroke, consequent to a significant 80% reduction in stroke risk reported in the EXPRESS Study.[40] Table 23.3 summarizes available guidelines for the long-term use of statin therapy for secondary prevention.

Atrial fibrillation

Atrial fibrillation (AF) is a common problem in older people, with prevalence rising steadily from 0.5% in the 50s to 8.8% in the 80s.[41] AF is associated with a fivefold increase in stroke risk.[42] While this risk remains static as people age, the relative contributions of other risk factors wanes,[43]

Table 23.3 Guidelines for statin therapy in the secondary prevention of ischaemic stroke

Guideline author	Publication year	When to intervene?	Threshold for intervention	How much reduction?	Agent	Ref
ASA	2014	Stroke/TIA with atherosclerosis	LDL >100 mg/dl	LDL<100 mg/dl	Statins	33
ESO	2009	Stroke			Atorvastatin Simvastatin	34
RCP	2016	Ischaemic stroke or TIA	TC >4.0 mmol/litre or LDL >2.0 mmol/litre	TC <4.0 mmol/litre or LDL <2.0 mmol/litre	Start Simvastatin 40 mg	7

ASA, American Stroke Association; ESO, European Stroke Organisation; RCP, Royal College of Physicians; TC, total cholesterol; LDL, low density lipoprotein.

highlighting the importance of AF in older people. Thus, older people are 16 times more likely to develop a cardioembolic stroke (compared to middle aged counterparts),[44] and AF-associated stroke constitutes 36% of all strokes in older people (vs. 20% in unselected cohorts).[45] Finally, AF-associated stroke is associated with higher mortality rates and significant disability in survivors. The importance of early AF identification (whether paroxysmal or persistent), risk stratification, and appropriate anticoagulation cannot be overemphasized.

A proportion of AF patients are asymptomatic, and screening with pulse checks in older people is essential, alongside health contacts for other reasons (e.g. flu vaccinations, blood pressure checks, and so on).[46] Any identified pulse irregularity should be confirmed by a standard 12-lead electrocardiogram. Where symptoms suggestive of paroxysmal AF (PAF) are reported, cardiac monitoring should be undertaken with a 24- or 48-hour cardiac monitor, and where appropriate more prolonged monitoring. There is also growing evidence to support cardiac monitoring in cryptogenic stroke patients, studies reporting higher prevalence of PAF with longer duration of monitoring (up to 3 years).[47]

While emergency AF management includes treatment of any life-threatening haemodynamic consequence of a tachyarrhythmia, potentially requiring rate and/ or rhythm control, the most important prevention step is an assessment of AF-associated embolism risk and the potential risk of anticoagulation-related bleeding, using objective scoring systems: CHA_2DS_2-VASC (1 point each for: congestive heart failure, hypertension, age 65–74 years, diabetes mellitus, vascular disease, and female sex category; and 2 points each for: prior stroke/TIA/thromboembolism and age $\geq$75 years—score range 0–9), and HAS-BLED (hypertension (uncontrolled systolic blood pressure >160 mmHg), abnormal renal and/or liver function, previous stroke, bleeding history, or predisposition, labile international normalized ratios, older people, and concomitant drugs and/ or alcohol excess).[48,49]

Anticoagulation should be initiated promptly in stable AF patients. Given the increased rate of drug side effects in older people, and a well-recognized association between age and increased risk of intracranial bleeding,[50] this decision should be individualized and include an informed discussion with the patient or their proxy. Finally, the majority of older patients with stable AF are managed with a rate-control strategy; however, cardiology referral to pursue rhythm control options may be considered in those with persistent symptoms despite rate control. *De novo* rhythm control strategy with cardioversion is not preferred given high rates of reverting to AF (up to 90%),[51] and has not been shown to reduce the risk of adverse clinical outcomes. Given the increased rate of side effects with drugs in older people, non-pharmacological options are attractive. However, interventional procedures like pulmonary vein isolation and atrioventricular node (AV) ablation have not been studied adequately in this population, and the net efficacy and safety remains unknown,[52] with some concern about high rates of procedural complications including cerebral embolism.[53] An ongoing trial (CABANA) is investigating the potential role of AF ablation.[54]

Low rates of warfarin use in older people have been well-documented,[55] despite reassuring data from clinical trials specifically studying older patients.[56] Barriers include: practical difficulties with monitoring, perceived high bleeding risk (e.g. recurrent falls), comorbidities, and international normalized ratio (INR) variability. Data from the GARFIELD Registry indicate that the advent of DOAC has increased the prevalence of patients with AF on anticoagulation from 57.4% to 71.1%, driven by an increase in DOAC use from 4.2% to 37.0%.[57] DOAC use has increasingly replaced both warfarin and aspirin for stroke prevention. Four DOACs are now available as an alternative to warfarin, with fixed-dosing regimen not requiring frequent monitoring. Several reviews of the clinical trials have demonstrated, compared to warfarin, at least similar efficacy in reducing systemic embolism, similar or lower rates of major bleeding, and consistently lower rate of intracranial haemorrhage, including in older subgroups.[58] Given that age is a well-recognized risk factor for intracranial haemorrhage, it is likely that DOACs will be attractive for use in this population. Care has to be taken to ensure compliance, dose adjustment in renal impairment, and avoidance in severe renal impairment, in line with the respective summary of product characteristics.

Where anticoagulation is genuinely contraindicated, a novel option is left atrial appendage occlusion (LAAO), which has been shown to be equivalent to warfarin therapy.[59] However, this study did not look at populations ineligible for anticoagulation, though the age distribution was generalizable with mean age of 72.[59]

Given the high absolute stroke risk in older people, the absolute benefits of anticoagulation are larger, and net benefit remains, though all efforts should be made to minimize bleeding risk by modifying risk factors enshrined in risk scores like HAS-BLED. In addition, it is important to be aware of the impact of general frailty and significant comorbid conditions on drug tolerance, ability to cope with monitoring requirements, and compliance. Focus may need to shift to quality of life rather than vascular events as the outcome of interest in some individuals.

Glycaemia

There is conclusive evidence that post-stroke hyperglycaemia is associated with worse outcomes.[60] However, a large RCT has shown no significant improvement in outcomes with intensive glycaemic control in acute stroke, with increased incidence of hypoglycaemia.[61] There is no evidence that glycaemic control in the acute stage improves outcomes.[62] Using a pragmatic approach, most guidelines recommend 'intervention' in acute stroke, if the glucose levels are persistently elevated above 10 mmol/litre.[7] However, macrovascular complications are not prevented by long-term glycaemic control, but diabetes marks out a group at high risk in whom vigorous vascular prevention is indicated.

The NICE guidelines for type 2 diabetes mellitus recommend a target HbA1c of less than 6.5%[63] in the long-term management of diabetes. A recent study of non-diabetic patients with insulin resistance (HOMA IR >3) reported a significant 2.8% absolute reduction in vascular events with pioglitazone, over 4.8 years of follow-up.[64] The clinical applicability of this finding remains unclear at present, and measurement of insulin resistance may need to be adopted into clinical practice. Despite no upper limit for age in the inclusion criteria, there was limited representation of older people (mean age 63.5, SD 10.7).[64]

Surgical intervention for carotid atheromatous disease

Two large RCTs (NASCET and ECST) demonstrated a significant benefit from carotid endarterectomy (CEA) in people with symptomatic severe carotid stenosis (>50% NASCET ~ >70% ECST).[65] The results are summarized in Table 23.4.

Early CEA (within 2 weeks) is much more effective than late CEA (at 3 months) for prevention of stroke (number needed to treat (NNT) 5 and 125, respectively).[65] Moreover, perioperative stroke or death rates were not increased with early surgical intervention in neurologically stable patients. Women only benefited from CEA if undertaken within 2 weeks of symptom onset.

Periprocedural stroke or death rate is higher in those receiving endovascular treatment (e.g. carotid artery stenting), the higher rate being restricted to those older than age 70 (double the risk), with no net benefit in under 70s. Thus, stenting is only advised when anatomical considerations limit CEA.

Most trials were undertaken before the advent of aggressive antihypertensive and statin therapy for carotid atheromatous disease, thus no RCT exists in the presence of modern risk factor

Table 23.4 Pooled analysis of carotid endarterectomy studies demonstrating stenosis and outcomes

Stenosis (ECST grading)	NNT to prevent one stroke over 5 years	Absolute risk reduction
Near occlusion	Harmful	
>=70%	6.3	16%
50–69%	22	4.6%
30–49%	No benefit	
<30%	Harmful	

ECST, European Carotid Surgery Trial; NNT, number needed to treat.

management. Nonetheless, there is likely to be incremental benefit from surgical intervention in symptomatic carotid disease. Conversely, best medical therapy is probably adequate for the majority of people with asymptomatic carotid stenosis, who have lower risk of stroke (compared to those with symptomatic disease)—3.6% over 5 years. The literature describes instances where surgery has been used in the presence of high-risk features (e.g. silent infarction on brain imaging; stenosis progression; hypoechoic plaques (GSM <15 mm^2); spontaneous embolization on transcranial Doppler (TCD); MR diagnosed intraplaque haematoma; plaque area more than 80 mm^2; irregular plaques, spontaneous embolization on TCD; juxtaluminal black area more than 10 mm^2, and tandem intracranial disease).[66] However, there was no evidence of benefit over the age of 75 years (Table 23.5).

Intracerebral haemorrhage

Intracerebral haemorrhage (ICH) accounts for 15% of all strokes.[67,68] Risk factors include hypertension, advancing age, cerebral amyloid angiopathy, anticoagulation, and a history of (ischaemic) cerebrovascular disease. ICH risk is highest from age 85 onwards.[50] A population-based study in Oxfordshire between 1981 and 2006 found increasing incidence of ICH in patients over 75 years of age, associated with anticoagulation and non-hypertensive lobar bleeds.[69] Case fatality increased with age with the highest fatality reported in the over 85-year-old group (30.9% CI 25.1–36.7%).[70]

Management of acute intracerebral haemorrhage involves discontinuation of anticoagulants and appropriate management of bleeding with consideration for anticoagulant-specific reversal agents. Whether these drugs can be restarted later on is still uncertain,[71] and under investigation (antiplatelet: RESTART)[72]; anticoagulant: SOSTART.[73] Elevated blood pressure can be lowered

Table 23.5 Guidelines for surgical therapy in carotid atheromatous disease

Guideline author	Publication year	When to intervene?	
ASA	2014	The diameter of the lumen of the internal carotid artery is reduced by >70% by non-invasive imaging or >50% by catheter-based imaging	[33]
ESO	2009	In patients with 70–99% stenosis. It may be indicated for certain patients with 50–69% stenosis: males with very recent hemispheric symptoms	[34]

ASA, American Stroke Association; ESO, European Stroke Organisation.

aggressively. While the ATACH study showed no benefit with BP lowering within 4.5 hours of ICH,[74] the INTERACT2 study demonstrated improvement in Rankin score with intensive BP lowering within 6 hours of ICH onset to a target systolic BP of less than 140 mmHg, though the primary outcome of death or major disability was not significantly reduced.[75] Therefore, the European Stroke Organisation (ESO) and American Stroke Association (ASA) guidelines now recommend early treatment with sustained control of systolic BP to less than 140 mmHg. Retrospective analysis also demonstrated an adverse effect of increasing BP variability,[68] though no intervention study of blood pressure variability (BPV) modulation has so far been undertaken.

With respect to long-term secondary prevention, most guidelines generally recommend a target BP of under 140/90.[34]

Summary

In summary, there is limited direct trial evidence for secondary prevention interventions in older stroke survivors. It is clear that more prospective trials are needed in both acute ischaemic stroke and intracerebral haemorrhage. Therefore, a pragmatic application of guidelines from the evidence base in younger populations is currently appropriate.

References

1. **O'Donnell MJ, Xavier D, Liu L,** et al. Risk factors for ischaemic and intracerebral haemorrhagic stroke in 22 countries (the INTERSTROKE study): a case-control study. *Lancet* 2010;**376**(9735):112–23.

2. **Shah RS & Cole JW.** Smoking and stroke: the more you smoke the more you stroke. *Expert Rev Cardiovasc Ther* 2010;**8**(7):917–32.

3. **Wolf PA, D'Agostino RB, Kannel WB, Bonita R, & Belanger AJ.** Cigarette smoking as a risk factor for stroke. The Framingham Study. *JAMA* 1988;**259**(7):1025–9.

4. **Ockene IS & Miller NH.** Cigarette smoking, cardiovascular disease, and stroke: a statement for healthcare professionals from the American Heart Association. American Heart Association Task Force on Risk Reduction. *Circulation* 1997;**96**(9):3243–7.

5. **Rice VH, Hartmann-Boyce J, & Stead LF.** Nursing interventions for smoking cessation. *Cochrane Database Syst Rev* 2013;**8**:CD001188.

6. **Gillum RF & Ingram DD.** Relation between residence in the southeast region of the United States and stroke incidence. The NHANES I Epidemiologic Followup Study. *Am J Epidemiol* 1996;**144**(7):665–73.

7. **Intercollegiate Stroke Working Party.** *National Clinical Guideline for Stroke*, 5th edition. London, UK: Royal College of Physicians, 2016.

8. **Knecht S, Rossmuller J, Unrath M, Stephan KM, Berger K, & Studer B.** Old benefit as much as young patients with stroke from high-intensity neurorehabilitation: cohort analysis. *J Neurol Neurosurg Psychiatry* 2016: **87**(5):526–30.

9. **Picorelli AM, Pereira LS, Pereira DS, Felicio D, & Sherrington C.** Adherence to exercise programs for older people is influenced by program characteristics and personal factors: a systematic review. *J Physiother* 2014;**60**(3):151–6.

10. **Graudal NA, Hubeck-Graudal T, & Jurgens G.** Effects of low sodium diet versus high sodium diet on blood pressure, renin, aldosterone, catecholamines, cholesterol, and triglyceride. *Cochrane Database Syst Rev* 2011;(**11**):CD004022.

11. **Skerrett PJ & Hennekens CH.** Consumption of fish and fish oils and decreased risk of stroke. *Prev Cardiol* 2003;**6**(1):38–41.

12. **Johnsen SP, Overvad K, Stripp C, Tjonneland A, Husted SE, & Sorensen HT.** Intake of fruit and vegetables and the risk of ischemic stroke in a cohort of Danish men and women. *Am J Clin Nutr* 2003;**78**(1):57–64.

13. **Diener HC, Cunha L, Forbes C**, et al. European Stroke Prevention Study 2. Dipyridamole and acetylsalicylic acid in the secondary prevention of stroke. *Lancet* 1996;**143**:1–13.

14. **CAPRIE Steering Committee.** A randomised, blinded, trial of clopidogrel versus aspirin in patients at risk of ischaemic events (CAPRIE). CAPRIE Steering Committee. *Lancet* 1996;**348**(9038):1329–39.

15. **Diener HC, Sacco RL, Yusuf S**, et al. Effects of aspirin plus extended-release dipyridamole versus clopidogrel and telmisartan on disability and cognitive function after recurrent stroke in patients with ischaemic stroke in the Prevention Regimen for Effectively Avoiding Second Strokes (PRoFESS) trial: a double-blind, active and placebo-controlled study. *Lancet Neurol* 2008;**7**(10):875–84.

16. **National Institute for Health and Care Excellence (NICE).** *Clopidogrel and Modified-Release Dipyridamole for the Prevention of Occlusive Vascular Events. NICE Technology Appraisal Guidance [TA210].* 2010. Available from: https://www.nice.org.uk/guidance/TA210 [Accessed: 31 July 2019].

17. **Antithrombotic Trialists' Collaboration.** Collaborative meta-analysis of randomised trials of antiplatelet therapy for prevention of death, myocardial infarction, and stroke in high risk patients. *BMJ* 2002;**324**(7329):71–86.

18. **Bhatt DL, Fox KA, Hacke W**, et al. Clopidogrel and aspirin versus aspirin alone for the prevention of atherothrombotic events. *N Engl J Med* 2006;**354**(16):1706–17.

19. **Johnston SC, Easton JD, Farrant M**, et al., **Clinical Research Collaboration, Neurological Emergencies Treatment Trials Network, and the POINT Investigators.** Clopidogrel and aspirin in acute ischemic stroke and high-risk TIA. *N Engl J Med* 2018;**379**:215–25.

20. **Wang Y, Wang Y, Zhao X**, et al., **CHANCE Investigators.** Clopidogrel with aspirin in acute minor stroke or transient ischemic attack. *N Engl J Med* 2013;**369**:11–19.

21. **Diener HC, Bogousslavsky J, Brass LM**, et al. Aspirin and clopidogrel compared with clopidogrel alone after recent ischaemic stroke or transient ischaemic attack in high-risk patients (MATCH): randomised, double-blind, placebo-controlled trial. *Lancet* 2004;**364**(9431):331–7.

22. **Jing J, Meng X, Zhao X**, et al. Dual antiplatelet therapy in transient ischemic attack and minor stroke with different infarction patterns. Subgroup analysis of the CHANCE randomized clinical trial. *JAMA Neurol* 2018;**75**(6):711–19.

23. **Bath PM, Woodhouse LJ, Appleton JP**, et al. Antiplatelet therapy with aspirin, clopidogrel, and dipyridamole versus clopidogrel alone or aspirin and dipyridamole in patients with acute cerebral ischaemia (TARDIS): a randomised, open-label, phase 3 superiority trial. *Lancet* 2018; **391**:850–9.

24. **Robinson TG, Potter JF, Ford GA**, et al. Effects of antihypertensive treatment after acute stroke in the Continue or Stop Post-Stroke Antihypertensives Collaborative Study (COSSACS): a prospective, randomised, open, blinded-endpoint trial. *Lancet Neurol* 2010;**9**(8):767–75.

25. **ENOS Trial Investigators, Bath PM, Woodhouse L**, et al. Efficacy of nitric oxide, with or without continuing antihypertensive treatment, for management of high blood pressure in acute stroke (ENOS): a partial-factorial randomised controlled trial. *Lancet* 2015;**385**(9968):617–28.

26. **Woodhouse LJ, Manning L, Potter JF**, et al., **for the Blood Pressure in Acute Stroke Collaboration.** Continuing or temporarily stopping prestroke antihypertensive medication in acute stroke an individual patient data meta-analysis. *Hypertension* 2017;**69**:933–41.

27. **Potter JF, Robinson TG, Ford GA**, et al. Controlling hypertension and hypotension immediately post-stroke (CHHIPS): a randomised, placebo-controlled, double-blind pilot trial. *Lancet Neurol* 2009;**8**(1):48–56.

28. **Sandset EC, Bath PM, Boysen G**, et al. The angiotensin-receptor blocker candesartan for treatment of acute stroke (SCAST): a randomised, placebo-controlled, double-blind trial. *Lancet* 2011;**377**(9767):741–50.

29. **The RIGHT-2 investigators.** Prehospital transdermal glyceryl trinitrate in patients with ultra-acute presumed stroke (RIGHT-2): an ambulance-based, randomised, sham-controlled, blinded, phase 3 trial. *Lancet* 2019;**393**:1009–20.

30. **PROGRESS Collaborative Group**. Randomised trial of a perindopril-based blood-pressure-lowering regimen among 6,105 individuals with previous stroke or transient ischaemic attack. *Lancet* 2001;**358**(9287):1033–41.

31. **Schrader J, Luders S, Kulschewski A**, et al. Morbidity and mortality after stroke, eprosartan compared with nitrendipine for secondary prevention: principal results of a prospective randomized controlled study (MOSES). *Stroke* 2005;**36**(6):1218–26.

32. **De Simoni A, Hardeman W, Mant J, Farmer AJ, & Kinmonth AL**. Trials to improve blood pressure through adherence to antihypertensives in stroke/TIA: systematic review and meta-analysis. *J Am Heart Assoc* 2013;**2**(4):e000251.

33. **Kernan WN, Ovbiagele B, Black HR**, et al. Guidelines for the prevention of stroke in patients with stroke and transient ischemic attack: a guideline for healthcare professionals from the American Heart Association/American Stroke Association. *Stroke* 2014;**45**(7):2160–236.

34. **European Stroke Organisation**. ESO Guidelines for Management of Ischaemic Stroke Update 2009—Translations. 2009.

35. **Amarenco P, Bogousslavsky J, Callahan A,3rd**, et al. High-dose atorvastatin after stroke or transient ischemic attack. *N Engl J Med* 2006;**355**(6):549–59.

36. **Goldstein MR, Mascitelli L, & Pezzetta F**. Hemorrhagic stroke in the stroke prevention by aggressive reduction in cholesterol levels study. *Neurology* 2009;**72**(16):1448; author reply 1448–9.

37. **Collins R, Armitage J, Parish S, Sleight P, Peto R, & Heart Protection Study Collaborative Group**. Effects of cholesterol-lowering with simvastatin on stroke and other major vascular events in 20536 people with cerebrovascular disease or other high-risk conditions. *Lancet* 2004;**363**(9411):757–67.

38. **Blanco M, Nombela F, Castellanos M**, et al. Statin treatment withdrawal in ischemic stroke: a controlled randomized study. *Neurology* 2007;**69**(9):904–10.

39. **National Institute for Health and Care Excellence (NICE)**. *Stroke and Transient Ischaemic Attack in Over 16s: Diagnosis and Initial Management. NICE guideline [CG68]*. 2008. Available from: https://www.nice.org.uk/guidance/ng128 [Accessed: 31 July 2019].

40. **Rothwell PM, Giles MF, Chandratheva A**, et al. Effect of urgent treatment of transient ischaemic attack and minor stroke on early recurrent stroke (EXPRESS study): a prospective population-based sequential comparison. *Lancet* 2007;**370**(9596):1432–42.

41. **Wolf PA, Abbott RD, & Kannel WB**. Atrial fibrillation as an independent risk factor for stroke: the Framingham Study. *Stroke* 1991;**22**(8):983–8.

42. **Lotze U, Liebetrau J, Malsch I**, et al. Medical treatment of patients with atrial fibrillation aged over 80 years in daily clinical practice: influence of age and CHADS(2) score. *Arch Gerontol Geriatr* 2010;**50**(1):36–41.

43. **Kannel WB, Abbott RD, Savage DD, & McNamara PM**. Coronary heart disease and atrial fibrillation: the Framingham Study. *Am Heart J* 1983;**106**(2):389–96.

44. **Ferro JM**. Cardioembolic stroke: an update. *Lancet Neurol* 2003;**2**(3):177–188.

45. **Wolf PA, Abbott RD, & Kannel WB**. Atrial fibrillation: a major contributor to stroke in the elderly. The Framingham Study. *Arch Intern Med* 1987;**147**(9):1561–4.

46. **Kearley K, Selwood M, Van den Bruel A**, et al. Triage tests for identifying atrial fibrillation in primary care: a diagnostic accuracy study comparing single-lead ECG and modified BP monitors. *BMJ Open* 2014;**4**(5):e004565.

47. **Camm AJ, Lip GY, De Caterina R**, et al. 2012 focused update of the ESC Guidelines for the management of atrial fibrillation: an update of the 2010 ESC Guidelines for the management of atrial fibrillation. Developed with the special contribution of the European Heart Rhythm Association. *Eur Heart J* 2012;**33**(21):2719–47.

48. **Lip GY, Nieuwlaat R, Pisters R, Lane DA, & Crijns HJ**. Refining clinical risk stratification for predicting stroke and thromboembolism in atrial fibrillation using a novel risk factor-based approach: the Euro heart survey on atrial fibrillation. *Chest* 2010;**137**(2):263–72.

49. **Pisters R, Lane DA, Nieuwlaat R, de Vos CB, Crijns HJ, & Lip GY.** A novel user-friendly score (HAS-BLED) to assess 1-year risk of major bleeding in patients with atrial fibrillation: the Euro Heart Survey. *Chest* 2010;**138**(5):1093–100.

50. **Fang MC, Chang Y, Hylek EM,** et al. Advanced age, anticoagulation intensity, and risk for intracranial hemorrhage among patients taking warfarin for atrial fibrillation. *Ann Intern Med* 2004 Nov 16;**141**(10):745–752.

51. **Elesber AA, Rosales AG, Herges RM,** et al. Relapse and mortality following cardioversion of new-onset vs. recurrent atrial fibrillation and atrial flutter in the elderly. *Eur Heart J* 2006;**27**(7):854–60.

52. **Calkins H, Kuck KH, Cappato R,** et al. 2012 HRS/EHRA/ECAS Expert Consensus Statement on Catheter and Surgical Ablation of Atrial Fibrillation: recommendations for patient selection, procedural techniques, patient management and follow-up, definitions, endpoints, and research trial design. *Europace* 2012;**14**(4):528–606.

53. **Blandino A, Toso E, Scaglione M,** et al. Long-term efficacy and safety of two different rhythm control strategies in elderly patients with symptomatic persistent atrial fibrillation. *J Cardiovasc Electrophysiol* 2013;**24**(7):731–8.

54. **CABANA Trial Group.** Catheter Ablation vs Anti-arrhythmic Drug Therapy for Atrial Fibrillation Trial (CABANA). 2015.

55. **Ogilvie IM, Newton N, Welner SA, Cowell W, & Lip GY.** Underuse of oral anticoagulants in atrial fibrillation: a systematic review. *Am J Med* 2010;**123**(7):638–45.e4.

56. **Mant J, Hobbs FD, Fletcher K,** et al. Warfarin versus aspirin for stroke prevention in an elderly community population with atrial fibrillation (the Birmingham Atrial Fibrillation Treatment of the Aged Study, BAFTA): a randomised controlled trial. *Lancet* 2007;**370**(9586):493–503.

57. **Kakkar AK, Mueller I, Bassand JP,** et al. Risk profiles and antithrombotic treatment of patients newly diagnosed with atrial fibrillation at risk of stroke: perspectives from the international, observational, prospective GARFIELD registry. *PLoS One* 2013;**8**(5):e63479.

58. **Sharma M, Cornelius VR, Patel JP, Davies JG, & Molokhia M.** Efficacy and harms of direct oral anticoagulants in the elderly for stroke prevention in atrial fibrillation and secondary prevention of venous thromboembolism: systematic review and meta-analysis. *Circulation* 2015;**132**(3):194–204.

59. **Healey JS, Crystal E, Lamy A,** et al. Left Atrial Appendage Occlusion Study (LAAOS): results of a randomized controlled pilot study of left atrial appendage occlusion during coronary bypass surgery in patients at risk for stroke. *Am Heart J* 2005;**150**(2):288–93.

60. **Capes SE, Hunt D, Malmberg K, Pathak P, & Gerstein HC.** Stress hyperglycemia and prognosis of stroke in nondiabetic and diabetic patients: a systematic overview. *Stroke* 2001;**32**(10):2426–32.

61. **Gray CS, Hildreth AJ, Sandercock PA,** et al. Glucose-potassium-insulin infusions in the management of post-stroke hyperglycaemia: the UK Glucose Insulin in Stroke Trial (GIST-UK). *Lancet Neurol* 2007;**6**(5):397–406.

62. **Bellolio MF, Gilmore RM, & Stead LG.** Insulin for glycaemic control in acute ischaemic stroke. *Cochrane Database Syst Rev* 2011;(9):CD005346.

63. **National Institute for Health and Care Excellence (NICE***). Type 2 Diabetes. NICE Guideline CG66.* 2008. [Updated and replaced by NICE guideline NG28]. Available from: https://www.nice.org.uk/guidance/CG66 [Accessed: 31 July 2019].

64. **Kernan WN, Viscoli CM, Furie KL,** et al. Pioglitazone after ischemic stroke or transient ischemic attack. *N Engl J Med* 2016;**374**:1321–31.

65. **Rothwell PM, Eliaszim M, Gutnikov SA,** et al. Analysis of pooled data from the randomised controlled trials of endarterectomy for symptomatic carotid stenosis. *Lancet* 2003;**361**:107–16.

66. **Naylor A R, Schroeder TV, & Sillesen H.** Clinical and imaging features associated with an increased risk of late stroke in patients with asymptomatic carotid disease. *Eur J Vasc Endovasc Surg* 2014;**48**(6):633–40.

67. **Sahni R & Weinberger J.** Management of intracerebral hemorrhage. *Vasc Health Risk Manag* 2007;**3**(5):701–9.

68. **Manning L, Hirakawa Y, Arima H**, et al. Blood pressure variability and outcome after acute intracerebral haemorrhage: a post-hoc analysis of INTERACT2, a randomised controlled trial. *Lancet Neurol* 2014;**13**(4):364–73.

69. **Lovelock CE, Molyneux AJ, Rothwell PM, Oxford Vascular Study**. Change in incidence and aetiology of intracerebral haemorrhage in Oxfordshire, UK, between 1981 and 2006: a population-based study. *Lancet Neurol* 2007 Jun;**6**(6):487–93.

70. **van Asch CJ, Luitse MJ, Rinkel GJ, van der Tweel I, Algra A, & Klijn CJ**. Incidence, case fatality, and functional outcome of intracerebral haemorrhage over time, according to age, sex, and ethnic origin: a systematic review and meta-analysis. *Lancet Neurol* 2010;**9**(2):167–76.

71. **Nielsen PB, Larsen TB, Skjoth F, Gorst-Rasmussen A, Rasmussen LH, & Lip GY**. Restarting anticoagulant treatment after intracranial hemorrhage in patients with atrial fibrillation and the impact on recurrent stroke, mortality, and bleeding: a nationwide cohort study. *Circulation* 2015;**132**(6):517–25.

72. **RESTART Trial**. *Results*. Available from: http://restarttrial.org/ [Accessed: 31 July 2019].

73. **SoSTRART Trial**. Available from: https://clinicaltrials.gov/ct2/show/NCT03153150 [Accessed: 31 July 2019].

74. **Qureshi AI, Palesh YY, Barsan WG**, et al. Intensive blood-pressure lowering in patients with acute cerebral haemorrhage. *N Engl J Med* 2016;**375**:1033–43.

75. **Anderson CS, Heeley E, Huang Y**, et al. Rapid blood-pressure lowering in patients with acute intracerebral hemorrhage. *N Engl J Med* 2013;**368**(25):2355–65.

Chapter 24

Hypertension in older people

Wayne Sunman

Introduction

If I had written this 15 years ago, I would have considered old to mean 65 or older, but more recently trials have been directed at, or at least included, patients aged 80 years or older. Formerly, people of this age were routinely excluded from trials, for fear of introducing too much variation due to comorbidities, variations in pharmacological sensitivities, polypharmacy, diminished homeostasis, and contamination of the mortality data as patients were at risk of dying of non-vascular causes.

Hypertension in old, and very old, patients is common, neglected, and important. Hypertension has a prevalence of over 60% in patients over 65 and yet higher in the over 75s (Health Survey for England 2006).[1] This problem will only increase as the world population ages and expands.[2] When it was reviewed by the American Heart Association in their 2011 report, while older patients were more likely to be aware they are hypertensive, they were less likely to have their blood pressure (BP) controlled.[3] In the Framingham Study, in those over 80 years old, only 23% of women and 38% of men had their BP treated to less than 140/90 mmHg.[4] Hypertension is important as it is a strong risk factor for the development of cardiovascular disease, the commonest cause of death worldwide and it is the most powerful, modifiable risk factor for stroke, which contributes over a third of those deaths (World Health Organization).

Background

This topic has been actively considered since at least 1895, when a lecture entitled 'Senile plethora or high arterial pressure in elderly persons' was presented to the Hunterian Society in London (Albutt, C. Lectures to the Hunterian Society, 1895).[5] He had treated five patients aged 65 to 80 years with mercurial diuretics and potassium iodide, successfully lowering their BP. Despite this, the prevailing view until quite recently was that high BP was required to ensure adequate target organ perfusion through narrowed and rigid vessels in older people. Reducing that pressure risked precipitating symptomatic cerebral hypoperfusion, ischaemia, and infarction. This view was supported by the ill-fated INWEST trial, in which patients randomised to intravenous infusion of a calcium channel blocker (CCB), nimodipine, early after ischaemic stroke, had worse functional and neurological outcomes at 21 days and 24 weeks than those given placebo; poor outcome correlated with early reductions in diastolic BP.[6] This effect was largely driven by those having less severe strokes which could extend in the same arterial distribution rather than strokes caused by complete, large vessel occlusion,[7] fuelling the thought that this could be due to extension of the stroke due to unselective vasodilatation diverting blood flow from diseased vessels. This is referred to as the vascular steal phenomenon.

Eleven small trials of antihypertensive treatment of older patients aged 60 to 70 years old conducted between 1972 and 1991 were analysed by Sanderson et al. in 1995,[8] establishing that both strokes and cardiac events were reduced significantly by a mean 19/9 mmHg reduction in BP and that the number needed to treat over 5 years for the whole group was smaller than for those who were younger. This encouraged trialists to actively investigate older patients and subsequently very old patients (those over 80 years old). Higher risk older patients contributed more cardiovascular events over a shorter time period, enabling positive trial results (or greater certainty) over a comparatively short timeframe.

This finding was confirmed by further meta analyses, notably a Cochrane Review in 1998,[9] which included trials following patients over 60 years old for over a year.

Differences in hypertension with age

In developed countries, systolic blood pressure (SBP) rises progressively with age, as illustrated in Fig. 24.1.[10] Diastolic pressure also rises with age until people are in their mid-50s and then falls. The effect of this is that pulse pressure rises with age dramatically from the mid-50s onwards and that the prevalence of isolated systolic hypertension (ISH) also increases dramatically, such that ISH predominates in the over 60s (Fig. 24.2).[11] Recent evidence has concentrated exclusively on systolic hypertension as isolated diastolic hypertension is almost exclusively the preserve of the young, who are at overall low risk, and for whom lifestyle advice and continued observation is the best strategy. This chapter will deal purely with systolic hypertension.

Two-year mortality rate in older people rises with systolic BP (Fig. 24.3).[12] Take a closer look at this figure. There are five lines on the graph each representing the relationship of mortality with systolic BP for patients with five different diastolic blood pressures. For a given SBP, *lower* diastolic blood pressure is associated with *higher* mortality. This would not be the case for a

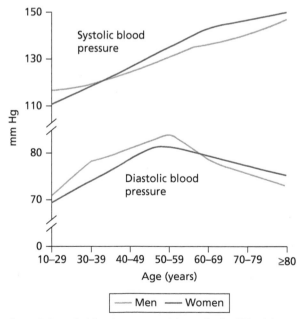

Fig. 24.1 Mean systolic and diastolic blood pressure with age in the US adult population.

Reproduced with permission from Burt VL, et al. Prevalence of Hypertension in the US Adult Population. *Hypertension*, 25(3), 305–313. Copyright © 1995, Wolters Kluwer Health. https://doi.org/10.1161/01.HYP.25.3.305

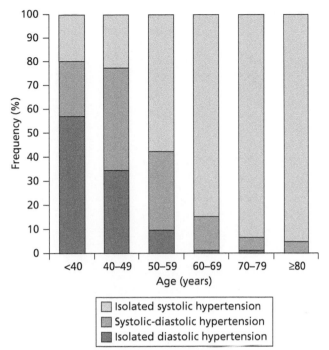

Fig. 24.2 Prevalence of isolated systolic hypertension, systolic-diastolic hypertension, and isolated diastolic hypertension in different age groups in American adults.

Reproduced with permission from Franklin SS, et al. Predominance of isolated systolic hypertension among middle-aged and elderly US hypertensives. *Hypertension*, 37(3), 869–874. Copyright © 2001, Wolters Kluwer Health. https://doi.org/10.1161/01.HYP.37.3.869

patient under 50 years old. Older patients develop higher SBPs and lower diastolic blood pressures for the same reason: their larger arteries have lost their elasticity. When the heart contracts and expels blood into the aorta, the pressure wave created travels more quickly than the blood is able to move. In younger people it might travel at 8 m/s, but when the arteries have lost their elasticity, it travels more quickly; about 12 m/s. This means that the pressure wave reflected from the smaller arterial branch points peripherally returns in late systole rather than mid-diastole as illustrated in the schematic in Fig. 24.4.[13] The central diastolic pressure is thus reduced and the peak central systolic pressure enhanced or augmented by the returning pressure wave. This augmented, central, systolic pressure increases the load on the heart and blood vessels and the lowered diastolic pressure reduces coronary perfusion as the coronary circulation is principally perfused during diastole.

Older patients are more sensitive to dietary salt. After salt loading, BP falls more when they are salt restricted and given a loop diuretic compared with younger hypertensives, perhaps because they are less efficient at excreting a salt load.[14,15] Re-analysis of patients included in double-blind trials of a sodium-restricted diet (10 g of salt vs. 5 g) revealed that for those with ISH mean age 63 years, there was a worthwhile 10/1 mmHg reduction.[16] Since there was a 1 month run-in period on low-sodium diet, little of this reduction could be accounted for by regression to the mean. In a small cross-over trial carried out in a long-term care facility with residents of mean age 85 years, a month of sodium-restricted diet reduced blood pressure significantly in all participants.[17]

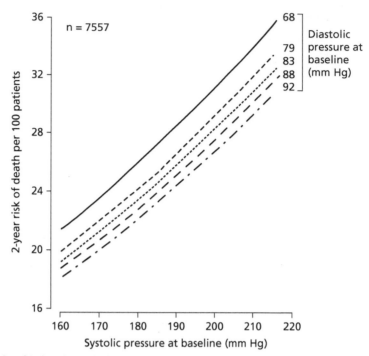

Fig. 24.3 Risks of isolated systolic hypertension in older people: meta-analysis of outcome trials.

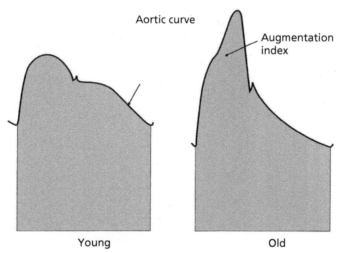

Fig. 24.4 In younger patients the reflected wave, travelling more slowly, arrives back during diastole (arrow), whereas in older patients with stiffer arteries it travels back quickly enough to augment central aortic systolic pressure. The augmentation index is the pressure difference between the late-systolic peak and the inflection on the early-systolic upstroke expressed as a fraction of the total pulse pressure. It is a measure of arterial stiffness.

Special situations

The case has been made for older patients with hypertension to be treated differently from their younger counterparts. The treatment of older patients is necessarily different from younger patients often being constrained by possibly drug interactions consequent on a high prevalence of polypharmacy, which in its turn relates to the multiple co-morbidities which is the lot of older patients. You should not prescribe a thiazide or thiazide-like diuretic for someone who necessarily takes loop diuretic for their heart failure, but you might decide to choose an angiotensin-converting enzyme (ACE) inhibitor instead. Similarly, you might choose a beta-blocker first-line in someone presenting with hypertension and associated angina and you might select a long-acting alpha adrenergic blocker if a man has symptoms of prostatic hypertrophy. In patients who are judged to be in their final illness, it would be hard to justify commencing an antihypertensive; it will probably be appropriate to withdraw some or all of their antihypertensives, if indicated purely for hypertension. However, beta-blockers should be tapered slowly so as not to exacerbate, sometimes occult, underlying ischaemic heart disease.

Thresholds and targets

It has also been suggested that older patients should have different therapeutic thresholds and different targets for antihypertensive treatment. This has created a great deal of confusion, which I hope to clarify by elaborating the results of three landmark studies.

The NICE hypertension guideline of 2019 (www.https://www.nice.org.uk/guidance/ng136) single out patients aged 80 years or over for different treatment. Drug treatment should be considered when their BP is consistently 150/90 mmHg or more and their treatment target should be less than 150/90. This is based on HYVET[18]; the first landmark trial. HYVET randomised 3845 patients, 80 years old or more, double-blind to either indapamide SR 1.5 mg OD (a thiazide-like diuretic), plus perindopril 2 mg or 4 mg, or matching placebo aiming for a BP of less than 150/80 mmHg. It was stopped early due to a significant, 21% reduction in all-cause mortality. At this point the BP difference between active treatment and placebo groups was 15/6 mmHg. There were significant associated reductions in death from stroke (39%) and heart failure (64%). These finding were present throughout all of the subgroups prespecified. There was no significant difference in plasma potassium, urate, glucose, and creatinine over the period of trial between the two groups. The investigators published a further paper showing that active treatment was associated with a lower fracture risk.[19] Unfortunately there were no data on falls.

The literature on this area is bedevilled by differing endpoints, differing sub-populations, and confounding. In the same edition of *Age & Ageing* there was a meticulously constructed and analysed case–control study drawing on a general practice database.[20] Allowing for all currently conceivable risk factors and co-morbidities, the authors were able to discern an increased probability of falling in the first few weeks after commencing a thiazide diuretic. This was not the case for other classes of antihypertensives. They had included all patients over 60 having their first fall, but the average age was 77 years, with 16% of patients over 80, so there was only a small age disparity between the two studies. Thiazides and thiazide-like diuretics do retain calcium within the body, so might reduce fracture risk after a fall, but would less than 2 years' treatment account for it? It is certainly possible that standard-formulation, thiazide diuretic differs from thiazide-like diuretic in falls risk and it is possible that the slow-release formulation and lower dose, employed in the HYVET trial could reduce falls risk and key the paradox. By selecting older people with falls, perhaps the case–control study considered a more frail population. The HYVET trial selected robust older patients. Perhaps frailty is the key?

Intriguingly, the latest American hypertension guideline advocates lifestyle measures and drug treatment for *all* adults with a BP of 130/80 mmHg or more and 10% or more 10 year risk of atherosclerotic cardiovascular events whether diabetic or not and irrespective of age, aiming for a BP of less than 130/80.[47] They based this on a network meta-analysis of 42 trials containing 144000 individuals, comparing the benefits of treating to more or less intensive BP targets. This showed that treatment benefits for prevention of stroke were lowest if the achieved SBP was 120–124 mmHg and somewhat lower for IHD. This relationship held true even if the largest and most recent study, the SPRINT trial, was excluded.[48] In SPRINT, my second landmark trial, over 9000 patients without prior history of stroke or diabetes mellitus were randomised to a target SBP of either less than 120 or less than 140 mmHg.[49] They achieved mean SBPs of 121 and 136 mmHG in the two arms of the trial and there was such a highly significant, 27% reduction in all-cause mortality and a 25% reduction in cardiovascular events with higher intensity treatment (at the cost of some extra adverse events) such that the trial was stopped early. BP was measured in the clinic using an automated BP machine, unaccompanied. The American guideline writers felt that clinic BPs were in general measured more rigorously in trials and so would be systematically lower and so in the their guideline the target, on-treatment BP was eased to become less than 130/80 mmHg.

The NICE 2019 guideline writers reached a different conclusion. They excluded the SPRINT trial from consideration as: it had included a high risk population, selected population, they were concerned that many patients were already on treatment when they were recruited and they did feel that taking measurements unaccompanied in clinic was unusual and would be difficult to correct for. When corrected for might mean that the mean SBP achieved in the more intense arm of the study (121 mmHg) and it was difficult to correct for the difference in the way the BP measurements were taken. In their view there was no compelling evidence to indicate a change to target BP for primary prevention of less than 140/90 mmHg, though they maintained a target of less than 130/80 for those with pre-existing cardiovascular disease. Their search strategy did not pick up the network meta-analysis, which had such decisive influence on the American guideline. The difference between multiple, automated, accompanied and unaccompanied clinic measurements has been neatly quantified by a meta-analysis in 2018.[50] Unaccompanied measurements were lower by 10/4 mmHg, making the mean achieved SBP of the intense treatment arm 131 mmHg.

Frailty

The issue was discussed in a leading article, once again in *Age & Ageing*,[21] making the case that despite the HYVET results, decisions to commence antihypertensives in older patients should take into account the frailty of the patient. The authors were responding to the Milan Geriatrics 75 + Cohort Study,[22] which found that for those 75 years old or older referred to hospital outpatients, the BP associated with the lowest mortality rate was 165/85 and for those with impaired cognition and impaired functional status, a lower systolic BP was associated with a higher mortality (Fig. 24.5). Within the HYVET population there was no evidence that increasing frailty reduced the benefits of treatment,[23] which is reassuring as far as it goes, but the trial had selected against particularly frail patients and so could only provide reassurance across a limited range. The HYVET authors derived a frailty index based on 60 comorbidities recorded at the outset of the trial. It was validated by comparison with frailty indices measured in population studies for people over 80 years.

It is worth recalling that BP falls in patients who are ill for any reason. Reverse causality as it is known is usually partially compensated for by checking that the relationship still pertains when reanalysed without the data from patients who died in the first year or so of entering the

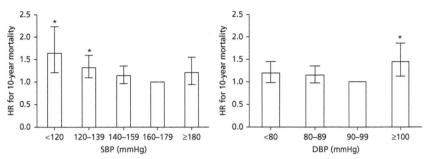

Fig. 24.5 Ten-year mortality rate in SBP and diastolic blood pressure (DBP) categories. Bars represent hazard ratios (95% confidence interval). The category of SBP 160–179 mmHg and the category of DBP 90–99 mmHg were set as references in the left and right graphs, respectively. The symbol * indicates a significant difference with the reference category.

Reproduced with permission from Ogliari G, et al. Blood pressure and 10 year mortality risk in the Milan Geriatrics 75+ Cohort Study: role of functional and cognitive status. *Age and Ageing*, 44(6), 932–937. Copyright © 2015, Oxford University Press. https://doi.org/10.1093/ageing/afv141

study. This was done in the Milan Geriatrics 75+ study, but we must infer that it did not change the findings as it is not specifically reported. The leading article also mentioned the PARTAGE study, which observed the outcomes of over a thousand frail people in their 80s and 90s in French nursing homes. They found that residents on two or more antihypertensives with a systolic BP less than 130 mmHg had a 2-year mortality rate of 78% greater than others in the study.[24] Orthostatic hypotension was no more prevalent in this group. Another study, this time conducted on Swedish nursing home residents, confirmed the excess mortality of patients whose systolic BP was less than 120 mmHg.[25] They had a higher risk of having or developing malnutrition and they also noted that mean BP for the residents fell over time. The Swedish authors concluded that the data is a powerful argument for frequent, systematic drug reviews of frail elderly people. Given that systolic BP drops over time in frail older people, cohort studies no matter how carefully constructed are always potentially confounded.

Fortunately, the SPRINT trialists deliberately recruited a high proportion of patients aged 75 years and above and collected data on comorbidities, which could be used to estimate frailty. Patients with diabetes or stroke were excluded from the study. They had an average age of 79 years at entry to the study, a moderate frailty index and mild cognitive impairment: MOCA score 22/30. There was good separation in achieved BPs between the two treatment strategies at 123/62 mmHg in intensive group, aiming for SBP less than 120 mmHG, versus a mean of 135/67 mmHG in the standard treatment group aiming for a SBP of less than 140 mmHg.[26] After 3 years there was a significant, 34% reduction in the primary composite of cardiovascular diseases, and a highly-significant, 33% reduction in all-cause mortality. Stratifying the outcomes by frailty index (FI) or by gait speed did not change the outcomes, indicating that increasing frailty whether measured by the presence or absence of a phalanx of comorbidities or by walking speed does not attenuate the beneficial effects of more intensive BP reduction.

Dementia and cognitive impairment

In the Milan Geriatrics 75+ study, higher systolic BPs were associated with lower mortality rates among participants with impaired cognition. Could dementia be a condition that merits a different approach to antihypertensive management? The possibility that antihypertensive treatment reduces cognition by reducing cerebral blood flow when autoregulation is impaired has been addressed in the DANTE Study. Cessation of all antihypertensives for 4 months, with a consequent rise in BP was not associated with any cognitive or functional improvement.[27,28]

Unfortunately, dementia, like frailty, is associated with falling BP as shown in the third landmark study. Observing people in Honolulu for a period of 32 years established that those developing dementia had a greater increase in their systolic BP over time, but did experience a fall to lower systolic BPs once they developed dementia and that this was more pronounced in those with vascular dementia than in those thought to have Alzheimer's type dementia.[29] It was found that current BP was not a risk factor for dementia, but that prior hypertension in middle age was; illustrating how reverse causation can confound cross-sectional studies.

This area has been very thoughtfully reviewed in 2016.[30] It was concluded that there was a lack of evidence in older patients with dementia for benefits from antihypertensive treatment, but that treatment should be tailored to the individual. They went on to advocate a pragmatic, randomised trial of deprescribing to support decision-making. They were somewhat dismissive of the SPRINT results, saying that the patients in the trial couldn't be frail as they had a low mortality rate. It could be that they had their BP and their associated vascular risk factors well-managed as treatment to less than 140 mmHg systolic is not routinely achieved in this age group. The SPRINT trialists have validated their FI, which used a deficit accumulation model,[31] finding that 27% of the recruits classified as frail by this index and that this group was 75% more likely to have an injurious fall (around 3% in the first year) and 145% more likely to be hospitalized (over 20% in the first year) than those classified as fit. The age-distribution of the FI in SPRINT matched that of large, unselected population studies. It can be concluded that this study did have sufficient frail elderly patients in to reassure us that the findings are applicable to them, but it did not include patients too immobile to attend clinic. A French study measured nursing home residents using a similar deficit accumulation scale, finding them to have a FI of 0.4.[32] This is outside the 99% CI for the FI in the SPRINT trial. The SPRINT results can be reasonably applied to the very old and frail, but there must be some uncertainty regarding the BP targets for patients who are sufficiently frail and immobile to require nursing home care.

Orthostatic hypotension (OH)

In the DANTE Study, 50% of patients with OH at the outset no longer had OH after 4 months off treatment.[28] Intriguingly, OH resolved in 38% of those who remained on treatment during the 16 weeks of the trial, indicating how variable OH is. This difference in incidence of OH between those off treatment and those continuing on treatment did not achieve significance in the intention to treat analysis (RR 1.31 (95% confidence interval (CI) 0.92–1.87); $P = 0.13$). In an 'on-treatment' analysis, there was a significant reduction in OH for those patients in whom it was possible to discontinue all medications. This excluded a group of patients in the intervention group whose blood pressure was too high to withdraw all medications. As higher systolic BP is associated with OH,[33] this approach is confounded and the finding unsafe.

Diabetes mellitus

Unfortunately, there was no analysis of the 6% of patients in HYVET that were diabetic, and diabetics were excluded from the SPRINT trial, so there is no trial evidence specific to the old or very old diabetic. However, the ACCORD trial recruited 4733 obese patients aged 40 to 79 years with long-standing type-2 diabetes mellitus and randomised them to intensive treatment of their diabetes or standard treatment: HbA1C <6% vs HbA1C 7 to 7.9%. They further randomised half of the overall group to intensive BP treatment, goal SBP less than 120 mmHg or standard BP treatment with a goal of less than 140 mmHg. The other half of the patients were randomised to intense or standard lipid-lowering therapy.[52] In the intensive SBP reduction group they achieved a mean SBP of 119 mmHg versus 133 mmHg on standard therapy. This was associated with a small reduction in stroke that was largely negated by a variety of serious adverse events, such that the primary endpoint of non-fatal stroke, non-fatal myocardial infarction, and cardiovascular death did not change significantly (1.87% in the intensive therapy group and 2.09% in the standard therapy group hazard ratio 0.88; 95% confidence interval 0.73–1.06; $P = 0.20$). It is possible that the combination of ACE inhibitor and angiotensin receptor blockers (ARB) used in 11% of the intensive treatment arm and only 3% of the standard treatment arm could account for some of the problems. This combination was shown to increase adverse events with no change in hard endpoints in the ONTARGET trail.[46] ACCORD was an open-label trial. It recruited a rather odd population in that trial patients had been diabetic for 10 years on average and were obese, with an average body mass index of 32. Most disturbing was that the intensive glycaemic control group had to be switched to usual diabetic therapy targets after 3.7 years when the data monitoring group reported a 22% increase in risk of death in that group.[54] The trial was continued to completion just over a year later, continuing to administer antihypertensives or cholesterol-lowering treatments as per protocol. Subsequent, pre-planned, subgroup analysis established that there was an improvement in the primary, endpoint, cadiovascular death, in patients treated to the standard glycaemic target with intensive BP treatment, but that there was no additional benefit derived from intensive BP control in those patients subject to intense diabetic control.[51] There is therefore an interaction between the treatments used in the 2x2 factorial design, which makes simple analysis by intensity of treatment of any one factor unsafe. This which was further explored by comparing the intense and standard BP control groups in the SPRINT and ACCORD trials, confirming that the intense BP target and intense glycaemic control subgroup of ACCORD failed to show expected benefit in cardiovascular outcomes.[53] Despite these concerns many of the guidelines on BP treatment targets in diabetics has advocated under 140/90 rather than under 130/80 mmHg as formerly.

Choice of antihypertensive

In patients over 80, a thiazide-like diuretic is the first-line drug of choice; however, in those aged 60–80 years there is evidence that CCBs are possibly a better choice. In the ACCOMPLISH trial, patients of average age 64 years were randomised to either an ACE inhibitor plus amlodipine (a long-acting CCB) or ACE inhibitor (ACEI) plus hydrochlorothiazide. Over 3 years of follow-up, both groups had very similar, well-controlled hypertension, but there was a significant reduction in the proportion of patients developing a cardiovascular endpoint to 9.6% in those on the ACEI-CCB combination compared to 11.8% in those treated with ACEI-thiazide.[37] So for older patients under 80 years old, a long-acting CCB could be a better choice, particularly if combined with ACEI. In the ALLHAT study of 33 000 patients over 5 years, treatment based on thiazide-like diuretic chlortalidone was equally as effective as treatment with ACEI-based and CCB-based drug regimens, and this effect was maintained in patients over 65 years.[38] Chlortalidone was more effective at reducing the frequency of heart failure. As the best evidence for benefit on treatment is with thiazide-like diuretics (chlortalidone and indapamide) rather than conventional thiazides such as hydrochlorothiazide and bendroflumethiazide, the National Institute for Health and Care Excellence (NICE) concluded thiazide-like diuretics should be used in preference.[39]

Post-stroke hypertension

The 2016 Royal College of Physicians of London (RCP) guideline on stroke,[40] in common with other guidelines from other countries, advises that blood pressure within the first week after an ischaemic stroke should only be treated if needed to attain a BP of less than 185/110 mmHg to enable a patient to be thrombolysed or if the patients has life-threatening complications of hypertension, for example: aortic dissection, hypertensive heart failure, eclampsia, pre-eclampsia, or hypertensive encephalopathy. There is no need or justification to vary this by age. I shall be concentrating on the management of blood pressure after the first week.

The RCP advised treating systolic BP levels of 130 mmHg or more and aiming for a BP of less than 130 systolic. Previous guidance, whether from the United States, Europe, or Scotland, while drawing on the same evidence base, drew a variety of different conclusions.

Stroke is a disease of old age. The average age of stroke patients passing through our stroke unit is 76 years, in common with other units in the United Kingdom. Trials examining only those patients under 80 years old are examining a skewed population, in which around 40% of patients have been excluded.

What is the evidence for managing hypertension longer-term after stroke in patients over 80 years old after stroke? No evidence is quoted in any of the guidelines in this specific population nor am I aware of any. There are, however, trials of treating stroke patients, many of whom are quite old and there are trials of treating very old patients who have hypertension, but no apparent end-organ damage which have already been discussed.

There are three trials of secondary prevention in stroke patients, which showed benefit in terms of the reduction of the risk of further stroke. In the PROGRESS trial over 6000 patients, average age 64 years, with prior stroke 2 weeks to 5 years earlier (median 8 months) were randomised to perindopril-based treatment or placebo.[34] At the individual trialist's discretion indapamide could be added to perindopril. After almost 5 years of follow-up there was a significant 28% reduction in the risk of developing a stroke in those given perindopril-based therapy compared to placebo. On further analysis, this benefit was confined to the 58% who were given perindopril and indapamide, but there was no benefit in the 42% given only perindopril. The beneficial effect was seen regardless of baseline blood pressure, even to those with a pretreatment as low as 115/75. The PATS trial was also a double-blind, randomised, trial comparing indapamide with placebo,[35] conducted in China. At total of 5665 patients of average age 60 years were treated for an average of 2 years, at which point the safety monitoring committee terminated the trial due to benefit on active treatment. A 6/3 mmHg reduction in blood pressure was associated with a significant 30% reduction in the primary endpoint of fatal and non-fatal stroke. Similar benefit was seen whether or not patients were over 60 years old or not and was also seen in those 16% who were normotensive (<140 mmHg systolic and <90 mmHg diastolic BP) at outset. The authors went on to incorporate the results into a metanalysis looking specifically at double-blind randomised, controlled trials with ACE inhibitors or ARBs and found an insignificant 7% reduction in risk of re-stroke versus placebo treatment compared with trials using thiazide diuretic (PATS, PROGRESS, and two smaller, older trials) in which there was a highly significant 37% reduction.

It is tempting to use CCBs. In primary prevention trials, long-acting oral CCBs perform as well as other agents.[38] Though they weren't exactly recommended in the latest RCP guidelines on management of stroke, they were the only class of drugs specifically mentioned in that section of the guideline. The American Heart Association (AHA) guideline on stroke prevention from 2014, gives advice conflicting with this.[41] It advocated use of thiazide-like diuretic and if needed ACE inhibitor and they suggested avoiding CCBs. Given early after stroke by intravenous infusion, CCBs are possibly harmful.[6,7] The AHA guideline referred to a metanalysis of 7665 patients from 29 trials of CCBs given within 14 days of a stroke, there was no benefit in terms of reduced mortality or dependency.[36] The RCP guideline referred instead to a large metanalysis compiled in 2016 of all trials of antihypertensives which had over a 1000 patient years of data published since 1966.[42] This did analyse by the presence and absence of previous cardiovascular disease by a variety of cardiovascular endpoints. It was also able to able to show that CCBs and ARBs were rather better than other drugs at preventing strokes. From the online appendix it is apparent that they were not able to analyse stroke trials by agent and that this analysis was, as far as can be told, *primary* prevention. This matters, as we have the results from a randomised, placebo-controlled trial in over 20 000 patients of an ARB after stroke or transient ischaemic attack lasting 2.5 years, which demonstrated no effect of the ARB on re-stroke (Fig. 24.6), despite the average BP being 3.8/2 mmHg lower in the treatment arm.[43] It is not safe to extrapolate from primary prevention data to guide decision-making in secondary prevention. A similar, highly influential metanalysis reported in 2009[44] concluded similarly that it was BP reduction that counted, rather than the agent used to reduce it, but that CCBs were superior in stroke prevention. This finding came from a mixture of primary and secondary prevention trials. They were able to carry out a comparison of agents used in secondary prevention by prior cardiovascular event. There were two trials listed as using CCBs after stroke in the online appendix. One was wrongly categorized and did in fact use thiazide diuretic. Although the remaining trial did show a significant ($P = 0.04$) reduction in strokes in patients with multi-infarct dementia during 6 month's treatment with nimodipine: 6 strokes were recorded on active treatment versus 17 for those on placebo,[45] 23 events is insufficient to power a between-trials comparison of two drug classes. It cannot be held to have established that CCBs have an equivalent effect to thiazide diuretics after stroke.

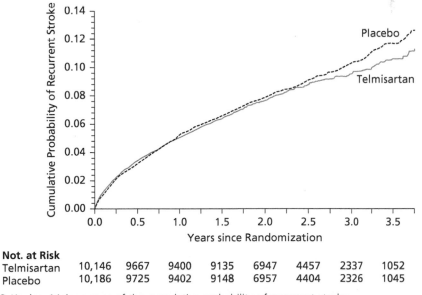

Fig. 24.6 Kaplan–Meier curves of the cumulative probability of recurrent stroke.

Table 24.1 Target BP and choice of antihypertensive by age and co-morbidity

Population	Target systolic BP (/mmHg)	1st line Rx	2nd line Rx
Age 60–80 yrs	<130	CCB or TLD*	ACEI
Type 2 DM	<130	ACEI	TLD
>80 yrs	<150	TLD	ACEI
Prior stroke	<130	TLD	ACEI

Notes: Use the lowest line in the table that applies to the patient. *TLD: thiazide-like diuretic.

Conclusions

It is possible that you are convinced by the evidence underpinning the American Guideline, in which case things are simple. For all those whose 10 year risk of developing cardiovascular disease is over 10% and whose BP is 130/80 mmHg offer drug treatment and aim for less than 130/80 mmHg. Very nearly everyone 60 years and over will exceed that 10 year risk.

For very old patients, it makes sense to adhere to the agents trialled. Based on HYVET, this means using indapamide and aiming for a BP of less than 150 mm systolic when possible, combining the indapamide with long-acting ACEI and, if needed, long-acting CCB. Comorbidities and other drug treatments will likely constrain or determine choice of agent. Limits will need to be interpreted in the light of what can be practically attained for less mobile and frailer older people such as those in nursing homes, for whom the evidence is sparse. Those in the age group 60–80 years will fare quite as well on treatment regimens based on long-acting CCBs as the first agent chosen as they will with a thiazide-like diuretic, particularly if the second agent is an ACEI (or possibly an ARB). In practical terms, to achieve targets, most patients (and particularly older patients with systolic hypertension) will need to be treated with a combination of two or more agents anyway. As diabetics were excluded from SPRINT, the target BP for diabetics 80 will have to remain under 150/90 mmHg based on HYVET. For those aged 60–80 without end-organ damage, the target should also be under 130 mmHg systolic based on the SPRINT results and the recent BP metanalysis[42] including those with type 2 diabetes, setting aside the results of the ACCORD trial.

For patients known to have had a previous stroke, the American guideline is best-evidenced for choice of antihypertensive agent and the weight of evidence is with using indapamide first, to which long-acting ACEI can be added. Long-acting CCB could be used third line. Once again, the target systolic BP should be less than 130 mmHg. Table 24.1 summarises this.

References

1. Craig R & Mindell J (eds.) *Health Survey for England—2006, CVD and risk factors for adults, obesity and risk factors for children*. **NHS Digital**. Available from: https://digital.nhs.uk/data-and-information/publications/statistical/health-survey-for-england/health-survey-for-england-2006-cvd-and-risk-factors-for-adults-obesity-and-risk-factors-for-children [Accessed: 31 July 2019].

2. He W, Goodkind D, & Kowal P. *U.S. Census Bureau, International Population Reports, P95/16–1, An Aging World: 2015*. Washington, DC: U.S. Government Publishing Office, 2016.

3. Roger Vl, Go AS, Lloyd Jones DM, et al. Heart disease and stroke statistics—2011 update. a report from the American Heart Association. *Circulation* 2011;**123**:e18–e209.

4. Lloyd-Jones DM, Evans JC, & Levy D. Hypertension in adults across the age spectrum. Current outcomes and control in the community. *JAMA* 2005;**294**(4):466–72.

5. **Albutt C.** 'Senile plethora or high arterial pressure in elderly persons'. *Lectures to the Hunterian Society* 27th February 1895, Lecture 1.

6. **Wahlgren NG, MacMahon DG, De Keyser J, Indredavik B, & Ryman T.** Intravenous Nimodipine West European Stroke Trial (INWEST) of nimodipine in the treatment of acute ischaemic stroke. *Cerebrovasc Dis* 1994;**4**:204–10.

7. **Ahmed N & Wahlgren NG.** Effects of blood pressure lowering in the acute phase of total anterior circulation infarcts and other stroke subtypes *Cerebrovasc Dis* 2003;**15**(**4**):235–43.

8. **Sanderson S.** Hypertension in the elderly: pressure to treat. *Health Trends* **28**:1996;117–21.

9. **Mulrow CD, Lau J, Cornell J, & Brand M.** Pharmacotherapy for hypertension in the elderly. *Cochrane Database Syst Rev* 1998;(2):CD000028.

10. **Burt V, Whelton P, Rocella EJ, et al.** Prevalence of hypertension in the U.S. adult population. Results from the third national health and nutrition examination survey, 1988–1991. *Hypertension* 1995;**25**:305.

11. **Franklin SS, Jacobs MJ, Wong ND, L'Italien GJ, & Lapuerta P.** Predominance of isolated systolic hypertension among middle-aged and elderly US hypertensives. Analysis based on National Health and Nutrition Examination Survey (NHANES) III. *Hypertension* 2001;**37**:869–74.

12. **Staessen JA, Gasowski J, Wang JG, et al.** Risks of untreated and treated isolated systolic hypertension in the elderly: meta-analysis of outcome trials. *Lancet* 2000; **355**:865–72.

13. **Safar ME & Jankowski P.** Central blood pressure and hypertension: role in cardiovascular risk assessment. *Clin Sci* 2009;**116**(**4**):273–82.

14. **Weinberger MH, Miller JZ, Luft FC, Grim CE, & Fineberg NS.** Definitions and characteristics of sodium sensitivity and blood pressure resistance. *Hypertension* 1986;**8**(Suppl II):127–34.

15. **Kawasaki T, Delea CS, Bartter FC, & Smith H.** The effect of high sodium and low sodium intakes on blood pressure and other related variables in human subjects with idiopathic hypertension. *Am J Med* 1978;**64**:193–8.

16. **He FJ, Markandu ND, & MacGregor GA.** Modest salt reduction lowers blood pressure in both isolated systolic hypertension and combined hypertension. *Hypertension* 2005;**46**:66–70.

17. **Palmer RM, Osterweil D, Loon-Lustig G, & Stern N.** The effect of dietary salt ingestion on blood pressure of old-old subjects. A double-blind, placebo-controlled, crossover trial. *J Am Geriatr Soc* 1989;**37**(10):931–6.

18. **Beckett NS, Ruth Peters, Fletcher AE, et al., for the HYVET Study Group.** Treatment of hypertension in patients 80 years of age or older. *N Engl J Med* 2008;**358**:1887–98.

19. **Peters R, Beckett NS, Burch L, et al.** The effect of treatment based on a diuretic (indapamide) ± ACE inhibitor (perindopril) on fractures in the Hypertension in the Very Elderly Trial (HYVET). *Age Ageing* 2010;**39**:609–16.

20. **Gribbin J, Hubbard R, Gladman JRF, Smith C, & Lewis S.** Risk of falls associated with antihypertensive medication: population-based case–control study. *Age Ageing* 2010;**39**:592–7.

21. **Van Den Wardt V.** Should guidance for the use of antihypertensive medication in older people with frailty be different? *Age Ageing* 2015;**44**:912–13.

22. **Ogliari G, Westendorp RG, Muller M, et al.** Blood pressure and 10 year mortality risk in the Milan Geriatrics 75 + Cohort Study: role of functional and cognitive status. *Age Ageing* 2015;**44**:932–7.

23. **Warwick J, Falaschetti E, Rockwood K, et al.** No evidence that frailty modifies the positive impact of antihypertensive treatment in very elderly people: an investigation of the impact of frailty upon treatment effect in the HYpertension in the Very Elderly Trial (HYVET) study, a double-blind, placebo-controlled study of antihypertensives in people with hypertension aged 80 and over. *BMC Med* 2015;**13**:78.

24. **Benetos A, Labat C, Rossignol P, et al.** Treatment with multiple blood pressure medications, achieved blood pressure and mortality in older nursing home residents. The PARTAGE study. *JAMA Intern Med* 2015;**175**(6):989–95.

25. Rådholm K, Festin K, Falk M, Midlöv P, Mölstad S, & Östgren CJ. Blood pressure and all-cause mortality: a prospective study of nursing home residents. *Age Ageing* 2016;**45**(6):826–32.

26. Williamson JD, Supiano MA, Applegate WB, et al., for the SPRINT Research Group. Intensive vs standard blood pressure control and cardiovascular disease outcomes in adults aged ≥75 years. A randomized clinical trial. *JAMA* 2016;**315**(24):2673–82.

27. Moonen JEF, Foster-Dingley JC, de Ruijter W, et al. Effect of discontinuation of antihypertensive treatment in elderly people on cognitive functioning—the DANTE Study Leiden. A randomized clinical trial. *JAMA Intern Med* 2015;**175**(10):1622–30.

28. Moonen JEF, Foster-Dingley JC, de Ruijter W, van der Grond J, de Craen AJM, & van der Mast RC. Effect of discontinuation of antihypertensive medication on orthostatic hypotension in older persons with mild cognitive impairment: the DANTE Study Leiden. *Age Ageing* 2016;**45**(2):249–55.

29. Stewart R, Xue Q-L, Masaki K, et al. Change in blood pressure and incident dementia. A 32-year prospective study. *Hypertension* 2009;**54**:233–40.

30. Harrison JK, Van Der Wardt V, Conroy SP, et al. New horizons: the management of hypertension in people with dementia. *Age Ageing* 2016;**45**(6):740–6.

31. Pajewski NM, Williamson JD, Applegate WB, et al., for the SPRINT Study Research Group. Characterizing frailty status in the systolic blood pressure intervention trial. *J Gerontol A Biol Sci Med Sci* 2016;**71**(5):649–55.

32. Fougère B, Kelaiditi E, Emiel O, et al. Frailty index and quality of life in nursing home residents: results from INCUR study. *J Gerontol A Biol Sci Med Sci* 2016;**71**(3):420–4.

33. Harris T1, Lipsitz LA, Kleinman JC, & Cornoni-Huntley J. Postural change in blood pressure associated with age and systolic blood pressure. The National Health and Nutrition Examination Survey II. *J Gerontol* 1991;**46**(5):M159–63.

34. PROGRESS Collaborative Group. Randomised trial of a perindopril-based blood-pressure-lowering regimen among 6105 individuals with previous stroke or transient ischaemic attack. *Lancet* 2001;**358**:1033–41.

35. Liu L, Wang Z, Gong L, et al., for the Post-stroke Antihypertensive Treatment Study (PATS) Investigators. Blood pressure reduction for the secondary prevention of stroke: a Chinese trial and a systematic review of the literature. *Hypertension Res* 2009;**32**:1032–40.

36. Horn J & Limburg M. Calcium Antagonists for Ischemic Stroke. A Systematic Review. *Stroke* 2001;**32**:570–6.

37. Jamerson K, Weber WA, Bakris GL, et al. for the ACCOMPLISH Trial Investigators. Benazepril plus amlodipine or hydrochlorothiazide for hypertension in high-risk patients. *N Engl J Med* 2008;**359**:2417–28.

38. The ALLHAT Officers and Coordinators for the ALLHAT Collaborative Research Group. Major outcomes in high-risk hypertensive patients randomized to angiotensin-converting enzyme inhibitor or calcium channel blocker vs diuretic: the Antihypertensive and Lipid-Lowering Treatment to Prevent Heart Attack Trial (ALLHAT). *JAMA* 2002;**288**(23):2981–97.

39. National Institute for Health and Care Excellence (NICE). *Hypertension in Adults: Diagnosis and Management. Clinical Guideline [CG127].* 2011. Available from: https://www.nice.org.uk/guidance/cg127 [Accessed: 31 July 2019].

40. Intercollegiate Stroke Working Party. *National Clinical Guideline for Stroke*, 5th edition. London, UK: Royal College of Physicians, 2016.

41. Kernan WN, Ovbiagele B, Black HR, et al. Guidelines for the prevention of stroke in patients with stroke and transient ischemic attack: a guideline for healthcare professionals from the American Heart Association/American Stroke Association. *Stroke* 2014;**45**:2160–236.

42. Ettehad D, Emdin CA, Kiran A, et al. Blood pressure lowering for prevention of cardiovascular disease and death: a systematic review and meta-analysis. *Lancet* 2016;**387**:957–67.

43. Yusuf S, Diener HC, Sacco RL, et al., for the PRoFESS Study Group. Telmisartan to prevent recurrent stroke and cardiovascular events. *N Engl J Med* 2008;**359**:1225–37.

44. **Law MR, Morris JK, & Wald NJ.** Use of blood pressure lowering drugs in the prevention of cardiovascular disease: meta-analysis of 147 randomised trials in the context of expectations from prospective epidemiological studies. *BMJ* 2009;**338**:b1665.

45. **Pantonia L, Bianchib C, Benekec M, Inzitaria D, Wallind A, & Erkinjuntti T.** The Scandinavian Multi-Infarct Dementia Trial: a double-blind, placebo-controlled trial on nimodipine in multi-infarct dementia. *J Neurol Sci* 2000;**175**:116–23.

46. **The ONTARGET Investigators.** Telmisartan, ramipril, or both in patients at high risk for vascular events. *N Engl J Med* 2008;**358**:1547–59.

47. **Whelton PK, Carey RM, Aronow WS,** et al. 2017 ACC/AHA/AAPA/ABC/ACPM/AGS/APhA/ASH/ASPC/NMA/PCNA guideline for the prevention, detection, evaluation, and management of high blood pressure in adults: a report of the American College of Cardiology/American Heart Association Task Force on Clinical Practice Guidelines. *Hypertension* 2018;**71**:e13–e115.

48. **Bundy JD, Li C, Stuchlik P,** et al. Systolic blood pressure reduction and risk of cardiovascular disease and mortality: a systematic review and network meta-analysis. *JAMA Cardiol* 2017;**2**:775–81.

49. **Wright JT Jr, Williamson JD, Whelton PK,** et al. A randomized trial of intensive versus standard blood-pressure control. SPRINT Research Group. *N Engl J Med* 2015;**373**:2103–16.

50. **Pappaccogli M, Di Monaco S, Perlo E,** et al. Comparison of Automated Office Blood Pressure With Office and Out-Of-Office Measurement Techniques. A Systematic Review and Meta-Analysis. *Hypertension* 2019;**73**:481–90.

51. **Margolis KL, O'Connor PJ, Morgan TM,** et al. Outcomes of Combined Cardiovascular Risk Factor Management Strategies in Type 2 Diabetes: The ACCORD Randomized Trial. *Diabetes Care* 2014;**37**:1721–8.

52. **Cushman WC, Evans GW, Byington RP,** et al. ACCORD Study Group. Effects of intensive blood-pressure control in type 2 diabetes mellitus. *N Engl J Med* 2010;**362**:1575–85.

53. **Beddhu S, Chertow GM, Greene T,** et al. Effects of Intensive Systolic Blood Pressure Lowering on Cardiovascular Events and Mortality in Patients With Type 2 Diabetes Mellitus on Standard Glycemic Control and in Those Without Diabetes Mellitus: Reconciling Results From ACCORD BP and SPRINT. *J Am Heart Assoc* 2018;**7**:e009326.

54. **Gerstein HC, Miller ME, Byington RP,** et al. Action to Control Cardiovascular Risk in Diabetes Study Group. Effects of intensive glucose lowering in type 2 diabetes. *N Engl J Med* 2008;**358**:2545–59.

Chapter 25

Post-stroke cognitive impairment

Sandeep Ankolekar and Michela Simoni

Introduction

Stroke and dementia are two of the most disabling conditions that affect older people. Their combined effects can be devastating and can have enormous implications for health and social care systems. Physical impairments following stroke are easily recognized, but cognitive consequences are less obvious, under-recognized, and neglected. Only 3 of 190 stroke trials published in English language literature from 1976 to 2003 had cognitive outcome measures.[1] Recent advances in stroke treatment mean that there will be an increasing number of stroke survivors with both physical and cognitive deficits, especially among older people where both are common.

In this chapter, we aim to outline the burden of post-stroke cognitive impairment, its pathological substrates, and clinical characteristics, and conclude by discussing some potential preventative and management strategies.

Definition

The presence of dementia following clinical stroke is known as post-stroke dementia (PSD), while post-stroke cognitive impairment (PSCI) refers to all cognitive symptoms following stroke, including those that do not meet the criteria for dementia. Acute stroke may cause specific cognitive deficits such as aphasia, apraxia, visuospatial problems, and agnosia, depending on the arterial territory that is affected. However, as age is the strongest risk factor for stroke, cerebrovascular disease, and neurodegenerative dementias such as Alzheimer's disease, in the older stroke patient, it is not uncommon to find additional cognitive deficits in the post-stroke period.

The term vascular cognitive impairment (VCI) and vascular dementia overlap with PSCI. VCI refers to cognitive deficits as a consequence of cerebrovascular disease irrespective of whether they were associated with a clinical stroke (Box 25.1 (a, b)). Criteria have been defined to describe the cerebrovascular processes causing cognitive impairment; these include the Diagnostic and Statistical Manual of Mental Disorders (DSM) 5 criteria for Major and Mild Vascular Neurocognitive disorder,[2] the International Classification of Disease-10 criteria for Vascular Dementia (VaD),[3] the International Workshop of the National Institute of Neurological Disorders and Stroke (NINDS), and the Association Internationale pour la Recherche et l'Enseignement en Neurosciences (AIREN),[4] commonly called the NINDS-AIREN criteria, for vascular dementia, the 2011 American Heart Association/American Stroke Association (AHA-ASA) criteria for vascular dementia and vascular mild cognitive impairment (VaMCI)[5] and, more recently, the 2014 International Society for Vascular Behavioural and Cognitive Disorders (VASCOG) Diagnostic criteria for vascular cognitive disorders: the VASCOG statement (Box 25.1a, b).[6]

The older criteria such as the NINDS-AIREN criteria, ICD-10, and the Diagnostic and Statistical Manual of Mental Disorders IV (DSM-IV)[7] required memory impairment as a prerequisite for the diagnosis of vascular dementia. With increasing recognition that progressive cerebrovascular

Box 25.1(a) VASCOG criteria for vascular cognitive disorders: proposed criteria for mild cognitive disorder and dementia (or major cognitive disorder)

Mild cognitive disorder

A. Acquired decline from a documented or inferred previous level of performance in *one or more* cognitive domains (listed in Box 25.1(b)) as evidenced by the following:
   a. Concerns of a patient, knowledgeable informant, or a clinician of mild levels of decline from a previous level of cognitive functioning. Typically, the reports will involve greater difficulty in performing the tasks, or the use of compensatory strategies; and
   b. Evidence of modest deficits on objective cognitive assessment based on a validated measure of neurocognitive function, (either formal neuropsychological testing or an equivalent clinical evaluation) in one or more cognitive domains listed in 2b. The test performance is typically in the range between 1 and 2 standard deviations below appropriate norms (or between the 3rd and 16th percentiles) when a formal neuropsychological assessment is available, or an equivalent level as judged by the clinician.

B. The cognitive deficits are not sufficient to interfere with independence (i.e. instrumental activities of daily living are preserved), but greater effort, compensatory strategies, or accommodation may be required to maintain independence.

Dementia* or major cognitive disorder:

A. Evidence of substantial cognitive *decline from a documented or inferred previous level of performance* in *one or more* of the domains outlined above. Evidence for decline is based on:
   a. Concerns of the patient, a knowledgeable informant, or the clinician, of significant decline in specific abilities; and
   b. Clear and significant deficits in objective assessment based on a validated objective measure of neurocognitive function (either formal neuropsychological testing or equivalent clinical evaluation) in one or more cognitive domains. These typically fall two or more standard deviations below the mean (or below the 3rd percentile) of people of similar age, sex, education, and sociocultural background, when a formal neuropsychological assessment is available, or an equivalent level as judged by the clinician.

B. The cognitive deficits are sufficient to interfere with independence (e.g. at a minimum requiring assistance with instrumental activities of daily living, i.e. more complex tasks such as managing finances or medications).

Box 25.1(b) VASCOG criteria for vascular cognitive disorders: Evidence for predominantly vascular aetiology of cognitive impairment

A. One of the following clinical features:

1. The onset of the cognitive deficits is temporally related to one or more cerebrovascular events (CVE). [Onset is often abrupt with a stepwise or fluctuating course owing to multiple such events, with cognitive deficits persisting beyond three months after the event. However, subcortical ischaemic pathology may produce a picture of gradual onset and slowly progressive course, in which case A2 applies]. The evidence of CVEs is one of the following:
   a. Documented history of a stroke, with cognitive decline temporally associated with the event
   b. Physical signs consistent with stroke (e.g. hemiparesis, lower facial weakness, Babinski sign, sensory deficit including visual field defect, pseudobulbar syndrome— supranuclear weakness of muscles of face, tongue, and pharynx, spastic dysarthria, swallowing difficulties, and emotional incontinence)
2. Evidence for decline is prominent in speed of information processing, complex attention, and/or frontal-executive functioning in the absence of history of a stroke or transient ischaemic attack. One of the following features is additionally present:
   a. Early presence of a gait disturbance (small step gait or marche à petit pas, or magnetic, apraxic–ataxic or parkinsonian gait); This may also manifest as unsteadiness and frequent, unprovoked falls
   b. Early urinary frequency, urgency, and other urinary symptoms not explained by urologic disease
   c. Personality and mood changes: abulia, depression, or emotional incontinence

B. Presence of significant neuroimaging (MRI or CT) evidence of cerebrovascular disease (one of the following):

1. One large vessel infarct is sufficient for mild vascular cognitive disorder (VCD), and two or more large vessel infarcts are generally necessary for VaD (or major VCD)
2. An extensive or strategically placed single infarct, typically in the thalamus or basal ganglia may be sufficient for VaD (or major VCD)
3. Multiple lacunar infarcts (> two) outside the brainstem; 1–2 lacunes may be sufficient if strategically placed or in combination with extensive white matter lesions
4. Extensive and confluent white matter lesions
5. Strategically placed intracerebral haemorrhage, or two or more intracerebral haemorrhages
6. Combination of the above

Box 25.1(b) VASCOG criteria for vascular cognitive disorders: Evidence for predominantly vascular aetiology of cognitive impairment *(continued)*

Exclusion criteria (for mild and major VCD)

1. History
   a. Early onset of memory deficit and progressive worsening of memory and other cognitive functions such as language (transcortical sensory aphasia), motor skills (apraxia), and perception (agnosia), in the absence of corresponding focal lesions on brain imaging or history of vascular events
   b. Early and prominent parkinsonian features suggestive of Lewy body disease
   c. History strongly suggestive of another primary neurological disorder such as multiple sclerosis, encephalitis, toxic or metabolic disorder, etc. sufficient to explain the cognitive impairment
2. Neuroimaging
   a. Absent or minimal cerebrovascular lesions on CT or MRI
3. Other medical disorders severe enough to account for memory and related symptoms
   a. Other disease of sufficient severity to cause cognitive impairment (e.g. brain tumour, multiple sclerosis, encephalitis)
   b. Major depression, with a temporal association between cognitive impairment and the likely onset of depression
   c. Toxic and metabolic abnormalities, all of which may require specific investigations
4. Other medical disorders severe enough to account for memory and related symptoms
   a. Other disease of sufficient severity to cause cognitive impairment (e.g. brain tumour, multiple sclerosis, encephalitis)
   b. Major depression, with a temporal association between cognitive impairment and the likely onset of depression
   c. Toxic and metabolic abnormalities, all of which may require specific investigations
5. [For research] The presence of biomarkers for Alzheimer's disease (cerebrospinal Aβ and pTau levels or amyloid imaging at accepted thresholds) exclude diagnosis of probable VCD, and indicate AD with CVD

---

disease is more likely to affect executive function than memory, the more recent criteria, namely the 2011 AHA-ASA criteria, 2013 DSM-5 criteria, and the 2014 VASCOG criteria, allow for the diagnosis of VCI and dementia to be made in the absence of memory impairment. In DSM-5, the term dementia has been replaced with neurocognitive disorder.

PSCI should be differentiated from post-stroke delirium. Delirium is an acute state of mental dysfunction characterized by alteration in awareness, attention, orientation, cognition, sleep cycle, and thought process that may also occur following stroke. It develops over a few hours to few days and is mostly due to systemic and medical complications that may affect the older stroke patient. Delirium symptoms often improve and potentially reverse with treatment of the underlying systemic and medical causes although some patients may not fully regain their mental abilities[8,9] and is a risk factor for PSCI.[10]

PSCI/PSD is a useful concept in the older stroke patient as cognitive impairment in such patients reflects the complex interplay of acute cognitive deficits from stroke on a background of pre-existing cognitive impairment from cerebrovascular and neurodegenerative brain disorders.

The problem

A quarter of stroke survivors show evidence of cognitive impairment. Diagnosing the cause of dementia is difficult and inaccurate in life, but up to a third of dementia cases may be attributed to cerebrovascular disease.[11]

Cognitive symptoms following an acute stroke may vary and fluctuate in the first few weeks before the core ischaemic/infarcted area stabilizes. The fluctuation may be more pronounced in older people due to post-stroke delirium. To allow for stabilization of cognitive deficits, PSCI is usually assessed 3 months or longer following a stroke.

The prevalence of dementia in the first year following stroke varies from 7.4% to 43%; most of the variability in estimates is explained by three main factors: presence of prestroke dementia, type of study (hospital vs. population-based), and presence of recurrent stroke.[12] Prestroke cognitive impairment, present in 9–14% of patients,[12] is an important contributor to PSCI. The incidence of dementia is 20% in the first 3–6 months and increases linearly by 3% each year in hospital based studies.[12] Due to shared pathophysiological processes, it is not surprising that cognitive impairment is also noted in patients who are seen after transient ischaemic attacks (TIAs),[13] although the TIA itself may not cause residual cognitive deficits.

Patients with PSD have a 2–6 times higher risk of death that is independent of stroke severity, recurrence, and comorbidities compared to patients with no dementia.[14,15] PSCI is also associated with increased disability, dependency, depression, and poor quality of life [16] and hence these patients are more likely to be institutionalized.[17]

Causes

Vascular dementia and Alzheimer's disease are responsible for 85–90% of all cases of dementia.[18] Among older people, cerebrovascular disease and Alzheimer's disease, and more likely a variable combination of these two pathologies, account for majority of the PSCI patients.

Cerebrovascular causes

Diseases of small and large blood vessels supplying the brain parenchyma due to a variety of vascular pathologies such as atherosclerosis, microatheromas, microaneurysms, lipohyalinosis, embolic blockage and several others can cause ischaemia, infarction, or haemorrhage of the brain. These processes lead to damage of both cortical and subcortical areas of the brain involved in cognitive processing.

Certain stroke related factors are a significant contributor to PSCI. These include: (a) recurrent stroke: the incidence of stroke rises after each recurrent stroke and the rate of dementia is three times higher in recurrent stroke compared to first ever stroke[12]; (b) severe strokes are associated with more cognitive impairment[16]; (c) multiple strokes; and (d) strategic infarcts—key areas of the brain involved in cognition such as the thalamus, basal forebrain, left inferior genu of the internal capsule, and inferior parietal cortex if involved in infarction or ischaemia increases the risk of cognitive impairment.

Silent small vessel disease without manifest stroke is an important contributor to PSCI; patients with leukoaraiosis are two and half times more likely to have PSD.[12] It is perhaps also responsible for the key feature of VCI—attentional deficits, executive dysfunction, and reduced information processing speed.[19] Small vessel disease most likely leads to cognitive impairment by causing disruption of neuronal circuits that connect key cortical frontal lobe areas like the dorsolateral prefrontal cortex, the orbitofrontal cortex, and the anterior cingulate cortex.

Cerebral amyloid angiopathy (CAA) is linked to Alzheimer's disease but commonly presents as stroke with recurrent and often multiple intracerebral haemorrhages. It occurs due to the deposition of beta-amyloid in the media and adventitia of small arteries, and less commonly the veins of the cerebral cortex and the leptomeninges. CAA is present in 10–30% of unselected brain autopsies of older patients but almost always in the presence of Alzheimer's disease.[20] CAA may lead to cognitive impairment independent of Alzheimer disease pathology,[21] via multiple cerebral microbleeds[22,23] and recurrent spontaneous intracerebral haemorrhages. However, CAA is also associated with cerebral micro infarcts[24] and white matter lesions[25] but it can also cause subacute progressive cognitive decline due to vascular and perivascular inflammation.[26]

Cerebral autosomal dominant arteriopathy with subcortical infarcts and leukoencephalopathy (CADASIL) is a hereditary cerebrovascular small vessel disease that can present with recurrent strokes and/or cognitive impairment.[27] It is due to missense mutation of the *Notch3* gene situated on the short arm of chromosome 19, resulting in accumulation of granular osmophilic material in the media of blood vessel wall leading to its degeneration. Most patients present with mood disturbances, cognitive impairment, and recurrent strokes in their 50s and 60s, and so it is unlikely to be a common cause of PSCI in older people. Other hereditary small vessel diseases such as cerebral autosomal recessive arteriopathy with subcortical infarcts and leukoencephalopathy (CARASIL) and familial cerebral amyloid angiopathies are rarer still, and unlikely to be relevant in the older stroke patient.

Unlike the gradually progressive course of neurodegenerative dementias such as Alzheimer's disease, the trajectory of vascular dementia varies. Patients may develop vascular dementia acutely following strategic strokes while others may have a stepwise decline in cognitive function due to recurrent stroke. Many patients also have progressive deterioration in cognitive function due to progressive small vessel cerebrovascular disease.

Alzheimer's disease

Alzheimer's disease is the most common cause of dementia. Hippocampal atrophy on imaging, a marker of Alzheimer's disease, is associated with an increased risk of PSD.[28] The estimates for cognitive impairment attributable to Alzheimer's disease vary from 19% to 41%.[15] Alzheimer's disease pathology compared to cerebrovascular disease may be less relevant as a cause of PSCI in the younger post-stroke patient.[29]

Combined cerebrovascular disease and Alzheimer's disease

In the older stroke patient, PSD is more likely to be due to a combination of both cerebrovascular and neurodegenerative pathologies; mixed Alzheimer's disease combined with VCI is common, followed by Alzheimer's with diffuse Lewy body disease (DLB); combined VCI and DLB is less common.[30–32] Neuropathological studies in older patients with dementia reveal that both Alzheimer's and vascular pathology coexist (mixed dementia) in up to 50% of patients.[33,34]

However, there is also accumulating evidence of the interaction between Alzheimer's disease pathology and cerebrovascular disease. First, epidemiological studies reveal that stroke patients have a 60% higher risk of developing Alzheimer's disease[35] and patients with Alzheimer's disease are at an increased risk of both ischaemic and haemorrhagic stroke compared to patients without

Alzheimer's disease, independent of vascular risk factors.[36] Second, neuropathological studies show that dementia in patients with Alzheimer's disease tends to occur earlier and is more severe when patients also have stroke.[37] Indeed, fewer lesions are needed to achieve the clinical diagnosis of Alzheimer's disease when patients had vascular lesions in the basal ganglia, thalamus, and deep white matter.[37] Third, both these conditions share common risk factors such as hypertension, diabetes, atherosclerosis, smoking, and atrial fibrillation.[38–44]

Several interactions between the two conditions occurs at the pathophysiological level: (a) deposition of beta-amyloid around small blood vessels can lead to ischaemia secondary to small vessel occlusion, and the chronic ischaemic process may then lead to further production and deposition of amyloid proteins; (b) ischaemia may promote amyloid-beta accumulation in the cerebrospinal fluid (CSF) by reducing its clearance[45,46]; (c) vascular amyloid-beta may promote ischaemia as it is a vasoconstrictor[47]; and (d) Alzheimer's disease-like pathology can occur in the blood vessels of the brain, causing haemorrhage.

Post-stroke delirium is common after stroke occurring in up to 12–48% of patients[48] and can contribute to long-term cognitive impairment after stroke.[10,49] It is important to recognize delirium after stroke as it independently carries a poor prognosis; patients with delirium have a longer stay in hospitals, are more likely to end up in nursing homes and die within 12 months.[48] In the absence of specific post-stroke delirium assessment scales, DSM-5 criteria,[2] Delirium Rating Scale,[50] or short Confusion Assessment Method (short CAM)[51] may be used to identify and diagnose post-stroke delirium. The Confusion Assessment Method for the Intensive Care Unit (CAM-ICU) has been validated in stroke patients to detect post-stroke delirium.[52]

Clinical characteristics

The clinical presentation of PSCI (see Table 25.1) will be contingent on the site, extent, evolution, and interaction of the various neuropathological processes.

Typical large vessel strokes involving the middle cerebral artery may cause problems with visuospatial processing, hemi-attention, apraxia, and neglect if affecting the right side and language problems if affecting the left side. Involvement of other key cognitive areas either by small or large vessel may cause problems with memory.[53] Of the three stages of memory formation—memory encoding, storage, and retrieval—vascular disease is more likely to affect memory retrieval rather than memory encoding deficits that are seen with Alzheimer's disease. Hence, memory impairments in VCI are more likely to improve with cuing strategies. Neuropsychiatric disturbances such as apathy and depression are also more common in VCI.[54] However, as silent small vessel disease involving subcortical neuronal circuits is a significant contributor, most patients with PSCI have problems with attention, speed of information processing, and executive function, which is a key feature of VCI. Patients harbouring associated Alzheimer's disease pathology will report cognitive symptoms mainly involving the domains of memory, executive function, and visuospatial function.

While key strategic infarcts or large strokes may cause acute PSCI, it usually occurs as a clinical or subclinical gradual decline in cognition, mainly causing problems with attention, information and speed processing, and executive function if vascular processes predominate and memory problems if Alzheimer's pathology is present.

Commonly, however, there is a variable involvement of several cognitive domains in the older patient due to mixed pathologies. Superimposed on this, clinical or asymptomatic strokes cause further deterioration in cognitive function in the domains of language, visuospatial abilities, and praxis in a stepwise fashion.

Table 25.1 Common cognitive deficits noted in post-stroke dementia

	Pathological process	Cognitive deficits
1.	Large vessel disease[1]	
	Left anterior cerebral artery[2]	Abulia and lack of initiative, impaired planning, transcortical motor aphasia, memory deficits
	Right anterior cerebral artery[2]	Abulia and lack of initiative, constructional apraxia, and sensory neglect
	Bilateral anterior cerebral artery	Akinetic mutism, apathy, and memory deficits
	Left middle cerebral artery[2]	Aphasia—expressive, receptive, mixed, transcortical, conduction, or global, alexia agraphia, acalculia, finger agnosia, left–right disorientation (Gerstmann's syndrome)
	Right middle cerebral artery[2]	Apraxia, neglect, hemi-inattention, anosognosia, delirium
	Left posterior cerebral artery	Alexia without agraphia, aphasia, and memory deficits with thalamic involvement
	Right posterior cerebral artery	Prosopagnosia, colour agnosia
	Bilateral posterior cerebral artery	Cortical blindness, anosognosia simultagnosia, oculomotor apraxia and optic ataxia (Balint syndrome)
	Right anterior choroidal artery[1]	Mild deficits of visual memory and perception, left spatial hemi-neglect, constructional apraxia, anosognosia, and motor impersistence
	Left anterior choroidal artery[2]	Minor language impairment
	Vertebrobasilar system	Language deficits, behavioural problems, and executive dysfunction
	Watershed stroke MCA[3]/ACA[4]	Transcortical motor aphasia preceded by mutism in dominant hemisphere, neglect, and anosognosia in non-dominant hemisphere
	Watershed stroke MCA/PCA[5]	Language deficits, transcortical sensory aphasia
2.	Small vessel disease[1] (leukoaraiosis, lacunar stroke, microbleeds)	Problems with working memory, memory retrieval, speed of information processing, abstract thinking, and mental flexibility. Complex attentional deficits and executive dysfunction
3.	Alzheimer's Disease	Problems with episodic memory encoding, word finding difficulty, semantic memory deficits, and visuospatial deficits. Executive dysfunction is less common
4.	Mixed Cognitive Impairment	Variable combination of the above

[1] In cerebral haemorrhage—deficits will depend on the area affected; [2] left dominant patients; [3] middle cerebral artery; [4] anterior cerebral artery; [5] posterior cerebral artery.

Cognitive assessments

On the stroke wards, it is often the occupational therapists who identify important cognitive deficits while they assess patients for functional tasks. Language problems are one of the commonest deficits after stroke and speech and language therapists (SALT) will be able to inform the clinician if patients have isolated aphasia or if there are additional cognitive deficits complicating the speech problem. However, detailed neuropsychological assessments are useful in identifying the most important and relevant cognitive deficits. The Neuropsychological Working Group of the National Institute of Neurological Disorders and Stroke—Canadian Stroke Network Vascular Cognitive Impairment Harmonization Standards Committee recommended three separate protocols[19] to serve different purposes in patients with VCI (Box 25.2). The 60-minute protocol is suggested for research studies and recommends tests in the four key cognitive domains of executive/attention, language, visuospatial, and memory in addition to tests for neurobehavioural change and mood. A 30-minute protocol is recommended to be used as screening tool for suspected VCI and tests are selected from within the 60-minute protocol. A 5-minute protocol is also suggested for potential use for primary care physicians, nurses, and other allied health professionals; it may help to identify and screen patients but is not suitable for diagnostic purposes.

In the older stroke patient, detailed cognitive testing may not be feasible and may cause considerable stress and anxiety to patients. Further problems may be encountered in patients with hearing difficulties, aphasia, neglect, and depression, and in those patients for whom English is not the first language. Some of the cognitive assessments address these difficulties. The Birmingham Cognitive Screen (BCoS)[55] may be used in patients with language difficulties and neglect and the Montreal Cognitive Assessment (MoCA) can be administered in several languages and more recently a version for hearing impaired patients has also become available (HI-MoCA).[56] Depression may cause cognitive symptoms and mood disturbances can occur in patients with cognitive impairment. Standard depression scales should be used to identify post-stroke depression. We discuss a few global cognition tests that have been studied in post-stroke patients and may take no more than 10–15 minutes to perform.

Information on prior memory and associated problems from a spouse, relative, or others may help to identify prestroke cognitive impairment and an informant-based questionnaire may be helpful to retrospectively assess for the presence of cognitive impairment. The Informant Questionnaire on Cognitive Decline in the Elderly (IQCODE)[57] is one such test that has been validated against standard cognitive assessments to detect dementia. It is usually completed by a relative, friend, or carer who knows the patient well and it takes 10–15 minutes. The informant is asked 26 questions (16 in the short form) related to change in cognitive function over a 10-year period but for stroke patients, a shorter timeframe such as a year may be used. Each question carries a score between 1 and 5, with higher values representing greater degrees of decline in cognitive function.

The overall score is derived by averaging the score for all the questions and ranges from 1 to 5. A score of 3 means that the patient is unlikely to have had prior dementia. A score range of 3.3–3.6 or higher is generally accepted as a cut-off for cognitive impairment.

The mini-mental status examination (MMSE) is a very popular test with a score range from 0 to 30 (30 is normal).[58] It is designed as a screening tool for dementia and a score of less than 24 is a cut-off score for diagnosing dementia.[59] It tests attention, orientation, memory, language, and visuospatial abilities. MMSE takes 5–10 minutes to perform, is easy to administer, and has been used widely as a cognitive outcome measure in several dementia trials. However, its main limitation is the lack of tests for executive function. Its use has also been hindered by copyright issues.[60]

The MoCA (Fig. 25.1) is becoming popular with stroke clinicians. It is a 30-point test assessing eight cognitive subdomains: visuospatial/executive function (5 points), naming (3 points), memory (5 points), attention (6 points), language (3 points), abstraction (2 points), and orientation (6 points). Higher scores mean better cognition. As it also tests executive function, MoCA is superior to the MMSE.[61] The test, instructions, and training are freely accessible at https://www.mocatest.org after a short registration. It is very dependent on visual and writing tasks, and

Box 25.2 The 2006 National Institute of Neurological Disorders and Stroke–Canadian Stroke Network Vascular Cognitive Impairment Harmonization Standards recommended 60-, 30-, and 5-minute neuropsychology protocols

60-minute test protocol

Executive/Activation

        Animal naming (semantic fluency)

        Controlled oral word association test

        WAIS-III digit symbol-coding

        Trail-making test

List learning test strategies

Future use: simple and choice reaction time

Language/Lexical retrieval

        Boston naming test 2nd edition, short form visuospatial

        Rey–Osterrieth complex figure copy memory

        Hopkins verbal learning test—revised

        Alternate: California verbal learning test–2

Supplemental: Boston naming test recognition

Supplemental: Digit symbol—coding incidental learning

Neuropsychiatric/Depressive symptoms

        Neuropsychiatric inventory questionnaire version

        Center for Epidemiological Studies—depression scale

Other tests

        Informant questionnaire for cognitive decline in older people

MMSE

30-Minute test protocol

Semantic fluency (animal naming)

Phonemic fluency (controlled oral word association test)

Digit symbol-coding from the Wechsler adult intelligence scale, third edition

Hopkins verbal learning test

Center for Epidemiologic Studies—depression scale

Neuropsychiatric inventory, questionnaire version (NPI-Q)

Supplemental tests: MMSE, trail-making test

5-Minute test protocol

MoCA subtests

5-word memory task (registration, recognition, and recall)

6 item orientation

1 letter phonemic fluency

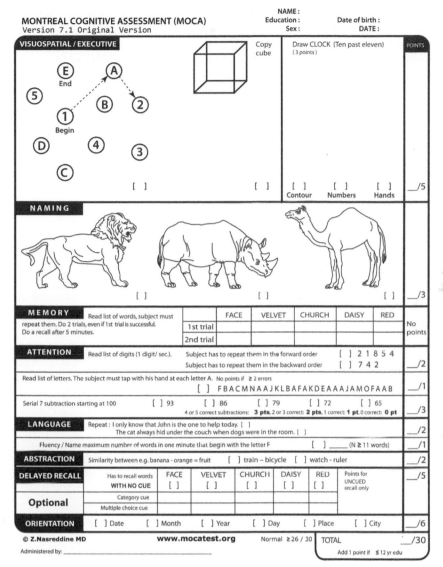

Fig. 25.1 Montreal Cognitive Assessment (MoCA) working sheet.

© Z. Nasreddine MD. Reproduced with permission. Copies are available at www.mocatest.org.

requires verbal responses, which can make it difficult. Alternative forms have been designed for long-term follow-up and for patients who are illiterate.

The Addenbrooke's cognitive examination is another useful but more detailed cognitive assessment that has good sensitivity (83%) and specificity (73%) for a cut-off score less than 94 in post-stroke patients.[62,63] The score range is 0–100 (normal cognition is 100) and it tests attention and orientation (18 points), memory (26 points), fluency (14 points), visuospatial function (16 points), and language (26 points). It takes 20–30 minutes to perform and is easy to administer. The test is freely available, and training is also available freely at https://www.mvls.gla.ac.uk/aceiiitrainer/.

The Birmingham Cognitive Screen (BCoS)[55,64] is a comprehensive cognitive screen that has been designed specifically for stroke patients. It tests several cognitive domains of language, mathematical/number abilities, praxis, memory, and attention and executive functions. Its main advantage is that it can be used in patients affected by neglect and aphasia. It can take up to an hour to administer but it is more time-efficient than the single domain specific cognitive test batteries. The test can be administered by non-neuropsychologists after training.

Investigations

Patients would be expected to have undergone the standard stroke work-up to assess for the likely cause and mechanism of stroke including neuroimaging, investigations, and assessments for hypertension, hypercholesterolemia, diabetes, atrial fibrillation, and other cardioembolic causes. These investigations should be reviewed to ensure that patients are optimally assessed and managed for cerebrovascular risk factors.

As up to 10% (although only 0.6% truly reversible) of patients with cognitive impairment may have a reversible component,[65] PSCI patients should be assessed and investigated for reversible conditions that include depression, delirium, side effects from medications, thyroid problems, vitamin deficiencies such as B_{12}, and excessive use of alcohol.

If patients have only had a computed tomography (CT) brain scan as part of stroke work, they should ideally undergo further MRI brain as it is better at assessing the extent of VCI, as well as cerebral atrophy. For MRI, T1-weighted imaging, T2-weighted, and T2*-weighted gradient recalled echo (GRE) or susceptibility-weighted sequences, diffusion-weighted imaging (and apparent diffusion coefficient map) for acute stroke, and FLAIR sequences should form part of the standard protocol to assess for the various cerebrovascular processes such as infarcts, haemorrhages, white matter disease, microbleeds, and acute ischaemic strokes. Coronal T1-weighted images can additionally help in assessing for hippocampal atrophy, a key finding in patients with concomitant Alzheimer's disease. The STandards for ReportIng Vascular changes on Euroimaging (STRIVE) lays down standards for research purposes but it can be useful in establishing an approach to cerebrovascular disease in clinical practice.[66]

Several biomarkers linked to Alzheimer's and cerebrovascular disease such as e4 allele of apolipoprotein E (APOE4), angiotensin-converting enzyme (ACE) DD allele,[67] beta-secretase enzyme (BACE1),[68] soluble receptor levels for advanced glycation end products (sRAGE),[68] and systemic inflammatory markers such as erythrocyte sedimentation rate (ESR), C-reactive protein (CRP), and interleukin-6 have been studied as potential biomarkers for PSCI but have failed to show convincing results.

Management

Lifestyle modifications

The Austrian Polyintervention Study to Prevent Cognitive Decline after Ischaemic Stroke (ASPIS) trial[69] studied 202 stroke patients to assess whether intensive control and motivation for better compliance with medication, regular blood pressure monitoring, diet changes, and physical activity over 2 years was better than standard stroke care to reduce cognitive decline. The study was neutral and cognitive decline occurred in 10.5% patients in the intervention group versus 12.0% in the standard group (relative risk reduction of 0.87; 95% confidence interval, 0.36–2.10), but was too small to exclude a moderately sized difference. Lifestyle advice that includes recommendations for a healthy diet with salt, sugar, and fat restriction, and generous proportions of fruit and vegetables, moderate physical activity and exercise, and smoking cessation, has positive effects on vascular disease, and patients with PSCI should also be actively advised about its benefits in vascular and brain health.

Treatment of vascular risk factors

Several large randomized blood pressure lowering trials, involving most of the standard antihypertensive agents, have assessed the effect of treating hypertension on cognitive function as a secondary outcome measure.[70] Three studies, Perindopril Protection Against Recurrent Stroke Study (PROGRESS),[71] Prevention Regimen For Effectively avoiding Second Strokes (PRoFESS),[72] and Secondary Prevention of Small Subcortical Strokes (SPS3) trial[73] included patients with previous stroke. While PROGRESS (n = 6105) showed positive effects on cognition with Perindopril, PRoFESS (n = 20 332) assessing telmisartan and SPS3 (n = 2916) and assessing intensive blood pressure lowering in recent lacunar stroke patients to less than 130 mmHg systolic, were neutral on cognition measures. However, a meta-analysis of studies involving BP lowering drugs (including those where the drugs were started post-stroke) studying cognition, was weakly positive.[70] The Prevention of Decline in Cognition After Stroke Trial (PODCAST) was designed to assess the benefits of intensive blood pressure and cholesterol lowering to prevent cognitive decline. The trial was stopped early as it did not achieve the desired recruitment rate and intensive blood pressure and cholesterol lowering did not alter cognition at 2 years.[74]

Two large randomized controlled trials, the Heart Protection Study (HPS)[75] and PROspective Study of Pravastatin in the Elderly at Risk (PROSPER),[76] have assessed lipid lowering with statins on cognition in patients with vascular disease but no dementia. The results were neutral and so were the studies assessing the effects of statins on Alzheimer's disease.[70]

Nevertheless, vascular risk factors including blood pressure and cholesterol should be treated and managed as per the current guidelines for secondary prevention of cerebrovascular disease to reduce recurrent stroke.

Cholinesterase inhibitors

Ascending cholinergic pathways may be affected in both Alzheimer's disease and cerebrovascular disease.[77] While cholinesterase inhibitors have a modest but clear benefit in patients with Alzheimer's disease, there is also some evidence of their usefulness in VCI.[70,78–80] These drugs may be used with caution in the appropriate elderly patients with PSCI. All such patients should be reviewed and medications should be stopped if there is no clear benefit.

Management of cognitive, behavioural, and psychological symptoms of dementia

A systematic review of cognitive rehabilitation strategies[81] noted that while attentional deficits, spatial neglect, and motor apraxia may improve immediately following treatment, this may not be sustained. Moreover, these trials have not shown significant change in day-to-day outcome other than for motor apraxia. Evidence for the benefits of memory rehabilitation, executive dysfunction, and perceptual problems is also lacking. While further studies and improving the quality of studies assessing the effects of cognitive rehabilitation is required, patients should be encouraged to participate in cognitive rehabilitation where appropriate.[81]

PSCI/PSD patients may suffer from several neurobehavioural symptoms including anxiety, depression, apathy, aggressive behaviour, wandering, agitation, and night-time disturbances. Appropriate advice should be sought from the neuropsychiatry and mental health services when necessary. Antipsychotic drugs may be used with caution and only under specialist supervision.

Patients with post-stroke delirium must be managed by a tailored multicomponent service that addresses the management of hypoxia, dehydration, pain, infection, nutrition, and also includes reorientation strategies. This approach may help in preventing delirium in susceptible individuals while also treating established delirium.[82] Sedation and antipsychotic drugs such as low-dose haloperidol or risperidone should be used sparingly.

Ongoing clinical trials

In the last 10 years, there has been a change in the PSCI research environment; there are now several ongoing clinical trials testing lifestyle modifications, vascular risk factor control and various pharmacological interventions in the management of PSCI either as a primary or secondary outcome measure[83] and their results are keenly awaited.

Supportive and symptomatic treatments

Patients with cognitive impairment benefit from comprehensive and active management of their condition by the healthcare team[84–86]; this includes the use of all available supportive and symptomatic treatment options, management of comorbidities and polypharmacy, multidisciplinary coordinated care from relevant healthcare providers including physicians, nursing staff, physiotherapists, occupational therapists, SALT, psychologists, dietitians, and caregivers, active encouragement of patient participation in social activities including adult day care programmes, and encouraging patients to be involved in support groups and services. This strategy should also be used for management of PSCI.

Patients with PSCI may need particular help with remembering to take their medications, arranging follow-up appointments, financial and legal affairs, help with basic and instrumental activities of daily living (IADLs), hiring and supervising their care, finding and using support services including day care centres, and to make necessary arrangements for assisted living or nursing home care.

Patients may undergo possible changes in their personality and behaviour, and as they increasingly rely on their relatives/caregivers for day-to-day activities, caregivers may undergo significant emotional and mental stress. Appropriate education about the disease, management of the behavioural symptoms, information about the resources and support services available, counselling services, and planned respite care may help in alleviating some of the stress experienced by caregivers.

Conclusion

Stroke and dementia occur commonly in the older patient and stroke is a significant risk factor for dementia. PSCI is most often due to cerebrovascular disease, Alzheimer's disease, or a variable combination of both. Lifestyle modifications, optimal management of vascular risk factors, and choline esterase inhibitors may all have a role in reducing the risk of cognitive decline.

References

1. **Anderson CA, Arciniegas DB, & Filley CM.** Treatment of acute ischemic stroke: does it impact neuropsychiatric outcome? *J Neuropsychiatry Clin Neurosci* 2005;**17**(4):486–488.
2. **American Psychiatric Association.** *Diagnostic and Statistical Manual of Mental Disorders*, 5th edition. Washington, DC: American Psychiatric Association, 2013.

3. **The World Health Organization**. *The ICD-10 Classification of Mental and Behavioural Disorders: Clinical Descriptions and Diagnostic Guidelines*. Geneva, Switzerland: World Health Organization, 1992.

4. **Roman GC, Tatemichi TK, Erkinjuntti T, et al.** Vascular dementia: diagnostic criteria for research studies. Report of the NINDS-AIREN International Workshop. *Neurology* 1993;**43**(2):250–60.

5. **Gorelick PB, Scuteri A, Black SE, et al.** Vascular contributions to cognitive impairment and dementia: a statement for healthcare professionals from the american heart association/american stroke association. *Stroke* 2011;**42**(9):2672–713.

6. **Sachdev P, Kalaria R, O'Brien J, et al.** Diagnostic criteria for vascular cognitive disorders: a VASCOG statement. *Alzheimer Dis Assoc Disord* 2014;**28**(3):206–18.

7. **American Psychiatric Association**. *Diagnostic and Statistical Manual of Mental Disorders*, 4th edition. Washington, DC: American Psychiatric Association, 2000.

8. **Inouye SK.** Delirium in older persons. *N Engl J Med* 2006;**354**(11):1157–65.

9. **Weber JB, Coverdale JH, & Kunik ME.** Delirium: current trends in prevention and treatment. *Int Med J* 2004;**34**(3):115–21.

10. **Melkas S, Laurila JV, Vataja R, et al.** Post-stroke delirium in relation to dementia and long-term mortality. *Int J Geriatr Psychiatry* 2012;**27**(4):401–8.

11. **Heart and Stroke Foundation of Canada.** *Mind the Connection: Preventing Stroke and Dementia 2016 Stroke Report*. 2016. Available from: https://www.heartandstroke.ca/-/media/pdf-files/canada/stroke-report/hsf-stroke-report-2016.ashx?la=en&hash=B84FFD2C434B4E3F5CF4585D9CB35713E6C406E5 [Accessed: 31 July 2019].

12. **Pendlebury ST & Rothwell PM.** Prevalence, incidence, and factors associated with pre-stroke and post-stroke dementia: a systematic review and meta-analysis. *Lancet Neurol* 2009;**8**(11):1006–18.

13. **van Rooij FG, Kessels RP, Richard E, De Leeuw FE, & van Dijk EJ.** Cognitive impairment in transient ischemic attack patients: a systematic review. *Cerebrovasc Dis* 2016;**42**(1–2):1–9.

14. **Tatemichi TK, Paik M, Bagiella E, Desmond DW, Pirro M, & Hanzawa LK.** Dementia after stroke is a predictor of long-term survival. *Stroke* 1994;**25**(10):1915–19.

15. **Leys D, Henon H, Mackowiak-Cordoliani MA, & Pasquier F.** Poststroke dementia. *Lancet Neurol* 2005;**4**(11):752–9.

16. **Ankolekar S, Renton C, Sare G, et al.** Relationship between poststroke cognition, baseline factors, and functional outcome: data from 'efficacy of nitric oxide in stroke' trial. *J Stroke Cerebrovasc Dis* 2014;**23**(7):1821–9.

17. **Brodaty H, Altendorf A, Withall A, & Sachdev PS.** Mortality and institutionalization in early survivors of stroke: the effects of cognition, vascular mild cognitive impairment, and vascular dementia. *J Stroke Cerebrovasc Dis* 2010;**19**(6):485–93.

18. **Plassman BL, Langa KM, Fisher GG, et al.** Prevalence of dementia in the United States: the aging, demographics, and memory study. *Neuroepidemiology* 2007;**29**(1–2):125–32.

19. **Hachinski V, Iadecola C, Petersen RC, et al.** National Institute of Neurological Disorders and Stroke—Canadian Stroke Network vascular cognitive impairment harmonization standards. *Stroke* 2006;**37**(9):2220–41.

20. **Jellinger KA.** Alzheimer disease and cerebrovascular pathology: an update. *J Neural Transm (Vienna)* 2002;**109**(5–6):813–36.

21. **Arvanitakis Z, Leurgans SE, Wang Z, Wilson RS, Bennett DA, & Schneider JA.** Cerebral amyloid angiopathy pathology and cognitive domains in older persons. *Ann Neurol* 2011;**69**(2):320–27.

22. **Werring DJ, Frazer DW, Coward LJ, et al.** Cognitive dysfunction in patients with cerebral microbleeds on T2*-weighted gradient-echo MRI. *Brain* 2004;**127**(Pt 10):2265–75.

23. **Qiu C, Cotch MF, Sigurdsson S, et al.** Cerebral microbleeds, retinopathy, and dementia: the AGES-Reykjavik Study. *Neurology* 2010;**75**(24):2221–8.

24. **Soontornniyomkij V, Lynch MD, Mermash S**, et al. Cerebral microinfarcts associated with severe cerebral beta-amyloid angiopathy. *Brain Pathol* 2010;**20**(2):459–67.

25. **Holland CM, Smith EE, Csapo I**, et al. Spatial distribution of white-matter hyperintensities in Alzheimer disease, cerebral amyloid angiopathy, and healthy aging. *Stroke* 2008;**39**(4):1127–33.

26. **Kinnecom C, Lev MH, Wendell L**, et al. Course of cerebral amyloid angiopathy-related inflammation. *Neurology* 2007;**68**(17):1411–16.

27. **Hara K, Shiga A, Fukutake T**, et al. Association of HTRA1 mutations and familial ischemic cerebral small-vessel disease. *N Engl J Med* 2009;**360**(17):1729–39.

28. **Cordoliani-Mackowiak MA, Henon H, Pruvo JP, Pasquier F, & Leys D**. Poststroke dementia: influence of hippocampal atrophy. *Arch Neurol* 2003;**60**(4):585–90.

29. **Lin JH, Lin RT, Tai CT, Hsieh CL, Hsiao SF, & Liu CK**. Prediction of poststroke dementia. *Neurology* 2003;**61**(3):343–8.

30. **Schneider JA, Arvanitakis Z, Bang W, & Bennett DA**. Mixed brain pathologies account for most dementia cases in community-dwelling older persons. *Neurology* 2007;**69**(24):2197–204.

31. **Schneider JA, Arvanitakis Z, Leurgans SE, & Bennett DA**. The neuropathology of probable Alzheimer disease and mild cognitive impairment. *Ann Neurol* 2009;**66**(2):200–8.

32. **Fernando MS, Ince PG, Function MRCC, & Ageing Neuropathology Study Group**. Vascular pathologies and cognition in a population-based cohort of elderly people. *J Neurol Sci* 2004;**226**(1–2):13–17.

33. **Wollenweber FA, Zietemann V, Rominger A**, et al. The Determinants of Dementia After Stroke (DEDEMAS) Study: protocol and pilot data. *Int J Stroke* 2014;**9**(3):387–92.

34. **Schneider JA**. High blood pressure and microinfarcts: a link between vascular risk factors, dementia, and clinical Alzheimer's disease. J Am Geriatr Soc. 2009;**57**(11):2146–2147.

35. **Honig LS, Tang MX, Albert S**, et al. Stroke and the risk of Alzheimer disease. *Arch Neurol* 2003;**60**(12):1707–12.

36. **Chi NF, Chien LN, Ku HL, Hu CJ, & Chiou HY**. Alzheimer disease and risk of stroke: a population-based cohort study. *Neurology* 2013;**80**(8):705–11.

37. **Snowdon DA, Greiner LH, Mortimer JA, Riley KP, Greiner PA, Markesbery WR**. Brain infarction and the clinical expression of Alzheimer disease. The Nun Study. JAMA. 1997;**277**(10):813–817.

38. **Ott A, Breteler MM, de Bruyne MC, van Harskamp F, Grobbee DE, & Hofman A**. Atrial fibrillation and dementia in a population-based study. The Rotterdam Study. *Stroke* 1997;**28**(2):316–21.

39. **Ott A, Stolk RP, van Harskamp F, Pols HA, Hofman A, & Breteler MM**. Diabetes mellitus and the risk of dementia: the Rotterdam study. *Neurology* 1999;**53**(9):1937–42.

40. **Hofman A, Ott A, Breteler MM**, et al. Atherosclerosis, apolipoprotein E, and prevalence of dementia and Alzheimer's disease in the Rotterdam Study. *Lancet* 1997;**349**(9046):151–4.

41. **Kivipelto M, Helkala EL, Laakso MP**, et al. Midlife vascular risk factors and Alzheimer's disease in later life: longitudinal, population-based study. *BMJ* 2001;**322**(7300):1447–51.

42. **Rusanen M, Kivipelto M, Quesenberry CP, Jr., Zhou J, & Whitmer RA**. Heavy smoking in midlife and long-term risk of Alzheimer disease and vascular dementia. *Arch Intern Med* 2011;**171**(4):333–9.

43. **Solomon A, Kivipelto M, Wolozin B, Zhou J, & Whitmer RA**. Midlife serum cholesterol and increased risk of Alzheimer's and vascular dementia three decades later. *Dement Geriatr Cogn Disord* 2009;**28**(1):75–80.

44. **Launer LJ, Ross GW, Petrovitch H**, et al. Midlife blood pressure and dementia: the Honolulu-Asia aging study. *Neurobiol Aging* 2000;**21**(1):49–55.

45. **Cirrito JR, Yamada KA, Finn MB**, et al. Synaptic activity regulates interstitial fluid amyloid-beta levels in vivo. *Neuron* 2005;**48**(6):913–22.

46. **Lewis H, Beher D, Cookson N**, et al. Quantification of Alzheimer pathology in ageing and dementia: age-related accumulation of amyloid-beta(42) peptide in vascular dementia. *Neuropathol Appl Neurobiol* 2006;**32**(2):103–18.

47. **Thomas T, Thomas G, McLendon C, Sutton T, & Mullan M.** Beta-amyloid-mediated vasoactivity and vascular endothelial damage. *Nature* 1996;**380**(6570):168–71.

48. **Shi Q, Presutti R, Selchen D, & Saposnik G.** Delirium in acute stroke: a systematic review and meta-analysis. *Stroke* 2012;**43**(3):645–9.

49. **Ojagbemi A & Ffytche DH.** Are stroke survivors with delirium at higher risk of post-stroke dementia? Current evidence and future directions. *Int J Geriatr Psychiatry* 2016;**31**(12):1289–94.

50. **Trzepacz PT, Baker RW, & Greenhouse J.** A symptom rating scale for delirium. *Psychiatry Res* 1988;**23**(1):89–97.

51. **Inouye SK, van Dyck CH, Alessi CA, Balkin S, Siegal AP, & Horwitz RI.** Clarifying confusion: the confusion assessment method. A new method for detection of delirium. *Ann Intern Med* 1990;**113**(12):941–8.

52. **Mitasova A, Kostalova M, Bednarik J,** et al. Poststroke delirium incidence and outcomes: validation of the Confusion Assessment Method for the Intensive Care Unit (CAM-ICU). *Crit Care Med* 2012;**40**(2):484–90.

53. **Akiguchi I, Ino T, Nabatame H,** et al. Acute-onset amnestic syndrome with localized infarct on the dominant side—comparison between anteromedial thalamic lesion and posterior cerebral artery territory lesion. *Jpn J Med* 1987;**26**(1):15–20.

54. **Nyenhuis DL, Gorelick PB, Geenen EJ,** et al. The pattern of neuropsychological deficits in vascular cognitive impairment-no dementia (vascular CIND). *Clin Neuropsychol* 2004;**18**(1):41–9.

55. **Birmingham Cognitive Screen. Birmingham, UK: University of Birmingham**, 2016. Available from: http://www.bcos.bham.ac.uk/index.html [Accessed: 31 July 2019].

56. **Lin VY, Chung J, Callahan BL,** et al. Development of cognitive screening test for the severely hearing impaired: Hearing-impaired MoCA. *Laryngoscope* 2017;**127** Suppl 1:S4–s11.

57. **Jorm AF & Korten AE.** Assessment of cognitive decline in the elderly by informant interview. *Br J Psychiatry* 1988;**152**:209–13.

58. **Folstein MF, Folstein SE, & McHugh PR.** 'Mini-mental state'. A practical method for grading the cognitive state of patients for the clinician. *J Psychiatr Res* 1975;**12**(3):189–98.

59. **Stuss DT, Meiran N, Guzman DA, Lafleche G, & Willmer J.** Do long tests yield a more accurate diagnosis of dementia than short tests? A comparison of 5 neuropsychological tests. *Arch Neurol* 1996;**53**(10):1033–9.

60. **Newman JC & Feldman R.** Copyright and open access at the bedside. *N Engl J Med* 2011;**365**(26):2447–9.

61. **Pendlebury ST, Cuthbertson FC, Welch SJ, Mehta Z, & Rothwell PM.** Underestimation of cognitive impairment by Mini-Mental State Examination versus the Montreal Cognitive Assessment in patients with transient ischemic attack and stroke: a population-based study. *Stroke* 2010;**41**(6):1290–3.

62. **Pendlebury ST, Mariz J, Bull L, Mehta Z, & Rothwell PM.** MoCA, ACE-R, and MMSE versus the National Institute of Neurological Disorders and Stroke—Canadian Stroke Network vascular cognitive impairment harmonization standards neuropsychological battery after TIA and stroke. *Stroke* 2012;**43**(2):464–9.

63. **Hsieh S, Schubert S, Hoon C, Mioshi E, & Hodges JR.** Validation of the Addenbrooke's Cognitive Examination III in frontotemporal dementia and Alzheimer's disease. *Dement Geriatr Cogn Disord* 2013;**36**(3–4):242–50.

64. **Humphreys GW, Bickerton WL, Samson D, & Riddoch MJ.** BCoS Cognitive Screen. London, UK: Psychology Press, 2012.

65. **Clarfield AM.** The decreasing prevalence of reversible dementias: an updated meta-analysis. *Arch Intern Med* 2003;**163**(18):2219–29.

66. **Wardlaw JM, Smith EE, Biessels GJ,** et al. Neuroimaging standards for research into small vessel disease and its contribution to ageing and neurodegeneration. *Lancet Neurol* 2013;**12**(8):822–38.

67. Szolnoki Z, Maasz A, Magyari L, et al. Coexistence of angiotensin II type-1 receptor A1166C and angiotensin-converting enzyme D/D polymorphism suggests susceptibility for small-vessel-associated ischemic stroke. *Neuromol Med* 2006;**8**(3):353–60.

68. Qian L, Ding L, Cheng L, et al. Early biomarkers for post-stroke cognitive impairment. *J Neurol* 2012;**259**(10):2111–18.

69. Matz K, Teuschl Y, Firlinger B, et al. Multidomain lifestyle interventions for the prevention of cognitive decline after ischemic stroke: randomized trial. *Stroke* 2015;**46**(10):2874–80.

70. Ankolekar S, Geeganage C, Anderton P, Hogg C, & Bath PM. Clinical trials for preventing post stroke cognitive impairment. *J Neurol Sci* 2010;**299**(1–2):168–74.

71. Tzourio C, Anderson C, Chapman N, et al. Effects of blood pressure lowering with perindopril and indapamide therapy on dementia and cognitive decline in patients with cerebrovascular disease. *Arch Intern Med* 2003;**163**(9):1069–75.

72. Diener HC, Sacco RL, Yusuf S, et al. Effects of aspirin plus extended-release dipyridamole versus clopidogrel and telmisartan on disability and cognitive function after recurrent stroke in patients with ischaemic stroke in the Prevention Regimen for Effectively Avoiding Second Strokes (PRoFESS) trial: a double-blind, active and placebo-controlled study. *Lancet Neurol* 2008;**7**(10):875–84.

73. Pearce LA, McClure LA, Anderson DC, et al. Effects of long-term blood pressure lowering and dual antiplatelet treatment on cognitive function in patients with recent lacunar stroke: a secondary analysis from the SPS3 randomised trial. *Lancet Neurol* 2014;**13**(12):1177–85.

74. Bath PM, Scutt P, Blackburn DJ, et al. Intensive versus guideline blood pressure and lipid lowering in patients with previous stroke: main results from the pilot 'Prevention of Decline in Cognition after Stroke Trial' (PODCAST) randomised controlled trial. *PloS One* 2017;**12**(1):e0164608.

75. MRC/BHF Heart Protection Study of cholesterol lowering with simvastatin in 20,536 high-risk individuals: a randomised placebo-controlled trial. *Lancet* 2002;**360**(9326):7–22.

76. Shepherd J, Blauw GJ, Murphy MB, et al. Pravastatin in elderly individuals at risk of vascular disease (PROSPER): a randomised controlled trial. *Lancet* 2002;**360**(9346):1623–30.

77. Roman GC & Kalaria RN. Vascular determinants of cholinergic deficits in Alzheimer disease and vascular dementia. *Neurobiol Aging* 2006;**27**(12):1769–85.

78. Birks J, McGuinness B, & Craig D. Rivastigmine for vascular cognitive impairment. *Cochrane Database Syst Rev* 2013(5):CD004744.

79. Malouf R & Birks J. Donepezil for vascular cognitive impairment. *Cochrane Database Syst Rev* 2004(1):CD004395.

80. Birks J & Craig D. Galantamine for vascular cognitive impairment. *Cochrane Database Syst Rev* 2013(4):CD004746.

81. Gillespie DC, Bowen A, Chung CS, Cockburn J, Knapp P, & Pollock A. Rehabilitation for post-stroke cognitive impairment: an overview of recommendations arising from systematic reviews of current evidence. *Clin Rehabil* 2015;**29**(2):120–8.

82. National Institute of Clinical Excellence (NICE). *Delirium in Adults. Quality Standard [QS63]*. 2014. Available from: https://www.nice.org.uk/guidance/qs63 [Accessed: 31 July 2019].

83. Brainin M, Tuomilehto J, Heiss WD, et al. Post-stroke cognitive decline: an update and perspectives for clinical research. *Eur J Neurol* 2015;**22**(2):229–38, e13–16.

84. Vickrey BG, Mittman BS, Connor KI, et al. The effect of a disease management intervention on quality and outcomes of dementia care: a randomized, controlled trial. *Ann Intern Med* 2006;**145**(10):713–26.

85. Grossberg GT, Christensen DD, Griffith PA, Kerwin DR, Hunt G, & Hall EJ. The art of sharing the diagnosis and management of Alzheimer's disease with patients and caregivers: recommendations of an expert consensus panel. *Prim Care Companion J Clin Psychiatry* 2010;**12**(1):PCC.09cs00833.

86. Voisin T & Vellas B. Diagnosis and treatment of patients with severe Alzheimer's disease. *Drugs Aging* 2009;**26**(2):135–44.

Chapter 26

Psychological and emotional issues after stroke

Reg C. Morris

Ageism, stigma, and pessimism

The focus of this book is stroke in older adults. The psychological, mental health, and social care needs of older people may, on average, exceed those of younger adults in numbers and complexity. But while the perception of psychological well-being and the expectations of psychological healthcare may be partly shaped by age and experience, psychological adjustment and perspectives are immensely variable and flexible. Moreover, few, if any, psychological conditions are the exclusive preserve of one age-group. Age-blindness in practitioners would be counterproductive, but above all, psychological care requires consideration of unique individual characteristics and needs, of which age-related needs and attributes form but one dimension. We should also exercise caution in assuming that outcomes and experiences following stroke are necessarily different in younger and older stroke survivors. Older and younger survivors share many of the same needs and issues.[1] In one study, age predicted functional scores at discharge, but the effect of age alone on *improvement* in functioning, after adjustment for initial level on admission, was small and accounted for less than 2% of variation.[2]

There is relatively little research into age differences in psychological conditions after stroke, but most people who have strokes are over 65 and consequently most research is conducted with typical stroke patients. Therefore, most of the evidence presented next will necessarily apply to older stroke patients. Where specific evidence about age difference is available it will be discussed, especially where it has implications for treatment.

Overview of psychological conditions

This chapter covers a selection of common psychological conditions after stroke, fatigue, cognitive problems, and apathy being covered in other chapters. Psychological conditions such as anxiety, depression, and fatigue are the most commonly reported problems following stroke in patients and carers,[3,4] being seen in around two-thirds of patients and in carers.[5] They hinder functional recovery[6] and present substantial additional costs to health services.[7,8] However, psychological conditions frequently go unrecognized and untreated[3,9]; in the United Kingdom specialist psychologists to assess and treat psychological conditions remain limited in hospitals and are even more scarce in the community settings.[10-12]

Common psychological conditions following stroke

The first three conditions described next will be familiar to all those working in stroke services, including those working in hospital services with patients soon after stroke. While emotionalism is usually a feature of the first few weeks or months, depression and anxiety can emerge at any stage, even up to 10 years or more after the stroke event.

Depression

Depression is common after stroke and is found in around one-third of stroke patients at any one time.[13] Moreover, the risk of depression remains constant in the years after stroke and 55% of stroke patients experience it at some stage.[14] The prevalence of depression has not declined over the past 20 years,[15] despite increased awareness and therapeutic attention. Depression is a significant factor for all age groups but is more common in those under 65.[16,17]

Depression after stroke predisposes to poor outcome. It is associated with poorer functional recovery[18] and lower quality of life.[19] It also impacts on the use of services, including impaired engagement in rehabilitation[20]; increased outpatient visits after discharge[21]; increased rate of rehospitalisation[22]; greater risk of institutionalization.[23]

To avoid such negative outcomes, it is vital that depression is identified soon after it occurs and that patients are offered appropriate treatment. It is not sufficient to screen only in the early stages of recovery; screening must be repeated at intervals over the succeeding years. This is best accomplished using a brief validated self-rating instrument such as the PHQ-9,[24] or, when there is communication impairment, an appropriate version of the carer-completed SADQ.[25] These screening instruments can be used by staff without specialist training. They can then refer on for specialist assessment and treatment where necessary, according to a screening protocol about which all relevant staff have received training from a psychologist.

In the United Kingdom, evidence-based guidelines for depression in the mental health context emphasize stepped care and cognitive behaviour therapy (CBT).[26] However, extrapolation from general mental health to the stroke population requires caution. To date there is no evidence for the effectiveness of CBT or stepped care after stroke, but brief psychological interventions, such as acceptance and commitment therapy, motivational interviewing or behaviour therapy may be helpful.[27–30] There is evidence that selective serotonin reuptake inhibitors (SSRIs) can reduce depression[31,32] and combining psychological treatment with antidepressant drug treatment may have some advantages.[33] But evidence for pharmacological therapy in the prevention of depression after stroke is equivocal.[34,35]

There is a self-management text, *Rebuilding your Life After Stroke*,[36] based on acceptance and commitment therapy that includes advice and practical exercises to manage depression after stroke. In England it is available free through the books on prescription scheme, available at https://reading-well.org.uk/books/books-on-prescription.

Anxiety

Anxiety prevalence estimates after stroke range from 18% to 38%[37] and during the first 10 years after stroke the cumulative incidence is 57%.[38] Anxiety is persistent,[39] more so than depression.[40] Anxiety is associated with poor social functioning,[41] lower quality of life,[42] and poorer functional ability.[43]

Anxiety can be screened with the self-report anxiety scale of the Hospital Anxiety and Depression Scale[44] or the Geriatric Anxiety Inventory,[45] or the General Anxiety Disorder 7 Item measure.[46] Where there are communication problems an alternative screen is the Behavioural Outcomes of Anxiety scale[46] which uses carer ratings.

Psychological interventions and/or drug treatments (SSRI or buspirone hydrochloride) may be useful in treating anxiety.[31,47] SSRIs reduce anxiety, but no one SSRI is superior to any other.[31]

Small randomized trials of a self-help relaxation CD[45,48] have demonstrated benefit for anxiety after stroke, but further research is needed with a large representative sample.[49]

For people with anxiety after stroke approaches to self-management may be found in the book, *Rebuilding your Life After Stroke*.[36]

Emotionalism

Emotional lability, or 'emotionalism', is excessive crying, or sometimes laughing, disproportionate to the emotional stimulus. It often occurs at the mention of personally significant people or events, or when family members visit. It affects about 20–25% of patients in the first 6 months after stroke but declines in frequency and severity so that by 12 months only around 10–15% of patients are affected.[50] A small number continue to experience symptoms beyond 12 months. But many of those affected at 12 months will not have experienced it for the whole year after stroke; few have persistent and severe problems. Emotionalism is distressing and embarrassing for patients and their families, and can interfere with rehabilitation and result in avoidance of social situations.

There are no specific assessments for emotionalism, and perhaps the most important indicator of severity and impact is the extent to which it produces distress for the individual and their immediate family.

Antidepressant drugs may reduce emotionalism, but the evidence is not conclusive and there is no basis to recommend choice of antidepressant.[50] The UK's Clinical Guidelines for stroke make recommendations for emotionalism based on consensus opinion. These propose specialist assessment (e.g. by a psychologist) and distraction from provoking stimuli with antidepressant treatment only if emotionalism is severe and enduring.[51] Patients with emotionalism, and their families, can be helped psychologically by explaining that it is a neurological consequence of the stroke and does not signify distress in the same way as 'normal' crying. This can help to alleviate distress and embarrassment. In addition, clinical experience suggests that training in controlled, regular breathing may be helpful in cases where severe bouts of crying persisted over several months. This may achieve its effect through distraction from the provoking event, or because controlled breathing is incompatible with crying. However, to date there have been no studies of psychological treatments for post-stroke emotionalism and controlled research trials are needed. As for anxiety and depression, the self-management book *Rebuilding your Life After Stroke*[36] offers guidance on how to manage emotionalism.

We will now consider some less well-delineated and researched areas that are nevertheless important aspects of psychological adjustment following stroke and have been identified by stroke survivors as areas particularly requiring assistance and support.[52]

Low self-efficacy, self-esteem, and confidence

Self-efficacy, self-esteem, and confidence are perceived as closely related by stroke survivors.[53] Self-efficacy has been defined as confidence in one's ability to perform a task or specific behaviour.[54] Self-esteem on the other hand is a person's sense of self-worth[55] and confidence has been defined as the belief one has in one's ability to do the things one tries to do.[53] Self-esteem has been shown to be impaired after stroke.[56] Although there is a validated measure of self-esteem after stroke,[57] at the time of writing there is no satisfactory measure of confidence after stroke, but Horne et al.[53] have identified its constituents in preparation for developing a measure.

Self-efficacy has been found to be positively associated with mobility, activities of daily living, and quality of life, and negatively associated with depression after a stroke.[58] Self-efficacy assumes importance due to its link with self-management which is a key approach for long-term conditions[59]: self-efficacy is a crucial element in the success of programmes that support self-management. Self-efficacy in stroke patients can be measured by the Stroke Self-efficacy Questionnaire[57] or the daily living self-efficacy scale.[60] It can be increased by interventions enabling people to challenge assumptions about threat and failure, identifying and challenging self-defeating strategies for compensating for poor self-esteem, and combating self-criticisms and enhancing self-acceptance by fostering a more positive self-percept. Furnishing examples of success and encouragement to strive to achieve goals are also helpful. Many useful techniques for building self-esteem and confidence are outlined in self-help text, *Overcoming Low Self-Esteem*.[61] The self-management text *Rebuilding your Life After Stroke*[36] offers guidance on valued-based living which is a key factor in the development of a positive self-image.

Altered self-identity or self-concept

Horne et al. (2014)[53] found that confidence, self-efficacy, self-esteem, and identity are closely associated constructs in the minds of stroke survivors. All are certainly aspects of the perception of self. However, identity is more closely aligned with global perceptions of personality and values than the other three constructs which are more concerned with capabilities and performance.

Reports of change or 'loss' of identity following brain injury, including stroke, are common[62,63] and the experience may persist over many years.[64] Identity change is the 'subjective discontinuity in their felt, embodied or social experience of who they are'.[65] Following stroke, it has been described as 'loss of me' and feeling distanced from the new self, which is perceived as strange and unfamiliar.[62] The self is often viewed more negatively after stroke to a degree unrelated to physical impairment.[63] Identity change crucially concerns brain injury survivors[66] and their families.[67] It engenders discomfort, grieving for the lost identity, and a striving to construct a new identity[68] which can be experienced as a struggle[69] that distracts from rehabilitation.[70] Change in identity, like identity itself, is associated with emotional problems,[71–73] social isolation,[74] pessimism about the future, and poorer quality of life.[70] Conversely, maintenance of social identity predicts well-being[75] and higher quality of life following brain injury.[76]

Identity after stroke can be assessed with Head Injury Semantic Differential Scale–III.[77] And change in identity can be gauged by asking patients to complete the scale as they were before stroke and comparing this with how they complete it for after their stroke. Interventions such as mindfulness based cognitive therapy[78] may be helpful in reducing discrepancies between current and prestroke self. Vickery et al. (2005)[76] described a self-concept group intervention for people with brain injury which produced significant overall improvement in self-concept. Narrative therapy approaches are yet unproven but have been proposed as an approach to issues of identity after stroke. For example, a person might be encouraged to construct their life story while highlighting valued aspects of themselves that are preserved following stroke,[79] or they might be helped to develop new self-narratives that emphasize positive aspects of their identity after stroke.[80,81] Throughout the goal should be to rebuild a sense of identity based on new possibilities, rather than to restore the preinjury self.[82] These approaches seem intuitively plausible, but caution should be exercised in the absence of evidence of effectiveness. More research into these important aspects of adjustment after stroke is required.

Post-traumatic stress and post-traumatic growth

No account of psychological adjustment to stroke would be complete without some reference to post-traumatic stress and the somewhat paradoxical related phenomenon of post-traumatic growth.

Stroke bears the hallmarks of a traumatic event, being unexpected, uncontrollable, and potentially life-threatening[83] and 10–31% of stroke survivors experience post-traumatic stress symptoms after stroke.[84–86] Post-traumatic stress reactions can be debilitating and include: re-experiencing (spontaneous memories of the traumatic event, recurrent dreams related to it, flashbacks); avoidance (distressing memories, thoughts, feelings, or external reminders of the event); negative cognitions and mood (persistent and distorted sense of blame of self or others, estrangement from others, diminished interest in activities, inability to remember the event); arousal (aggressive, reckless, or self-destructive behaviour, sleep disturbances, hypervigilance).[87] Post-traumatic stress can be assessed with the post-traumatic diagnostic scale (PDS).[88]

It is important to be aware of post-traumatic stress since it has been related to non-adherence to medication and adverse clinical outcomes in heart disease.[89] Merriman et al. (2007)[85] found that symptoms decreased naturally over time and therefore NICE guidance suggests that it is prudent to wait to determine if post-traumatic stress symptoms resolve before intervening.[90] However, in cases where symptoms persist this NICE guidance recommends a course of trauma-focused cognitive behavioural therapy or eye movement desensitization and reprocessing.

The other side of the post-traumatic stress coin is the paradoxical but robust finding that posttraumatic growth (PTG) commonly follows trauma[91,92] and can create 'an increased appreciation for life in general, more meaningful interpersonal relationships, an increased sense of personal strength, changed priorities, and a richer existential and spiritual life'.[93] It represents an experience of profound positive change which goes beyond pretrauma levels of psychological functioning[93,94] and is commonly found following illnesses including stroke.[95–97] It can be assessed with the post-traumatic growth inventory.[98]

The literature on positive psychology suggests that the kinds of positive emotions found in PTG confer benefits other than just 'feeling good', and include improved health, success, and social engagement.[99] It has been suggested that PTG should be considered in clinical practice,[100] through increasing awareness of the potential for PTG, listening out for news of growth when working with stroke survivors, and using reflective listening skills to focus on narratives of PTG during therapy. There is also emerging evidence to suggest that peer support, for example, through peer support groups, can facilitate the development of PTG after illness.[101]

Delivery of psychological care

When to assess psychological factors

Stroke services, with their emphasis on rapid response and early intervention for physiological damage, can facilitate a similar approach to psychological problems. But while there are undoubtedly psychological conditions that are a direct and immediate consequence of stroke, such as communication and cognitive impairments, most psychological conditions are secondary consequences of the impact of stroke on a person's experience, relationships, and life. As such they do not necessarily require the same emphasis on early assessment and intervention and can emerge at any stage after stroke. For example:

◆ Depression/absence of depression early on does not predict later depression (between 1 and 3 months after stroke).[102]

◆ Anxiety occurs at different times after stroke[37]; 40% of those who experience anxiety at some time in 10 years are not anxious at 3 months.[38]

◆ Cognitive function does not remain stable after stroke.[103]

◆ Patients often report that psychological problems start after discharge.[104]

Indeed, in the case of cognitive impairment as well as mood, early assessment may not be predictive of subsequent psychological status and early screening may be counterproductive[105,106] and watchful monitoring of psychological state may be the optimal strategy.

Models of psychological care

There are several models for the delivery of psychological care:

◆ Stratified or matched care is hierarchical, moving from low- to high-intensity interventions, but patients' needs determine the initial intervention level.

◆ Collaborative care has four key elements: collaborative patient and professional identification of problems; collaborative goal-planning; self-management training and support to facilitate the success of interventions, behaviour change, and emotional coping; active follow-up.

◆ Stepped care involves all individuals starting treatment with the lowest intensity interventions ('least intervention first'). The system allows individuals to be 'stepped up' to more intensive or comprehensive interventions if they do not respond to lower intensity interventions.

Stepped care has been recommended for stroke.[51,107] In practice, stepped care requires a level 1 in which the whole stroke team, including ancillary staff, are trained in the management of basic psychological reactions. At level 2 assistant psychologists or other therapists in the stroke team, trained in specific psychological therapies, work under the supervision of a psychologist to deliver therapies for those patients who require more than level 1 support. Finally, at level 3 a psychologist or psychiatrist manages the more complex cases who do not respond at level 2. However, no stroke-specific evidence for the model exists. Although evidence from general mental health suggests that stepped care may be effective, even in this context the evidence is limited and inconclusive.[108,109]

Moreover, it has been suggested that stepped care is:

◆ Overly rigid and prescriptive and does not allow patient choice about treatment.

◆ Psychologically harmful for those with more complex problems through the demoralizing experience of failure at the lower levels before being 'stepped up'.

◆ Impracticable to implement in stroke services unless there is funding for: (a) psychological therapist training and time at level 2; and (b) for specialist psychology input at the higher level—which is only available at all in around 60% of stroke units in the United Kingdom, and even then, is usually part-time.[10,11]

Approaches to meeting demand for psychological care

The issue of providing psychological care to meet the immense level of demand among stroke patients[5] and to reduce the social and economic impact of psychological morbidity[7,8] is challenging.

Clearly an initial step is to ensure that the guidelines for the inclusion of psychologists in the stroke team are followed.[51,110] The British Psychological Society recommend one consultant and one junior psychologist and one assistant psychologist post dedicated to stroke in each typical general hospital catchment of 500 000.[111] With these levels of staffing, a psychology service would deliver a net saving of around £39 000 to the NHS and adult social care over 2 years.[8] This equates to a saving of around £10 million over 2 years for the NHS and social care across the United Kingdom, while improving services.

In planning the services that psychology provides, it is important to consider the very high level of need and demand. Based on a stroke prevalence rate of 2% and an annual incidence rate of 135 per 100 000 with 75% of patients surviving stroke and 60% having a carer, we can make some predictions for a catchment area of 500 000. There will be:

- 16 000 people affected by stroke (10 000 patients and 6000 carers).
- 800 carers and survivors will be adjusting to a recent stroke (within 1 year).

Based on the prevalence figures available, within the 10 000 stroke survivors:

- 3300 will have clinical depression at any one time[13] and 5000 at some point after stroke.[14]
- 2000 will experience clinical anxiety at any one time[36] and 5800 at some time after stroke.[38]
- 3800 will have other emotional problems (e.g. anger and frustration).[3]
- 5000–6000 will have fatigue; about 1900 will need help with it.[3,112]
- 4000 will have significant cognitive problems.[3]

Even allowing for multiple problems in the same individuals, we can expect around 5000 to have psychological problems at any one time.

If only 20% of the 6000 carers have psychological problems at any time[4] there will be 1200 carers with psychological problems. So, in total there will be 6200 people affected by stroke with psychological problems at any one time.

Service demands of this magnitude require innovative approaches, and it is arguable whether one-to-one therapy, except in the most serious cases, is a good use of psychologist's time. In England government funding has been forthcoming for a scheme called 'Improving Access to Psychological Therapies' (IAPT). This uses a stepped-care approach (with elements of matched care for more serious conditions) and most treatment is provided by graduates who have been trained in low or high-intensity therapies based on the cognitive behavioural approach. It has been successful in several mental health contexts,[113] and it may be appropriate to refer stroke patients with less severe psychological problems into such schemes. However, the practitioners will have training in general mental health, principally in treating depression and anxiety with cognitive behavioural therapy and will not have knowledge of how to adapt approaches to the needs of the stroke population.

Another strategy is for psychologists to train and supervise other stroke team staff in the delivery of psychological care. This is the approach used in stepped care for stroke[107] and has potential for the management of milder psychological problems at level 1 of stepped care. It may also be possible to develop level 2 of stepped care for more serious psychological problems that do not respond at level 1. But unless there is additional funding for this it would deplete other functions of the stroke team if, for example, physiotherapists or nurses delivered psychological therapy.

Alternatively, psychologists may develop psychoeducation and therapy programmes that can be delivered in a cost-effective group format. Controlled studies have shown that group interventions after stroke can be both effective in terms of outcomes and reduced costs.[114,115] In the current climate of economic stringency in healthcare, there is increasing interest in group delivery and it is finding application in areas other than psychology (e.g. physiotherapy). A promising therapy that can be delivered in groups is acceptance and commitment therapy,[116] which is a transdiagnostic approach that can help both patients and carers with a range of different symptoms such as anxiety, depression, emotionalism, or low self-esteem. Acceptance and commitment therapy teaches patients that acceptance is sometimes a better strategy than struggling to 'fix' symptoms or to get back to how they were before the stroke. It helps them to combat thinking errors that make life seem bleak and empty and distorts their experience and mood. It teaches techniques such as mindfulness for dealing with stress and anger, as well as helping patients and their carers to identify their core values and translate these into goals for recovery and life after stroke. Variants of acceptance and commitment therapy have been shown to be beneficial in other health conditions, including epilepsy[117,118] and for dementia carers,[119] and can be delivered in a cost-effective group format[120] and it has now been demonstrated to be effective in improving mood in a stroke population.[28]

Recently, forms of self-management for stroke, that require only limited staff time, have become popular and may encompass goal setting, skills training, action planning, and monitoring, and educational programmes with follow-up and support. Self-management has been defined as;

> The actions individuals and carers take for themselves, their children, their families, and others to stay fit and maintain good physical and mental health . . . and maintain health and wellbeing after an acute illness or discharge from hospital.[121]

Such programmes empower stroke survivors and carers to improve outcomes, quality of life, and experience through education or training to improve skills, knowledge, attitudes, and access to resources. Self-management has a growing evidence-base in stroke.[122–124] Interventions aimed at promoting self-management may take several forms and encompass aspects of many current intervention programmes such as education and provision of support workers. De Silva (2011)[59] identified four key targets that self-management programmes should address; information provision, development of skills, promotion of self-efficacy, and support for behaviour change. Lorig and Holman[125] have complemented these proposals by identifying five key elements that facilitate self-management: problem solving; decision-making; resource utilization; forming partnership with healthcare providers; and taking necessary actions. Bolstering self-efficacy or confidence is a core component of any programme designed to promote self-management.

One highly cost-effective self-management approach is book prescription or 'bibliotherapy'.[126] As noted earlier, there is a now a self-management book[36] based on acceptance and commitment therapy specifically designed for stroke survivors and carers that is available through the books on prescription scheme in England https://reading-well.org.uk/books/books-on-prescription/long-term-conditions/stroke/16840135. In addition, there are over a dozen books written by stroke patients or carers providing accounts of recovery from stroke. Many of those affected by stroke find reading these engenders hope and offers practical tips for dealing with the aftermath of stroke. National stroke charities in the United Kingdom and elsewhere publish inspiring patients' and carers' stories on their websites and may also provide booklists including stroke patients' and carers' books which are also available on their websites (e.g. The Stroke Association).

Other promising general approaches include the use of peer support; former stroke patients and carers join groups of more recent stroke patients to offer psychological and practical support. In this way the experiential knowledge of the former patients, sometimes referred to as 'experts by experience', is harnessed in helping more recent patients to address their own psychological issues. Initial qualitative results suggest this is a feasible and helpful strategy,[127,128] but properly controlled clinical trials are required as well as a greater theoretical understanding of the mechanisms and principles by which peer support achieves its benefits.

Summary

This selective overview has covered some of the most common psychological conditions after stroke. Others such as fatigue and cognitive problems are covered in other chapters. A range of screening and assessment tools exist for each of the conditions, as well as several approaches to treatment. Treatments for anxiety and depression have the best evidence base, whereas treatments for other conditions tend to be based on expert opinion. When considering psychological conditions, it is important to realize that many develop some time after stroke. In addition, the high prevalence rate requires psychological treatments that can be delivered in a cost-effective manner.

References

1. **Pringle J, Hendry C, & McLafferty E.** A review of the early discharge experiences of stroke survivors and their carers. *J Clin Nurs* 2008;**17**:2384–97.

2. **Bagg S, Pombo AP, & Hopman W.** Effect of age on functional outcomes after stroke rehabilitation. *Stroke* 2002;**33**:179–85.

3. **McKevitt C, Fudge N, Redfern J**, et al. *The Stroke Association UK Stroke Survivor Needs Survey.* London, UK: The Stroke Association, 2010.

4. **Low JT, Payne S, & Roderick P.** The impact of stroke on informal carers: a literature review. *Soc Sci Med* 1999;**49**:711–25.

5. **The Stroke Association.** *Feeling Overwhelmed: The Emotional Impact of Stroke.* London, UK: The Stroke Association, 2013.

6. **West R, Hill K, Hewison J**, et al. Psychological disorders after stroke are an important influence on functional outcomes: a prospective cohort study. *Stroke* 2010;**41**:1723–7.

7. **Naylor C, Parsonage M, McDaid D**, et al. (2012). *Long-term Conditions and Mental Health: The Cost of Co-morbidities.* London, UK: The King's Fund.

8. **Gillham S, Carpenter M, & Leathley M.** (2012). *Psychological Care After Stroke: Economic Modelling of a Clinical Psychology Led Team Approach.* Leicester, UK: NHS Improvement.

9. **The Comptroller and Auditor General/The National Audit Office.** *Progress in Improving Stroke Care.* Norwich, UK: The National Audit Office, 2010.

10. **Royal College of Physicians.** *Sentinel Stroke National Audit Programme: Acute Organisational Audit Report 2014.* London, UK: Royal College of Physician, 2014.

11. **Royal College of Physicians.** *Sentinel Stroke National Audit Programme: Post-acute Organisational Audit Report 2015.* London, UK: Royal College of Physician, 2015.

12. **Care Quality Commission.** *Supporting Life After Stroke. A Review of Services for People Who Have Had a Stroke and Their Carers.* London, UK: Care Quality Commission, 2011.

13. **Hackett ML, Yapa C, Parag V, & Anderson CS.** Frequency of depression after stroke: a systematic review of observational studies. *Stroke* 2005;**36**:1330–40.

14. **Ayerbe L, Ayis S, Crichton S, Wolfe CD, & Rudd AG.** The natural history of depression up to 15 years after stroke: the South London Stroke Register. *Stroke* 2013;**44**:1105–10.

15. **Hackett ML & Pickles K.** Part I: frequency of depression after stroke: an updated systematic review and meta-analysis of observational studies. *Int J Stroke* 2014;**9**:1017–25.

16. **McCarthy MJ, Sucharew HJ, Alwell K**, et al. Age, subjective stress, and depression after ischemic stroke. *J Behav Med* 2016;**39**:55–64.

17. **Broomfield NM, Quinn TJ, Abdul-Rahim AH, Walters MR, & Evans JJ.** Depression and anxiety symptoms post-stroke/TIA: prevalence and associations in cross-sectional data from a regional stroke registry. *BMC Neurol* 2014;**14**:198.

18. **Morris PLP, Raphael B, & Robinson RG.** Clinical depression is associated with impaired recovery from stroke. *Med J Aust* 1992;**157**:239–42.

19. **Bays CL.** Quality of life of stroke survivors: a research synthesis. *J Neurosci Nurs* 2001;**33**: 310–16.

20. **Gillen R, Tennen H, McKee TE, Gernert-Dott P, & Affleck G.** Depressive symptoms and history of depression predict rehabilitation efficiency in stroke patients. *Arch Phys Med Rehabil* 2001;**82**:1645–9.

21. **Jia H, Damush TM, Qin H**, et al. The impact of poststroke depression on healthcare use by veterans with acute stroke. *Stroke* 2006;**37**: 2796–801.

22. **Ghose SS, Williams LS, & Swindle RW.** Depression and other mental health diagnoses after stroke increase inpatient and outpatient medical utilization three years poststroke. *Med Care* 2005;**43**:1259–64.

23. **Kotila M, Numminen H, Waltimo O, & Kaste M.** Post-stroke depression and functional recovery in a population-based stroke register: the Finnstroke study. *Eur J Neurol* 1999;**6**:309–12.

24. **Meader N, Moe-Byrne T, Llewellyn A, & Mitchell AJ.** Screening for poststroke major depression: a meta-analysis of diagnostic validity studies. *J Neurol Neurosurg Psychiatry* 2014;**85**:198–206.

25. **Sutcliffe LM & Lincoln NB.** The assessment of depression in aphasic stroke patients: the development of the Stroke Aphasic Depression Questionnaire. *Clin Rehabil* 1998;**12**:506–13.

26. **National Institute for Health and Clinical Excellence (NICE).** *Depression in Adults with Chronic Physical Health Problem: Recognition and Management.* Clinical Guideline [CG91]. Leicester, UK: NICE, 2009. Available from: https://www.nice.org.uk/guidance/cg91 [Accessed: 1 August 2019].

27. **Graham CD, Gillanders D, Stuart S, & Gouick J.** An acceptance and commitment therapy (ACT)–based intervention for an adult experiencing post-stroke anxiety and medically unexplained symptoms. *Clin Case Stud* 2014;**14**(2):83–97. https://doi.org/10.1177/1534650114539386

28. **Majumdar S, & Morris R.** The efficacy of and ACT-based group for stroke survivors. *Brit J Clin Psychol* 2019;**58**(1):70–90. doi:10.1111/bjc.12198

29. **Watkins CL, Wathan JV, Leathley MJ, et al.** The 12-month effects of early motivational interviewing after acute stroke: a randomized controlled trial. *Stroke* 2011;**42**:1956–61.

30. **Thomas SA, Walker MF, Macniven JA, Haworth H, & Lincoln NB.** Communication and low mood (CALM): a randomized controlled trial of behavioural therapy for stroke patients with aphasia. *Clin Rehabil* 2013;**27**:398–408.

31. **Mead GE, Hsieh CF, Lee R, et al.** Selective serotonin reuptake inhibitors (SSRIs) for stroke recovery. *Cochrane Database Syst Rev* 2012;(11):CD009286.

32. **Hackett, ML, Anderson CS, House A, & Xia J.** Interventions for treating depression after stroke. *Cochrane Database Syst Rev* 2008;(4):CD003437.

33. **Mitchell PH, Veith RC, Becker KJ, et al.** Brief psychosocial–behavioral intervention with antidepressant reduces poststroke depression significantly more than usual care with antidepressant. Living well with stroke: randomized, controlled trial. *Stroke* 2009;**40**:3073–8.

34. **Hackett ML, Anderson CS, House A, et al.** Interventions for preventing depression after stroke. *Cochrane Database Syst Rev* 2008;(3):CD003689.

35. **Tsai C-S, Wu C-L, Chou S-Y, Tsang H-Y, Hung T-H, & Su J-A.** Prevention of poststroke depression with milnacipran in patients with acute ischemic stroke: a double-blind randomized placebo-controlled trial. *Int Clin Psychopharmacol* 2011;**26**:263–7.

36. **Morris R, Falck M, Miles T, Wilcox J, & Fisher-Hicks S.** *Rebuilding Your Life After Stroke: Positive Steps to Wellbeing.* London, UK: Jessica Kingsley, 2017.

37. **Campbell Burton CA, Murray J, Holmes J, Astin F, Greenwood D, & Knapp P.** Frequency of anxiety after stroke: a systematic review and meta-analysis of observational studies. *Int J Stroke* 2013; **8**:545–59.

38. **Ayerbe L, Ayis S, Crichton S, Wolfe CD, & Rudd AG.** Natural history, predictors and associated outcomes of anxiety up to 10 years after stroke: the South London Stroke Register. *Age Ageing* 2013;**43**:542–7.

39. **Astrom M.** Generalised anxiety disorder in stroke patients: a 3-year longitudinal study. *Stroke* 1996;**27**:270–5.

40. **Morrison V, Pollard B, Johnston M, & MacWalter R.** Anxiety and depression 3 years following stroke: demographic, clinical, and psychological predictors. *J Psychosom Res* 2005;**59**:209–13.

41. **Shimoda K & Robinson RG.** Effects of anxiety disorder on impairment and recovery from stroke. *J Neuropsych Clin Neurol* 1998;**10**:34–40.

42. **Jeong BO, Kang HJ, Bae KY, et al.** Determinants of quality of life in the acute stage following stroke. *Psychiatry Investig* 2012;**9**:127–33.

43. **D'Alisa S, Baido S, Mauro A, & Miscio G.** How does stroke restrict participation in long term post-stroke patients? *Acta Neurologica Scandinavica* 2005;**112**:157–62.

44. **Zigmond AS & Snaith RP.** Hospital anxiety and depression scale. *Acta Psychiatrica Scandinavica* 1983;**67**:361–70.

45. **Kneebone II, Fife-Schaw C, Lincoln NB, & Harder H.** A study of the validity and the reliability of the Geriatric Anxiety Inventory in screening for anxiety after stroke in older inpatients. *Clin Rehabil* 2016;**30**:1220–8.

46. **Eccles A, Morris R, & Kneebone I.** Psychometric properties of the behavioural outcomes of anxiety questionnaire in stroke patients with aphasia. *Clin Rehabil* 2017;**31**:369–78.

47. **Campbell Burton CA, Holmes J, Murray J, et al.** Interventions for treating anxiety after stroke. *Cochrane Database Syst Rev* 2011;(12):CD008860.

48. **Golding K, Kneebone I, & Fife-Schaw C.** Self-help relaxation for post-stroke anxiety: a randomised, controlled pilot study. *Clin Rehabil* 2015;**30**:174–80.

49. **Willson R & Veale D.** *Overcoming Health Anxiety: A Self-help Guide Using Cognitive Behavioural Techniques*. London, UK: Robinson, 2009.

50. **Hackett ML, Yang M, Anderson CS, Horrocks JA, & House A.** Pharmaceutical interventions for emotionalism after stroke. *Cochrane Database Syst Rev* 2010;(2):CD003690.

51. **Intercollegiate Stroke Working Party.** *National Clinical Guidelines for Stroke*, 5th edition. London, UK: Royal College of Physicians, 2016.

52. **Pollock A, St George B, Fenton M, & Firkins L.** Top ten research priorities relating to life after stroke. *Lancet Neurol* 2012;**11**:209.

53. **Horne J, Lincoln NB, Preston J, & Logan P.** What does confidence mean to people who have had a stroke?—a qualitative interview study. *Clin Rehabil* 2014;**28**:1125–35.

54. **Bandura A.** Self-efficacy. In: Ramachaudran VS (ed.) *Encyclopedia of Human Behavior*, Vol. 4, pp. 71–81. New York, NY: Academic Press, 1994. (Reprinted in Friedman H (ed.) *Encyclopedia of Mental Health*. San Diego, CA: Academic Press, 1998).

55. **Rosenberg M.** *Conceiving the Self*. Malabar, FL: Krieger Publishing, 1979.

56. **Keppel CC & Crowe SF.** Changes to body image and self-esteem following stroke in young adults. *Neuropsychol Rehabil* 2000;**10**:15–31.

57. **Jones F, Partridge C, & Reid F.** The Stroke Self-Efficacy Questionnaire: measuring individual confidence in functional performance after stroke. *J Clin Nurs* 2008;**17**:244–52.

58. **Korpershoek C, Van Der Bijl J, & Hafsteinsdóttir TB.** Self-efficacy and its influence on recovery of patients with stroke: a systematic review. *J Adv Nurs* 2011;**67**:1876–94.

59. **De Silva D.** *Helping People Help Themselves: A Review of the Evidence Considering Whether it is Worthwhile to Support Self-Management*. London, UK: The Health Foundation, 2011.

60. **Maujean A, Davis P, Kendall E, Casey L, & Loxton N.** The daily living self-efficacy scale: a new measure for assessing self-efficacy in stroke survivors. *Disabil Rehabil* 2014;**36**:504–11.

61. **Fennel MJV.** *Overcoming Low Self-Esteem: A Self-Help Guide Using Cognitive Behavioural Techniques*. London, UK: Robinson, 2009.

62. **Murray C & Harrison B.** The meaning and experience of being a stroke survivor: an interpretative phenomenological analysis. *Disabil Rehabil* 2004;**26**:808–16.

63. **Ellis-Hill CS & Horn S.** Change in identity and self-concept: a new theoretical approach to recovery following a stroke. *Clin Rehabil* 2000;**14**:279–87.

64. **Pallesen H.** Body, coping and self-identity: a qualitative 5-year follow-up study of stroke. *Disabil Rehabil* 2014;**36**:232–41.

65. **Yeates GN, Gracey F, McGrath JC.** A biopsychosocial deconstruction of 'personality change' following acquired brain injury. *Neuropsychol Rehabil* 2008;**18**:566–89.

66. **Ben-Yishay Y.** Foreword. *Neuropsychol Rehabil* 2008;**18**:513–21.

67. **Landau J & Hissett J.** Mild traumatic brain injury: impact on identity and ambiguous loss in the family. *Fam Syst Health* 2008; **26**:69–85.

68. **Moldover JE, Goldberg KB, & Prout MF.** Depression after traumatic brain injury: a review of evidence for clinical heterogeneity. *Neuropsychol Rev* 2004;**14**:43–154.

69. **Morris D.** Rebuilding identity through narrative following traumatic brain injury. *J Cogn Rehabil* 2004;**22**:15–21.

70. **Cloute K, Mitchell A, & Yates P.** Traumatic brain injury and the construction of identity: a discursive approach. *Neuropsychol Rehabil* 2008;**18**:651–70.

71. **Cantor JB, Ashman TA, Schwartz ME, et al.** The role of self-discrepancy theory in understanding post–traumatic brain injury affective disorders: a pilot study. *J Head Trauma Rehabil* 2005;**20**: 527–43.

72. **Carroll E & Coetzer R.** Identity, grief and self-awareness after traumatic brain injury. *Neuropsychol Rehabil* 2011;**21**:289–305.

73. **Wright JC & Telford R.** Psychological problems following minor head injury: a prospective study. *Br J Clin Psychol* 1996;**35**:399–412.

74. **Engberg AW & Teasdale TW.** Psychosocial outcome following traumatic brain injury in adults: a long-term population-based follow-up. *Brain Injury* 2004;**18**:533–45.

75. **Haslam C, Holme A, Haslam SA, Iyer A, Jetten J, & Williams WH.** Maintaining group memberships: social identity continuity predicts wellbeing after stroke. *Neuropsychol Rehabil* 2008;**18**:671–91.

76. **Vickery CD, Gontkovsky ST, & Caroselli JS.** Self-concept and quality of life following acquired brain injury: a pilot investigation. *Brain Injury* 2005;**19**:657–65.

77. **Tyerman A & Humphrey M.** Changes in self-concept following severe head injury. *Int J Rehabil Res* 1984;**7**:11–23.

78. **Crane C, Barnhofer T, Duggan DS, Hepburn S, Fennell M, & Williams MG.** Mindfulness-based cognitive therapy and self-discrepancy in recovered depressed patients with a history of depression and suicidality. *Cogn Ther Res* 2008;**32**:775–87.

79. **Hinojosa R, Boylstein C, Rittman M, Hinojosa MS, & Faircloth CA.** Constructions of continuity after stroke. *Symbolic Interaction* 2008;**31**:205–24.

80. **Ellis-Hill C, Payne S, & Ward C.** Using stroke to explore the life thread model: an alternative approach to understanding rehabilitation following an acquired disability. *Disabil Rehabil* 2007;**30**(2):150–9.

81. **Nochi M.** Reconstructing self-narratives in coping with traumatic brain injury. *Soc Sci Med* 2000;**51**:1795–804.

82. **Hill H.** Traumatic brain injury: a view from the inside. *Brain Injury* 1999;**13**(11):839–44.

83. **Field EL, Norman P, & Barton J.** Cross-sectional and prospective associations between cognitive appraisals and posttraumatic stress disorder symptoms following stroke. *Behav Res Ther* 2008;**46**(1):62–70.

84. **Bruggimann L, Annoni JM, Staub F, Von Steinbüchel N, Van der Linden M, & Bogousslavsky J.** Chronic posttraumatic stress symptoms after nonsevere stroke. *Neurology* 2006;**66**(4):513–16.

85. **Merriman C, Norman P, & Barton J.** Psychological correlates of PTSD symptoms following stroke. *Psychol Health Med* 2007;**12**(5):592–602.

86. **Sembi S, Tarrier N, O'Neill P, Burns A, & Faragher B.** Does post-traumatic stress disorder occur after stroke: a preliminary study. *Int J Geriatr* 1998;**13**(5):315–22.

87. **American Psychiatric Association.** *Diagnostic and Statistical Manual of Mental Disorders*, 5th edition. Washington, DC: APA, 2013.

88. **Foa EB, Cashman L, Jaycox L, & Perry K.** The validation of a self-report measure of post-traumatic stress disorder. The post-traumatic diagnostic scale. *Psychol Assess* 1997;**9**:445–51.

89. **Shemesh E, Yehuda R, Milo O, et al.** Posttraumatic stress, non-adherence and adverse outcomes in survivors of a myocardial infarction. *Psychosom Med* 2004;**66**:521–6.

90. National Institute for Health and Care Excellence (NICE). *Post-traumatic Stress Disorder: Management: Clinical Guideline [CG26].* 2005. [Available from: https://www.nice.org.uk/guidance/cg26 [Accessed: 1 August 2019] [This guidance has been updated and replaced by NICE guideline NG116.]

91. **Tedeschi RG. & Calhoun LG.** *Trauma and Transformation: Growing in the Aftermath of Suffering.* Thousand Oaks, CA: Sage Publications, 1995.

92. **Park CL & Helgeson V.** Introduction to the special section: growth following highly stressful life events--current status and future directions. *J Consult Clin Psychol* 2006;**74**(5):791-6.

93. **Tedeschi RG & Calhoun LG.** Posttraumatic growth: conceptual foundations and empirical evidence. *Psychological Inquiry* 2004;**15**(1):1-18.

94. **Schaefer JA & Moos RH.** Life crises and personal growth. In: Carpenter BN (ed.) *Personal Coping: Theory, Research and Application,* pp. 149-70. Westport, CT: Greenwood Publishing, 1992.

95. **Gangstad B, Norman P, & Barton J.** Cognitive processing and posttraumatic growth after stroke. *Rehabil Psychol* 2009;**54**(1):69-75.

96. **Gillen G.** Positive consequences of surviving a stroke. *Am J Occupat Ther* 2005;**59**(3):346-50.

97. **Kuenemund A, Zwick S, Rief W, & Exner C.** (Re-) defining the self–enhanced posttraumatic growth and event centrality in stroke survivors: a mixed-method approach and control comparison study. *J Health Psychol* 2014;**21**:679-89.

98. **Tedeschi RG & Calhoun LG.** The posttraumatic growth inventory: measuring the positive legacy of trauma. *J Traumatic Stress* 1996;**9**(3):455-71.

99. **Lyubomirsky S, King L, & Diener E.** The benefits of frequent positive affect: does happiness lead to success? *Psychol Bull* 2005;**131**(6):803-55.

100. **Joseph S & Linley PA.** Growth following adversity: theoretical perspectives and implications for clinical practice. *Clin Psychol Rev* 2006;**26**:1041-53.

101. **Morris BA, Campbell M, Dwyer M, Dunn J, & Chambers SK.** Survivor identity and post-traumatic growth after participating in challenge-based peer-support programmes. *Br J Health Psychol* 2011;**16**(3), 660-674.

102. **Townend BS, Whyte S, Desborough T,** et al. Longitudinal prevalence and determinants of early mood disorder post-stroke. *J Clin Neurosci* 2007;**14**:429-34.

103. **Hurford R, Charidimou A, Fox Z, Cipolotti L, & Werring DJ.** Domain-specific trends in cognitive impairment after acute ischaemic stroke. *J Neurol* 2013;**260**:237-41.

104. **Lincoln NB, Kneebone II, Macniven J, & Morris R.** *The Psychological Management of Stroke.* Chichester (UK): Wiley International, 2012, Chapter 1.

105. **Lees R & Broomfield NM.** Post-stroke cognitive screening: the good, the bad and the unknown. *Int J Ther Rehabil* 2014;**21**:8-9.

106. **Lees R, Stott DJ, Terence J, Quinn TJ, Niall M, & Broomfield NM.** Feasibility and diagnostic accuracy of early mood screening to diagnose persisting clinical depression/anxiety disorder after stroke. *Cerebrovasc Dis* 2014;**37**:323-9.

107. **Gillham S & Clarke L.** *Psychological Care After Stroke—Improving Stroke Services for People with Cognitive and Mood Disorders.* Leicester, UK: NHS Improvement, 2011.

108. **Frith N, Barkham M, & Kellett S.** The clinical effectiveness of stepped care systems for depression in working age adults: a systematic review. *J Affect Dis* 2015;**170**:119-30.

109. **van Straten A, Hill J, Richards DA, & Cuijpers P.** Stepped care treatment delivery for depression: a systematic review and meta-analysis. *Psychol Med* 2015;**45**:231-46.

110 **Department of Health.** *National Stroke Strategy.* London, UK: Department of Health, 2007.

111. **Division of Neuropsychology/Division of Clinical Psychology.** *Psychological Services for Stroke Survivors and their Families Briefing Paper 19.* Leicester, UK: British Psychological Society, 2009.

112. **Duncan F, Wub S, & Mead GE.** Frequency and natural history of fatigue after stroke: a systematic review of longitudinal studies. *J Psychosom Res* 2012;**73**:18-27.

113. **Fonagy P & Clarke D.** Update on the improving access to psychological therapies programme in England. *BrJPsych Bull* 2015;**39**:248–51.

114. **Johansson B, Bjuhr H, & Ronnback I.** Mindfulness-based stress reduction (MBSR) improves long-term mental fatigue after stroke or traumatic brain injury. *Brain Injury* 2012;**26**:1621–8.

115. **Harrington R, Taylor G, Hollinghurst S, Reed M, Kay H, & Wood VA.** A community-based exercise and education scheme for stroke survivors: a randomized controlled trial and economic evaluation. *Clin Rehabil* 2010;**24**:3–15.

116. **Hayes SC.** *Acceptance and Commitment Therapy: An Experiential Approach to Behavior Change.* New York & London: Guilford Press, 1999.

117. **Lundgren T, Dahl J, Melin L, & Kies B.** Evaluation of acceptance and commitment therapy for drug refractory epilepsy: a randomized controlled trial in South Africa—a pilot study. *Epilepsia* 2006;**47**:2173–9.

118. **Lundgren T, Dahl J, Yardi N, & Melin L.** Acceptance and commitment therapy and yoga for drug-refractory epilepsy: a randomized controlled trial. *Epilepsy & Behavior* 2008;**13**:102–8.

119. **Losada A, Marquez-Gonzalez M, Romero-Moreno1 R, et al.** Cognitive behavioral therapy (CBT) versus acceptance and commitment therapy (ACT) for dementia family caregivers with significant depressive symptoms: results of a randomized clinical trial. *J Consult Clin Psychol* 2015;**83**:760–72.

120. **Luciano JV, Guallar JA, Aguado J, et al.** Effectiveness of group acceptance and commitment therapy for fibromyalgia: a 6-month randomized controlled trial (EFFIGACT study). *Pain* 2014;**155**:693–702.

121. **Department of Health.** *Self-care—A Real Choice.* London, UK: Department of Health, 2005.

122. **Parke HL, Epiphaniou E, Pearce G, et al.** Self-management support interventions for stroke survivors: a systematic meta-review. *PLoS One* 2015;**10**(7):e0131448.

123. **Lennon S, McKenna S, & Jones F.** Self-management programmes for people post stroke: a systematic review. *Clin Rehabil* 2013;**27**:867–78.

124. **Warner G, Packer T, Villeneuve M, Audulv A, & Versnel J.** A systematic review of the effectiveness of stroke self-management programs for improving function and participation outcomes: self-management programs for stroke survivors. *Disabil Rehabil* 2015;**37**:2141–63.

125. **Lorig KR & Holman HR.** Self-management education: history, definition, outcomes, and mechanisms. *Ann Behav Med* 2003;**26**, 1–7.

126. **Fanner D & Urquhart C.** Bibliotherapy for mental health service users part 1: a systematic review. *Health Info Libr J* 2008;**25**: 237–52.

127. **Morris R. & Morris P.** Participants' experiences of hospital-based peer support groups for stroke patients and carers. *Disabil Rehabil* 2012;**34**:347–54.

128. **Dorning H, Davies M, Ariti C, Allen K, & Georghiou T.** *Knowing You're Not Alone: Understanding Peer Support for Stroke Survivors.* London, UK: Nuffield Trust, 2016.

Chapter 27

Stroke care in the community and long-term care facilities

Adam L. Gordon and Phillipa A. Logan

Introduction

Stroke is the leading cause of severe activity limitation (disability) and participation restriction (handicap) in developed economies. In the United Kingdom, for example, just over a third of the 152 000 patients with strokes occurring each year are discharged home with persistent stroke-related disability. This prevalence has changed, and will change over time, in response to improvements in rehabilitation and recovery trajectories following improved hyper- and subacute care. On the other hand, case fatality has fallen, and more severely affected patients now survive when they might not have done so previously.

One consequence, however, of such improved care is that more stroke patients have less profound disabilities and are able to receive rehabilitation in less specialized settings closer to home, sooner in their clinical course. Whether the need for community stroke care will rise or fall over time will depend upon whether the fall in disability is compensated for by earlier discharge and more community, rather than hospital, based rehabilitation. It is, likely, however that an increasing proportion of rehabilitation will be delivered ever closer to home over time and that the need for well-developed community-based stroke teams will persist.

Much of the management of patients with stroke-related disability in the community is governed by conceptual models of what represents good holistic, person-centred care for long-term conditions. The prevailing considerations are around having an appropriate mix of staff, with appropriate skills, who are empowered to work as a team, focused around patient and carer needs, with an infrastructure designed to support continuous quality improvement and models of funding which recognize, incentivize, and reward each of these domains. These concepts have been summarized in the House of Care Model (see Fig. 27.1).

This chapter will consider organizational and institutional aspects of community-based care for patients with stroke-related disability, before describing models of health and well-being, and models of care delivery, that underpin effective care delivery in the community.

Organizational or institutional aspects of care

A number of innovative services have emerged in the United Kingdom to support patients with stroke in the community in recent years. These are largely incorporated within models of intermediate care, where intermediate care is defined as outlined in Box 27.1.[1,2]

Intermediate care can take place in community or subacute rehabilitation hospitals, long-term care facilities (care homes), or the patient's own home. Where it takes place within long-term care facilities, intermediate care is usually managed separately from the normal long-term care workload. Residents receiving intermediate care in long-term care facilities pass through these for rehabilitation on a recovery trajectory that it is anticipated will conclude with the patient's discharge

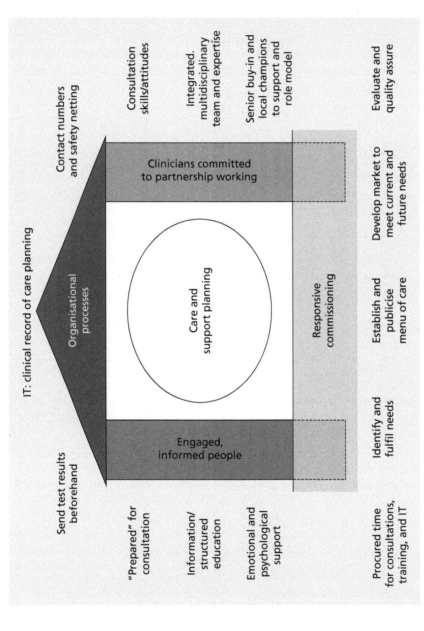

Fig. 27.1 The National Health Service House of Care Model.

Box 27.1 Definition of intermediate care as used in the UK national audit of intermediate care

What is intermediate care?

Intermediate care services are provided to patients, usually older people, after leaving hospital, or when they are at risk of being sent to hospital. The services offer a link between hospitals and where people normally live, and between different areas of the health and social care system—community services, hospitals, general practitioners, and social care. There are three main aims of intermediate care, and they are to:

- help people avoid going into hospital unnecessarily;

- help people be as independent as possible after a stay in hospital; and

- prevent people from having to move into a residential home until they really need to.

Reproduced with permission from Young J, et al. The second national audit of intermediate care. *Age Ageing*, 44(2), 182–4. Copyright © 2014, Oxford University Press. https://doi.org/10.1093/ageing/afu174

to their own home. Intermediate care can, occasionally, be used as a venue to further assess patients whose recovery trajectory is uncertain, where it is possible that placement in a long-term care facility will be the ultimate outcome, but it is felt that more time is needed prior to drawing this conclusion. Intermediate care has been shown, in a number of randomized controlled trials, to be broadly equivalent to acute hospital-based rehabilitation in terms of outcomes.[3–5] The venue of care, which is less hospital-like and geographically closer to home, is generally preferred by patients and their relatives. The health-economics governing intermediate care have not been well delineated, but it is likely that these settings provide care which is at least marginally cheaper than subacute rehabilitation provided in acute hospital settings.

Although governed by the conceptual models of intermediate care, community stroke teams tend to be organizationally separated from more generic intermediate care services. This is, in part, a consequence of the high prevalence of stroke-related disability, which generates sufficient demand to allow condition-specific services to be operationally and economically feasible. Another important consideration, though, is that many of the care requirements of patients with stroke-related disability are quite specialized and therefore a team with specific competencies— over and above those required of more generic frailty-focused intermediate care teams—is required. Three-quarters of those with persistent disability after stroke have limb weakness, just under half have swallowing difficulties, a third aphasia, or depression, and one in ten are affected by emotionalism that persists beyond 6 months.[6]

Patients with strokes also make up a significant proportion of older people living in long-term care facilities. In the United Kingdom, 31% of those in institutional long-term care have had a stroke, which compares with 11% in the United States and 18% in Ireland.[7–9] The reasons for patients moving into institutional long-term care, as opposed to receiving long-term care within their own homes, are manifold and differ from country to country depending on the threshold for admission to such facilities, the funding arrangements in place and the types of nursing and medical support available. Institutional long-term care is, however, frequently triggered by difficulty managing frequent or troublesome nocturnal symptoms—particularly those related to behavioural disturbance, or double incontinence—which families can struggle to support at home.

Admission rates to long-term care, and hence thresholds for admission of individual patients, are influenced by broader societal and political concerns. Admission rates tend to be higher when patients are socially isolated, in societies where geographically dispersed nuclear families are the norm, and where state-funding for long-term institutional care is generous.[10] This has historically led to higher rates of institutional long-term care in Northern European countries, for example, when compared with Mediterranean states. The societal factors governing these admission rates are, however, changing over time in most countries. Many countries which have traditionally had generous funding of long-term institutional care are reconsidering these arrangements in light of rising costs driven by demographic shifts towards older, more dependent populations, while other states that have traditionally seen care provided by cohabiting extended families are witnessing cultural and economic changes which are leading to increased dispersal and consequent loss of social infrastructure.

The way in which long-term care is delivered to older patients with stroke in long-term care institutions also varies between countries.[11] In some administrations, for example the Netherlands, care is coordinated by qualified nurses in conjunction with doctors who are employed by, and who work full-time within, nursing homes. Care home companies in the Netherlands often directly employ broader multidisciplinary teams to meet the requirements for physical, occupational, dietetic, and speech and language therapies. In other countries, for example, the United Kingdom, care is delivered by social care staff who have rudimentary care qualifications with specific nursing tasks, such as complex medication administration, specialist continence care, and wound dressings, conducted either by in-reach National Health Service teams in residential homes and care home-employed nursing teams in nursing homes. All medical care in UK care homes is provided on an in-reach basis by general practitioners. Multidisciplinary input is, for the most part, provided by the NHS but a significant proportion of care home residents are unable to directly access therapy services which would be available to their community-dwelling counterparts.[12] This exclusion from care has largely been by accident, rather than design, with the failure to recognize that many care home residents require structured multidisciplinary input to support ongoing management of their disabilities. Access to these services is improving over time as the gaps are identified and filled. In other countries, a spectrum of care models exists between the highly medicalized and structured care seen in the Netherlands and the more ad hoc socialized care seen in the United Kingdom, an example of an intermediate model being the medical director-led model of care used in nursing homes in the United States. It is important to realize that the care arrangements described are provided by generalist doctors and nurses with competencies in generic management of long-term conditions, multimorbidity, and frailty. More specialized aspects of stroke care, for example, management of complex aphasia or spasticity, may still require stroke specialist input, even in the setting of long-term care facilities.

Holistic models of health and well-being as drivers of good care

Regardless of how the team and/or institution providing care are structured, the principles of good care for patients with stroke in the longer term are the same. Broad models of health and well-being are particularly important. The World Health Organization (WHO) defines health as 'a state of complete physical, mental and social well-being and not merely the absence of disease or infirmity'.[13] Operationalizing such a definition involves moving away from a medical diagnostic paradigm of healthcare to one driven by broader considerations around activity and participation. A useful framework to do so is the International Classification of Functioning, Disability, and

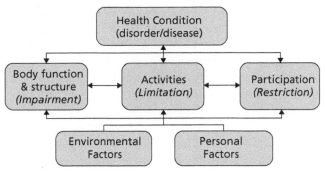

Fig. 27.2 Schematic representation of the International Classification of Functioning, Disability, and Health.

Health (or ICF for short).[14] This superseded the previous WHO International Classification of Impairments, Disabilities and Handicaps (ICIDH) in 2001. It is summarized in Fig. 27.2.

The ICF includes a comprehensive coding structure incorporating impairments of body structures, body functions, activity, participation, environmental, and social factors. The coding structure can be viewed in full on the website of the WHO. At a clinical level, the ICF is useful because it provides a framework for describing health which takes account of the interplay between environment, personal, and social factors, individual impairments of body structure and function, and how these influence activity limitation and participation restriction.[15] By considering health in this way, it becomes clear that longer-term care requires an approach that can account for each of these domains. In addition it provides a means of conceptualizing and thus explaining to patients, their carers, and other health professionals how rehabilitation to maximize activity and participation needs to focus not just upon restoration of body structure and function—restorative rehabilitation—but also compensatory measures taking account of social, environmental, or personal issues—adaptive rehabilitation.

An understanding of health well-being shaped by the ICF can be used to frame rehabilitation goals and discussions around these. For example, a patient who has persistent hemiplegia despite intensive physiotherapy can be encouraged to see effective incorporation of aids and appliances into their daily regimen as a means of enabling independent performance of activities of daily living—a rehabilitation success. Another patient might be encouraged to see participation in an activity which they value highly, for example, attendance at regular religious or social gatherings which are integral to their personal identity, as the ultimate goal of rehabilitation, even if they require significant support from carers in order to achieve this. Clearly goal setting in such circumstances should be highly individualized and driven by the values of an individual patients and their carers—concepts of person and relationship-centred care are key here—but the ICF represents a way to open up such discussions to broad and higher-level concepts of health and well-being.

Structuring care delivery to take account of broad models of care

Implicit in broad models of health and well-being is that a care team is employed which has the prerequisite expertise to be able to complete assessments and interventions which take account not just of impairments of body structure and function but also broader issues around environmental, social, and personal factors. The list of staff who could be required to support such a model is extensive and a widely taken pragmatic approach to this has been to structure community-based stroke teams around a core team of healthcare professionals (physiotherapist, occupational therapist, nurse, and doctor) with mechanisms in place to readily consult other allied health professionals (e.g. speech and language therapy, psychology, dietetics, orthotics, dentistry) as necessary.

Useful unifying concepts come from the literature on comprehensive geriatric assessment (CGA).[16] CGA is a model of healthcare which accommodates broad models of health and well-being by assessing older people against five domains (physical, psychological, functional, environmental, and social), through the coordinated activity of a multidisciplinary team (see Fig. 27.3).

Physical assessment involves listing active diagnoses and geriatric syndromes. Psychological assessment includes assessment of cognition and, if relevant, behavioural symptoms, as well as a broader mental state assessment incorporating affect. Functional assessment involves assessing capabilities, with particular reference to ability to conduct basic and extended activities of daily living. Environmental assessment involves looking at how patients interact with their living environment and the extent to which environmental issues act as barriers or facilitators to participation. Social assessment involves consideration of social networks and how family and friends are able to facilitate the patient in terms of recovery, rehabilitation, and future living.

CGA then uses the insights from these multidomain assessments to establish a stratified problem list and management plan. Stratification of the problem list is based upon both logic (e.g. treating constipation before removing a catheter inserted for retention of urine) and upon patient priorities (e.g. by factoring potential social embarrassment caused by incontinence at a forthcoming social event into decision-making about the timing of trial removal of catheter). It is important that each problem is associated with a management strategy, even if the strategy is simply watchful waiting while other, more pressing management issues are addressed. By doing this, it avoids the risk of problems being accidentally omitted from the problem list over time and multiple iterations of CGA.

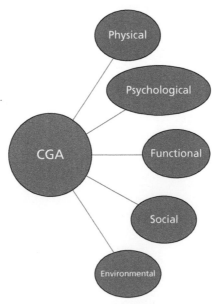

Fig. 27.3 The domains of comprehensive geriatric assessment.

Management strategies should be accompanied by treatment goals which are SMART (specific; measurable; achievable; realistic; and time-delimited). Goals should, where possible, be objective so that they can be evidenced. It is often useful for rehabilitation goals, in particular, to be measured using objective scales, for example, by using the timed-up-and-go test or Berg Balance Scale to measure progress with gait and balance, respectively. This enables progress over time to be mapped, and for goals to be iterated forward in a progressive way—for example, by using progressively higher target Berg Balance Scores over a number of weeks to demonstrate progress with balance objectives. It can, however, be acceptable to use categorical or dichotomous variables to demonstrate objective progress where these map to patient objectives—for example, a patient may stipulate that they wish to be free of cough following cessation of an ACE-inhibitor and the intervention be regarded as successful only when this is achieved. It is important that, where time-delimited objectives are specified, they are followed up at the relevant interval and future goals specified in light of progress. Thus, CGA gets iterated forward over time (see Fig. 27.4).

Clearly these models of working are only achievable in the context of care teams with the prerequisite balance of professional expertise and where professionals act together as a functional team. This can prove more challenging in the community than in hospital-based settings. Rehabilitation in a hospital ward environment, particularly slow-stream rehabilitation over a number of weeks, provides opportunities for resident teams to sit down at multidisciplinary meetings to plan care. At these meetings, multiple professionals can hear directly from each other, if necessary, in the presence of the patient or their carers, and collective decisions can be made. Staff in the community have more geographically dispersed workloads that make physical face-to-face meetings more challenging. Even where these are able to occur, for example, at weekly case conferences, it is not always possible to involve the patients or their carers directly in these discussions, as they are frequently held at centralized healthcare offices. Multiple agencies and employing organizations with competing priorities can lead to, for example, primary care doctors, rehabilitation teams, care agency, or care home staff each with different patterns of working which mean that some, but not all, professionals can sit down together regularly.

Some of these issues can be addressed by technology, for example, using shared electronic care records, remote video conferencing and, as the market expands, remote monitoring of healthcare data from patients and their relatives. Of much greater importance, however, is that teams are

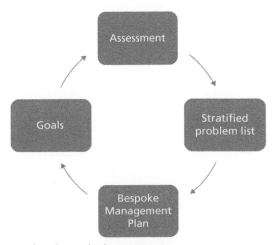

Fig. 27.4 Iteration in comprehensive geriatric assessment.

structured to enable 'virtual' multidisciplinary working. This requires, in practice, that one professional is recognized by the rest of the team as coordinating or managing care for the patient, that the coordinating professional recognizes themselves as doing so and that they are made aware of all changes in assessments, management plans, and treatment goals by other members of the team.

General vs. specialist care

It is clear from the previous points that many aspects of stroke care in the community can be accommodated by general practitioners and other community-based generic healthcare staff such as district nurses and community matrons, with intermittent input by a more specialized team on an as required basis. The usual trajectory of specialist involvement is of intensive, stroke-specific, multidisciplinary input for initial rehabilitation following discharge from the acute hospital setting. In many regards, limiting such input to a rigid timeframe is illogical and the duration of multidisciplinary input should be determined by individual patient needs. The multidisciplinary team should provide input until such time as it is clear that further ongoing support is unlikely to yield further improvement against established objectives. This can mean that individual members of the multidisciplinary team (MDT) withdraw from the supporting the patient at different times. A patient might quite rapidly find themselves able to mobilize independently outdoors, such that ongoing physiotherapy and occupational therapy is no longer required but they may have prolonged issues with post-stroke depression, or difficult to manage post-stroke epilepsy, or aphasia, that requires ongoing input from a community mental health nurse, stroke specialist doctor, or speech and language therapist, respectively. In practice many stroke teams offer more strictly time-limited rehabilitation services (in parts of the United Kingdom, for example, such offers may be limited to 6 weeks) but it important to realize that these arrangements are not evidence-based and are a consequence of resource constraints. They do not represent an example of individualized patient-centred care.

Many stroke therapists and nurses are entirely based in the community. It is much less common for stroke specialist doctors, whether geriatricians or neurologists, to practice exclusively in this setting. Much discussion of whether such specialists should perform home visits has focused upon the perceived inefficiencies of a doctor travelling by car or public transport to a single patient's home. This may take up much of an afternoon and the specialist might be able to see many patients in clinic in the same time interval. Deciding about which patients require a domiciliary visit can be well addressed by the approach of restricting such attention to those patients who 'can't come, shouldn't come, or won't come' to hospital.

◆ Can't come—these are patients who are physically very dependent. Perhaps bed bound, perhaps patients who required complex hoist transfers into a specialized wheelchair. Ambulance transfers for such patients can be exhausting, painful, and it can, on balance, be better for the doctor to visit the patient rather than vice versa. This must be balanced, however, against personal goals and rehabilitation objectives. The need to attend clinic can be a potent incentive for an anxious and agoraphobic patient, for example, to travel out of doors and can, in itself, be a rehabilitation intervention allowing the patient to normalize the requirement to mobilize outside of the home. If necessary, community-based stroke rehabilitation therapists can support visits to hospital as part of a broader rehabilitation strategy.

◆ Shouldn't come—these are patients for whom meaningful diagnostic information can best be gleaned by seeing them in their community setting. Perhaps particular activities during the daily routine trigger muscle spasms, or pain, in a way that can only be understood by seeing the patient conduct activities in their home environment, with access to their own equipment.

Patients resident in long-term care facilities frequently fit into this category. Seeing them with senior members of the care facility staff on hand, with full access to their care records, their medication administration sheets, and understanding how environment and the care team impact upon their health status are important gains which should not be overlooked. If such patients are made to attend hospital, it is not always possible for care home staff to attend with them for logistical reasons and vital diagnostic information may be lost as a consequence.

♦ Won't come—sometimes patients don't attend their outpatient appointments. The traditional response of the medical profession to such a situation has been to discharge the patient back to primary care. Non-attendance, however, can be a sign of ongoing stroke-specific symptoms that make attendance at clinic difficult. Or it can be a sign of deterioration. At the very least non-attendance at clinic should trigger collateral history taking from the patient, their family, their community-based therapy team, and their primary care doctor. If there is evidence of stroke-specific issues contributing to deterioration, a domiciliary visit may represent a more ethical and effective use of physician time than allowing them to deteriorate to such a point that they require admission to hospital.

It is important when community-based rehabilitation teams withdraw from care that they establish with the patient, their family or carers, and the primary care team taking the case forward what parameters should trigger subsequent referral back to the stroke team. Patients can find that their physical functioning deteriorates over time as they adopt less rigorous approaches to lifestyle and activities of daily living than they did during the rehabilitation phase. Personal circumstances can change resulting in decompensation due to altered social or environmental circumstances. Intercurrent illness, such as infection, depression, or dehydration can result in deterioration of stroke symptoms such that specialist input becomes necessary again. Initial decompensation in one aspect of functioning can result in more generic decline if not attended to. For example, deteriorating swallow due to general deconditioning following a chest-infection can result in dehydration, with loss of gait and balance ability due to orthostatic hypotension. More severe functional decline can then set in as the patient takes to bed. Prompt re-escalation to a community-based stroke team familiar with the patient's case, with rapid response and early intervention, can be an effective intervention in such a situation. A brief period of thickened fluids and fork-mashable diet could be an effective intervention in the scenario described, if doing so allows them to maintain oral intake until they start to recover postinfection. In such circumstances, brief step-up admission to intermediate care facilities can enable institution-based rehabilitation to take place but it is important that such admissions are accompanied by SMART treatment goals. Intermediate care should be seen as an active intervention, otherwise patients may stagnate requiring long-term admission to a care facility.

New focal neurological deficit, or sudden recrudescence of old stroke symptoms, may of course represent a new vascular event. General practitioners can find themselves uncertain as to whether, or how rapidly, to escalate care in such situations. Telephone advice from a stroke physician can be a very helpful decision-support when uncertainties are triggered and such services are an established part of many community stroke teams. Where general practitioners are geographically remote from specialist stroke advice, telehealth solutions can enable a stroke physician in a specialist centre to provide care remotely.

Conclusion

Much of what has been described in this chapter may seem like 'good common-sense care'. The technical aspects of stroke rehabilitation and maintenance of function in the community are, in many ways, the same as for hospital settings. The organization of care, meanwhile, is influenced by many jurisdiction- and healthcare system-specific issues that mean that overarching principles of care can only be stated in general terms.

It should not be inferred from this, however, that care in the community is straightforward. Working to patient-centred treatment goals in non-clinical settings requires adaptability, improvisational skills, and the ability to accommodate sometimes imperfect compromises into management plans. Ethical dilemmas can be presented about when to champion individual patient needs and when to accept the pragmatic limitations of real-world settings. Acting as a functional multidisciplinary team when staff members may be employed by different, geographically dispersed, agencies requires attention to detail and robust models of working and communication. Deciding who should see a patient, when, and where, requires a highly individualized approach to care that can be difficult to protocolize. Negotiating the boundaries of rehabilitation—when it should start and stop and if/when it should recommence in the event of functional deterioration—requires skill. All of these require stroke-specific training and experiential learning to establish the community-specific competencies required to deliver high-quality specialist care. Simplicity is in the eye of the beholder and is often only witnessed when care is delivered by highly specialised teams who understand the very demanding nuances of providing care within such settings.

References

1. **Eaton S, Roberts S, & Turner B.** Delivering person centred care in long term conditions. *BMJ* 2015;**350**:h181.

2. **Young J, Gladman JRF, Forsyth DR**, et al. The second national audit of intermediate care. *Age Ageing* 2015;**44**:182–4.

3. **Griffiths PD, Edwards MH, Forbes A**, et al. Effectiveness of intermediate care in nursing-led in-patient units. *Cochrane Database Syst Rev* 2007;**18**(2):CD002214.

4. **Young J, Green J, Forster A**, et al. Postacute care for older people in community hospitals: a multicenter randomized, controlled trial. *J Am Geriatr Soc* 2007;**55**:1995–2002.

5. **Gladman J, Forster A, & Young J.** Hospital- and home-based rehabilitation after discharge from hospital for stroke patients: analysis of two trials. *Age Ageing* 1995;**24**:49–53.

6. **The Stroke Association.** *Stroke Statistics 2015–16.* Available from: https://www.stroke.org.uk/sites/default/files/stroke_statistics_2015.pdf [Accessed: 15 December 2016].

7. **Gordon AL, Franklin M, Bradshaw L**, et al. Health status of UK care home residents: a cohort study. *Age Ageing* 2014;**43**(1):97–103.

8. **Cowman S, Royston M, Hickey A**, et al. Stroke and nursing home care: a national survey of nursing homes. *BMC Geriatr* 2010;**10**:4.

9. **US Centre for Disease Control.** *Prevalence of Stroke Among Residential Care Residents, by Sex and Age Group—National Survey of Residential Care Facilities, United States, 2010.* Available from: https://www.cdc.gov/mmwr/preview/mmwrhtml/mm6321a7.htm [Accessed: 1 August 2019].

10. **Kraus M, Czypionka T, Riedel M**, et al. *How European Nations Care for Their Elderly. A New Typology of Long-erm Care Systems.* Available at: *ENEPRI Policy Br no 7.* 2011. Available from: https://www.ceps.eu/ceps-publications/how-european-nations-care-their-elderly-new-typology-long-term-care-systems/ [Accessed: 1 August 2019].

11. **Sanford AM, Orrell M, Tolson D**, et al. An international definition for 'nursing home'. *JAMDA* 2015;**16**(3):181–4.

12. **Iliffe S, Davies SL, Gordon AL**, et al. Provision of NHS generalist and specialist services to care homes in England: review of surveys. *Prim Health Care Res Dev* 2015;**17**(2):1–16.

13. **World Health Organization.** Preamble to the Constitution of the World Health Organization as adopted by the International Health Conference. *Off Rec World Heal Organ* 1948;**2**:100.

14. **World Health Organization.** *International Classification of Functioning, Disability and Health.* Geneva, Switzerland: WHO, 2001.

15. **Gladman JRF.** The international classification of functioning, disability and health and its value to rehabilitation and geriatric medicine. *J Chin Med Assoc* 2008;**71**:275–8.

16. **Welsh TJ, Gordon AL, & Gladman JR.** Comprehensive geriatric assessment—a guide for the non-specialist. *Int J Clin Pract* 2014;**68**(3):290–3.

Chapter 28

Readmission to hospital after stroke

Mohana Maddula and Sunil K. Munshi

Introduction

+ How common are stroke readmissions?
+ What are the causes of readmissions?
+ How can we prevent readmissions?
+ Implications for patients and healthcare providers

There is a significant resource implication and consequent economic burden from stroke hospitalization, especially if this becomes a recurrent issue. While there is no doubt that readmissions are necessary in a cohort of patients who require urgent and specialized hospital care, we would premise that a significant proportion of readmissions of stroke survivors may be preventable.

Older people, at least in the developed world, represent the largest group of hospital users.[1] Patients over the age of 65 occupy two-thirds of general and acute hospital beds in England.[1] Older people in general are more likely to be readmitted than their younger counterparts.[2] The vast majority of strokes occur in older people, who may be vulnerable to hospital readmissions as a consequence of general frailty, comorbid conditions, and social circumstances. Some of these issues may be unrelated to the stroke itself. We shall explore the evidence and complex dynamics that are involved in the issue of readmissions for stroke survivors.

Older people have reported feeling depressed and frustrated about being readmitted, with a perception of not being in control of at the time of emergency readmissions.[3]

How common are stroke readmissions?

The evidence and limitations

Most of the information about readmissions comes from administrative databases, such as US healthcare insurance schemes and registries. The observational nature of such research therefore has implications for the quality of evidence at our disposal. Table 28.1 illustrates the proportions of stroke survivors who were readmitted at varying intervals following their index stroke admission. Taking into account the *caveat* of heterogeneity in the studies, about 38% of stroke patients had been rehospitalized by 1 year.

There are several factors that we need to consider when understanding these figures. First, there is significant variation in the definition of what constitutes a readmission. For instance, should we only consider admissions to acute hospitals and disregard those to community or subacute institutions? Additionally, some studies also only looked at readmissions to their own institution, and were not set up to pick up admissions to hospitals in other cities or states. Furthermore, a limitation of research that comes out of administrative databases is that there is often little

Table 28.1 Incidence of readmission after a stroke

28 days – 1 month	90 days	1 year	5 year	Stroke type	Author
		37.1%		All strokes	Johansen, 2005[31]
10.7%		40%		IS	Bravata, 2007[7]
		15%		ICH	Christensen, 2008[32]
		10.8%		IS	
		49.6%		All strokes all TIAs	Tseng, 2009[33]
14.1%	29.2%	55.3%		IS	Fonarow, 2010[26]
		49%	83%	IS	Lakshminarayan, 2011[34]
9.9%				IS and TIAs	Bhattacharya, 2011[35]
10%	17%	36%		All strokes	Lin, 2011[36]
6.4%				All strokes	Nahab, 2012[4]
	18%			All strokes	Ottenbacher, 2012[37]
		29%		All strokes and TIAs	Lee, 2013[38]
9%				IS	Suri, 2013[39]
6.5%				All strokes	Kilkenny, 2013[40]
14.4%				IS	Litchman 2013[11]
		32.2%		All strokes	Lainay, 2014[27]
15.2%				IS	Burke, 2014[5]
12.8%				All strokes	Keyhani, 2014[41]
21%	35%	55%		IS	Fehnel 2015[18]
		42%		All strokes and TIAs	Kilkenny 2015[42]
10.6%				All Strokes	Slocum, 2015[17]
	18.8%			IS	Bjerkreim, 2015[29]
		40.6%		ICH	Bjerkreim, 2016[43]

IS, ischaemic stroke; ICH, intracerebral haemorrhage; TIAs, transient ischaemic attacks.

information about the index stroke admission, such as stroke severity, or the causes of subsequent readmissions.

Another important factor is the stroke type. While most studies looked at all strokes or only ischaemic strokes, some studies included only haemorrhagic strokes, including subarachnoid haemorrhages, or transient ischaemic attacks. We know that patients with intracerebral haemorrhage generally have poorer outcomes and may therefore form a patient group more vulnerable to readmissions, and mortality. The follow-up periods also varied, with some studies only looking at readmissions in the first month, and others up to 5 years. Finally, on the issue of whether some readmissions are preventable, some studies classified elective readmissions for carotid revascularization as 'avoidable'.[4] Presumably such patients were discharged after their index stroke admission to reduce length of stay, and were then readmitted on a planned basis for carotid revascularization.

Variations in healthcare

Health and social care has different shapes and forms across the world. Even within the United States there is great variability in readmission rates between hospitals.[5] A significant proportion of this variation may be explained by hospital practices which were not specifically evaluated, such as care coordination after discharge or stroke severity. The effectiveness of secondary prevention strategies such as anticoagulation, where appropriate, may be important in reducing recurrent stroke rates. We know already that time spent in the therapeutic range varies significantly in different countries. Subtherapetic anticoagulation can increase the risk of recurrent stroke, requiring readmission.

The quality of community care and support may have a large bearing on readmissions for older people. There are regional and local variations in the proportion of older people living in the area, the availability of out-of-hours general/family practitioners, socioeconomic status, affordability and accessibility to healthcare, and the provision of hospital avoidance or 'crisis' teams, tasked with the aim to support older people in their own homes who may experience functional deterioration due to whatever reason.

There is some evidence from large registries that readmissions of stroke patients are becoming less frequent.[6] This may reflect improved secondary prevention strategies, or better discharge planning and community support.

A vulnerable population

Bravata et al. (2007) discovered that more than one-quarter of stroke patients were admitted at least once in the year leading up to the index stroke admission.[7] This suggests that there may be a predisposition to the requirement for hospital care in at least a proportion of stroke survivors. It is also unsurprising that hospitalization prior to a stroke correlates positively with the risk of being readmitted following the index event.[8] Stroke survivors form a frail and susceptible group who are at high risk of developing new illness, or suffer the aggravation of known diseases, with resultant functional decline and poor outcomes.

What are the causes of readmissions?

Persistent neurological symptoms with resultant functional limitations and disability, combined with medical, mental, and social issues can all be factors in explaining the high readmission rates for stroke survivors. Recurrent stroke and respiratory infections are the two most common reasons (Box 28.1). The latter may be related to stroke-induced immunodepression, or dysphagia leading to aspiration.

In our own experience, older stroke patients with residual neurological impairment are particularly prone to being readmitted when they endure a change in their environment, in combination with perhaps an intercurrent illness. The case vignette described in Box 28.2 is not uncommon, and illustrates the vulnerability of frail older people to hospitalization when multiple factors come together. Had the patient been at home with his usual carer (his wife) and had he been reviewed by his usual general/family practitioner, acute hospitalization may have been avoided. Establishing baseline level of function and continuity of care among caregivers is important. Often admissions are prompted when new carers have come to look after the patient, or the patient has been temporarily admitted to a new care setting for whatever reason (e.g. respite for family carers). This issue is often compounded by the patient's impaired cognitive function, and as result the patient may be unable to give a good history, thereby making it difficult to determine if the noticed neurological deficit is new or residual from a previous stroke.

Box 28.1 Reasons for readmissions to hospital in stroke survivors

Respiratory infections

Other infections (e.g. urinary infections)

Falls and mobility issues

Recurrent stroke and TIA

Recurrent stroke and TIA

Cardiac problems

Chest pain and acute MI

Dysrhythmias (e.g. atrial fibrillation)

Heart failure

Seizures

Syncope

Polypharmacy and side effects of medications

Confusion or change in mental state

Psychosocial problems

Not able to cope at home

Illness of caregiver

Depression

Worsening of stroke symptoms due to intercurrent illness

Suboptimal discharge planning

Insufficient adaptations made to home environment

Patients require higher level of care

Patient's perception that they were discharged too early

Unaddressed or unresolved or new medical issues (e.g. diabetes-related issues, urinary retention, blockage or displacement of feeding tubes, gastrointestinal bleed, haematuria, alcohol excess, hypertension, acute kidney injury, gout, constipation, subdural haematoma)

The expectations of the family or caregivers are important. Not uncommonly, inadequate explanations may have been provided by healthcare professionals about the patient's stroke severity and prognosis; or it is possible that things have simply not 'sunk in' for the family, with the consequence that unrealistic expectations of recovery are harboured. Clear and effective communication with regular updates may help to clarify things. Equally it is important to adequately 'prepare' family members or carers for the task of looking after stroke survivors.[9]

Particular mention should also be made about the effects of polypharmacy on older people. Apart from being a well-known risk factor for falls, older people are particularly susceptible to the sedative effects of analgesics or the anticholinergic burden from a number of medications. Overtreatment with antihypertensives to meet target blood pressure criteria may also lead to falls through postural hypotension.

Box 28.2 Case study

Mr R is a frail older person with a history of stroke and residual left-sided weakness who was transferred to a residential home from his own house for respite purposes, when his wife (main carer) was herself admitted for an elective procedure. He has several comorbidities and took multiple analgesics for chronic pain, which include opiates and neuroleptics. The staff in the residential home noticed one morning that Mr R was leaning to one side and therefore sought urgent medical opinion from the out-of-hours general/family practitioner.

Mr R was reviewed by Dr S who has never met him before. Dr S was concerned about the apparent new left-sided weakness. The patient was drowsy and confused, and as a result was unable to provide a good history. Dr S arranged for urgent admission to an acute hospital for a suspected new stroke. Upon review in hospital by a specialist it was deduced that Mr R had functional deterioration of his prior neurological impairment due to a urinary tract infection (UTI) and sedative effects of his analgesics. There was no convincing evidence of another stroke.

How can we prevent readmissions?

In a large retrospective analysis of all emergency readmissions to NHS hospitals, about 30% of readmissions were felt to be 'potentially preventable'.[10]

Litchman et al. (2013)[11] applied the criteria developed by the US Agency for Healthcare Research and Quality and identified that a small proportion of readmissions after ischaemic stroke were preventable (e.g. pneumonia). It is also possible that medical issues had been left unaddressed at the time of discharge. For instance, the severity of dysphagia and resultant silent aspiration may not have been identified and adequately addressed.

Acute hospitals may not be the best places for frail, older adults with accompanying risks such as delirium, falls, and nosocomial infections. It is not an uncommon scenario where an older person is admitted for a minor ailment and then develops delirium, leading to wandering around the ward at night in an unfamiliar environment, resulting in a fall and hip fracture. Hospitalization for an older person may also lead to loss of independence and functional deterioration. It is therefore incumbent upon healthcare professionals to ensure robust processes are in place to avoid hospitalization where it is unnecessary. Equally, those patients who are readmitted may be in need of expert and specialist hospital services, and it is an opportunity for healthcare staff to optimize the patients' treatment with a view to improving their health.

Identifying patients at risk of readmissions

Those with more severe strokes with resultant high disability seem to be more vulnerable to being readmitted (Box 28.3). Increasing age (Table 28.1) is also a predictor of rehospitalization. Prestroke functional status and hospitalizations is another risk factor for readmissions. Patients who have spent longer in hospital at their index stroke admission have increased risk, presumably a marker of stroke severity or a complicated post-stroke period. Lewsey et al. looked at stroke readmissions and found that hospitalizations due to infection, gastrointestinal problems, and immobility were more common in deprived areas.[12]

The management of stroke survivors is complex and requires specialist medical, nursing, and therapy input in a coordinated way. Stroke survivors in the United States who are looked after

---

Box 28.3 Characteristics of stroke survivors with increased risk of being readmitted

Severe strokes

High NIHSS stroke severity score

Greater disability

Patients who required tracheostomy and mechanical ventilation[44]

Discharge to nursing home

Longer index length of stay

Prior hospitalizations and ED presentations

Poor prestroke functional status

Older patients

Severe adverse events and complications during index hospitalization

Comorbidities and higher burden of vascular risk factors

Coronary artery disease

Diabetes

Atrial Fibrillation

Atherosclerotic aetiology of index stroke

Availability of social support

Socioeconomic factors

Unemployment

Educational qualifications

Poverty

Patients who were looked after by non-specialists (e.g. medical specialties other than stroke units) at index admission

NIHSS, National Institute of Health Stroke Scale; ED, emergency department.

---

by medical specialists other than neurology or neurosurgery have an increased risk of being re-admitted. Obese stroke patients are less likely to be readmitted compared to a matched non-obese stroke cohort.[13]

Predicting the risk of readmission

In the general (not stroke-specific) population methods of predicting risk of readmission to hospitals at an individual level have been developed, and with reasonable sensitivity and specificity.[14] There is however limited data on the predictors of hospital readmission for stroke survivors. A systematic review by Litchman et al. (2010) did not identify any statistical models for predicting readmissions after stroke.[15] It was also noted that there was considerable variability in case definitions, analytic approaches, outcome definitions, follow-up periods, and model covariates. However, the inclusion of age, stroke severity, sex, comorbid conditions, and vascular risk factors in models for predicting outcomes (such as readmissions) has been suggested.[16]

In the group of patients readmitted to acute care from an inpatient stroke rehabilitation setting, a statistical model based on functional status and age showed better predictive ability than models based on medical comorbidities.[17] In the cohort of stroke survivors admitted to acute hospitals from nursing homes, higher levels of social engagement (a marker of nursing home quality) was found to independently reduce odds of admissions.[18] Finally, in one of the rare randomized controlled trials, a 4-week postdischarge transitional care programme in Hong Kong was shown to reduce rehospitalization after stroke. Participants randomized to intervention arm had better spiritual-religion-personal measures, higher satisfaction, lower depression levels, and reduced disability scores. The 4-week long nurse-led intervention was based on the assessment-intervention-evaluation Omaha system framework.[19]

Strategies for prevention of readmissions

In the drive to vacate hospital beds to accommodate increasing demand, there is a risk of discharging stroke survivors prematurely without adequate planning and preparation. In older people as a whole there has been an increase in the proportion of rehospitalizations that occur within 0–1 day of the index admission, raising the possibility that some patients are being discharged too quickly.[2] In another study the risk of readmission was found to be greater for stroke patients who had a shorter index admission length of stay, although the authors felt there was insufficient evidence to suggest that reductions in length of stay were not associated with increased risk of readmission.[20]

Nevertheless, rehospitalization can be detrimental to the health of older patients, and it is the duty of healthcare professionals to ensure there are robust processes in place to prevent unnecessary readmissions (Box 28.4). A key factor is good discharge planning, and working closely with patients' family or carers. Equally, postdischarge care is very important especially when patients leave the supported environment of acute hospitals to live in their own homes, sometimes by themselves. This is sometimes quite a major transition. In an earlier randomized controlled trial, comprehensive interdisciplinary postdischarge care management was found to result in significantly better health profiles for stroke survivors.[21] Hospitals with higher use of occupational therapists (OTs) were also found to have fewer readmissions.[5] While input from such specialists may be beneficial at the patient level, it is also possible that hospitals that use more OTs may also have better systems in place such as more intensive, earlier therapy assessment and better discharge planning.

Intensive rehabilitation in the acute setting and at home has also been shown to reduce rehospitalization in stroke survivors.[22,23] Another randomized trial showed reductions in rehospitalization through discharge coordination, and education, medicines reconciliation, and follow-up appointments. Patients also felt more prepared for discharge through this intervention.[24]

Medical interventions such as influenza and pneumococcal vaccinations may reduce respiratory infections, which are a major cause for readmissions in older stroke patients. Adherence to modified diet, oral hygiene and mouth care, and regular speech and language therapy input in the community may also be of beneficial to stroke survivors with dysphagia. Lastly there is also some evidence that treatment with statins for ischaemic strokes can reduce readmission rates and improve survival.[25]

> ## Box 28.4 Ways to reduce risk of readmissions in older stroke survivors
>
> Preventing pneumonia and respiratory illness through
> - Vaccinations against influenza and pneumococcal infections
> - Oral hygiene, and adherence to modified diet and fluids as recommended by SALT
>
> Secondary prevention of vascular risk factors to reduce risk of stroke recurrence
>
> Multidisciplinary and comprehensive assessment of stroke patients with involvement of family and carers in discharge planning
>
> Availability of adequate support at home (e.g. family or social services)
>
> Good handover to community services
>
> Postdischarge care coordination and transitional care models
>
> Continuing rehabilitation in the community
>
> Early follow-up in outpatient clinic
>
> Assess falls risk carefully prior to discharge
>
> Avoidance of polypharmacy
>
> SALT, speech and language therapist.

Implications for patients and healthcare providers

What does this mean for patients?

Fonarow et al. (2011) found that those patients readmitted within the first 30 days of discharge are more likely to die in the first year of their stroke.[26] Similar results were echoed in the Dijon Stroke registry study which found that hospitalization was negatively associated with being alive after one year in patients who have had a stroke.[27] Additionally, stroke patients who are readmitted in the first month have reduced survival and higher total healthcare expenditure over the next year. Researchers in the same study also noticed that those stroke patients with multiple readmissions were from a lower socioeconomic class, suggesting that stroke survivors in this category may need more support at home to reduce readmissions.[28] Overall, it appears readmissions after stroke seem to be an indicator of post-stroke well-being at the very least.

What does this mean for healthcare?

Although Martin et al. (2016)[20] felt there was insufficient evidence to implicate reductions in length of stay with readmissions, a Norwegian study[29] into readmissions of patients with ischaemic stroke found that early readmissions were associated with shorter index length of stay. This suggests that there may have been unaddressed medical issues at time of discharge.

There is a balance that needs to be met between keeping stroke patients in acute hospitals for as long as inpatient care appears to be beneficial to their recovery, and premature discharge leading to adverse patient outcomes from unaddressed medical issues or inadequate inpatient rehabilitation.

The question arises as to whether readmissions of stroke patients should be a marker of quality of care. Such a measure of hospital quality of care is patient-centred, since it is that individual who has to experience the consequences (clinical, social, or financial) of being rehospitalized.

Readmissions may also be an indicator of the quality of discharge processes, planning, and transition of care to the community. We may also presume that some readmissions are preventable. Reducing potentially unnecessary readmissions may help redirect healthcare resources elsewhere. Some acute hospitals therefore endure financial penalties for what are deemed as preventable readmissions, with the intention that this would be a driver for improving care and efficiency.[30]

The accreditation for centres looking after stroke patients was thought to be important for readmissions, however, Litchman et al. (2010)[15] found no different in readmission rates between accredited stroke centres and others. Interestingly, supposed latent measures of quality of hospital care, such as use of intravenous alteplase, have not been found to reduce readmission at the hospital level.[5]

At present there are limitations with data and level of our understanding on the complex issue of stroke readmissions. Nevertheless it is certain that a proportion of stroke readmissions are avoidable, and the challenge for healthcare providers is to tackle this effectively without compromising patient care. There is a need for high-quality research to help target interventions in the right areas and on groups of patients who may be at higher risk of readmissions. The ageing population worldwide with resultant greater demand on acute medical services is compelling enough for healthcare institutions to make the necessary reforms.

Conclusions

Readmissions rates in stroke survivors are high, and those patients who are readmitted have poorer outcomes. The underlying mechanisms are not well understood but nonetheless, readmissions in stroke survivors may be an indicator of their general well-being. While a proportion of readmissions in stroke survivors are necessitated by the requirement for urgent and specialist hospital care, there is no doubt that some readmissions are avoidable. Some readmissions may have resulted from suboptimal discharge planning, not enough support at home, and insufficiently addressed or unidentified medical issues. It is incumbent upon healthcare providers to identify areas of improvement and focus targeted intervention on the specific groups of stroke survivors at higher risk of being readmitted.

References

1. **Department of Health**. *Improving Care and Saving Money*. 2010. Available from: https://lemosandcrane.co.uk/resources/DoH%20-%20Improving%20care%20and%20saving%20money.pdf [Accessed: 1 August 2019].

2. **Cornwell J, Levenson R, Sonola L**, et al. *Continuity of Care for Older Hospitalised Patients. A Call for Action*. London, UK: Kings Fund, 2012.

3. **Lawrie M & Battye F.** *Older People's Experience of Emergency Hospital Readmission*. London, UK: Age UK, 2012.

4. **Nahab F, Takesaka J, Mailyan E**, et al. Avoidable 30-day readmissions among patients with stroke and other cerebrovascular disease. *Neurohospitalist* 2012;2(1):7–11.

5. **Burke JF, Skolarus LE, Adelman EE**, et al. Influence of hospital-level practices on readmission after ischemic stroke. *Neurology* 2014;**82**:2196–204.

6. **Krumholz HM, Normand SL, & Wang Y.** Trends in hospitalizations and outcomes for acute cardiovascular disease and stroke. *Circulation* 2011;**130**(12):966–75.

7. **Bravata DM, Ho SY, Meehan TP, Brass LM, & Concato J.** Readmission and death after hospitalization for acute ischemic stroke. 5-year follow-up in the medicare population. *Stroke* 2007;**38**:1899–904.

8. **Strowd RE, Wise SM, Umesi UN**, et al. Predictors of 30-day hospital readmission following ischemic and hemorrhagic stroke. *Am J Quality* 2015;**30**(5):441–6.

9. White CL, Brady TL, Saucedo LL, et al. Towards a better understanding of readmissions after stroke: partnering with stroke survivors and caregivers. *J Clin Nurs* 2014;**24**:1091–100.

10. Blunt I, Bardsley M, Grove A, et al. Classifying emergency 30-day readmissions in England using routine hospital data 2004–2010: what is the scope for reduction? *Emerg Med J* 2014;**32**(1):44–50.

11. Litchman JH, Leifheit-Limson EC, Jones SB, et al. Preventable readmissions within 30 days of ischemic stroke among medicare benefiaries. *Stroke* 2013;**44**:3429–35.

12. Lewsey J, Ebueku O, Jhund PS, et al. Temporal trends and risk factors for readmission for infections, gastrointestinal and immobility complications after an incident hospitalisation for stroke in Scotland between 1997–2005. *BMC Neurol* 2015;**15**:3.

13. Barba R, Marco J, Ruiz J, et al. The obesity paradox in stroke: impact on mortality and short-term readmission. *J Stroke Cerebrovasc Dis* 2015;**24**(4):766–70.

14. Billings J, Dixon J, Mijanovich T, et al. Case finding for patients at risk of readmission to hospital: development of algorithm to identify high risk patients. *BMJ* 2006;**333**(7563):327.

15. Litchman JH, Leifheit-Limson EC, Jones SB, et al. Predictors of hospital readmission after stroke: a systematic review. *Stroke* 2010;**41**(11):2525–33.

16. Katzan IL, Spertus J, Bettger JP, et al. Risk adjustment of ischemic stroke outcomes for comparing hospital performance. A statement for healthcare professionals from the American Heart Association/ American Stroke Association. *Stroke* 2014;**45**:918–44.

17. Slocum C, Gerrard P, Black-Schaffer R, et al. Functional status predicts acute care readmissions from inpatient rehabilitation in the stroke population. *PLoS One* 2015;**10**(11):e0142180.

18. Fehnel CR, Lee Y, Wendell LC, et al. Post-acute care data for predicting readmission after ischemic stroke: a nationwide cohort analysis using the minimum data set. *J Am Heart Assoc* 2015;**4**(9):e002145.

19. Wong FK & Yeung SM. Effects of a 4-week transitional care programme for discharged stroke survivors in Hong Kong: a randomised controlled trial. *Health Soc Care Community* 2015;**23**(6):619–31.

20. Martin S, Street A, Han L, et al. Have hospital readmissions increased in the face of reductions in length of stay? Evidence from England. *Health Policy* 2016;**120**(1):89–99.

21. Allen KR, Hazelett S, Jarjoura D, et al. Effectiveness of a postdischarge care management model for stroke and transient ischemic attach: a randomised controlled trial. *J Stroke Cerebrovasc Dis* 2002;**11**(2):88–98.

22. Andrews AW, Li D, & Freburger JK. Association of rehabilitation intensity for stroke and risk of hospital readmission. *Phys Ther* 2015;**95**(12):1660–7.

23. Langstaff C, Martin C, Brown G, et al. Enhancing community-based rehabilitation for stroke survivors: creating a discharge link. *Top Stroke Rehabil* 2014;**21**(6):510–19.

24. Jack BW, Chetty VK, Anthony D, et al. A reengineered hospital discharge to decrease rehospitalization. A randomized trial. *Ann Intern Med* 2009;**150**(3):178–87.

25. Arevalo-Lorido JC, Carretero-Gomez J, Fernandez-Recio JM, et al. Lowering C-reactive protein with statins after ischemic stroke avoid mortality and readmissions. A prospective cohort study. *Ann Med* 2015;**47**(3):226–32.

26. Fonarow GC, Smith EE, Reeves MJ, et al. Hospital-level variation in mortality and rehospitalisation for medicare beneficiaries with acute ischemic stroke. *Stroke* 2011;**42**:159–66.

27. Lainay C, Benzenine E, Durier J, et al. Hospitalization within the first year after stroke. The Dijon Stroke Registry. *Stroke* 2015;**46**:190–6.

28. King AJH, Smith MA, & Liou JI. The price of bouncing back: one-year mortality and payments for acute stroke patients with thirty day bounce-backs. *J Am Geriatr Soc* 2008;**56**(6):999–1005.

29. Bjerkreim AT, Thomassen L, Brogger J, et al. Causes and predictors for hospital readmission after ischemic stroke. *J Stroke Cerebrovasc Dis* 2015;**24**(9):2095–101.

30. Betts P. *The Impact of Non-Payment for Acute Readmissions.* **NHS Confederation** 2011. Available from: http://www.chks.co.uk/userfiles/files/The%20impact%20of%20non-payment%20for%20acute%20 readmissions%20FINAL%20FOR%20WEB.pdf [Accessed: 1 August 2019].

31. **Johanesen HL. Wielgosz AT, Nguyen K,** et al. Incidence, comorbidity, case fatality and readmission of hospitalized stroke patients in Canada. *Can J Cardiol* 2006;**22**(1):65–71.

32. **Christensen MC & Munro V.** Ischemic stroke and intracerebral haemorrhage: the latest evidence on mortality, readmissions and hospital costs from Scotland. *Neuroepidemiology* 2008;**30**(4):239–46.

33. **Tseng MC & Lin HJ.** Readmission after hospitalization for stroke in Taiwan: results from a national sample. *J Neurol Sci* 2009;**284**(1–2):52–5.

34. **Lakshminarayan K, Schissel C, Anderon DC,** et al. Five-year rehospitalisation outcomes in a cohort of patients with acute ischemic stroke: medicare linkage study. *Stroke* 2011;**42**(6):1556–62.

35. **Bhattacharya P, Khanal D, Madhavan R,** et al. Why do ischemic stroke and transient ischemic attack patients get readmitted? *J Neurol Sci* 2011;**307** (1–2):50–4.

36. **Lin HJ, Chang WL, & Tseng MC.** Readmission after stroke in a hospital-based registry: risk, etiologies, and risk factors. *Neurology* 2011;**76**(5):438–43.

37. **Ottenbacher KJ, Garaham JE, Ottenbacher AJ,** et al. Hospital readmission in persons with stroke following postacute inpatient rehabilitation. *J Gerontol A Biol Sci Med Sci* 2012;**67**(8):875–81.

38. **Lee HC, Chang KC, Huang YC,** et al. Readmission, mortality and first-year medical costs after stroke. *J Chin Med Assoc* 2013;**76**(12):703–14.

39. **Suri MF & Qureshi AI.** Readmissions within 1 month of discharge among patients with acute ischemic stroke: results of the University Health System Consortium Stroke Benchmarking study. *J Vasc Interv Neurol* 2013;**6**(2):47–51.

40. **Kilkenny MF, Longworth M, Pollack M,** et al. Factors associated with 28-day hospital readmission after stroke in Australia. *Stroke* 2013;**44**(8):2260–8.

41. **Keyhani S, Myers LJ, Cheng E,** et al. Effect of clinical and social risk factors on hospital profiling for stroke readmissions: a cohort study. *Ann Intern Med* 2014;**161**(11):775–84.

42. **Kilkenny MF, Dewey HM, Sundararajan V,** et al. Readmissions after stroke: linked data from the Australian stroke clinical registry and hospital databases. *MJA* 2015;**203**(2):102–7.

43. **Bjerkreim AT, Thomassen L, Waje-Andreassen U,** et al. Hospital readmission after intracerebral haemorrhage. *J Stroke Cerebrovasc Dis* 2016;**25**(1):157–62.

44. **Lahiri S, Navi BB, Mayer SA,** et al. Hospital readmission rates among mechanically ventilated patients with stroke. *Stroke* 2015;**46**(10):2969–71.

Chapter 29

Research trials in the older stroke patient

Kailash Krishnan and Nikola Sprigg

Introduction

Stroke primarily affects older people. As the 'baby boom generation' get older, the usefulness of any treatment or intervention will need validation in this rapidly increasing population.[1] Clinical trials are the most conservative and valid methodology to test effects but have trended to include participants who are young, healthier, and take few medications.[2] Anxiety among healthcare professionals about comorbidity or perceived lack of benefit has prevented those who are older from participating in studies testing new treatments or intervention.[3, 4] As for the frail and even less able, the numbers are even fewer.[5] Thus, the challenge in stroke management lies in narrowing the gap between complex real-world patients representative of those seen in clinical practice and those participating in clinical trials.[6] This chapter defines the challenge of ageism in treatment of older stroke patients, efforts taken by recent studies to address the issue and highlights gaps in current knowledge. A discussion on barriers to recruitment and retention and potential solutions in this important group follows.

Defining the challenge

The evidence that ageism exists in acute stroke is well known:

Data from the UK national sentinel audit showed that older adults were less likely to be treated in a stroke unit than younger individuals ($\geq$ 85 vs. <65, risk ratio = 0.82, 95% CI = 0.75–0.90), and neuroimaging within 24 hours was performed in nearly three-quarters of individuals younger than 65, but just over half of those aged 85 or older.[7]

A systematic review of 27 trials involving 10 187 participants examining thrombolytic agents for acute stroke reported that less than 1% were of age above 80 years.[8]

The average age of patients included in 49 trials of interventional studies in acute stroke was 65; even in trials with no upper age limit the mean age was only 67 years.[9]

While it might be tempting to extrapolate results from trials involving the young, this approach might not be appropriate. Older patients experience higher rates of complications and side effects compared to their younger counterparts.[10] Furthermore, pathophysiological changes in organ systems associated with ageing will affect response.[11]

Acute treatment

Intravenous thrombolysis

Although thrombolysis using intravenous alteplase (r-tPA) as treatment for acute ischaemic stroke is licensed up to 4.5 hours and pooled analysis of data from the randomized controlled trials demonstrated a reduction in death or major disability, uncertainties remained about the benefits of t-PA in the very elderly and those who presented in later time windows.[12, 13] Fewer than 100 patients included in the completed trials were older than 80 years, although 30% of all acute strokes occur in this age group.[8,14,15] Furthermore, the evidence was lacking in patients with multiple comorbidities including diabetes mellitus, hypertension, or previous stroke. With this background, the International Stroke Trial (IST-3) was initiated in 2000 and included patients presenting within 6 hours of stroke onset who were allocated to alteplase or control.[16,17] To date, IST-3 is the largest randomized controlled trial of alteplase (3035 patients) in acute stroke and the majority of patients were older than 80 years.[17] The primary outcome was the number of patients who were alive and dependent at 6 months defined by the Oxford Handicap Score (OHS).[17] Although IST-3 was neutral on its primary outcome, ordinal analysis showed a significant shift in those treated with alteplase (common OR 1.27; 95%CI 1.10–1.47; $P = 0.001$).[17] Furthermore, the odds of survival increased in those treated very early.[18] A recent meta-analysis of patient level data from all randomized trials in acute ischaemic stroke showed that irrelevant of age or stroke severity, alteplase given within 4.5 hours significantly improves the odds of good outcome, with earlier treatment leading to more clinical benefit.[19] No differential effect of treatment was seen in those with a history of cerebrovascular disease, diabetes, and hypertension suggesting withholding treatment in these groups is not justified.[17,20] Despite the evidence, clinicians continue to withhold treatment with alteplase in eligible older patients[21,22] making implementation in real-world practice challenging.

There is emerging evidence that cerebral amyloid angiopathy (CAA), which can cause brain haemorrhage (CAAH), may contribute to or directly cause thrombolysis associated intracranial haemorrhage (TICH).[23,24] Sporadic CAA is common in the older people, caused by progressive deposition of β-amyloid in the lobar vessels in the brain.[25] CAA has a predilection for cortical brain regions and is associated with transient focal neurological episodes (TFNE) called 'amyloidspells'[26] and is associated with dementia.[23,25] To date, the underlying mechanisms are confined to anecdotal clinico-post-mortem correlations[24] and therefore prospective studies to understand the effects of CAA in patients with TICH are urgently needed.

Endovascular therapy

Fewer than 5% of acute ischaemic stroke patients are eligible for r-tPA, mainly due to the delay in presentation or at risk of systemic haemorrhage (high international normalized ratio (INR), recent major surgery, previous intracerebral haemorrhage).[27,28] The utility of intravenous r-tPA alone has also been shown to be limited by the size of clot, clot composition, and location of vessel occlusion.[29,30] In one retrospective analysis, only a third of an occluded proximal middle cerebral artery occlusions recanalized with r-tPA implying that a large proportion of treated patients were left disabled.[31] Similar results[32,33] led onto the search and development of additional effective therapies for acute ischaemic stroke.

Catheter directed intra-arterial thrombolysis demonstrated use in extended time windows, drug delivery to the site of clot reducing systemic exposure, and greater rates of recanalization.[34,35] Thrombectomy devices open occluded vessels but trials in the last decade failed to demonstrate better clinical outcomes; the reasons attributed to inappropriate patient selection including those with lack of clear vessel occlusion and late treatment windows.[36–38] In 2015, five randomized controlled trials demonstrated clear evidence of improved outcomes in patients with large artery occlusion (distal internal carotid or proximal middle cerebral artery, M1).[39–43] Patients were carefully selected: those with minimal brain ischaemia with salvageable penumbra, confirmed anterior circulation vessel occlusion, and randomized to thrombectomy immediately without waiting for response to intravenous thrombolysis.[39–43] Clinical characteristics were comparable: median NIH Stroke Scale (NIHSS) scores of 17 (interquartile range, 13–21), mean age of 66 years, ASPECTS of 9 (range, 6–10) and the majority of participants received r-tPA.[39–43] Although the extent and time to recanalize varied across the trials, a significant difference favouring good outcomes was observed in the group randomized to endovascular treatment in addition to intravenous t-PA compared to standard treatment alone (14–31%; numbers needed to treat (NNT) for one additional good outcome ~4).[44] A systematic review examining for treatment effects by age (>80 years vs. <80 years) found no significant differences in the odds of good outcome indicating that endovascular thrombectomy should be considered for those presenting within 6 hours with occlusion of a proximal anterior circulation vessel, regardless of age.[45]

What further work in this area is now needed? Favourable outcomes reported in the recent trials were in those treated under conscious sedation whereas general anaesthesia was associated with worse outcomes.[44,46] This would impact patients that are older with multiple comorbidities; more research in this area is needed. Patients who are more than 80 years old also constitute the majority of wake-up ischaemic strokes and assessment of whether this group stand to gain from thrombectomy is needed.

Acute blood pressure lowering

The relative risks and benefits of lowering blood pressure in the acute phase has remained an enigma for clinicians as highlighted in a report first published in the 1980s.[47] Arguments favouring blood pressure reduction are based on preventing rebleeding in acute intracerebral haemorrhage, and haemorrhagic transformation of infarction, and reduction of cytotoxic oedema. Those against cite pathophysiological evidence of impaired cerebral autoregulation and worsening brain ischaemia.[48,49] In acute stroke, blood pressure is usually lowered if there is evidence of end-organ compromise (e.g. hypertensive encephalopathy, aortic dissection, or congestive cardiac failure).[50] To date, limited evidence exists on which agents are more appropriate for use in older people or actual level of blood pressure reduction that might benefit. Recently, two large trials of blood pressure lowering in predominantly acute ischaemic stroke were completed, one showing worsening stroke progression in those treated with candesartan[51] and the other neutral with transdermal glyceryl trinitrate.[52] A systematic review including these and 22 other trials involving 17 011 patients reported that blood pressure lowering did not improve death or disability.[53] In this review, the authors reported that very few older patients (>80) were included and to assume the effects of changing blood pressure observed in younger patients may be inappropriate.[53] Clinical practice is, therefore, to accept hypertension in patients who are not candidates for thrombolysis, although recent evidence that early blood pressure reduction after acute intracerebral haemorrhage might improve outcome is changing management of patients with this condition.[50,54]

Decompressive hemicraniectomy in acute ischaemic stroke

In acute stroke, 'malignant' middle cerebral artery infarction (MMI) is associated with high mortality and survivors left with long-term disability.[55] The causes are usually from thrombosis or embolic occlusion of the internal carotid or proximal middle cerebral artery and the pathophysiological hallmark is persistent formation of early cytotoxic and late vasogenic and interstitial edema.[56] Consequently, brain swelling occurs peaking around the second to the fifth day after stroke onset.[56] The rationale underlying decompressive hemicraniectomy (DHC) is to allow external expansion of oedematous tissue, thereby preventing fatal internal displacement of the cerebral hemispheres and subsequent herniation.[57] Although a lesser proportion (4 in 10 of patients with MMI) are aged over 80, one-third of all hemicraniectomy procedures are performed in this group.[58] In all except one randomized trial (Decompressive Surgery for the Treatment of Malignant Infarction of the Middle Cerebral Artery, DESTINY II) patients up to age of 80 were included.[59] A total of 112 patients with MMI were assigned to DHC within 48 hours of stroke onset or standard care in an intensive care setting.[59] At 6 months, more patients who underwent surgery survived (57% vs. 24%) without severe disability compared to those randomized to standard care (mRS 38% vs. mRS 18%; NNT5).[59] Older patients also reported similar or better quality of life than those who were younger patients.[59] It is debatable whether a life needing assistance is 'favourable' but nonetheless, disabled people and carers manage better compared with healthy subjects in comparable situations especially after a near-fatal experience with MMI. At the least these results, along with a meta-analysis,[60] indicate that older patients with MMI should be considered for DHC.[58]

Secondary prevention

Cardioembolism

The risk of stroke and vascular events increase with age and concerns about bleeding have led to undertreating of the older people with oral anticoagulation. Such patients are usually prescribed antiplatelet agents, most commonly aspirin.[61] A recent meta-analysis of involving hospitalized older patients with atrial fibrillation (4136 patients $\geq$75 years; of those: 85 to 90 years, n = 819 and >90 years, n = 386) found that treatment with vitamin K antagonists (VKAs) was associated with a significant reduction in the composite endpoint of stroke/thromboembolism with the effect maintained with increasing age.[62] Moreover, the risk of major bleeding in older people did not increase when compared to younger patients.[62] The positive effects are consistent in two well-documented studies undertaken in primary care, the Birmingham AF Treatment of the Aged Study (BAFTA) and Warfarin versus Aspirin for stroke prevention in octogenarians trial.[63, 64] Even for those with a history of falls and/or early dementia, the superiority of VKAs including warfarin compared to aspirin in reducing thromboembolism were distinct.[65,66]

It should also be remembered that aspirin use has also its own problems; in one study of octogenarians with AF, aspirin was associated with more serious adverse events than warfarin.[64]

The direct anticoagulants (DOACS) (dabigatran, apixaban, rivaroxaban, edoxaban) are increasingly used in prevention after stroke in older people with the advantages of not needing regular monitoring, or diet or drug interactions. Although the efficacy is known in the general population,[67,68] it was not clear until a recent systematic review about the effects in older patients taking multiple medications and comorbidity. In 31 418 elderly patients recruited to 11 trials, the risk reduction of stroke in AF was similar or superior with DOACS compared to VKAs.[69] A significantly lower risk of major bleeding was observed for apixaban and edoxaban, but not rivaroxaban and dabigatran.[69]

Carotid endarterectomy

Extracranial carotid artery stenosis is a significant cause of ischaemic stroke and more prevalence in the older patient.[70] Carotid endarterectomy (CEA) was introduced in the 1950s and since then around 4500 CEA operations are performed in the United Kingdom each year.[71] Since CEA as a means to prevent stroke prevention in symptomatic carotid stenosis has been validated, there is interest in establishing who benefits most and those who are at significant perioperative risk. A report including 1961 patients undergoing CEA listed increasing age as a risk factor of poor prognosis after CEA (postoperative stroke and death of 3.5% vs. 1.5% in younger patients) and therefore clinicians became less inclined to refer older patients.[72] However, pooled analysis including the two largest randomized trials of CEA–European Carotid Surgery Trial[73] and North American Symptomatic Carotid Endarterectomy Trial,[74] revealed benefit for those aged more than 75 years.[75] Subgroups including male patients, those with hemispheric symptoms, irregular plaque morphology, contralateral carotid occlusion, intracranial disease, and no collaterals have been shown to benefit from surgery.[75] In terms of timing, early intervention favours good outcome and guidelines recommend CEA in severe patients (70–99%) within 2 weeks from onset of symptoms.[76,77] For symptomatic patients with severe stenosis in whom CEA is not feasible (e.g. postradiation-induced carotid stenosis, restenosis after surgery) carotid stenting is an alternative.[76]

The optimal treatment strategy for patients with asymptomatic carotid stenosis remains unclear and no consensus exists on which treatment modality is appropriate in older people. Options include CEA, percutaneous carotid angioplasty, and stenting (both in combination with medical therapy) or medical therapy alone.[78] Enthusiasm for intervening is highest among surgeons, radiologists, and cardiologists, citing case series and in countries driven by 'fee for service' but lowest in 'conservative' neurologists and stroke physicians citing prohibitively high morbidity and mortality data.[78,79] So why are clinicians polarized in their opinions? The answers are complex and may relate to concerns of periprocedural complications (such as myocardial infarction (MI), stroke) and expert opinion that 'best' medical treatment alone is sufficient in preventing further vascular events.[78–80] A systematic review of 47 trials comparing medical therapy alone, CEA plus medical therapy, or carotid angioplasty and stenting (CAS) with medical therapy for asymptomatic carotid stenosis found that patients randomized to medical therapy alone received suboptimal treatment, making the results unbalanced.[81] Further studies are therefore needed in these groups of patients to inform future clinical decision-making.

Lipid lowering

The most effective treatment of hypercholesterolemia is using HMG-COA reductase inhibitors or statins, and this section will focus on these agents. Many trials have shown the efficacy of statins for primary and secondary prevention of coronary artery disease but because these studies have not been specifically oriented towards older people, the value of such treatment has been questioned. The first study aimed at reducing first-ever strokes, included 5804 older patients (between 70 and 82 years of age) with cardiovascular risk factors/disease and failed to show reduction in cerebrovascular events. The results were attributed to several factors, including overestimate of the effect and shorter duration of follow-up (just over 3 years, previous trials followed up for 5–6 years).[82] Nonetheless, meta-analysis including nine trials of 19 569 patients showed that statins reduced the risk of stroke by 25% (RR 0.75; 95%CI 0.56–0.94) with NNT of 28.[83] Importantly, this analysis and another demonstrated that the side effects of statins were no different in those aged over 65 years and under 65 years.[83,84]

In patients with a history of cerebrovascular disease, the benefit of statins was first shown in the Heart Protection Study with a significant reduction in total vascular events.[85] However, it was not until 4 years later in 2006 that stroke prevention by aggressive reduction in cholesterol levels was demonstrated.[86] In this study, patients with a non-disabling stroke or transient ischaemic attack (TIA) and no history of coronary artery disease or hypercholesterolemia were assigned randomly to 80 mg of either atorvastatin or placebo.[86] In a subgroup of 2249 elderly patients, the mean age was 72 years and 30% of these were aged 70 or older.[87] Although the 10% reduction in the primary endpoint of fatal and non-fatal strokes was not significant, there were significant reduction in risk of stroke and TIA (HR 0.79; $P = 0.01$) and major coronary events (HR 0.61; $P = 0.0006$).[86] Atorvastatin had no benefit in those without carotid stenosis and almost non-significant effect in those with carotid stenosis indicating that no definite conclusions can be drawn.

Antihypertensive therapy

Treating hypertension has been shown to decrease stroke recurrence by about 30%.[88,89] Few trials have included patients with a history of cerebrovascular event above the age of 75, although this group would be expected to have a higher baseline risk and possibly derive greater benefit from treatment. The Perindopril Protection Against Recurrent Stroke Study (PROGRESS) had a mean age of 64 years, the Morbidity and Mortality After Stroke, Eprosartan Compared With Nitrendipine for Secondary Prevention Study (MOSES) had a mean age of 68 years, and in the Post-stroke Antihypertensive Treatment Study (PATS), the average age was 60, highlighting that more trials in older people are clearly needed.[90–92]

Experts recommend a target of less than 140/90 mmHg in most stroke patients and less than 130/80 mmHg with diabetes or chronic kidney disease using a combination of thiazide-type diuretic and an angiotensin-converting enzyme inhibitor[93] offset by risk of orthostatic hypotension or syncope. Like cardiac tissue, peripheral blood vessels become stiffer with old age and so older patients are less responsive to blood pressure modulation. A case in point is a large randomized controlled trial of spironolactone, which revealed significantly positive outcomes in heart failure patients.[94] With the publication of the results came an increase in spironolactone prescriptions but a subsequent increase in hospital admissions and mortality from hyperkalaemia; admissions increase from 2.4 per 1000 patients in 1994 to 11.0 per 1000 patients in 2001, the associated mortality arose from 0.3 per 1000 to 2.0 per 1000 patients.[94] One key reason for the observed effect was those who were treated with spironolactone were older patients, with a higher prevalence of diabetes and renal failure in comparison to the study population.

Most blood pressure lowering trials included very few patients with TIA or minor stroke and these patients represent a large majority of referrals to cerebrovascular clinics.[95] The number and proportion of older patients attending such services will increase, as the population ages so more research in this area is needed. There is also little information about the effects about acute blood pressure lowering on long-term survival, as most trials to date performed final follow-up at 3 months. The SCAST investigators recently published data on functional outcome at 1 year, indicating that the hazards of candesartan were sustained beyond 3 months[96]; however, information on other agents is still awaited. That is not to say that the one drug will be better than the others, but simply the data does not exist and more research in this area is needed. Such information will be very useful in understanding the impact on health economics. Evidence has also shown that blood pressure variability has been shown to have prognostic implications in the acute stroke.[97,98] The effect of this phenomenon in the older patient needs further research.

Challenges in recruiting older patients to stroke trials and potential solutions

Although the conduct and quality of clinical trials have significantly improved in the last few decades, the evidence base for older stroke patients remains work in progress. The gap is even wider in those with the added burden of frailty. Several factors contribute and one commonly cited is that there is no consensus or clear strategy in how to recruit older participants.[4,10,99] Socioeconomic state and personal temperament are also factors but the direct impact is not known.[100] Older people as such, do not actively seek clinical trials and few are informed about their availability.[99] One solution is to have a flexible approach and adapt methods to engage this group of patients. Telephone calls, radio announcements, and newspaper advertisements have been shown to be useful[101,102] while websites, flyers, and emails do not to have much yield.[99] Perception of trial efficacy is an issue and older people are more likely to consent to a study if it relates to their own health condition.[4,103] A case in example would be a cancer trial where nearly a half of patients initially declined but later participated in a study comparing standard treatment with a novel agent.[103] About 20% of those patients consent to take part because they felt that at the least they would receive standard treatment.[103] This view of apparent no clinical benefit can be challenging and patient education might alleviate this concerns.[104] Reassuring potential participants that studies are subject to external institutional and ethics committee review might also help.[104] Researchers also should clearly explain to patients of the option to out for any reason and at any time. Older patients generally prefer making their own decisions about their own treatment (autonomy)[4] and this approach will mean that they will not lose their decision-making capacity. Once recruited, older people tend to report positive experiences of participation in a study even if outcomes are not positive.[4,105]

Acute stroke patients can be challenging to recruit to research owing to their illness from altered consciousness, severe neurological deficit or aphasia, and may not be to provide informed consent.[106,107] Research on the provision of informed consent in this population has revealed that on average, only a third of patients are able to give consent themselves.[99,106] Factors such as poor eyesight, cognitive impairment, or poor concentration might make this even more complicated. It is therefore useful for researchers to be trained to assess capacity and refer uncertainty to treating clinicians. In the United Kingdom it is not legal to undertake research on people lacking mental capacity if the research question could be answered by studying those with mental capacity, but the law aims to be inclusive, enabling recruitment if necessary. The law rightfully protects incapacitated patients from coercion (but to whom any potential benefit may arise from taking part in a study), but agreement may be obtained from a family member (surrogate consent).[108,109] In the United Kingdom, research ethics committees (RECs) decide whether research can be undertaken in those patients who are unable to consent and lack mental capacity. RECs also consider whether such patients stand to benefit considering the condition under investigation. It is therefore vital that RECs are informed about any potential major and minor hazards involved in a study. From an early stage, meeting and discussing with patient representatives to formulate solutions helps.[107] If a proxy consent is necessary, investigators should attempt to obtain assent from the participant together with surrogate agreement from the proxy.[106,109] An example is a haemostatic trial of acute intracerebral haemorrhage where consent can be obtained from a relative if the potential participant is assessed to be eligible but unable to consent.[110] This approach has avoided excluding an appropriate sample of patients lacking capacity due to their acute illness but important to the study in question. As in all studies with emergency consent procedures, a participant (or their legal representative) can subsequently withdraw consent at any stage.[110]

Some medical aspects are specific to older people: they are more likely to become unwell to continue or dropout due to hospitalization, institutionalization, or may not survive trials spanning many years. Although there are no easy answers, efforts are needed towards designing clinical trials enabling a broad spectrum of patients to participate while at the same time limiting exclusions only to those relevant to that study.[111] For example, an investigator could consider the cognitive and physical performance required to take part in an observational study rather than explicitly state all health conditions that should not be present. Another would be in case of a study of intervention, when it might be justified to explain why certain categories of older adults are not to be included. Where possible, investigators could combine potential treatments (pharmacological and non-pharmacological) and test multiple domains of ageing such as cognitive impairment, cardiovascular disease, or osteoporosis.[112] When a single disease is the subject of research, therapies aimed at different pathophysiological targets could be attempted.[112] An example of such an innovative design could be a trial of acute haemorrhagic stroke combining blood pressure lowering, haemostasis with or without surgical decompression. Such a factorial design would make it more justifiable, allow pharmacodynamic and pharmacokinetic analysis, identify biomarkers, and measure endpoints and safety aspects specific to older people. Moreover, this approach would need fewer participants, prevent dropouts, and avoid high costs.

The first few days of a hospital admission can be stressful for older patients to concentrate and understand the researcher's information sheet and consent forms. Listing the purpose, design, conduct, risks, and benefits using simple language might minimize barriers.[6] It would be useful to have audiovisual supplements in case of either visual or hearing impairment.[99, 113] Lack of understanding trial protocols could be managed with researchers with excellent interpersonal skills and knowledge.[10] A good example is a study of exercise intervention in older women, which reported excellent recruitment from good communication provided by the research team.[114] Researchers will also need to build good working relationships with members of the clinical team and ensure they are aware of potentially eligible patients for the study that they are covering.[99, 114] To overcome bias,[105,112] it is important for treating clinicians to recognize that the study is relevant and the treatment or intervention offered might benefit. Regular training days and group presentations could ensure that trial recruitment becomes a part of routine care and not unusual ward activity.[112]

It is not uncommon for older participants wanting to take into account the views of the family or carer before deciding to take part in a study.[105] Efforts to include them at the very beginning would then be pivotal.[99] If the family member or carer recognizes the value of the study, they are more likely to support trial participation, especially if any benefit might be observed at a personal level.[107,113] Having written leaflets or face-to-face meetings might also be useful.[113] It is important for the research team to remain flexible and reinforce that participation (or non-participation) will not affect patient care or discharge in any way.[105]

Logistical factors present challenges when following-up older stroke patients participating in clinical trials.[2,99,105] These include difficulty accessing research sites from a large distance or geography, lack or problem in maintaining a driver's licence, absence of private or public transport, and morbidity from neurological impairment or fatigue.[105] One way to overcome these would be to provide transport or offer financial compensation to cover costs.[2] An alternative would be to invite the participant to a support network (e.g. Stroke Association UK).

When following-up participants, it is important to remember that the frail, older patient might miss an evaluation and trial protocols should allow return for future assessments.[10,113] Alternatively, offering a home visit or a brief 'essential' assessment might overcome the issue of timely assessment but might need additional staff and more resources.[99] It is important for trialists to remember that outcomes relevant to older stroke patients need to be recorded and reported: health-related quality of life, functional status, cognitive decline, feeding status, institutionalization and, where relevant, death. When a participant is not able to self-report, provisions can be made to allow an informant or relative to provide information. Recent trials have headed in this direction and should continue.[17,40,42,52]

While such innovative thinking to recruit and retain older patients is needed at a practical level, a shift is also needed at other aspects. For example, journal editors could encourage authors to report results stratified by age to help understand the effects of the intervention.[113] The publication should detail the eligibility, screening, enrolment, consenting, and study implementation. This will help to identify the effects of morbidity and mortality. Grant sponsors need to recognize the additional resources required to recruit and enrol older patients and offer funding consistent with those needs. Regulatory bodies have published guidance and recommended not to set an upper age limit and to include participants representative of the population intended to treat.[115,116]

Conclusions

Older patients should not be excluded from research in acute stroke and trialists have increasingly started to focus on this important group. Efforts to promote recruitment and retention include broadening inclusion criteria (including those lacking mental capacity but relevant to the study) and lowering logistical barriers. Methodological improvements in trial design are needed to evaluate efficacy in this group where side effects and complications are common. Researchers need to be flexible and creative as there is no single recruitment and retention strategy. Communication with patients and families is key and presents opportunities to explore any patient-centred barriers. More efforts are needed to convince physicians that excluding frail patients with comorbidity in clinical trials limits generalisability of results and best practice in this population. Until then, treating the majority users of our healthcare systems will be based on opinion and not on conclusive robust data. Although this chapter quotes examples in drug and interventional trials in acute stroke, the relevance in nursing or behavioural intervention should not be overlooked.

References

1. **Madouros V.** *Labour Force Projections 2006–2020.* London, UK: Office for National Statistics, 2006.
2. **Cherubini A, Del Signore S, Ouslander J, Semla T, & Michel J.** Fighting against age discrimination in clinical trials. *J Am Geriatr Soc* 2010;**58**:1791–6.
3. **Kemeny MM, Peterson BL, Kornbltih AB,** et al. Barriers to clinical trial participation by older women with breast cancer. *J Clin Oncol* 2003;**21**:2268–75.
4. **Denson AC & Mahipal A.** Participation of the elderly population in clinical trials: barriers and solutions. *Cancer Control* 2014;**21**:209–14.
5. **Azad N, Molnar F, & Byszewski A.** Lessons learned from a multidisciplinary heart failure clinic for older women: a randomised controlled trial. *Age Ageing* 2008;**37**:281–7.
6. **McMurdo ME, Witham MD, & Gillespie ND.** Inclusion of older people in clinical research. *BMJ* 2005;**331**:1036–7.
7. **Rudd AG, Hoffman A, Down C, Pearson M, & Lowe D.** Access to stroke care in England, Wales and Northern Ireland: the effect of age, gender and weekend admission. *Age Ageing* 2007;**36**:247–55.
8. **Wardlaw JM, Murray V, Berge E, & del Zoppo GJ.** Thrombolysis for acute ischaemic stroke. *Cochrane Database Syst Rev* 2009;(7):CD000213.
9. **Hadbavna A & O'Neill D.** Ageism in interventional stroke studies. *J Am Geriatr Soc* 2013;**61**(11): 2054–5.
10. **McMurdo MET, Roberts H, Parker S,** et al. Improving recruitment of older people to research through good practice. *Age Ageing* 2011;**40**:659–65.
11. **Bernabei R, Gambassi G, Lapane K,** et al. Management of pain in elderly patients with cancer. Systematic assessment of geriatric drug use via epidemiology. *JAMA* 1999;**279**:1877–82.
12. **Hacke W, Donnan G, Fieschi C,** et al. Association of outcome with early stroke treatment: pooled analysis of ATLANTIS, ECASS, and NINDS RT-PA stroke trials. *Lancet* 2004;**363**:768–74.
13. **Lees KR, Bluhmki E, von Kummer R,** et al. Time to treatment with intravenous alteplase and outcome in stroke: an updated pooled analysis of ECASS, ATLANTIS, NINDS, and EPITHET trials. *Lancet* 2010;**375**:1695–703.
14. **Marini C, Baldassare M, Russo T, De Santis F, Sacco S, & Ciancarelli I.** Burden of first-ever ischemic stroke in the oldest old: evidence from a population-based study. *Neurology* 2004;**62**:77–81.
15. **Di Carlo A, Baldereschi M, Gandolfo C,** et al. Stroke in an elderly population: incidence and impact on survival and daily function. Italian longitudinal study on aging. *Cerebrovasc Dis* 2003;**161**:141–50.
16. **Sandercock P, Lindley R, Wardlaw J,** et al. The third international stroke trial (ist-3) of thrombolysis for acute ischaemic stroke. *Trials* 2008;**9**:37.

17. **Sandercock P, Wardlaw JM, Lindley RI**, et al. The benefits and harms of intravenous thrombolysis with recombinant tissue plasminogen activator within 6 h of acute ischaemic stroke (the third international stroke trial [ist-3]): a randomised controlled trial. *Lancet* 2012;**379**:2352–63.

18. **Sandercock P, Wardlaw JM, Dennis M**, et al. Effect of thrombolysis with alteplase within 6 h of acute ischaemic stroke on long-term outcomes (the third international stroke trial ist-3): 18-month follow-up of a randomised controlled trial. *Lancet Neurol* 2013;**12**:768–76.

19. **Emberson J, Lees KR, Lyden P**, et al. Effect of treatment delay, age, and stroke severity on the effects of intravenous thrombolysis with alteplase for acute ischaemic stroke: a meta-analysis of individual patient data from randomised trials. *Lancet* 2014;**384**:1929–35.

20. **Gensicke H, Strbian D, Zinkstok SM**, et al. Intravenous thrombolysis in patients dependent on the daily help of others before stroke. *Stroke* 2016;**47**:450–6.

21. **Wahlgren N.** Systemic thrombolysis in clinical practice: what have we learned after the safe implementation of thrombolysis in stroke monitoring study? *Cerebrovasc Dis* 2009;**27**:168–76.

22. **Lees KR, Ford GA, Muir KW**, et al. Thrombolytic therapy for acute stroke in the United Kingdom: experience from the safe implementation of thrombolysis in stroke (sits) register. *Q J Med* 2008;**101**:863–9.

23. **Charidimou A, Nicoll JA, & McCarron MO.** Thrombolysis-related intracerebral hemorrhage and cerebral amyloid angiopathy: accumulating evidence. Front Neurol 2015;**6**:99.

24. **McCarron MO & Nicoll JA.** Cerebral amyloid angiopathy and thrombolysis-related intracerebral haemorrhage. *Lancet Neurol* 2004;**3**:484–92.

25. **Viswanathan A & Greenberg SM.** Cerebral amyloid angiopathy in the elderly. *Ann Neurol* 2011;**70**:871–80.

26. **Greenberg SM, Vonsattel JP, Stakes JW, Gruber M, & Finklestein SP.** The clinical spectrum of cerebral amyloid angiopathy: presentations without lobar hemorrhage. *Neurology* 1993;**43**:2073–9.

27. **Barber PA, Zhang J, Demchuk AM, Hill MD, & Buchan AM.** Why are stroke patients excluded from tpa therapy? An analysis of patient eligibility. *Neurology* 2001;**56**:1015–20.

28. **Deng YZ, Reeves MJ, Jacobs BS**, et al. IV tissue plasminogen activator use in acute stroke: experience from a statewide registry. *Neurology* 2006;**66**:306–12.

29. **Meunier JM, Wenker E, Lindsell CJ, & Shaw GJ.** Individual lytic efficacy of recombinant tissue plasminogen activator in an in vitro human clot model: rate of 'nonresponse'. *Acad Emerg Med* 2013;**20**:449–55.

30. **Colucci M, Scopece S, Gelato AV, Dimonte D, & Semeraro N.** *In vitro* clot lysis as a potential indicator of thrombus resistance to fibrinolysis—study in healthy subjects and correlation with blood fibrinolytic parameters. *Thromb Haemo* 1997;**77**:725–9.

31. **Linfante I, Llinas RH, Selim M**, et al. Clinical and vascular outcome in internal carotid artery versus middle cerebral artery occlusions after intravenous tissue plasminogen activator. *Stroke* 2002;**33**:2066–71.

32. **Molina CA, Montaner J, Arenillas JF, Ribo M, Rubiera M, & Alvarez-Sabin J.** Differential pattern of tissue plasminogen activator-induced proximal middle cerebral artery recanalization among stroke subtypes. *Stroke* 2004;**35**:486–90.

33. **Christou I, Burgin WS, Alexandrov AV, & Grotta JC.** Arterial status after intravenous tpa for ischaemic stroke. A need for further interventions. *Int Angiol* 2001;**20**:208–13.

34. **Bourekas EC, Slivka AP, Shah R, Sunshine J, & Suarez JI.** Intraarterial thrombolytic therapy within 3 hours of the onset of stroke. *Neurosurgery* 2004;**54**:39–44.

35. **Wolfe T, Suarez JI, Tarr RW**, et al. Comparison of combined venous and arterial thrombolysis with primary arterial therapy using recombinant tissue plasminogen activator in acute ischemic stroke. *J Stroke Cerebrovasc Dis* 2008;**17**:121–8.

36. **Broderick JP, Palesch YY, Demchuk AM**, et al. Endovascular therapy after intravenous t-pa versus t-pa alone for stroke. *N Engl J Med* 2013;**368**:893–903.

37. **Kidwell CS, Jahan R, Gornbein J,** et al. A trial of imaging selection and endovascular treatment for ischemic stroke. *N Engl J Med* 2013;**368**:914–23.

38. **Ciccone A, Valvassori L, Nichellati M,** et al. Endovascular treatment for acute ischemic stroke. *N Engl J Med* 2013;**368**:2433–4.

39. **Berkhemer OA, Fransen PS, Beumer D,** et al. A randomized trial of intra-arterial treatment for acute ischemic stroke. *N Engl J Med* 2015;**372**:11–20.

40. **Goyal M, Demchuk AM, Menon BK,** et al. Randomized assessmen of rapid endovascular treatment for acute ischemic stroke. *N Engl J Med* 2015;**372**:1019–30.

41. **Campbell BC, Mitchell PJ, Kleinig TJ,** et al. Endovascular therapy for ischemic stroke with perfusion-imaging selection. *N Engl J Med* 2015;**372**:1009–18.

42. **Saver JL, Goyal M, Bonafe A,** et al. Stent-retriever thrombectomy after intravenous t-pa vs t-pa alone in stroke. *N Engl J Med* 2015;**372**:2285–95.

43. **Tobin TG, Chamorro A, Cobo E,** et al. Thrombectomy within 8 hours after symptom onset in ischemic stroke. *N Engl J Med* 2015;**372**:2296–306.

44. **Grotta JC & Hacke W.** Stroke neurologist's perspective on the new endovascular trials. *Stroke* 2015;**46**:1447–52.

45. **Yarbrough CK, Ong CJ, Beyer AB, Lipsey K, & Derdeyn CP.** Endovascular thrombectomy for anterior circulation stroke: systematic review and meta-analysis. *Stroke* 2015;**46**:3177–83.

46. **Abou-Chebl A, Yeatts SD, Yan B,** et al. Impact of general anesthesia on safety and outcomes in the endovascular arm of interventional management of stroke (IMS) III trial. *Stroke* 2015;**46**:2142–8.

47. **Hachinski V.** Hypertension in acute ischaemic strokes. *Arch Neurol* 1985;**42**:1002.

48. **Bath PMW.** How to manage blood pressure in acute stroke. *Journal of Hypertension* 2005;**23**:1135–6.

49. **Bath PMW.** High blood pressure as risk factor and prognostic predictor in acute ischaemic stroke: when and how to treat it? *Cardiovasc Dis* 2004;**17**:51–7.

50. **Intercollegiate Stroke Working Party.** *National Clinical Guideline for Stroke*, 4th edition. 2012. London, UK: Royal College of Physicians.

51. **Sandset EC, Bath PM, Boysen G,** et al. The angiotensin-receptor blocker candesartan for treatment of acute stroke (SCAST): a randomised, placebo-controlled, double-blind trial. *Lancet* 2011;**377**: 741–50.

52. **Bath PMW, Woodhouse L, Scutt P,** et al. Efficacy of nitric oxide, with or without continuing antihypertensive treatment, for management of high blood pressure in acute stroke (ENOS): a partial-factorial randomised controlled trial. *Lancet* 2015;**385**:617–28.

53. **Bath PM & Krishnan K.** Interventions for deliberately altering blood pressure in acute stroke. *Cochrane Database Syst Rev* 2014;**10**:CD000039.

54. **Hemphill 3rd JC, Greenberg SM, Anderson CS,** et al. Guidelines for the management of spontaneous intracerebral hemorrhage. *Stroke* 2015;**46**:2032–60.

55. **Hacke W, Schwab S, Horn M, Spranger M, DeGeorgia M, & von Kummer R.** 'Malignant' middle cerebral artery territory infarction—clinical course and prognostic signs. *Arch Neurol* 1996;**53**: 309–15.

56. **Ng LK & Nimmannitya J.** Massive cerebral infarction with severe brain swelling: a clinicopathological study. *Stroke* 1970;**1**:158–63.

57. **Staykov D & Gupta R.** Hemicraniectomy in malignant middle cerebral artery infarction. *Stroke* 2011;**42**:513–16.

58. **Neugebauer H & Juttler E.** Hemicraniectomy for malignant middle cerebral artery infarction: current status and future directions. *Int J Stroke* 2013;**9**:460–7.

59. **Juttler E, Unterberg A, Woitzik J, Bosel J, Amiri H, & Sakowitz OW.** Hemicraniectomy in older patients with extensive middle-cerebral-artery stroke. *N Engl J Med* 2014;**370**:1091–100.

60. **Lu X, Huang B, Zheng J,** et al. Decompressive craniectomy for the treatment of malignant infarction of the middle cerebral artery. *Sci Rep* 2014;**4**:7070.

61. Lubitz SA, Bauer KA, Benjamin EJ, et al. Stroke prevention in atrial brillation in older adults: existing knowledge gaps and areas for innovation: a summary of an American federation for aging research seminar. *J Am Geriatr Soc* 2013;**61**:1798–803.

62. Lip GY, Clementy N, Pericart L, Banerjee A, & Fauchier L. Stroke and major bleeding risk in elderly patients aged ≥75 years with atrial fibrillation: the Loire Valley Atrial Fibrillation Project. *Stroke* 2015;**46**:143–50.

63. Mant J, Hobbs FD, Fletcher K, et al. Warfarin versus aspirin for stroke prevention in an elderly community population with atrial brillation (the Birmingham Atrial Fibrillation Treatment of the Aged Study, BAFTA): a randomised controlled trial. *Lancet* 2007;**370**:493–503.

64. Rash A, Downes T, Portner R, Yeo WW, Morgan N, & Channer KS. A randomised controlled trial of warfarin versus aspirin for stroke prevention in octogenarians with atrial fibrillation (WASPO). *Age Ageing* 2007;**36**:151–6.

65. Garwood CL & Corbett TL. Use of anticoagulation in elderly patients with atrial fibrillation who are at risk of falls. *Ann Pharmacother* 2008;**42**:523–32.

66. Jacobs LG, Billett HH, Freeman K, Dinglas C, & Jumaquio L. Anticoagulation for stroke prevention in elderly patients with atrial fibrillation, including those with falls and/or early-stage dementia: a single-center, retrospective, observational study. *Am J Geriatr Pharmacother* 2009;**7**:159–66.

67. Castellucci LA, Cameron C, Le Gal G, et al. Efficacy and safety outcomes of oral anticoagulants and antiplatelet drugs in the secondary prevention of venous thromboembolism: systematic review and network meta-analysis. *BMJ* 2013;**347**:f5133.

68. Ruff CT, Giugliano RP, Braunwald E, et al. Comparison of the efficacy and safety of new oral anticoagulants with warfarin in patients with atrial fibrillation: a meta-analysis of randomised trials. *Lancet* 2014;**383**:955–62.

69. Sharma M, Cornelius VR, Patel JP, Davies JG, & Molokhia M. Efficacy and harms of direct oral anticoagulants in the elderly for stroke prevention in atrial fibrillation and secondary prevention of venous thromboembolism: systematic review and meta-analysis. *Circulation* 2015;**132**:194–204.

70. O'Leary DH, Polak JF, Kronmal RA, Kittner SJ, Bond MG, & Wolfson Jr SK. Distribution and correlates of sonographically detected carotid artery disease in the cardiovascular health study. The CHS collaborative research group. *Stroke* 1992;**23**:1752–60.

71. Halliday AW, Lees T, Kamugasha D, et al. Waiting times for carotid endarterectomy in UK: observational study. *BMJ* 2009;**338**:b1847.

72. Sundt TM, Sandok BA, & Whisnant JP. Carotid endarterectomy. Complications and preoperative assessment of risk. *Mayo Clin Proc* 1975;**50**:301–6.

73. European Carotid Surgery Trial investigators. Randomised trial of endartectomy for recently symptomatic carotid stenosis: final results of the MRC European Carotid Surgery Trial (ECST). *Lancet* 1998;**351**:1379–87.

74. Ferguson GG, Eliasziw M, Barr HW, et al. The North American Symptomatic Carotid Endarterectomy Trial: surgical results in 1415 patients. *Stroke* 1999;**30**:1751–8.

75. Rerkasem KRP. Carotid endarterectomy for symptomatic carotid stenosis. *Cochrane Database Syst Rev* 2017;**6**:CD001081.

76. Ricotta JR, AbuRahma A, Ascher E, Eskandari M, Faries P, & Lal BK. Updated society for vascular surgery guidelines for management of extracranial carotid disease. *J Vasc Surg* 2011;**54**:e1–e31.

77. Brott TG, Halperin JL, Abbara SA, Bacharach JM, Barr JD, & Bush RL. Guideline on the management of patients with extracranial carotid and vertebral artery disease: executive summary. *Circulation* 2011;**124**:489–532.

78. Spence JD. Management of asymptomatic carotid stenosis. *Neurol Clin* 2015;**33**:443–57.

79. Naylor AR, Gaines PA, & Rothwell PM. Who benefits most from intervention for asymptomatic carotid stenosis: patients or professionals? *Euro J Vasc Endovasc Surg* 2009;**37**:625–32.

80. **Divya KP, Sandeep N, Sarma S, & Sylaja PN.** Risk of stroke and cardiac events in medically treated asymptomatic carotid stenosis. *J Stroke Cerebrovasc Dis* 2015;**24**:2149–53.

81. **Raman G, Moorthy D, Hadar N, Dahabreh IJ, O'Donnell TF, & Thaler DE.** Management strategies for asymptomatic carotid stenosis: a systematic review and meta-analysis. *Ann Int Med* 2013;**158**:676–85.

82. **Shepherd J, Blauw GJ, Murphy MB,** et al. Pravastatin in elderly individuals at risk of vascular disease (PROSPER): a randomised controlled trial. *Lancet* 2002;**360**:1623–30.

83. **Baigent C, Keech A, Kearney PM,** et al. Efficacy and safety of cholesterol-lowering treatment: prospective meta-analysis of data from 90,056 participants in 14 randomised trials of statins. *Lancet* 2005;**366**:1267–78.

84. **Afialo J, Duque G, Steele R, Jukema JW, de Craen AJM, & Eisenberg MJ.** Statins for secondary prevention in elderly patients. A hierarchical Bayesian meta-analysis. *J Am Coll Cardiol* 2008;**51**:37–45.

85. **Heart Protection Study Collaborative Group.** MRC/BHF heart protection study of cholesterol lowering with simvastatin in 20536 high-risk individuals: a randomised placebo-controlled trial. *Lancet* 2002;**360**:7–22.

86. **The Stroke Prevention by Aggressive Reduction in Cholesterol Levels (SPARCL) Investigators.** High-dose atorvastatin after stroke or transient ischemic attack. *N Engl J Med* 2006;**355**:549–59.

87. **Chaturvedi S, Zivin J, Breazna A,** et al. Effect of atorvastatin in elderly patients with a recent stroke or transient ischemic attack. *Neurology* 2009;**72**:688–94.

88. **Chalmers J, Beilin L, Mancia G, Whitworth J, & Zanchetti A.** International Society of Hypertension (ISH): statements on blood pressure and stroke. *Journal of Hypertension* 2003;**21**:649–50.

89. **SHEP Cooperative Research Group.** Prevention of stroke by antihypertensive drug treatment in older persons with isolated systolic hypertension. Final results of the systolic hypertension in the elderly program (SHEP). JAMA 1991;**265**(24):3255–264.

90. **PROGRESS Collaborative Group.** Randomised trial of a perindopril-based blood-pressure-lowering regimen among 6105 individuals with previous stroke or transient ischaemic attack. *Lancet* 2001;**358**:1033–41.

91. **Schrader J, Luders S, Kulschewski A,** et al. Morbidity and mortality after stroke, eprosartan compared with nitrendipine for secondary prevention. Principal results of a prospective randomised controlled study (MOSES). *Stroke* 2005;**36**:1218–26.

92. **PATS Collaborating Group.** Post-stroke antihypertensive treatment study. A preliminary result. *Chin Med J* 1995;**108**:710–17.

93. **Chobanian AV, Bakris GL, Blakc HR,** et al. The seventh report of the joint national committee on prevention, detection, evaluation, and treatment of high blood pressure. *J Am Med Assoc* 2003;**289**:2560–72.

94. **McMurray JV & O'Meara E.** Treatment of heart failure with spironolactone—trial and tribulations. *N Engl J Med* 2004;**351**:526–8.

95. **Rothwell PM.** Blood pressure in acute stroke: which questions remain? *Lancet* 2015;**385**:582–5.

96. **Hornslein AG, Sandset EC, Igland J,** et al. Effects of candesartan in acute stroke on vascular events during long-term follow-up: results from the Scandinavian Candesartan Acute Stroke Trial (SCAST). *Int J Stroke* 2015;**10**:830–5.

97. **Manning L, Hirakawa Y, Arima H,** et al. Blood pressure variability and outcome after acute intracerebral haemorrhage: a post-hoc analysis of interact2, a randomised controlled trial. *Lancet Neurol* 2014;**13**:364–73.

98. **Lau KK, Wong YK, Teo KC,** et al. Long-term prognostic implications of visit-to-visit blood pressure variability in patients with ischemic stroke. *Am J Hypertens* 2014;**27**:1486–94.

99. **Ridda I, MacIntyre CR, Lindley RI, & Tan TC.** Difficulties in recruiting older people in clinical trials: an examination of barriers and solutions. *Vaccine* 2010;**28**:901–6.

100. **Atchley RC.** Respondents vs. refusers in an interview study of retired women: an analysis of selected characteristics. *J Gerontol* 1969;**24**:42–7.

101. **Adams J, Silverman M, Musa D, & Peele P.** Recruiting older patients for clinical trials. *Control Clin Trials* 1997;**18**:14–26.

102. **Harris TJ, Carey IM, Victor CR, Adams R, & Cook DG.** Optimising recruitment into a study of physical activity in older people: a randomised controlled trial of different approaches. *Age Ageing* 2008;**37**:659–65.

103. **Jenkins V, Farewell V, Farewell D, et al.** Drivers and barriers to patient participation in RCTS. *Br J Cancer* 2013;**108**:1402–7.

104. **Williams SG.** How do the elderly and their families feel about research par- ticipation? Nurses conducting research among the elderly should know what concerns the patient and the family. *Geriatr Nurs* 1993;**14**:11–14.

105. **Knechel NA.** The challenges of enrolling older adults into intervention studies. *Yale J Biol Med* 2013;**86**:41–7.

106. **Rose DZ & Kasner SE.** Informed consent: the rate-limiting step in acute stroke trials. *Front Neurol* 2011;**2**:65.

107. **Mendyk AM, Labreuche J, Henon H, et al.** Which factors influence the resort to surrogate consent in stroke trials, and what are the patient outcomes in this context? *BMC Med Ethics* 2015;**16**:1–9.

108. **World Medical Association.** Declaration of Helsinki: ethical principles for medical research involving human subjects. *J Int Bioethique* 2004;**15**:124–9.

109. **Flaherty ML, Karlawish J, Khoury JC, Kleindorfer D, Woo D, & Broderick JP.** How important is surrogate consent for stroke research? *Neurology* 2008;**71**:1566–71.

110. **TICH-2 investigators.** *Tranexamic Acid for Intracerebral Haemorrhage (TICH-2).* ISRCTN Registry. 2013. Available at: http://www.isrctn.com/ISRCTN93732214?q=tich%202&filters=&sort=&offset=1&totalResults=3&page=1&pageSize=10&searchType=basic-search [Accessed: 2 August 2019].

111. **Ferruci L, Guralnik JM, Studenski S, Fried LP, Cutler Jr GB, & Walston JD.** Designing randomized, controlled trials aimed at preventing or delaying functional decline and disability in frail, older persons: a consensus report. *J Am Geriatr Soc* 2004;**52**:625–34.

112. **Witham MD & George J.** Clinical trial design for older people—time for a rethink. *QJM* 2014;**107**:15–16.

113. **Herrera AP, Snipes SA, King DW, Torres-Vigil I, Goldberg DS, & Weinberg AD.** Disparate inclusion of older adults in clinical trials: priorities and opportunities for policy and practice change. *Am J Public Health* 2010;**100**:S105–12.

114. **Resnick B, Concha B, Burgess JG, et al.** Recruitment of older women: lessons learned from the Baltimore hip studies. *Nurs Res* 2003;**52**:270–3.

115. **Diener L, Hugonot-Diener L, Alvino S, et al.; European Forum for Good Clinical Practice: Geriatric Medicine Working Party.** Medical research for and with older people in Europe: proposed ethical guidance for good clinical practice: ethical considerations. *J Nutr Health Aging* 2013;**17**(7):625–7.

116. **U.S. Department of Health and Human Services FaDA.** *E7 Studies in Support of Special Populations: Geriatrics, Questions and Answers.* 2012. Available from: https://www.fda.gov/regulatory-information/search-fda-guidance-documents/e7-studies-support-special-populations-geriatrics-questions-and-answers [Accessed: 2 August 2019].

Chapter 30

End-of-life care in stroke

Declan O'Kane

Introduction

Improvements in care have meant that stroke death rates in the United States and the United Kingdom have declined over the past 20 years, but it still remains the fifth leading cause of death in the United States[1] and the fourth in the United Kingdom.[2] Approximately 11% of all deaths in England and Wales are due to stroke.[3] In the United Kingdom, approximately 15% of all patients admitted with stroke will die in the first 30 days, half within the first 7 days. Mortality for those with intracerebral haemorrhage or total anterior circulation strokes is high at about 40% at 30 days.[4] Stroke is, therefore, one of the most lethal acute conditions in healthcare. Both stroke incidence and mortality increase with age.

A typical hyperacute stroke service admitting 1000 stroke patients per annum will usually have on average between two to four patients needing end-of-life care at any one time. In 2010 out of all stroke deaths, more than 80% occurred in those over the age of 75.[5] Older patients frequently have additional life-threatening comorbidities with frailty and cognitive decline, as well as cardiorespiratory disease and malignancy. As the population ages, the challenge of managing high-quality end-of-life care for these patients will become an increasingly important role for the stroke team. It is important that those looking after older patients with stroke have the skills, time, and support to provide the appropriate care for the patient and their family.

Good end-of-life care should allow a patient to die with comfort, compassion, and dignity in the place of their choosing. In most healthcare systems there will never be enough palliative care specialists to manage these needs 24/7. The fundamental aspects of palliative management should be a core competency for any stroke physician.[6] Stroke physicians are in the best place to detect and respond to ever-changing clinical events and to recognize when a patient is dying and inform and support those close to the patient. Unfortunately, it is a topic often ignored in the leading stroke texts.[7]

On an international perspective, the access to quality palliative care for those with stroke is variable and often lacking.[8] End-of-life care involves difficult religious, moral, cultural and ethical considerations. It is an emotive subject and public perception may have been shaped by misinformation and misunderstandings, as demonstrated by the controversies into the implementation of the Liverpool Care Pathway (LCP) in the United Kingdom and the issues around so-called 'death panels' in the United States. There is a need for ongoing active and informed national debate into the issues around death and dying so that patients can get the best care and families the best information and support.

In this discussion, we use the following as interchangeable or equivalent terms: 'those important to' or those 'close to' the patient or 'family' to mean those who through their prior closeness to the patient can best represent the views and wishes of the patient who is incapacitated. Unless they have a formal legally recognized role, their input is primarily to reflect any known views of the patient to help determine what represents the patient's best interest.

Specific challenges in stroke

Palliative care in the setting of acute stroke is particularly challenging. Stroke is by its nature sudden and unexpected. The prognosis may be uncertain. For some patients, the stroke at presentation may be catastrophic and rapidly fatal. But all too often the clinical state remains precarious and dying can become drawn out over days and weeks, especially in those who are already frail and elderly. For many of these patients, a stroke is the beginning of the end and futile interventions should be minimized. The patient is often comatose, hemiplegic, and/or dysphasic, and/or hemianopic. They may have pre-existing or new cognitive impairment. Mental capacity may be lost and so best interests decisions must be made by others.[9] The availability of an advanced care plan is uncommon[10] and this again places key decision-making with others.

For many family members, the potential loss of a parent or spouse with a life threatening stroke will be their first close experience of the issues around death and dying. The family have not only to deal with the emotional aspects of the new threat to their loved one but for them, there is often a need for quality and accurate prognostic information specific to the patient when the clinical state is uncertain. They may have differing concerns and often complex needs. The opportunity for an appropriately paced, careful, compassionate, and sensitive discussion that can be afforded those with other more chronic end-of-life conditions is simply not possible. We need to find ways to allow time for such significant conversations in comprehensive stroke services where clinical time is competing with assessing patients for thrombolysis and thrombectomy and other urgent demands.

Identifiers of poor outcome

The early presence of coma which persists in the first few days suggests a poor outcome. The National Institutes of Health Stroke Scale (NIHSS) score strongly predicts recovery after stroke. An initial NIHSS ≥16 forecasts a high probability of death or severe disability.[11] A continuing high NIHSS >16 in the first 10 days suggests a very poor outcome.[12] The worst outcomes are seen in those with proximal middle cerebral artery infarcts, large bihemispheric infarcts, extensive posterior circulation infarcts involving the basilar artery or bilateral vertebral arteries, and those with haemorrhagic stroke. Other poor prognostic factors include prestroke frailty and disability, a history of hypertension or ischaemic heart disease, congestive cardiac failure, male sex, age over 85, and admission hyperglycaemia.[13,14]

Patients with large volume haemorrhagic stroke, bleeding into ventricles,[15] midline shift, and obstructive hydrocephalus do worse. Investigators identified poorer outcomes with haemorrhages into the posterior limb of the internal capsule, thalamus, and infratentorial sites.[16] Cerebellar and brainstem haemorrhage differ in their clinical characteristics and prognosis, with the latter being associated with higher case fatality,[17] the exception being cerebellar bleeding associated with severe hydrocephalus.

The IScore is a tool which has been designed as a predictive model of stroke mortality in those with ischaemic stroke. Multivariable predictors of 30-day and 1-year mortality included older age, male sex, severe stroke, non-lacunar stroke subtype, glucose ≥7.5 mmol/litre (135 mg/dl), history of atrial fibrillation, coronary artery disease, congestive heart failure, cancer, dementia, kidney disease on dialysis, and dependency before the stroke.[18]

All of these factors are red flags to prompt the staff to initiate conversations to prepare the family for the uncertainty of recovery and to discuss the care the patient would have wished for. There will always be exceptions to any predictive evaluation of who will survive and so all early advice should be guarded and emphasize uncertainty.

Effective communication

Initial contact with the patient and family may be in the emergency department or hyperacute stroke unit (HASU). For those with markers of poor prognosis who are not imminently dying, the 'uncertainty of outcome' should be the message. Resuscitation status can be discussed. If the stroke is large and disabling but death is not imminent it is important to discuss the likelihood that survival may be associated with significant disability requiring all care and a marked reduction in life expectancy in the following months. The prognosis in the older often frail patient is even more bleak. These discussions should occur in an unhurried manner in the first few days. It may be useful to get the family to think and reflect on issues from the patient's perspective: 'What would they want us to do? What gave value to their life? How would they regard this new situation?'. The evidence base around end-of-life care in stroke is sparse. Much is extrapolated from the care of patients with cancer which is often not transferrable. The suddenness of stroke means that support for patients and families in this regard is often much less than for oncology patients.[19]

Families may have little personal experience or knowledge of issues around end-of-life care in stroke. A structured conversation may help to ensure that all the main issues are covered and documented (Box 30.1). These might include discussions on resuscitation, ceilings of care, feeding, and nutrition, use of antibiotics and palliative medications, and final place of care. Studies looking at the needs of families show that they appreciate an active dialogue with professionals even after a more palliative direction is taken.[20] Once a patient has started end-of-life care, the family will often need even more support. Clinicians should not fall into the trap of disengagement at this time when their skills and advice are badly needed.

Deaths and stroke

Deaths occur by various mechanisms and at various times. Some deaths are predictable and others less so. Possible causes and mechanisms change with time. These are shown in Table 30.1.

Decision-making

The practice of end-of-life care starts with a presumption in favour of prolonging life but, as the UK General Medical Council (GMC)[21] states, there is no absolute obligation to prolong life irrespective of the consequences for the patient. Decisions must respect known patient views. Doctors should offer treatments where the likely benefits outweigh burdens or associated risks. If the patient lacks capacity, as is usually the case in patient dying from the effects of a stroke, then his/her interests may be represented by a legal surrogate or by legally valid decisions to refuse treatment. Without this, those close to the patient must help clinicians to respect and represent the patient's best interest. There is a strong emphasis on establishing a consensus. At times it may be useful or even mandatory in some countries to involve an Advocate to help represent the patient's best interests.

The uncertainty phase

In those patients who do not suffer a catastrophic stroke with death within the first 1–2 days, there are those with a large stroke who enter a state where the patient is neither improving but also not felt to be in the 'dying phase' and in whom short-term survival is uncertain. This may be termed the 'uncertainty phase' when the immediate survivability of the stroke is in question. This may continue for days or even the first few weeks.

Concerns over errors in prognostication are always a concern for clinicians as well as the patient and families. There is a constant balance to be struck over prematurely diagnosing dying

Box 30.1 The ideals in end-of-life care in stroke

Initial admission and assessment

- Stroke is diagnosed early and quickly, and appropriate care is given.
- The risk of dying is highlighted early on and information communicated with family.
- Any advanced directive is respected, and the legal surrogate is involved.
- End-of-life care is not started early unless the futility of active treatment is clear.
- Decisions are made in the best interests of the patient and no one else.
- Those important to the patient are kept updated and kept involved in the care.

Uncertainty phase

- There is a daily review of clinical status with feedback from the stroke team and family.
- Supportive care is given and time allowed to see if the trend is for improvement.

Dying phase

- Dying is diagnosed and explained sensitively to those close to the patient.
- Dying is not drawn out or prolonged needlessly.
- Avoidance of futile actions—DNACPR, surgery, antibiotics, gastrostomies, drips, nasogastric tubes.
- Families receive an explanation of all the positive actions that the end-of-life care plan brings with it in terms of care, compassion, observation, and symptom control.
- The explicit advice that the goal is for the patient not to suffer.
- All distressing symptoms will be actively managed and, if possible, prevented.
- The patient is kept clean, dry, and warm in a quiet area with full access for family.
- The patient is cared for by the correct skill mix and numbers of healthcare staff.
- Staff are trained in end-of-life care and supported by specialist palliative services.
- Patients are only moved if it enhances care, privacy, dignity, and the family updated.
- A sensibly estimated prediction of when death may occur is given within its margins of error.
- If the desired place of final care was other than a hospital that this is respected and expedited.
- Cultural, spiritual, and personal needs should be met and respected.
- Patients are seen and evaluated daily by the stroke team and family supported.

After death

- Care after death is timely and appropriate and information is given.
- Family can speak openly to the ward staff about any issues and can achieve some closure and that there is support for the grieving process and a process by which families, carers, and those important to the patient can come back to discuss and understand issues that are troubling to them.
- There is an open transparent and auditable process by which healthcare professionals involved in end of life can continue to have feedback to develop and further improve care and reflect upon what went well and what did not.
- Families understand that such care is complex, unpredictable, and difficult, and that even in the best centres' imperfections are possible but that centres wish to learn and strive to do their best.

DNACPR, do not attempt cardiopulmonary resuscitation.

Source data from Holloway RG, et al. (2014). Palliative and End-of-Life Care in Stroke. *Stroke*, 45(6), 1887–1916. https://doi.org/10.1161/STR.0000000000000015

Table 30.1 Trajectories of dying after a stroke

Time	End-of-life care
Die early <24 hrs	Significant intracerebral haemorrhage too ill for intervention. Fixed pupils, Cheyne–Stokes breathing. Often will go straight onto palliative EOL care within 24 hrs. Die in ED or ITU or soon after arriving on the HASU.
Death <7 days	Massive infarction often with midline shift and oedema which may be complicated by spontaneous or thrombolysis-related haemorrhagic transformation. Coexisting cardiopulmonary disease. Often go onto EOL care after 1–2 days. Fluids/hydration may be stopped. Infection may also contribute. There is a general decline over 48 hrs and death in days.
Death <30 days but this may be drawn with months of decline	Significant stroke on the background of multiple comorbidities with significant premorbid issues and modified Rankin >2, often elderly (85+). Bedbound, all care, feeding issues, medical input prolonging living or dying. Suffering. When to stop actively managing? Difficult. Stroke often a final event in a frail older person. Death by aspiration pneumonia, nutritional issues. Early or delayed EOL care. Unlikely to survive the admission. May takes time to accept the prognosis.
Death unexpected within the hospitalization	Unpredictable. Aspiration pneumonia, arrhythmia, Pulmonary embolism, re-bleeding with ICH, haemorrhagic transformation, acute coronary syndrome. May be unrelated to stroke severity.

ED, emergency department; EOL, end of life; ICH, intracerebral haemorrhage; ITU, intensive therapy unity; HASU, hyperacute stroke unit; PE, pulmonary embolism

against continuing futile treatments and prolonging a dying phase and potential suffering. An expectant approach is often appropriate with frequent clinical reassessments by staff and updates with family. A 'hope for the best but to be prepared for the worst' strategy is useful in this setting. It is a key time to share the uncertainties of outcome with family. It can be challenging for stroke physicians and shared decision making can be helpful.

During this period active treatment and supportive management are continued. In this phase, in the older patient there are often issues with worsening frailty, muscle wasting, fatigue, dysphagia, skin care, mood, pain, weight loss, feeding, hydration, recurrent urinary tract and chest infection, aspiration, and fever, as can be seen in Box 30.2. Feeding can be challenging, needing repeated swallow assessments and trials of nasogastric feeding. The patient often remains bedbound and drowsy, and unsuitable for even the most basic therapy assessments. Some patients appear to simply 'give up' and it is important to try to look for and manage low mood (e.g. move a patient out of a side-room, manage pain, or a trial of antidepressant drugs).

There have been concerns that an early overly pessimistic outlook can prejudice outcomes. End-of-life decisions should probably be delayed in all but the most severe cases within the first 24 hours unless there are overriding comorbidities.[22] This time may also allow those close to the patient to visit and seek information and understand the situation and determine best interests. However, for some patients, it is clear early on that the patient is dying and palliation is appropriate.

For some death is not the only feared outcome. Patients may have expressed a preference to not survive such an event rather than face what would likely be a shortened life of complete dependency which they may have regarded as undignified and intolerable especially in their later years. Others may desire life at all costs, though life expectancy may have been markedly reduced. This is made more complex by studies that some adapt to a new state.[23] Some patients with 'locked-in' syndromes, notably, those who can still communicate their views, report a relatively satisfactory quality of life level that stays stable over time.[24] It is more difficult to judge quality when lasting

---

Box 30.2 Communication issues for families

Meeting agenda—tick and sign if covered
Introduction of who is who and record this ☐
Explore family understanding of current status ☐
Medical recap of how we got to here ☐
Review notes/show imaging if helpful ☐
Express concerns over the uncertainty of recovery ☐
Explore patient's wishes if they were known about dying ☐
Discuss the preferred place of final care ☐
Discuss Hospital DNAR +/– Community DNAR ☐
Discuss treatment escalation plan and ceiling of care ☐
Discuss AMBER* pathway ☐
Diagnosis of dying ☐
Discuss personalized care plan for the dying ☐
Explain the need for frequent monitoring of symptoms ☐
Focus on a high level of personal care and comfort ☐
Symptom control (pain) ☐
Symptom control (agitation, anxiety) ☐
Symptom control (respiratory secretions) ☐
Symptom control (breathlessness) ☐
Discuss the role of clinically assisted hydration ☐
Cultural issues/spiritual support ☐
Communication with GP ☐
Role and use of hospice at home services ☐
Role and use of hospice services ☐
Involvement of palliative care ☐
Plan further meetings ☐
Information booklet ☐

---

*AMBER care: a care plan for situations where the outcome is uncertain.

---

damage permanently affects cognition, vision, hearing, memory, and the ability to understand or produce language with loss of all forms of communication.

Commencing end-of-life care

Despite the best care, patients may fail to improve or worsen and enter what is known as the 'dying phase'. This transition should not be on the basis of a snapshot assessment of a patient. It should be made only after repeated assessments by an experienced clinician and repeated discussions with family and the nursing staff and other carers.

There are a few caveats; those who are intubated and ventilated can only be assessed once sedation and muscle relaxants have been discontinued and true neurology assessed. Alternative causes of persisting coma should be considered. These may include non-convulsive status, sedation, opiates, raised intracranial pressure, hypoglycaemia, acute infection, or isolated bilateral thalamic infarcts with initial somnolescence who may need time to recover. There is rarely much harm waiting for 12–24 hours and then reassessing. The key is repeated assessments. Even the most experienced and careful clinician can be surprised by unexplained improvements, which if persisting can place the patient back in the uncertainty phase.

If end-of-life care is commenced then it is key that medical staff remain involved and the patient should be seen daily. It is often useful if rounds occur when the family who should be allowed open visiting are in attendance. It shows care and consideration and allows them to raise issues and concerns and avoid misunderstandings and it allows clinicians to sensitively explain the current aims of care and expectations. Families often need increasing support, especially when the dying phase is prolonged.

One of the uses of a formal personalized care plan for the dying is that there is clear explicit documentation of the discussions with family and decisions made when the patient enters the dying phase.

It is important to always emphasize that end-of-life care is not simply a list of interventions denied to a patient, but a change in direction with a focus on high-quality nursing care, frequent assessment for anxiety, distress, pain, breathlessness, and use of palliative medications to ensure that the patient is always comfortable. Some ideal qualities of end-of-life care have been listed in Box 30.3.

Role of resuscitation

Modern resuscitation in the medical setting was developed primarily to deliver the benefits of defibrillation in the context of ventricular arrhythmias in the acute coronary syndrome or other

---

Box 30.3 Challenging training needs for healthcare staff

- How to have conversations about the uncertainty of prognosis, time of death.
- Conversations on the trajectory of dying and giving bad news.
- Dealing with anxious, distressed, or aggressive relatives.
- Communication within MDT and recording information from conversations.
- Conversations about feeding and hydration.
- Managing unrealistic expectations.
- Conversations about stopping futile treatment.

MDT, multidisciplinary team.

Reproduced with permission from Bailey F, et al. *Difficult conversations with families and patients about end of life care after stroke: what are the educational needs of health care professionals?* Copyright © 2015, NHS National Services Scotland. Available at https://www.palliativecarescotland.org.uk/content/publications/11.-Difficult-conversations-with-families-and-patients-about-end-of-life-care.pdf

proarrhythmic states who could then survive well. It was not designed to increase longevity for those elderly patients with a large disabling stroke dying a natural and often non-arrhythmic death.

Resuscitation has little merit in the dying stroke patient. It is fundamentally a decision for healthcare professionals but the law in England is quite specific that consultation with an explanation of the decision and reasons for it must be made to the patient or those close to the patient. This must take place before a do not attempt cardiopulmonary resuscitation (DNACPR) decision, to ensure that it is legally valid. Case law shows that this is mandatory even to the practical extent of contacting family overnight[25] and not doing so is a breach of human rights. If those close to the patient are unavailable despite reasonable attempts at contact, then a documented multidisciplinary decision is advised. Making isolated decisions should be discouraged. In the United Kingdom it is not enough to simply sign a DNACPR order and pass this duty on to someone else to contact the family at some point in the future.

There will be some patients for whom attempting cardiopulmonary resuscitation (CPR) is clearly inappropriate; for example, an elderly patient with massive intracerebral haemorrhage where death is imminent and unavoidable and CPR would not be successful, but in whom time has not allowed a formal CPR decision. In such case, a carefully considered and balanced decision not to start CPR should be supported by senior colleagues, employers, and professional bodies. But where possible, all reasonable efforts should be made to make contact with those important to the patient.[26]

Clinically assisted hydration and nutrition

Patients who are dying with stroke are usually comatose and unable to take nutrition or hydration. Options for nutrition include nasogastric tube or gastrostomy but these are all considered as invasive medical treatments and are usually withheld or withdrawn on the grounds of futility and the obvious discomfort and risks of aspiration in the dying patient. Feeding supine patients with little airways protection will mean an accumulating reservoir of acidic gastric contents that can reflux into the airways with resultant chemical pneumonitis and dyspnoea, chest pain and discomfort, and then chest sepsis. Feeding may lead to osmotic diarrhoea. In the dying phase, ongoing artificial feeding is futile and possibly harmful.

Artificial hydration is the use of parenteral fluids (intravenous or subcutaneous) to provide hydration and is considered in most jurisdictions as a medical intervention.[27] There are arguments both for and against the uses of artificial hydration in patients dying from a stroke. Families and clinicians often find this a difficult area.

The National Institute for Health and Care Excellence (NICE) guidance for end-of-life care[28] suggests a 'trial' of hydration, which, if felt to be beneficial for symptoms can be continued. A Cochrane review[29] assessed the evidence for medically assisted hydration in palliative care and found no clear evidence either way. However, this was based predominantly on those with cancer. Stroke care is very different, as in the dying phase patients are usually comatose with markedly reduced awareness and sentience.

Artificial hydration may lead to fluid overload and local as well as generalized oedema. Replacing lines may cause some discomfort and cause local irritation, discomfort, and infection. The hydration given may be less than the physiological needs for life and it becomes slow dehydration with little justification rather than a genuine attempt to achieve euvolaemia, which would require strict fluid balance management and blood tests. Elderly patients often appear to have much-reduced awareness of thirst. It is not uncommon to see an older patient with significant physical and biochemical evidence of severe water deprivation with no thirst. Mouth care is key for comfort and can be provided with sponges and sprays. It can be carried out by carers and family. If fluids are stopped, then care can be given in any setting and discharge home or to a nursing home may be easier. These are difficult subjects and family often need time to consider options.

When fluids are stopped in the dying patient there is a usually a further reduction in the level of consciousness after several days and death usually comes within 7–10 days. Some generic personalized care plans for end-of-life care suggest that death may come sooner in 3–4 days but this is not usually the case for stroke. The lack of hydration can lessen cerebral oedema and patients may appear to show mild improvements after a day. This may lead to a re-evaluation of the appropriateness of end-of-life care and recommencing fluids. This can then lead to a return to the *status quo ante* but for some improvements may persist.[30] There are rare incidences when an unexpected improvement occurs in a patient on end of life care which must be reevaluated and can lead to a discussion with these close to the patient and for some a reinstitution of standard care for the time being until the prognosis is more established.

There is no ethical or legal distinction between withholding and withdrawing life-sustaining treatment. Some staff may feel reluctant to remove a nasogastric tube but prefer to allow the tube to come out accidentally or remove it if it is blocked or causing local irritation or agitation.

The personalized plan records decisions on resuscitation, hydration, nutrition, oral intake, and preference for the final place of care as well as a daily review and can provide useful guidelines that allows staff to monitor and record symptoms and corresponding actions. It should be used to share information among those caring for the patient.

It is not uncommon that the patients have previously expressed wishes of where they wish to die. If family are supportive it is not uncommon to expedite discharge to home or back to a nursing home if there is a rapid response service that can provide the community support needed. This is often best anticipated in discussions in the transition phase so that the move is done as early as possible when end-of-life care is started.

Occasionally families are placed in the intolerable position of either being asked to take sole responsibility for decisions on resuscitation and withdrawing life-sustaining care or believing wrongly that this is their role. It should always be made clear that these are primarily medical decisions made by the medical team but that discussion with those close to the patient to achieve consensus to do what is in the patient's best interest is the goal.[31]

Symptom control

Mazzocato and colleagues[32] looked at stroke deaths and symptoms and their control. The mean NIHSS on admission was 21. The main symptoms recorded were dyspnoea (81%) and pain (69%). Other symptoms included dry mouth (62%), constipation (38%), anxiety/sadness (26%), and delirium (14%). There was an inability to communicate due to dysphasia or low level of consciousness in 93% of patients. Patients received antimuscarinic drugs (52%) and opioids (33%). The pain was mainly treated by opioids (69%). In the final 48 hours, over 80% of patients were free of pain and 48% of respiratory distress.

Pain is difficult to assess in the dying patient and staff should be aware of pain behaviours— head holding, distressed expressions, agitation, negative verbalizations, rubbing of the body, and grimacing. These may be more apparent to those doing close personal care or family who must feel encouraged to raise concerns and observations with staff (Table 30.2).

It is important to have pre-emptive (anticipatory) prescribing of palliative care medications to ensure no delay when needed and that the drugs are available. If a particular symptom has required acute drug management more than once in 24 hours, then a syringe driver providing a basal level of the drug(s) should be considered. There are usually few problems with mixing any of the palliative care drugs listed as follows for the standard 24-hour period but the syringe driver

Table 30.2 Specific management of palliative symptoms

Symptoms	Practical management as per British National Formulary
Dyspnoea	Assess whether there is a role for chest physiotherapy to aid expectoration but this requires patient cooperation and so is often not appropriate. Suctioning may help to reduce upper airways secretions. Assess if the patient has heart failure and consider stopping any artificial hydration. Consider drug management with diamorphine 2.5–5 mg SC/IM/IV or morphine 5–10 mg SC/IM/IV. Consider a syringe drive if more than one episode in 24 hrs.
Pain	Diamorphine 2.5–5 mg SC/IM/IV or morphine 5–10 mg SC/IM/IV. Consider a syringe drive if more than one episode in 24 hrs.
Agitation and anxiety	Haloperidol reduces agitation but is less sedating. Given as an SC infusion dose of 5–15 mg/24 hours. Midazolam provides sedation and may be combined with haloperidol in a very restless patient; Give 10–20 mg SC infusion over 24 hours. Doses up to 60 mg/24 hours are given.
Mouth dryness	Oral care with wet sponges. Good mouth care, moisten the mouth at least once an hour with water from a water spray, dropper, or sponge stick or ice chips placed in the mouth. To prevent cracking of the lips, smear petroleum jelly (e.g. Vaseline®) on the lips. However, if a person is on oxygen apply a water-soluble lubricant (for example K-Y Jelly®). When the weather is dry and hot, if possible, use a room humidifier or air conditioning.
Respiratory Secretions	Glycopyrronium 0.6–1.2 mg/24 hours by subcutaneous infusion may also be used to treat excessive respiratory secretions.
Seizures and Myoclonus	Midazolam is the drug of choice for continuous subcutaneous infusion, and it is given initially in a dose of 20–40 mg/24 hours.
Constipation	Enemas for those distressed by constipation.
Bowel colic with pain	Hyoscine hydrobromide reduces bowel colic and is sedative and does reduce respiratory secretions. It is given in a subcutaneous infusion dose of 1.2–2 mg/24 hours.

SC, subcutaneous; IM, intramuscular; IV, intravenous.

Source: data from Joint Formulary Committee, British National Formulary, Copyright (2018), Pharmaceutical Press and NICE Palliative care—oral. (https://cks.nice.org.uk/palliative-care-oral#!scenario:7).

should be inspected regularly to ensure that the subcutaneous site is not inflamed and that the needle is not displaced and that the rate of flow is appropriate and the remaining drug is what is expected. The syringe itself should be checked for any precipitates which cause discolouration.

After death and grieving

Stroke-related deaths in the older patient can have a huge impact on those close to the patient, especially with the complex issues involved. For some patients and their families death is a taboo subject that has never been discussed. Grief may be overwhelming and can lead to intense anger and blame which can often surface months later, even over what some would regard as less important issues or over misunderstandings that were not addressed at the time. It is often unpredictable and needs to be managed with openness, tolerance, and sympathy, even when reactions appear to be disproportionate.[33] It underlines the need to be very available and engaged during the dying phase and actively seek issues of worry and concern among those close to the patient.

Some family members may appreciate the option to discuss any issues after death. Concerns and worries and guilt may persist that even a supportive phone call might assuage.

Staff and carers

The provision of training in palliative care is often patchy. Staff have listed the issues that they find challenging and suggested as themes for learning (see Box 30.3). It is important not to underestimate the impact on staff. Most of the time the relationship between the stroke team with families is excellent and supportive. However it is an incredibly emotive time and occasionally grief and worry is manifest by families as blame and anger and in these cases medical and nursing staff need support. There should be mechanisms for staff to be debriefed and supported. Those who care for the dying have needs too. Complaints are not uncommon around end-of-life care and can be troubling to staff who may be directly or indirectly blamed and need to be supported. The response should be to demonstrate that the best care was given and if not to address the issues and apologize and implement change. It is important to demonstrate that the service has a robust ethos of transparency, candour, continual reflective practice and organisational improvement that learns from events.

References

1. **Centers for Disease Control and Prevention (CDC).** Vital signs: recent trends in stroke death rates—United States, 2000–2015. *MMWR* 2017;**66**(35):933–9.
2. **Stroke Association**. *State of the Nation. Stroke Statistics February 2018*. Available from: https://www.stroke.org.uk/resources/state-nation-stroke-statistics [Accessed: 2 August 2019].
3. **Intercollegiate Stroke Working Party**. *National Clinical Guideline for Stroke*, 5th edition. London, UK: Royal College of Physicians. 2016
4. **Aguilar MI & Brott TG.** Update in intracerebral hemorrhage. *Neurohospitalist* 2011;**1**(3):148–59.
5. **Townsend N, Wickramasinghe K, Bhatnagar P**, et al. (2012). *Coronary Heart Disease Statistics*. London, UK: British Heart Foundation, 2012, p. 19
6. **Holloway RG, Arnold RM, Creutzfeldt CJ**, et al. Palliative and end-of-life care in stroke. a statement for healthcare professionals from the American Heart Association/American Stroke Association. *Stroke* 2014;**45**(6):1887–916.
7. **Grotta JC.** *Stroke: Pathophysiology, Diagnosis, and Management*. 6th edition. Philadelphia, PA: Elsevier Inc., 2016.
8. **Worldwide Palliative Care Alliance.** *Global Atlas of Palliative Care at the End of Life*. Geneva, Switzerland: World Health Organization, 2014.
9. **Editorial.** Palliative and end-of-life care should not be last or least. *Lancet Neurol* 2014;**13**(5):439.
10. **Alonso A, Dörr D, & Szabo K.** Critical appraisal of advance directives given by patients with fatal acute stroke: an observational cohort study. *BMC Med Ethics* 2017;**18**:7.
11. **Adams HP, Davis PH, Leira EC**, et al. Baseline NIH Stroke Scale score strongly predicts outcome after stroke. A report of the Trial of Org 10172 in Acute Stroke Treatment (TOAST). *Neurology* 1999;**53**(1): 126.
12. **Frankel MR.** Predicting prognosis after stroke: a placebo group analysis from the National Institute of Neurological Disorders and Stroke rt-PA Stroke Trial. *Neurology* 2000;**55**(7):952.
13. **Wood AD, Gollop ND, Bettencourt-Silva JH**, et al. A 6-Point TACS score predicts in-hospital mortality following total anterior circulation stroke. *J Clin Neurol* 2016;**12**(4):407–13.
14. **Myint PK, Bachmann MO, Loke YK**, et al. Important factors in predicting mortality outcome from stroke: findings from the Anglia Stroke Clinical Network Evaluation Study. *Age Ageing* 2017;**46**(1):83–90.

15. **Chan E.** Significance of intraventricular hemorrhage in acute intracerebral hemorrhage: intensive blood pressure reduction in acute cerebral hemorrhage trial results. *Stroke* 2015;**46**(3):653–8.

16. **Delcourt C, Sato S, Zhang S,** et al. Intracerebral hemorrhage location and outcome among INTERACT2 participants. *Neurology* 2017;**88**(15):1408–14.

17. **Chen R, Wang X, Anderson CS,** et al. **INTERACT Investigators.** Infratentorial intracerebral hemorrhage. *Stroke* 2019;**50**:1257–9.

18. **Saposnik G, Kapral MK, Liu Y,** et al. IScore: a risk score to predict death early after hospitalization for an acute ischemic stroke. *Circulation* 2011;**123**:739–49.

19. **Eriksson H, Milberg A, Hjelm K,** & **Friedrichsen M.** End of life care for patients dying of stroke: a comparative registry study of stroke and cancer. *PLoS One* 2016;**11**(2):e0147694.

20. **Majesko A, Hong SY, Weissfeld L,** et al. Identifying family members who may struggle in the role of surrogate decision maker. *Crit Care Med* 2012;**40**:2281–6.

21. **General Medical Council (GMC).** *Treatment and Care Towards the End of Life: Good Practice in Decision Making.* Available from: https://www.gmc-uk.org/ethical-guidance/ethical-guidance-for-doctors/treatment-and-care-towards-the-end-of-life [Accessed: 2 August 2019].

22. **National Hospice and Palliative Care Organization.** *Medical Guidelines for Determining Prognosis in Selected Non-Cancer Diseases,* 2nd edition. Alexandria, VA: National Hospice and Palliative Care Organization, 1996.

23. **Broderick, J, Connolly S, Feldmann E,** et al. Guidelines for the management of spontaneous intracerebral hemorrhage in adults: 2007 update: a guideline from the American Heart Association/ American Stroke Association Stroke Council, High Blood Pressure Research Council, and the Quality of Care and Out. *Stroke* 2007;**38**:2001–23.

24. **Creutzfeldt CJ** & **Holloway RG.** Treatment decisions after severe stroke: uncertainty and biases. *Stroke* 2012;**43**:3405–8.

25. **Payne S, Burton C, Addington-Hall J,** & **Jones A.** End of life issues in acute stroke care: a qualitative study of the experiences and preferences of patients and families. *Palliat Med* 2010;**24**(2):146–53.

26. **Joint Statement.** *Decisions Relating to Cardiopulmonary Resuscitation. Guidance from the British Medical Association, the Resuscitation Council (UK) and the Royal College of Nursing,* 3rd edition (1st revision), 2016.

27. **Winspear v City Hospitals Sunderland NHS Foundation Trust.** [2015] 2015 EWHC 3250 (QB), [2015] MHLO 104.

28. **McIlmoyle J** & **Vernon MJ.** Artificial nutrition and hydration: science, ethics and law. *Clin Med (Lond)* 2003;**3**(2):176–8.

29. **National Institute for Health and Care Excellence (NICE).** *Care of Dying Adults in the Last Days of Life. NICE Guideline [NG31].* 2015. Available from: https://www.nice.org.uk/guidance/ng31 [Accessed: 2 August 2019].

30. **Good P, Richard R, Syrmis W,** et al. Medically assisted hydration for adult palliative. *Cochrane Database Syst Rev* 2014;**(4):**CD006273

31. **Baumstarck K, Alessandrini M, Blandin V, Billette de Villemeur T,** & **Auquier P.** *Orphanet J Rare Dis* 2015;**10**:88.

32. **Guy's and St Thomas' NHS Foundation Trust.** *The AMBER Care Bundle.* Available from: http://www.ambercarebundle.org [Accessed 15 April 2017].

33. **Mazzocato C, Michel-Nemitz J, Anwar D,** & **Michel P.** The last days of dying stroke patients referred to a palliative care consult team in an acute hospital. *Eur J Neurol* 2009;**17**(1):73–7.

Name Index

Tables and figures are indicated by *t* and *f* following the page number

For the benefit of digital users, indexed terms that span two pages (e.g., 52–53) may, on occasion, appear on only one of those pages.

Subject Index

Tables, figures and boxes are indicated by *t*, *f* and *b* following the page number

For the benefit of digital users, indexed terms that span two pages (e.g., 52–53) may, on occasion, appear on only one of those pages.